The Routledge Handbook of Visual Impairment

W0113159

The Routledge Handbook of Visual Impairment examines current debates as well as cross-examining traditionally held beliefs around visual impairment. It provides a bridge between medical practice and social and cultural research drawing on authentic investigations.

It is the intention of this Handbook to provide an opportunity to engage with academic researchers who wish to ensure a coherent and rigorous approach to research construction and reflection on visual impairment that is in collaboration with, but sometimes beyond, the medical realm.

This Handbook is divided into ten thematic areas in order to represent the wide range of debates and concepts within visual impairment. The ten themes include:

- cerebral visual impairment;
- education;
- sport and physical exercise;
- assistive technology;
- understanding the cultural aesthetics;
- socio-emotional and sexual aspects of visual impairment;
- orientation, mobility, habitation and rehabilitation;
- recent advances in "eye" research and sensory substitution devices;
- ageing and adulthood.

The 27 chapters that explore the social and cultural aspects of visual impairment can be taken and used in a variety of different ways in order to promote research and generate debate among practitioners and scholars who wish to use this resource to inform their practice in supporting and developing positive outcomes for all.

John Ravenscroft, PhD (Chair of Childhood Visual Impairment) is a psychologist, educationalist and lectures a little in philosophy. He has vast experience of inclusive education, and has advised various governments, locally, nationally and internationally on promoting inclusive education. Professor Ravenscroft is also Head of the Scottish Sensory Centre, which is a national centre that provides career-long professional development for teachers of children with sensory impairment, including those with cerebral visual impairment. He is also the current editor-in-chief of the *British Journal of Visual Impairment* and lectures on inclusive education, visual impairment, as well as on areas of virtue epistemology and ontology. He has published widely on visual impairment, disability and research methods.

Routledge International Handbooks

For more information about this series, please visit: www.routledge.com/Routledge-International-Handbooks/book-series/RIHAND

The Routledge Handbook of Visual Impairment

Edited by John Ravenscroft

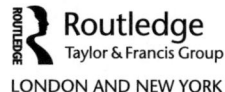

Routledge
Taylor & Francis Group

LONDON AND NEW YORK

First published 2020
by Routledge
2 Park Square, Milton Park, Abingdon, Oxon OX14 4RN

and by Routledge
605 Third Avenue, New York, NY 10017

Routledge is an imprint of the Taylor & Francis Group, an informa business

2019 selection and editorial matter, John Ravenscroft; individual
chapters, the contributors

The right of John Ravenscroft to be identified as the author of the
editorial material, and of the authors for their individual chapters, has
been asserted in accordance with sections 77 and 78 of the
Copyright, Designs and Patents Act 1988.

All rights reserved. No part of this book may be reprinted or
reproduced or utilised in any form or by any electronic, mechanical,
or other means, now known or hereafter invented, including
photocopying and recording, or in any information storage or
retrieval system, without permission in writing from the publishers.

Trademark notice: Product or corporate names may be trademarks
or registered trademarks, and are used only for identification and
explanation without intent to infringe.

British Library Cataloguing in Publication Data
A catalogue record for this book is available from the British Library

Library of Congress Cataloging in Publication Data
Names: Ravenscroft, John, author.
Title: The Routledge handbook of visual impairment / John
    Ravenscroft.
Description: Milton Park, Abingdon, Oxon ; New York, NY :
    Routledge, 2019. | Series: Routledge international handbooks |
Includes bibliographical references and index.
Identifiers: LCCN 2018051608| ISBN 9781138085411 (hardback) |
    ISBN 9781315111353 (ebook)
Subjects: LCSH: Vision disorders. | Vision disorders—Case studies.
Classification: LCC RE91 .R38 2019 | DDC 617.7—dc23
LC record available at https://lccn.loc.gov/2018051608

ISBN: 978-1-138-08541-1 (hbk)
ISBN: 978-0-367-67059-7 (pbk)
ISBN: 978-1-315-11135-3 (ebk)

Typeset in Bembo
by Swales & Willis Ltd, Exeter, Devon, UK

Contents

Contents

Contents

Figures

Figures

Tables

Contributors

Carla J. Abbott, BOptom, PhD, is an optometrist with a research interest in retinal and optic nerve disease, including translational clinical research. Her research career has focused on evaluating the structure and function of the retina in disease. She is currently at the Centre for Eye Research Australia and Department of Ophthalmology in Melbourne, Australia, involved in safety and efficacy testing of pre-clinical bionic eye devices and evaluating a visual prosthesis for patients with inherited eye disease.

Penelope J. Allen, MBBS, FRANZCO, is an ophthalmologist and vitreoretinal surgeon at the Royal Victorian Eye and Ear Hospital and the Centre for Eye Research Australia. She is the lead surgeon and principal investigator for the Melbourne-based suprachoroidal prosthesis trials. Dr Allen is also an expert on intraocular infection (endophthalmitis) and vitreoretinal surgical techniques.

Vassilios Argyropoulos, PhD, is Associate Professor at the University of Thessaly (UTH), Greece, in the area of visual impairment since 2003. Previously, he had taught in the Center of Education and Rehabilitation for the Blind in Athens for ten consecutive years. He has participated in a number of national, Erasmus+ and Horizon projects in the areas of special education and he runs as a coordinator an Erasmus+ programme since 2014. He serves the International Council for Education of People with Visual Impairments (ICEVI) as the contact person in Balkan countries. He is also a member of the Committee of the Disability Centre at the UTH, which supports students who have disabilities and special educational needs during their studies.

Lauren N. Ayton, BOptom PhD, is an optometrist and academic with special interests in retinal disease, low vision and vision restoration. From 2010 to 2017 she was the clinical team leader of the Bionic Vision Australia consortium, who completed a first-in-human study of a suprachoroidal prosthesis. She has recently taken on the role of Director of Clinical and Regulatory Affairs at Bionic Eye Technologies in Ithaca, New York, who are developing a subretinal prosthesis. Dr Ayton is passionate about utilising new technologies to assist people with different sensory challenges.

Corinna M. Bauer, PhD, is Instructor of Ophthalmology at Massachusetts Eye and Ear Infirmary at the Harvard Medical School in Boston, Massachusetts. Her research focuses on understanding how the visual dysfunctions observed in individuals with cerebral/cortical visual impairment (CVI) relate to underlying brain structure and function.

Duncan E. Crombie is an early career researcher at CERA and the University of Melbourne, with a focus on automation of methods for stem cell research.

Maciej Daniszewski is a PhD student at the University of Melbourne. His research focuses on the large-scale modelling of primary open-angle glaucoma using patient-specific induced pluripotent stem cells.

Lil Deverell, PhD, is a Certified Orientation and Mobility Specialist (COMS) based in Melbourne, Australia. She works with research partners internationally, developing functional assessment tools that measure what matters to clients. She also works with colleagues both locally and internationally to develop and maintain professional standards in orientation and mobility. Lil has written two children's activity books about low vision/blindness and a manual for trainee O&M specialists.

Graeme Douglas, PhD, is Professor of Disability and Special Educational Needs in the School of Education at the University of Birmingham, UK. He has carried out research in the area of vision impairment and education since 1993. He is a co-director of the Vision Impairment Centre for Teaching and Research (VICTAR) and head of the Department of Disability Inclusion and Special Needs (DISN).

Gordon N. Dutton is a paediatric ophthalmologist with multiple academic interests, including the many cerebral visual impairments (CVI), their origin, diagnosis, characterisation, impact and life-long management (primarily through empowerment of those affected, their parents and carers). He has contributed to a wide range of ophthalmic literature and is a co-editor and contributor to a number of textbooks addressing the topic of CVI.

David Feeney, PhD, is a Lecturer in Disability and Education at Liverpool Hope University and is a core member of Hope's Centre for Culture and Disability Studies. He previously worked as a lecturer and service manager at the University of Edinburgh, as art review manager at Edinburgh College of Art and as an access facilitator at the John Hansard Gallery, Southampton. He has written and presented extensively on visual impairment and aesthetics, including an interdisciplinary monograph on representations of blindness in modern drama.

Jennifer C. Fielder, received her BSc (Hons) in Psychology from the University of Bath. She is a research apprentice in the Crossmodal Cognition Lab working with Dr Proulx. She previously worked with Professor Susan Carey at the Harvard University Laboratory for Developmental Studies as co-lab manager and as a research assistant.

Frances Gentle, PhD, is a Lecturer with the Royal Institute for Deaf and Blind Children's Renwick Centre in Sydney, Australia. She holds conjoint positions with the University of Newcastle and Macquarie University. Frances is President of the International Council for Education of People with Visual Impairment (ICEVI), Co-President of the South Pacific Educators in Vision Impairment (SPEVI), Executive Member of the World Blind Union and a member of the editorial boards of the ICEVI and SPEVI journals. Frances has 30 years of experience as an educator and lecturer in the field of disability in Australia and internationally, with over 20 years of specialisation in education of children with blindness and low vision.

Contributors

Gregory L. Goodrich, PhD, trained in experimental psychology at Washington State University, specialising in visual sensory perception. He has over 40 years of experience in visual impairment research in low vision, blindness and brain injury-related visual impairment. He is currently an independent research consultant and associate editor for the *Journal of Visual Impairment and Blindness*. He has written numerous peer-reviewed publications, book chapters, as well as national and international presentations. Among his research awards is the US Department of Veterans Affairs Olin E. Teague Award, which recognises extraordinary research beneficial to war-injured veterans.

Justin A. Haegele, PhD, CAPE, is an Assistant Professor in the Department of Human Movement Science at Old Dominion University in Norfolk, Virginia. His research interests are situated in the field of adapted physical activity and focus on examining how individuals with disabilities, including those with visual impairments, experience physical activity and what factors influence decisions to be active among these populations. His research spans leisure-time and school-based physical activity contexts.

Simon Hayhoe, PhD, is a Reader in the Department of Education at the University of Bath. He is also a Special Research Associate in the Centre for the Philosophy of Natural and Social Science, London School of Economics, and has written widely about blindness and the arts. He is the author of five books on blindness and visual culture and has researched this field for the past 25 years.

Rachel Hewett, PhD, is a Birmingham Fellow working in the Vision Impairment Centre for Teaching and Research (VICTAR) in the Department of Disability Inclusion and Special Needs (DISN) at the University of Birmingham. Rachel's research interests in the field of vision impairment include young people's transition experiences from compulsory education through to the labour market and inclusion in higher education. She is a member of the University of Birmingham's Inclusive Education Committee.

Hyvärinen Lea, MD, PhD, is Honorary Professor in the Faculty of Rehabilitation Sciences, Technische Universität Dortmund, Dortmund, Germany. Her main research interest areas are atypical vision, causes and structure, early intervention and rehabilitation and development of assessment methods.

Gaylen Kapperman, PhD, holds the rank of Professor Emeritus in the Visual Disabilities Program located at Northern Illinois University, DeKalb, Illinois. His research interests in the field of blindness have included the use of assistive technology with a focus on strategies for the study of mathematics and foreign languages and improvement in methods for the provision of sex education instruction.

Jill Keeffe, OAM, PhD, is a member of the faculty at L.V. Prasad Eye Institute in Hyderabad, India. Her current work involves research, project development and teaching. She currently holds the position of Chair of the International Agency for Prevention of Blindness Low Vision Working Group and has worked with the World Health Organization (WHO) on many projects on eye care. Jill is a technical advisor to Lions Clubs International Foundation's SightFirst programme and Convenor of the Diabetes Working Group. She received an Order of Australia Medal in 2007 for services to eye care education and practice.

Stacy M. Kelly, EdD, TVI, COMS, CATIS, is an Associate Professor in the Northern Illinois University Visual Disabilities Program in DeKalb, Illinois. Her research interests include assistive technology for people with visual impairments, implications of instruction in the expanded core curriculum for students with visual impairments and secondary analysis of large-scale databases pertaining to people with visual impairments.

John M. Kennedy, FRSC, was born in Belfast and attended Rosetta Primary, followed, after passing the 11-Plus, by the august Royal Belfast Educational Institution. He obtained an MA in Psychology at Queens University Belfast, before going on to study at Cornell with the remarkable J.J. Gibson, which led to his PhD on outline pictures and the prediction that blind people should understand pictures. John taught visual and tactile perception and psycholinguistics and child development at Harvard and then at Toronto. In 2002 the *New York Times* said that he "offers ideas that change the way we think".

Grace E. Lidgerwood is an early career researcher at CERA and the University of Melbourne. She models aspects of inflammation in the retina using human pluripotent stem cell–derived retinal cells.

Lauren J. Lieberman, PhD, is a Distinguished Service Professor at the College at Brockport, State University of New York (SUNY). She teaches undergraduate and graduate courses in Adapted Physical Education. She earned her PhD at Oregon State University. She taught in the Deafblind programme at the Perkins School for the Blind. She is the founder and director of Camp Abilities: an educational sports camp for children with visual impairments. She has published over 125 peer-reviewed articles and published 18 books related to inclusion and on physical activity and sport for children with sensory impairments.

Amanda Hall Lueck, PhD, is Professor Emerita in Special Education at San Francisco State University where she conducts teaching, research and curriculum development activities. At the Low Vision Clinic, University of California, Berkeley School of Optometry, Dr Lueck participated in low vision research and practice across the lifespan. Amanda is the author of numerous articles, chapters and curricular materials related to low vision, cerebral visual impairment and visual impairments, her books include *Vision and the Brain: Understanding Cerebral Visual Impairment in Children* (2015), *Functional Vision: A Practitioner's Guide to Evaluation and Intervention* (2004), and *Developmental Guidelines for Infants with Visual Impairments, Birth to 2 Years* (1998).

Nicola McDowell works as a senior tutor in the Institute of Education at Massey University, New Zealand. She is the coordinator of the Blind and Low Vision endorsement of the joint Massey/Canterbury Specialist Teaching Programme. Previously Nicola has worked as a Developmental Orientation and Mobility (DOM) Specialist and a Resource Teacher Vision (RTV). Nicola is currently undertaking doctoral research in education, focusing on supporting children with cerebral visual impairment.

Mike McLinden, PhD, is co-director of the Vision Impairment Centre for Teaching and Research (VICTAR) in the Department of Disability Inclusion and Special Needs (DISN) at the University of Birmingham and programme lead for the professional development courses in visual impairment. Mike's research interests in the field of vision impairment education include the role of touch in the learning experiences of learners with complex needs, literacy development and early intervention approaches in low- and middle-income countries.

Natalie Martiniello is a Certified Vision Rehabilitation Therapist with expertise in braille and assistive technology training. She earned a bachelor's degree in English and Educational Studies from McGill University and a master's degree in Vision Science (Visual Impairment and Rehabilitation) from the University of Montreal. She is a PhD candidate in Vision Science (Visual Impairment and Rehabilitation) at the University of Montreal. Her research focuses on the impact of aging on braille acquisition, the influence of refreshable braille on reading performance and the development of evidence-based approaches for adult and senior braille learners. She also conducts research related to assistive technology usage and employment of the visually impaired. She is the President of Braille Literacy Canada.

Alice Pébay, PhD, is head of the regeneration research unit at the Centre for Eye Research Australia and principal research fellow at the University of Melbourne. Her laboratory focuses on the use of human pluripotent stem cells to model degenerative diseases of the eye and brain. She has published over 28 peer-reviewed articles and book chapters in the last five years and is on the editorial board of four international stem cell journals.

Matthew A. Petoe, PhD, is a biomedical engineer with a keen interest in human perception, neuroscience and clinical research. His research career has aimed to improve clinical outcomes in a range of patient groups, such as the congenitally deaf and patients with motor deficits following a stroke. His current position is at the Bionics Institute in Melbourne, Australia, overseeing the fitting and evaluation of a visual prosthesis for patients with inherited eye disease.

Michael J. Proulx, PhD, is Reader in Psychology and director of the Crossmodal Cognition Lab at the University of Bath. He is also co-director of the Mixed and Augmented Reality and Virtual Environments Lab and part of the Centre for Digital Entertainment in the Department of Computer Science. He received his BSc in Psychology from Arizona State University and his PhD in Psychological and Brain Sciences from Johns Hopkins University. He is a Fellow of the Society for Experimental Psychology and Cognitive Science of the American Psychological Association and was honoured as a torchbearer for the London 2012 Paralympic Games.

Samir Qasim, PhD, is an Assistant Professor of Adapted Physical Activity and Martial Arts with the Department of Sport Sciences at Yarmouk University in Jordan. He received his PhD from the University of Edinburgh in 2015. His research interests include analysing psychosocial health of individuals with visual impairment as well as determining the effectiveness of exercise interventions to improve psychological health, inclusion and physical fitness of individuals with disabilities.

Joao Roe, PhD, is an experienced teacher of children with visual impairment and head of a sensory support service based in Bristol. Joao has combined research and practice and her main areas of interest are social emotional development, play, early years and literacy through braille. She is involved in the training of teachers of children with visual impairment in a range of UK universities and is Honorary Lecturer in Psychology at the University of Bath.

Louise A Rooney is a research assistant at the Centre for Eye Research Australia (CERA). Her work concentrates on using stem cell-derived organoids to study neurodegeneration.

Peter Simcock is a Senior Lecturer in Social Work at Birmingham City University, UK. Prior to working in social work education, he was a specialist social worker with d/Deaf and deafblind people. Peter has a long-standing practice and research interest in dual sensory loss, particularly as experienced by older people. He is currently undertaking doctoral studies at King's College London, focusing on the lived experience of vulnerability among older deafblind people.

Wendy Timmons is Programme Director of the MSc Dance Science and Education at the University of Edinburgh. She has experience teaching and training professional dancers and dance teachers. Wendy has published in both dance science and education journals, her research includes the development and validation of technology for dance and she has two patents. Wendy is a member of the editorial board for the *Research in Dance Education* journal and is an editorial advisor for the *Scottish Journal for Performance*. She is also vice chairperson for the Traditional Dance Forum of Scotland.

Siu Yue-Ting, PhD, is a teacher of students with visual impairments (TVI) and coordinator of the Program in Visual Impairments at San Francisco State University. Her research focuses on TVIs' ongoing professional development via online communities of practice as mediated by social media. Ting's ultimate mission is to align technology developments and universal design with classroom implementation for optimal accessibility for all students.

Karl Wall, PhD, is a Senior Research Fellow in the UCL Centre for Inclusive Education at the UCL Institute of Education, London. Trained as a biologist and developmental psychologist, he has been a teacher, lecturer, practitioner-trainer and researcher, focusing on special educational needs and disabilities and specifically visual impairment and habilitation. As principle investigator for the UK Government-funded "Mobility21 Project" (directed by Dr Olga Miller) he developed the first national habilitation training and delivery standards in the UK. He also developed a training course with his practitioner team that remains the only specialist training route for new habilitation practitioners in the UK. He advises on and researches habilitation nationally and internationally.

Walter Wittich, PhD, is an Assistant Professor at the School of Optometry at the University of Montreal, in Montreal, Quebec, Canada. Following his master's degree in Psychology (Concordia University) and a PhD in Visual Neuroscience (McGill University), he completed a Postdoctoral Fellowship in Audiology at the University of Montreal. Coming from a background in low vision rehabilitation, he now conducts research in dual sensory impairment and acquired deafblindness. He is the inaugural chair of the Deafblind International Research Network, a Fellow of the American Academy of Optometry and is Quebec's first Certified Low Vision Therapist.

Karen E. Wolffe, PhD, manages a private practice as a career counsellor and consultant in Austin, Texas. She coordinates content for the World Blind Union's employment resources website, Project Aspiro, consults with organisations and schools worldwide on employability skills training and transition programming for individuals with disabilities and teaches distance education courses via Salus University (formerly Pennsylvania College of Optometry) and Fitchburg University through the Perkins eLearning program. Dr Wolffe has written extensively on the importance of careers and employment, social skills development, self-determination and transition in the lives of people with vision disabilities.

Acknowledgements

I have been extremely honoured and privileged to have been able to collaborate and work with all of the contributors in this book. I am extremely grateful to them all, my learning in visual impairment has significantly increased due to their expertise and knowledge and I cannot thank them enough for their help and support in developing this Handbook. They have worked tirelessly and have responded with great grace to my many queries and comments, which sometimes I am aware have been contradictory. All the authors therefore have my enormous respect.

I would like to say particular thanks to all of the people that have helped me to conceptualise the book, from the reviewers of the original proposal to Aline Nardo who supported me in helping to create the themes and areas the book needed to cover. To all of my colleagues at the University of Edinburgh that have had to, on a daily basis, listen to me talk about the compiling of this compendium. I would also like to thank the many international colleagues who I have met at conferences and other meetings for their guidance and support, particularly Amanda Lueck, Lauren Lieberman and Lea Hyvärinen.

Marion Linden provided the clerical support need to keep me calm in those final weeks, this was very much needed – thank you. And a special thank you goes to Routledge for being the first publishing house to agree to publish a non-medical based handbook on visual impairment, something that I have been trying to get agreement for several years now.

I must pay particular attention and thanks to all of the people, families and children that have participated in the various research activities described in the book. Thank you.

Finally, it is my family, Elaine and Euan, that have shown the utmost patience with me and have tirelessly supported me in all of my efforts. It hasn't gone unnoticed.

Abbreviations

ADL	activities of daily living
AFB	American Foundation for the Blind
AMD	age-related macular degeneration
APH	American Printing House for the Blind
BaLM	Basic Assessment of Light and Motion
CCTVs	closed-circuit television magnification systems
CNIB	Canadian National Institute for the Blind
CRPD	United Nations Convention on the Rights of Persons with Disabilities
CVI	cerebral visual impairment
CYPVN	children and young people with visual needs
DALYs	disability-adjusted life years
ECC	expanded core curriculum
EFD	Employers' Forum on Disability
ELSA	English Longitudinal Study of Ageing
FFA	fusiform face area
GSE	global self-esteem
hESC	human embryonic stem cell
hPSC	human pluripotent stem cell
HRQOL	health-related quality of life
IADL	instrumental activities of daily living
ICD	International Classification of Diseases
IDEA	Individuals with Disabilities Education Act
ILD	interaural loudness difference
iPSC	induced pluripotent stem cell
ITD	interaural time difference
LHON	Leber hereditary optic neuropathy
LOtv	lateral occipital tactile vision area
LoVADA	Low Vision Assessment of Daily Activities
MOI	mobility, orientation and independent living
MSVI	moderate and severe vision impairment
NCD	non-communicable diseases
NEET	not in employment, education or training
NVDA	NonVisual Desktop Access
O&M	orientation and mobility
OCR	optical character recognition
OMI	orientation, mobility and independent living

OMO	O&M outcomes
OVI	ocular visual impairment
PCS	Perceived Competence Scale for Children
Project ISSSL	International Study of Support and Sensory Loss Project
PSPCSA	perceived competence and social acceptance
RESC	Refractive Error Studies in Children
RGC	retinal ganglion cell
RLF	retrolental fibroplasia
ROP	retinopathy of prematurity
RPE	retinal pigmented epithelium
rTMS	repetitive transcranial magnetic stimulation
SBC	Screen Braille Communicator
TAPE	Tool to Assess Preparedness for Employment
TDU	tongue display unit
TGMD	Test for Gross Motor Development
TVI	teacher of students with visual impairments
UI	Uncertainty Interval
USABA	United States Association of Blind Athletes
VN	visual need
VROOM	vision-related outcomes in O&M
WABDL	World Association of Bench Press and Dead Lifters Association
WBU	World Blind Union
WHO	World Health Organization
YLD	years lived with a disability

Introduction and synthesis of themes

The editor's perspective

John Ravenscroft

Introduction

Books on visual impairment,[1] with a particular focus on social and cultural factors, have not proliferated the academic arena as have more traditional medical notions of visual impairment, However, as a journal editor where I constantly review journal publications, chapters and conference proceedings in visual impairment, I have noticed that there has been a significant development and even a consolidation of practice for the last five years. As such, I have felt the time has come to distil the research and explore these exciting international avenues of practice.

This new Handbook of visual impairment was put together with the aim of examining current debates as well as cross-examining traditionally held beliefs around visual impairment. This book aims to provide a bridge between medical practice and social and cultural research drawing on authentic investigations. It is the intention of the Handbook to provide an opportunity to engage with academic researchers who wish to ensure a coherent and rigorous approach to research construction and reflection on visual impairment that is in collaboration with but sometimes beyond the medical realm.

If research is to have meaning and value, it is hoped that this text will enable the researcher to make informed choices and sound decisions about research direction and design, by demonstrating complex ideas and theoretical framing needed to underpin more advanced research in visual impairment. It is, therefore, one of the main objectives in putting this Handbook together to provide insights into the ways in which this foundational knowledge of research and research processes can then be applied in order to build further coherent, relevant and rigorous outcomes for people with visual impairment.

Some medical and pedagogical challenges within visual impairment have been stale in moving on from traditional beliefs in that visual impairment should only be the focus of optical eye damage, that is, visual impairment is a result of damage or functional limitation of the eyes. However, in the past decade we now know that this is not the case and that, particularly in children, in developed economic countries visual impairment is due mainly to damage or functional limitation of the brain (Kong et al., 2012). This book will reflect this changing view of visual impairment and all the authors that have contributed to this Handbook fully understand this relationship between the eye and the brain.

Contributors to the Handbook provide an international perspective, with contributions coming from Canada, America, the United Kingdom, Jordan, Australia, Finland, Greece and New Zealand. The editor does note that one of the shortcomings of the book is the limitation of space and at least a doubling of contributions could have been included, thus indicating the revised research interest of areas identified in the book. The Handbook is therefore not meant to be exhaustive, but rather it is a collection of chapters that each of the authors have provided to illustrate and highlight with numerous examples how positive and successful outcomes for people with visual impairment can best be achieved.

The Handbook is divided into ten parts, each covering different thematic areas in order to represent the wide range of debates and concepts within visual impairment, in a structure that hopefully continuously builds and interlinks with each other. Note though, there were countless ways in which this book could have been thematically assembled but the editor's decisions to construct the book was driven by the complexity of the topic as well as a ride range of theoretical positions and conceptual arguments relating to social and cultural outcomes for people with visual impairment. These drivers reflect the changing research landscape within visual impairment and taken together hopefully has resulted in a new collection that provides a comprehensive, high-level review of debate and research that has intrinsic value but also can provide the catalyst for further research.

The ten themes within the book explore our recent understanding and representation of how people with visual impairment explore and interact with the world as well as focus on aspects of technology that have recently come to the forefront of assisting people of all ages with visual impairment. In addition the Handbook examines the important role of education and career education while also looking at the socio-emotional aspects of visual impairment and ends with a discussion of aging and adulthood.

The first theme of the book in Part I aims to identify and understand the profile, sociological and psychological impact of visual impairment explores. In Chapter 2, Keeffe presents some interesting data from the 2015 Global Burden of Disease publications and shows there has been a decrease in the prevalence of both vision impairment and blindness but an increase in the numbers of people with vision loss, which generally can be put down to the increase in life expectancy, in most countries. Chapter 2 is therefore also linked to the final theme in Part X and the last two chapters on aging and adulthood (Chapters 26 and 27). The third chapter within this initial theme explores the importance of the visual experience for cognitive processes, with a particular focus on perception of the environment. In other words, it provides us with an understanding from a psychological and neuroscience perspective on how people with no vision "see" the world. Fielder and Proulx's chapter (Chapter 3) links to Hayhoe's chapter (Chapter 15) in Part VI on understanding the cultural aesthetics, as well as Siu's chapter (Chapter 14) in Part V on assistive technology. In order for us to perhaps begin to understand the sociological impact of being blind, a personal account is necessary. Kapperman's own narrative of "On being blind" (Chapter 4) provides us with a very open and honest account of what it is like growing up as a person with visual impairment in the United States. He outlines some of the expected and not so expected challenges throughout his life and how he has overcome these challenges, particularly as he transitioned into college and university life.

Part I provides us with this general overview of a social and cultural perspective, and an understanding of the nature of representation of people with visual impairments. We know that "seeing" the world might be different for those with visual impairments compared to those with vision, but that their perception is just as rich and varied (Fielder and Proulx, Chapter 3 this volume).

The concept of trying to understand the unique individual world we each occupy, and how, where and why it is different from others, is key to understanding how, where, when and what support and accommodations need to be made with people with visual impairment is continued in the next three chapters in Part II, amalgamated under the second theme of cerebral visual impairment (CVI). It is important to always remember when reading these three chapters that CVI is not a single diagnosis, for it has commonly become known as an umbrella term for "all types of visual impairment due to brain damage or dysfunction" (Chokron and Dutton, 2016). Dutton and Bauer's chapter (Chapter 5) provides our first introduction to CVI and reinforces how vision is created by the brain and that this creation is unique to every individual and that "we must never use our own perceptions, to guide our educational approach to children with CVI, we must always use theirs" (Dutton and Bauer, Chapter 5 this volume). It is interesting to compare the next chapter by McDowell (Chapter 6), who provides us with another personal account of being visually impaired, but instead of describing life with an ocular impairment as Kapperman does (Chapter 4), McDowell explains how living with CVI has equally affected her quality of life. It is worth reading these two chapters side by side and noting the similarities and differences.

By Chapter 7 I hope the objective of understanding how the concept of individual representation of vision loss has been successfully messaged. An additional way of examining this is through having an understanding of how the assessment of visual processing functions and disorders occurs and this is exactly what Hyvärinen highlights (Chapter 7). The three case studies in this chapter show why acuity is not the determining factor for a child's visual function and that a thorough and detailed assessment process needs to be conducted to identify each individual's level of functioning. Hyvärinen rightly informs us in the chapter that visual acuity values should not be used to limit educational or medical services for students with visual processing disorders . . . each student's functioning, participation and environment should be thoroughly assessed to find the strengths and weaknesses of functions and available compensatory strategies.

This is, in part, why I have not started this introduction to the Handbook with the more traditional opening of trying to define exactly what visual impairment is. World health definitions are included in several of the chapters, and in terms of CVI no one adopted definition currently exists, although there have been recent attempts (Sakki et al., 2018). As such I wanted to ensure that acuity measures, which are the foundation of many traditional definitions of visual impairment, which are important, are not necessarily the sole or main driver to understand the nature of each person's visual impairment. As we read through the book it is clear that much more information is needed to understand the world in which people with visual impairment inhabit. By demonstrating the complex nature of visual impairment in these first seven chapters, it is hoped that the Handbook is successful in demonstrating that in order to create the right enabling conditions for rich social and cultural experiences, a holistic approach to understanding visual impairment and blindness is need.

Holistic approaches are often found within education. As McLinden et al. (2017) suggest, qualified teachers of pupils with visual impairment can be understood to qualify and work within a holistic ecological framework. Approaches in the education of children with visual impairment have changed over several decades, so in order to contextualise this change and to see the progressive development of the education of pupils with visual impairment, the first chapter in Part III, covering the theme of education, takes an interesting holistic, historical American perspective. This chapter highlights the elements that have shaped the delivery of low vision education services to pupils. It shows how the influences from a range of areas – medical and educational discoveries, population changes, technological innovations, as well as legislation, funding and differing approaches to teacher education programmes – have all combined to influence our modern day practice. Chapter 9, written by Argyropoulos and Gentle, continues this theme and considers formal and informal approaches within education for pupils with visual impairment and or multiple disabilities and vision impairment. The chapter successfully links these approaches to micro- and macro-perspectives and as with the previous chapter we see just how important current technological, cultural, societal and political changes need to be taken into account when we start to examine the formal and informal contemporary "educational landscape" of pupils with visual impairment and for those with multiple disabilities.

Transition as any child, parent and educational professional will testify is an extremely important phase of the child's life. So the third chapter in this theme (Chapter 10) by Douglas, Hewett and McLinden focuses upon the transition from school into higher education by young people with vision impairment. The authors make a distinction between "access to learning" and "learning to access". The former focuses upon inclusive practice and environmental adjustments, while the latter focuses upon developing a young person's agency and independence. Using a holistic ecological framework, several key messages merge that highlight the importance of good support structures, an inclusive environment and the utility of the young person's own agency. Obtaining a positive destination after school such as higher and further education and or employment is critical. One way for that person to obtain this goal is through the importance of career education. In the last of the education-themed chapters, Wolffe (Chapter 11) introduces what are the internal and external barriers that impede career development. However, and importantly, the chapter offers several solutions to overcome these barriers as well as directing readers to a series of assessment toolkits that can be used by the practitioner to support the pupil in obtaining the positive destination they seek. What comes across within these two latter transition chapters is the interweaving of the importance of personal agency by the young person themselves, but in order for the young person to have this agency, the role afforded by the practitioner in supporting and developing the young person's independence and determinism is also key.

The area of sport and physical exercise for people with visual impairment has often been a neglected area of research. However, coinciding with the growth of the Paralympics and the rights of people with visual impairment to have equal access to sport, this has slowly changed. Part IV covers the theme of sport and physical exercise for people with visual impairment and reflects this change, identifying the recent research and debates around sport and physical exercise, as well as providing a practical focus on sport and physical exercise for people with visual impairment and multiple disabilities. Chapter 12, for example, specifically focuses on children who are deafblind and Chapter 13 examines the role of movement and the need for physical activities for children with visual impairment. These two chapters, by Lieberman and Haegele, link very closely to Chapter 18 by Timmons and Ravenscroft, which examines expressive movement, and also to Chapters 19 and 20 by Roe and Qasim, which focus on socio-emotional aspects of people with visual impairment and self-esteem.

As technology appears to advance daily, there is a notion of always playing catch-up when researching within this area. However, to have a *Handbook of Visual Impairment* without specific reference to research with access technology would not do the book any justice. As such, the sole chapter by Siu in Part V on the theme of assistive technology (Chapter 14) provides us with a timely solution to this problem. Siu outlines a very interesting conceptual framework for approaching research in this area and suggests that part of the solution is that the research must be action-oriented. In a rapidly changing, technological environment, the development and implementation of assistive technology has become increasingly complex, the focus then is perhaps to consider more the implications of a research project as it will distil the purpose of any proposed agenda and advise investigators on designing a meaningful study. This approach could perhaps be adopted far beyond the visual impairment field and even beyond disability studies.

The four chapters in Part VI on the theme of understanding the cultural aesthetics provide a collection of research and conceptual ideas that in some sense connect all the way through the Handbook. As already noted, Chapter 15 by Hayhoe on philosophies on blindness and cross modal transfer links to the first theme discussed in Part I, but so too does Chapter 16 by Kennedy where he examines how tactile pictures make sense to people with no vision. Kennedy critically evaluates the opposing view that touch and pictures are a contradiction in terms – ontologically impossible. Through a nuanced argument with specific real-life examples he takes us through a journey of the nature of representation and explores how tactile outline drawings have become the main access point for accessing the arts for people with visual impairment. Feeney, on the other hand (Chapter 17), takes us into a different direction regarding the aesthetic value of art produced by artists with visual impairments. His exploration of the role of "gatekeepers" has currency throughout the Handbook and one that researchers, academics and professionals should keep returning too. Linking to self-esteem and socio-emotional factors as well as physical education, Chapter 18 by Timmons and Ravenscroft sits happily within this theme with an exploration of kinaesthetic empathy in movement and dance. It can also be linked with Siu's chapter on technology (Chapter 14), as the role of access through haptic touch is explored within kinaesthesia and kinaesthetic experiences.

Part VII discusses the theme of socio-emotional and sexual aspects of visual impairment, as it is so important to the lives of people with visual impairment. Roe's analysis in Chapter 19, supported by the voice of young people themselves, of the impact of vision impairment on social emotional development, illustrates from an early age what adults need to be aware of when promoting development in this area. The environment where different people are valued and the way language is used, are some of the important factors in determining the self-agency of children and young people with visual impairment. Without directly identifying the negative role that "gatekeepers" may play, Roe highlights support strategies that promote independence and lead to a positive sense of self-efficacy and well-being. People with visual impairment have conventionally been considered to have low self-esteem (Pinquart and Pfeiffer, 2011). But, if we accept Qasim's argument (Chapter 20) that self-esteem should be seen as a multidimensional hierarchical concept that provides subjective evaluation of self, children and adolescents with visual impairment actually record similar self-esteem levels as their sighted peers. The chapter identifies the need to improve the importance of some "self-domains" and argues that this is not a matter of notation but rather it is about the identification of a range of self-esteem domains that become important for people with visual impairment. The result then is to focus on decreasing those domains that continuously result in affording low self-esteem and increase the domains that lead to positive self-esteem. The last chapter in this theme by Kapperman and Kelly (Chapter 21) is the first ever exploration of "mate selection" from an evolutionary psychological perspective with respect to visual impairment. Kapperman and Kelly provide a very interesting approach (with the use of the dating app Tinder), to examine the possible relationships of adults with and without vision.

Themes of technology, self-esteem, education, activity, among others are also found throughout Part VIII on orientation, mobility, habilitation and rehabilitation. Wall (Chapter 22) outlines some of the research practices in habilitation and rehabilitation research that have hindered research in this particular area but one should read these as an extension to research in vision impairment as a whole. The chapter frames a historical overview as to why habilitation and rehabilitation is more than orientation and mobility and importantly challenges all researchers to not necessarily rely on the compendious publications that summarise much of the current literature around children and young people's habilitation needs. Instead Wall alerts us to the need to explore national literatures (often web-based) and go beyond our reluctance to explore journals in anything other than English. In Chapter 23, Deverell takes a constructivist approach to measuring functional vision and orientation and mobility. She reinforces the held belief discussed in the Handbook that measures of acuity alone do not provide sufficient information on the everyday impact of vision impairment. Rather, she calls for a suite of person-centred measures to generate this evidence and to use this evidence collaboratively with the person with vision impairment to design, develop and review approaches to enhance quality of life.

The Handbook's intention has been to clearly focus on the social and cultural aspects of living with vison impairment. However, in putting together this collection, and in particular Proulx's earlier chapter in combination with Kapperman, McDowell, Hayhoe and Siu, challenges the field to consider "what if" specific advances that are being made in terms of stem cell research and in technologies for vision impairment namely bionic eyes and other technological sensory substitution devices changes the nature of psychological representation? This is a question that I had not really considered. Although this question is not directly addressed in Part IX, which discusses recent advances in "eye" research and sensory substitution devices, I am extremely grateful for the two chapters in this theme (Chapter 24, Rooney et al. and Chapter 25, Ayton et al.) as they provide a clear understanding as to the current state of the art in this new developing area and enable us to start to ask some of these psychological and philosophical epistemological questions around their nature of representation regarding people who will use these devices or have benefitted from enhanced vision through stem cell developments.

The first chapter in Part X on the theme of aging and adulthood has obvious links to Chapter 11 by Wolffe, and could be read directly afer it, enhancing both positions put forward by all the authors. Martiniello and Wittich (Chapter 26) immediately highlight the issues by noting the rate of employment for people with visual impairments in developed countries is around between 25% and 40%, with 70% of adults with visual impairments either unemployed or underemployed or working in positions that do not reflect their qualifications. Research in this area is critical and again the two authors in this chapter highlight (as do Wall, Siu and Deverell in their respective chapters) the current deficits in research on employment that need to be addressed. The last chapter in the Handbook by Wittich and Simcock (Chapter 27) gives an overview of deafblindness research. Linkages again between the other chapters are clearly apparent with a discussion of the psycho-social impact of deafblindness being at the forefront of this chapter, as well as a clear call for the need for more a specific measurement tool to capture the clinical outcomes of rehabilitation interventions. An extremely interesting end to the chapter brings us back again to the nature of representation. The authors of this chapter specifically note deafblindness is a multiplicative impairment "that goes beyond the addition of vision loss plus hearing loss, [for it] creates a new and more severe entity because the absence of the second sense impairs the capacity to compensate".

Conclusion

The Handbook is therefore divided up into ten themes with 27 chapters that explore the social and cultural aspects of visual impairment. However, it is equally clear that the book could have also been divided into several other themes such as the nature of representation, conceptual research frameworks, definitions, quality of life and personal agency, which also run through the book. As such it is hoped that the Handbook can be taken and used in a variety of different ways in order to promote research, generate debate among practitioners and scholars who wish to use this resource to inform their practice in supporting and developing positive outcomes for all.

Note

1 The terms visual impairment and vision impairment are used interchangeably within the Handbook.

References

Chokron, S. and Dutton, G.N. 2016. Impact of cerebral visual impairments on motor skills: Implications for developmental coordination disorders. *Frontiers of Psychology*, 7, 1471.

Kong, L., Fry, M., Al-Samarraie, M., Gilbert, C. and Steinkuller, P.G. 2012. An update on progress and the changing epidemiology of causes of childhood blindness worldwide. *Journal of American Association for Pediatric Ophthalmology and Strabismus*, 16(6), 501–507.

McLinden, M., Ravenscroft, J., Douglas, G., Hewett, R. and Cobb, R. 2017. The significance of specialist teachers of learners with visual impairments as agents of change: Examining personnel preparation in the United Kingdom through a bioecological systems theory. *Journal of Visual Impairment and Blindness*, 111(6), 569–584.

Pinquart, M. and Pfeiffer, J.P. 2011. Bullying in German adolescents: Attending special school for students with visual impairment. *British Journal of Visual Impairment*, 29(3), 163–176.

Sakki, H.E.A., Dale, N.J., Sargent, J. and Perez-Roche, T. 2018. Is there consensus in defining childhood cerebral visual impairment? A systematic review of terminology and definitions. *British Journal of Ophthalmology*, 102, 424–432.

Part I

Introducing and understanding the profile, sociological and psychological impact of visual impairment

2

Global data on vision loss

Implications for services

Jill Keeffe

Introduction to global prevalence and causes of vision loss

The Global Burden of Disease team collected and analysed data and published papers including the review and meta-analysis of 333 diseases and injuries for 195 countries and territories from 1990 to 2016 (Murray et al., 2017). All the findings may be accessed on the Institute of Health Metrics and Evaluation website (www.healthdata.org.). Over that time period healthy life expectancy increased by 6.04 years but the number of disability-adjusted life years (DALYs) remained largely unchanged (www.healthdata.org/search?search_terms=DALYs). DALYs are a measure of the rating of the effect of a disability and the years lived with a disability. While the rates of some causes of disability are lower over the past few decades, the length of time lived with a disability has increased due to increased life expectancy in most countries (www. healthdata.org/data-visualization/life-expectancy-probability-death).

Within the Global Burden of Disease team a Vision Loss Expert Group was formed that has published global, regional and national data on the causes, prevalence and numbers of people with vision impairment or blindness for 1990, 2010 and 2015 (Bourne et al., 2017; Flaxman et al., 2017). For the 2015 papers the data were sourced from 288 relevant published papers with data from 98 countries. The data from those papers were analysed and modelled to provide data on the causes, prevalence and numbers of people with blindness and vision impairment from 190 countries in 7 regions and 21 subregions. The results are available on the International Agency for Prevention of Blindness (IAPB) website in the 2017 Vision Atlas (IAPB, 2017).

The papers from 1990 and 2010 presented data for blindness (visual acuity <3/60) and moderate and severe vision impairment (MSVI) (<6/18–3/60). For the 2015 data the category of mild vision impairment (<6/12–6/18) was added as was near vision impairment (presenting near vision worse than N6 or N8 at 40 cm) (Bourne et al., 2017). Results were provided for people of all ages and the group where vision impairment is most common is that of those aged ≥50 years. As an example, Figure 2.1 shows the distribution of the causes and numbers of people blind in the North America high-income region. The pattern of the increase in the older ages is similar in other regions but the high-income regions have the greatest numbers in the older age groups. Globally the burden of vision impairment is greatest in the ≥50 years age group with 31 million (86%) of the 36 million who were blind, 172.3 (80%) of the 216.6 million with MSVI

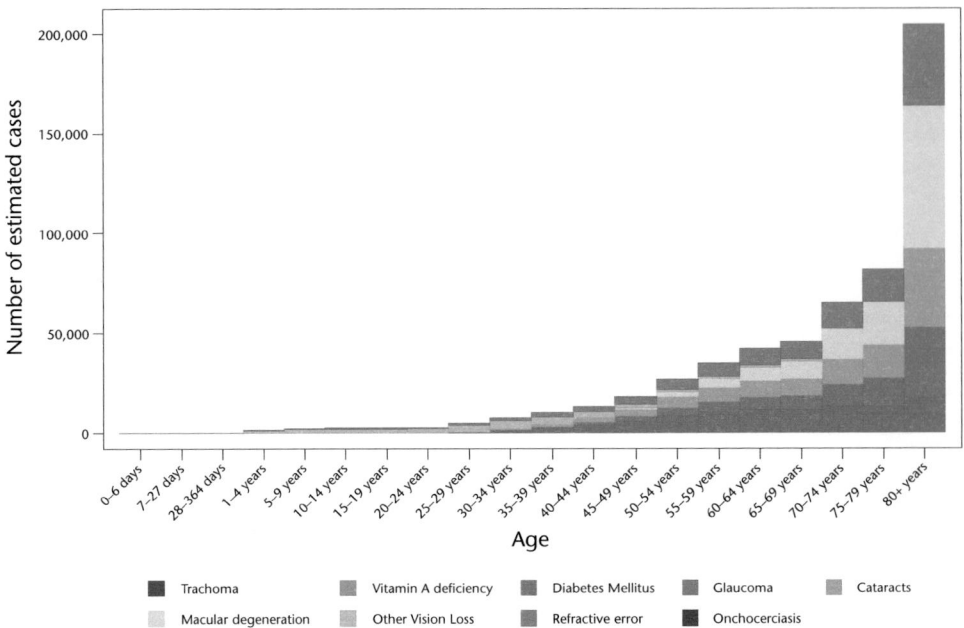

Figure 2.1 The number of people and causes of blindness in North America in 2010 from birth to ≥80 years.

and 140.3 million (74%) of the 188.5 million with mild vision impairment in that oldest age group (Table 2.1). There was a slightly lower proportion of those with functional presbyopia (near vision impairment) with 666.7 (61%) of the 1094.7 million in that age category (Bourne et al., 2017). The predictions for the numbers blind in 2020 are 38.5 million abd 114.6 million with MSVI.

Overall, the prevalence of blindness and vision impairment worldwide has decreased since the early results from 1990. The global age-standardised prevalence of blindness for all ages decreased from 0.75% (Uncertainty Interval (UI) 0.25%–1.41%) in 1990 to 0.48% (UI 0.17%–0.87%) in 2015 and age-standardised prevalence of MSVI for all ages decreased from 3.8% (UI 1.66%–6.42%) in 1990 to 2.9% (UI 1.31%–4.8%) in 2015. All the 21 subregions showed reduced prevalence in both males and females but there was significant variation from high- to low-income regions with the highest prevalence rates in African, South Asian and Oceania regions.

Despite the reduced prevalence of vision impairment and blindness in all regions between 1990 and 2015, the numbers of people have increased (Table 2.1). This increase in numbers is primarily due to the increased life expectancy of the population with greater proportions of people in older age groups where the prevalence of vision impairment is higher with 80% of vision impairment in people 50 years of age and older. The decrease is associated with:

- overall socio-economic development;
- concerted public health action including awareness and early detection;
- increased availability and accessibility of eye care services;
- awareness in the general population about seeking care for the problems related to vision impairment such as cataract surgery and glasses for refractive error.

Table 2.1 The number of people in the world blind or vision impaired from 1990 to 2010.

	Blind (million)	MSVI (million)	Mild VI (million)	Near VI (million)
1990	31.8	172		
2010	32.4	191		
2015	36.0	216.6	188.5	1,094.75

Note: MSVI = moderate and severe vision impairment; VI = vision impairment

To assist in increasing awareness, knowledge and continued use of services the World Health Organization (WHO) has developed a new programme using messaging via mobile phones that aims to increase access to and use of services to work towards universal health coverage. This is now feasible in most countries with the availability of mobile phones including in rural areas. Messages are transmitted by mobile phones to assist in disease prevention and management to ensure treatment compliance, to change behaviours and manage chronic diseases so that people seek health care, maintain function and live independently (WHO, 2014). The World Health Organization mHealth programme provides messages across many areas of health including diabetes (mDiabetes) and ageing (mAgeing), the latter including areas such as vision and hearing, mobility, cognitive impairments and depressive symptoms.

While the prevalence has reduced and the number of people with vision impairment has increased there are only quite small changes in the proportions of the main causes of vision loss (Table 2.2). One important change has been in the proportion of people with cataracts globally, which has reduced particularly in the MSVI category from 26.6% to 18.4%. There are now only very small proportions of the global population with trachoma, as programmes to eliminate trachoma have been successful with the global proportions reducing from 2.8% of vision loss to 1% in 2015. Corneal opacity has also seen a reduction. Age-related macular degeneration has seen a small decline but the proportions of vision loss due to glaucoma and diabetic retinopathy have changed very little.

In South Asia the preventable causes of vision loss, cataracts and uncorrected refractive error (URE) made up a substantial total of 74.3% of blindness in 1990 and 73% in 2015. The proportions of MSVI due to cataracts and URE are similar with 90.4% in 1990 and the total of 91.6% in 2015 (Table 2.2).

Table 2.2 Causes of blindness and moderate and severe vision impairment (MSVI) in adults ≥50 years with percentages of each of the causes globally and in the South Asian region.

	Cataracts	URE	AMD	Glaucoma	DR	Corneal opacity	Trachoma	Other
Blindness								
1990	36.6	19.6	8.0	8.6	0.9	4.8	2.8	18.8
World	38.8	35.5	3.1	6.0	0.1	3.9	0.2	12.4
South Asia								
2015	35.2	20.3	6.0	8.5	1.1	3.2	1.0	25.0
World	36.6	36.4	2.4	5.8	0.2	2.4	0.04	16.1
South Asia								
M/S VI								
1990	26.6	51.1	6.0	2.1	1.0	1.8	2.0	9.7
World	25.8	64.6	1.8	1.1	0.1	1.3	0.1	5.2
South Asia								
2015	18.4	52.9	4.4	2.2	1.3	1.1	0.6	13.0
World	25.2	66.4	1.3	1.1	0.2	0.8	0.03	6.7
South Asia								

While the proportions of the causes have changed very little over the 25 years, the numbers have increased (Table 2.1). The increase is related to the ageing of the population over the last few decades. Many countries have experienced an increase of 5 to 10 years in life expectancy in the two decades from 1990. The increase in the population over that period was 30% with an increase in numbers with vision impairment of 2% for blindness and 11% for vision impairment due to the decrease in prevalence of both blindness and MSVI.

An example of the use of the Global Burden of Disease data has been published for China (Wang et al., 2017). The age-standardised prevalence of the causes of vision loss were similar between 1990 and 2015. There was a very small increase in the rates of glaucoma and age-related macular degeneration but trachoma was much lower due to an intensive programme for its elimination. In addition to the data on prevalence and numbers of people with vision impairment an important measure is the years lived with a disability (YLD). YLDs increased in China from 2,047,000 to 3,800,000 from 1990 to 2015 with a global ranking of second at each time behind India. The rates per 100,000 for 19 of the G20 countries were also presented for 1990 and 2015 with China ranking tenth. The countries with the highest ranking of the rates per 100,000 in the population in 2015 were India, South Africa, Mexico, Saudi Arabia and Indonesia (Muhit et al., 2018). India had top ranking at both times for the numbers of people with YLD. The countries with the lowest rankings in the G20 group were the rates for Canada, USA, UK, France and Australia.

Vision impairment in children

While there are excellent data from many publications on the prevalence of vision impairment and blindness in adults, there are very few population-based studies on children especially those that cover all ages from 0 to 15 years. There have been many studies to determine the prevalence and causes of vision loss conducted in primary and/or secondary schools and schools for the blind but they do not cover all ages and especially those children out of school. Other studies report data from children attending hospitals or clinics but also do not cover the whole population of children with vision loss. As there were few reliable studies on vision loss in children, the World Health Organization developed estimates for the rates of blindness in children based on the under 5 years mortality rates for countries. The World Health Organization estimates range from 1.2 per 1,000 children who were blind (visual acuity <3/60) in low-income countries where under 5 mortality rates were highest to 0.2 per thousand in high-income regions. The numbers of children with low vision was estimated to be three times the rate of blindness.

Studies were often conducted in schools for the blind to determine the causes and estimated number of children with vision impairment or blindness. In most countries now a relatively small proportion of children with blindness and vision impairment attend special schools with many in inclusive education settings at primary and secondary levels.

A study in Fiji, a small island country in the Pacific region, in 2006–2007 utilised multiple methods to estimate the causes and prevalence of vision impairment and blindness from non-refractive causes (Cama, Sikivou and Keeffe, 2010). As there were no published population-based studies in that region, the sample size was calculated using the World Health Organization prevalence estimates, which were based on under 5 years mortality rates (WHO/IAPB, 2000). The results for causes and prevalence were sourced from screening programmes in primary schools, records from the Fiji School for the Blind and the Fiji Society for the Blind community-based programme, the country's main hospital and key informants such as community-based health nurses. Surveys were conducted as part of the study in secondary schools and schools for children with hearing, physical and intellectual disabilities. The rate of blindness was 0.39 per thousand and 0.8 per 1,000 for low vision, double the rate of blindness, not three times as the World Health Organization estimates. The World Health Organization estimate of the rate of blindness based on the Fiji under 5 mortality was 0.4 per 1,000 thus almost the same as the estimate from the survey (WHO, 1992). The three main causes were retinal diseases, cataracts and cortical and whole globe anomalies. In previous decades observations at the Fiji School for the Blind there were children with vision loss from corneal disease related to vitamin A deficiency. In the 2006–2007 study the youngest child with corneal-related vision loss was aged 15. The proportion of children with multiple disabilities including vision was 26%. Of all the children included in this study 12% were from a school for the blind or clinics thus representing a small proportion of all children with blindness or MSVI.

As the name suggests the Refractive Error Studies in Children (RESC) were designed to determine the prevalence of vision loss focusing on refractive error in children aged 5–15 years to plan services for children requiring eye care (Gilbert et al., 2008). The surveys were population-based clusters of children from villages who were screened and then examined based on the results of the screening. The sample sizes required for surveys were based on the estimated prevalence of refractive errors, thus the numbers of children with vision loss from non-refractive error were quite small with corneal disease and retinal disorders most common (Dandona et al., 2002). While the age of the population sampled in the study by Dandona et al. (2002) (7–15 years) was school-age children, only approximately half of the children examined were attending school with others screened in the community. The study showed that conducting studies only in schools will not cover the whole population of children in an area.

Studies need to be population-based with very large sample sizes to gain reliable data on the prevalence and causes given the relatively low prevalence of blindness in children. A population-based study in southern India started by screening 23,100 children in villages and towns (Kemmanu et al., 2016) to list the causes of ocular morbidities. Those detected with eye-related problems were then examined by an ophthalmologist. The most common causes of blindness were retinal, lens diseases and whole globe anomalies. Two current population-based studies are being conducted on children in a similar area of southern India with sample sizes of over 50,000 children aged 0–15 years. The sample sizes are considerably larger than the Kemmanu et al. (2016) study that was conducted almost ten years ago and will therefore provide reliable prevalence data.

Implications and challenges

Almost two decades ago Vision 2020 set the aim to eliminate avoidable blindness by 2020. While there have been some positive changes in the reduction in the prevalence of blindness and MSVI, the main avoidable causes of vision loss, cataracts and refractive error are still the main causes of vision loss. Targeted cataract programmes have been successful in reducing the prevalence of vision loss due to cataracts in many regions but there still is much to be done to increase cataract surgical coverage in many areas and populations. With knowledge on barriers to awareness and accessibility to eye care, countries need to target programmes to overcome existing barriers such as accessibility and gender differences in access to and use of services.

While these factors have had an impact there are still many barriers such as availability and access to services related to infrastructure, equipment and the health workforce. Where an adequate number of quality services exists, barriers include knowledge that eye problems can be treated and in some cases vision restored or vision loss prevented. In most countries the data show marked differences in the prevalence of vision loss between men and women with the highest rates in women (Bourne et al., 2017). A recent study in African and Asian countries showed significant inequity with use of cataract surgical services favouring boys in settings in both regions (Reddy et al., 2018). Cataracts are usually one of the top three causes of vision loss in children and critical as it is a preventable cause of vision loss. The study showed that community-based case finding is necessary to identify children needing cataract surgery.

There is now a focus on non-communicable diseases (NCD) across all areas of health. This is similar in eye care with a focus on the NCD categories of vision loss, specifically age-related macular (AMD) degeneration, diabetic retinopathy and glaucoma. Figure 2.1 shows the increase in these three causes of vision loss from about 50 years of age but can occur prior to that in some people. It is not only the numbers of people that create a challenge in providing eye care and rehabilitation services but it is the length of time that people have vision loss from these causes. With life expectancy now very common beyond 70 years and over 80 years in some countries, people will have vision loss for perhaps 20 to 30 years or occasionally more. Regular visits, often annually but occasionally more frequently to an eye care provider are necessary to prevent vision loss or monitor conditions. This means that planning of eye care and rehabilitation services needs not only to count the number of people with vision loss due to NCDs who require services but also to estimate the number of visits needing to be provided. Low vision and rehabilitation services are likely to be required long term due to vision changes over time, but also if vision does not deteriorate rehabilitation needs to be changed as a person's needs change.

Conclusion

The World Health Organization has stated in the Global Action Plan 2014–2019 that countries should assess the magnitude and causes of vision impairment and blindness to plan services and monitor the changes over time (WHO, 2013). The data that have been published recently from the Global Burden of Disease Vision Loss Expert Group can be accessed on the International Agency for Prevention of Blindness Atlas website, so are readily available to any country that may not have or be aware of the data (IAPB, 2017).

References

Bourne, R.R.A., Flaxman, S.R., Braithwaite, T., Cicinelli, M.V., Das, A., Jonas, J.B., Keeffe, J., Kempen, J.H., Leasher, J., Limburg, H., Naidoo, K., Pesudovs, K., Resnikoff, S., Silvester, A., Stevens, G.A., Tahhan, N. and Taylor, H.R., on behalf of the Vision Loss Expert Group. 2017. Magnitude, temporal trends, and projections of the global prevalence of blindness and distance and near vision impairment: A systematic review and meta-analysis. *Lancet Global Health*, 5(9), 888–897.

Cama, A.T., Sikivou, B. and Keeffe, J. 2010. Childhood vision impairment in Fiji. *Archives of Ophthalmology*, 128(5), 608–612.

Dandona, R., Dandona, L., Srinivas, M., Sahare, P., Narsaiab, S., Munoz, S.R., Pokharel, G.P. and Ellwein, L.B. 2002. Refractive error in children in a rural population in India. *Investigative Ophthalmology and Vision Science*, 43, 616–622.

Flaxman, S.R., Bourne, R.R.A., Resnikoff, S., Ackland, P., Braithwaite, T., Cicinelli, M.V., Das, A., Jonas, J.B., Keeffe, J., Kempen, J.H., Leasher J., Limburg, H., Naidoo, K., Pesudovs, K., Resnikoff, S., Silvester, A., Stevens, G.A., Tahhan, N. and Taylor, H.R., on behalf of the Vision Loss Expert Group. 2017. Global causes of blindness and distance vision impairment 1990–2020: A systematic review and meta-analysis. *Lancet Global Health*, 5(12), 1221–1234

Gilbert, C.E., Ellwein, L.B. and the Refractive Error Study Group. 2008. Prevalence and causes of functional low vision in school-age children: Results from standardized population-based surveys in Asia, Africa, and Latin America. *Investigative Ophthalmology and Vision Science*, 49, 877–881.

International Agency for Prevention of Blindness. 2017. IAPB Vision Atlas [e-resource]. Accessed July 2018. www.iapb.org/news/iapb-vision-atlas-book-published.

Kemmanu, V., Hedge, K., Gillyar, S.K., Shetty, B.K., Kumaramanichavel, G. and McCarty, C.A. 2016. Prevalence of childhood blindness and ocular morbidity in a rural pediatric population in southern India: The Pavagada Pediatric Eye Disease Study-1. *Ophthalmic Epidemiology*, 23, 187–192.

Muhit, M., Karim, T., Islam, J., Hardianto, D., Muhiddin, H.S., Purwanta, S.A., Suhardjo, S., Widyandana, D. and Khandaker, G. 2018. The epidemiology of childhood blindness and severe visual impairment in Indonesia. *British Journal of Ophthalmology*, 102(11), 1543–1549. http://dx.doi:10.1136/bjophthalmol-2017-311416

Murray, C.J.L., the GBD 206 DALYs and HALE contributors. 2017. Global, regional, and national disability-adjusted life years (DALYs) for 333 diseases and injuries and healthy life expectancy (HALE) for 195 countries and territories, 1990–2016: A systematic analysis for the Global Burden of Disease Study. *Lancet*, 390(10100), 1260–1344.

Reddy, P.A., Kishiki, E.A., Thapa, H.B., Demers, L., Geneau, R. and Bassett, K. 2018. Interventions to improve utilization of cataract surgical services by girls: Case studies from Asia and Africa. *Ophthalmic Epidemiology*, 25, 199–206.

Wang, B., Congdon, N., Bourne, R., Li, Y., Cao, K., Zhao, A., Yusufu, M., Done, W., Zhou, M. and Wang, N. 2017. Burden of vision loss associated with eye disease in China 1990–2020: Findings from the Global Burden of Disease Study 2015. *British Journal of Ophthalmology*, 102(2), 310–333.

World Health Organization. 1992. *Management of low vision in children: Report of a WHO consultation*. Bangkok, 23–24 July. Accessed July 2018. WHO/PBL/93.27 http://apps.who.int/iris/handle/10665/61105.

World Health Organization. 2013. *Universal eye health: Global action plan 2014–2019* [e-resource]. Accessed July 2018. www.who.int/blindness/AP2014_19_English.pdf.

World Health Organization. 2014. *Be He@lthy be mobile: New horizons for health through mobile technology* [e-resource]. Accessed July 2018. www.who.int/nmh/publications/be-healthy-be-mobile/en.

World Health Organization and International Agency for Prevention of Blindness. 2000. *Preventing blindness in children: Report of a WHO/IAPB scientific meeting*. World Health Organization, WHO/PBL/00.77. Geneva: WHO.

3

Psychological representation of visual impairment

Perception and how visually impaired people "see" the world

Jennifer C. Fielder and Michael J. Proulx

Introduction

Despite living in a highly visual environment, our perceptual experience of the world is richly multisensory (Ghazanfar and Schroeder, 2006; Spence, 2011). We are able to extract information derived from one sensory modality to inform another; we may know a shape by touch and identify it by sight or know a violin by touch and identify it by sound. This chapter focuses on how blind people perceive the world using different sensory modalities. Comparing congenitally blind, late blind and sighted individuals enables the role of visual experience for cognition (at psychological and neural levels) to be explored. This sheds light on how the "blind brain" may differ from the sighted brain, which is important to establish for developing interventions, such as assistive technology and sensory substitution devices (Proulx et al., 2016; Scheller, Petrini and Proulx, 2018), and could benefit employment and educational practice (Metatla et al., 2015; Metatla et al., 2016). Furthermore, if congenitally blind and late blind individuals significantly differ on cognitive tasks, this suggests visual input during the first few years of life plays a role in cognitive development, reflecting a critical period in neural and psychological terms. How "critical" critical periods are for visual development is also important to establish because blind individuals who can be treated (for example if their blindness is due to cataracts) sometimes remain untreated due to the assumption that they would not develop sight later in life because they have missed a critical period for visual development, for example 40% of blind children in India (Kalia et al., 2017). This chapter explores the importance of visual experience for cognitive processes, with particular focus on their perception of the environment and subsequently how blind individuals "see" the world.

Compensatory hypothesis

There is a substantial body of physiological and behavioural research that suggests that blind individuals have enhanced sensitivity of their remaining sensory modalities since they rely on these to a greater extent than sighted individuals. This reflects a phenomenon known as "compensatory plasticity" in which individuals cope with the loss of vision by developing supranormal skills when using one of the remaining senses (Kupers and Ptito, 2011). It has been hypothesised that these enhancements depend on the high plasticity of the visual cortex (Merabet and Pascual-Leone, 2010; Merabet et al., 2005). For example, it has been found that the visual cortex in blind individuals is recruited to carry out non-visual tasks such as braille reading (Burton, Sinclair and Agato, 2012; Cohen et al., 1997) and sound localisation (Gougoux et al., 2005; Leclerc et al., 2000).

Auditory processing

Audition is argued to be the most studied sensory modality in blind individuals (Kupers and Ptito, 2014). Gougoux et al. (2004) tested early blind and sighted participants on a pitch discrimination task, in which participants had to decide whether the pitch between two tones was rising or falling. They found that nearly blind individuals performed significantly better than sighted controls in this task, even when the speed of change was ten times faster than that perceived by controls. This supports the compensatory hypothesis since it provides evidence of increased auditory perceptual abilities in blind individuals. However, one could argue that enhanced auditory capacities in blind individuals may depend on their usually greater musical experience, rather than due to differences in vision loss per se (Cattaneo et al., 2011). Rokem and Ahissar (2009) accounted for this by comparing congenitally blind individuals with sighted controls matched on musical training, as well as on age and education. They found superior auditory frequency discrimination and superior speech perception measured by resilience to noise among the congenitally blind individuals. Wan et al. (2010) also consider musical experience by controlling for musical training and absolute pitch (the ability to recreate or recognise a musical note without a reference tone) when comparing auditory perception skills in blind and sighted individuals. They found that congenitally (but not late) blind subjects outperformed the sighted controls in pitch discrimination and pitch-timbre categorisation (making judgements on both pitch and timbre) but not in pitch working memory (listening to a series of tones and determining whether the first and last tones were the same). This suggests that visual deprivation onset early in life does not lead to superior performance in all auditory tasks, and that the enhancement of auditory acuity related to pitch stimuli in the blind is restricted to basic perceptual skills rather than extending to higher-level processes such as working memory.

It is also important to consider auditory perception in more naturalistic settings such as processing speech sounds, yet only a few studies do so (Kupers and Ptito, 2014). Hugdahl et al. (2004) investigated consonant-vowel syllable discrimination via headphones in a dichotic listening task in which participants were instructed to pay attention to the right ear stimulus, left ear stimulus or no specific instruction was given. Fourteen congenitally or early blind individuals were compared with 129 sighted individuals. The blind individuals outperformed sighted individuals in correctly identifying syllables. Furthermore, when instructed to pay attention to the left ear stimulus and only report from the attended channel, they were significantly better than sighted controls. The typical finding in this paradigm is a right ear advantage, which indicates better processing of the consonant-vowel syllable stimuli in the left hemisphere. The results from Hugdahl et al. (2004) therefore suggest that there is hemispheric reorganisation in blind individuals in the auditory modality that may enable enhanced speech processing. In contrast however, Gougoux et al. (2009) found no behavioural differences in voice recognition between congenitally blind, late blind and sighted participants.

Contrasting results on how visual experience impacts auditory processing is being revealed by an increasing number of studies in the domain of spatial cognition; for a review see Scheller et al. (2018). Auditory localisation is key for many behaviours and normally is a cross-modal or multisensory task incorporating vision. Blind individuals can show normal or even supranormal auditory localisation performance in the far space as well as near space in a number of studies (Fieger et al., 2006; Lessard et al., 1998; Voss et al., 2004). However, other studies reported that early or congenitally blind individuals compared to sighted individuals have a compromised representation of auditory space in the vertical (sagittal) plane (Finocchietti, Cappagli and Gori, 2015). This might be due to a disruption of audio-visual multisensory calibration (Gori et al., 2014a), where visual perception early in life serves as a mechanism for multisensory "glue" that calibrates the other senses (Pasqualotto and Proulx, 2012). Auditory localisation in the horizontal plane in the visually impaired provides accurate or even superior results because cues used by the brain to decode sound source location (interaural loudness difference (ILD) and interaural time difference (ITD)) are still available without vision. Other studies have also found supranormal sound localisation in the horizontal plane (Lessard et al., 1998; Voss et al., 2004). Sound location in the vertical plane can only be mapped based on the pinna-related spectral shape cues, which are less accurate than interaural time or loudness differences, unless one has specially adapted pinna such as the barn owl (Konishi, 2000). Interestingly, the superior auditory localisation performance of blind individuals is observed mainly in the lateral perceptual field but not in the centre, perhaps suggesting a monaural mechanism for such superior performance rather than standard auditory localisation binaural cues (Roder et al., 1999). The age of onset of blindness seems to play a critical role as well. While, in the study by Finocchietti et al. (2015), early blind individuals showed impaired audio localisation in the lower sagittal plane, late blind individuals did not. This group's responses were similar to those of sighted participants. This might indicate that multisensory calibration builds up the foundations for understanding physical properties in the environment at an early age, when plasticity is high (Pasqualotto and Proulx, 2012; Proulx, Brown et al., 2014; Scheller et al., 2018).

Somatosensory processing

The ability of touch provides a great deal of information about the environment, for example recognising everyday objects. For blind individuals especially, utilising the sensory modality of touch enables them to read and write in braille, thus facilitating vital communication. It is therefore unsurprising to propose that their tactile perceptual abilities used to "see" the world may be enhanced given their increased reliance on tactile information. Indeed, Van Boven et al. (2000) compared 15 early blind braille readers with 15 sighted subjects in a grating orientation discrimination task used to measure psychophysical limits of spatial acuity. They found that the blind individuals had a significantly lower mean grating orientation discrimination threshold compared to the sighted group, and that their index finger (braille reading finger) had a significantly lower threshold than the other fingers. This suggests that blind individuals may have enhanced tactile spatial acuity due to adaptive changes. This higher tactile acuity in blind individuals has also been supported by subsequent research (Goldreich and Kanics, 2003; Legge et al., 2008).

However, not all touch is improved in the absence of visual experience. Other studies do not find significant differences between blind and sighted subjects in tactile pressure sensitivity (Pascual-Leone and Torres, 1993; Sterr, Green and Elbert, 2003; Sterr et al., 1998) or spatial-acuity-dependent grating orientation discrimination (Grant, Thiagarajah and Sathian, 2000). Wong, Gnanakumaran and Goldreich (2011) tested whether improved tactile acuity was due to their reliance on tactile experience (tactile experience hypothesis), or due to the loss of vision itself driving increased tactile acuity (visual deprivation hypothesis). They tested spatial acuity on the index, middle and ring finger of each hand as well as the lips, comparing 28 blind individuals with 55 sighted individuals. They found that the blind individuals significantly outperformed the sighted group in all fingers, but not on the lips, consistent with the tactile experience hypothesis. Furthermore, within the blind participants, proficient braille readers outperformed non-readers on their preferred reading index finger, and within the proficient braille readers, their preferred index finger outperformed their opposite index finger, and this was correlated with weekly reading time. These results suggest that enhanced tactile acuity is due to increased tactile experience rather than the actual loss of vision. This is further supported by studies that use a visual-tactile sensory substitution device known as the tongue display unit (TDU), which translates visual information into electro-tactile stimulation applied to the tongue. When training both congenitally blind and matched sighted control subjects, both performed equally well in discriminating orientation (Ptito et al., 2005), motion (Matteau et al., 2010) and shapes (Ptito et al., 2012). This therefore suggests that blind individuals have enhanced tactile perception due to their increased experience and reliance on tactile information to see the world, such that practice makes perfect (Sathian, 2000).

Olfaction

The sense of smell is important for almost all species, from finding the right food to choosing a mate (Kupers et al., 2011), and can evoke strong emotions and vivid memories (Gottfried, 2006). While it is believed that humans have a less refined sense of smell than animals, they are nonetheless able to distinguish between thousands of different odours. Like in auditory and tactile processing, it has been proposed that blind individuals, given their loss of vision, have enhanced olfactory performance. For example, Cuevas et al. (2009) found that blind individuals were better than sighted controls in the free identification of odours and odour discrimination. Furthermore, Beaulieu-Lefebvre et al. (2011) found that blind subjects have a lower odour detection threshold and report being more aware of their olfactory environment. Like with enhanced auditory and tactile perception, this is proposed to be due to cross-modal plasticity, since the olfactory bulb in the forebrain is very plastic (Li et al., 2006). Indeed, Rombaux et al. (2010) found that superior olfactory performance in blind subjects was related to increased volume of the olfactory bulb. Moreover, Kupers et al. (2011) found that congenitally blind subjects activated higher-order olfactory bulb areas more strongly than blindfolded sighted subjects.

However, there is also evidence that shows comparable performance in blind and sighted individuals in terms of olfactory thresholds, discrimination abilities and cued smell identification (Cuevas et al., 2009; Kupers et al., 2011; Rombaux et al., 2010; Rosenbluth, Grossman and Kaitz, 2000). The discrepancy in results possibly reflects limited sample sizes of congenitally blind participants, such as Cuevas et al. (2009) and Beaulieu-Lefebvre et al. (2011), or in combining congenital, early and late blind individuals into one group, a persistent problem in the literature (Pasqualotto and Proulx, 2012). Addressing these limitations, Sorokowska (2016) studied congenitally blind (n = 43), late blind (n = 41) and sighted (n = 84) participants matched for age and gender, with sample sizes that are extraordinarily rare in neuroscience and psychology research on the topic of visual impairment. Sorokowska found no significant difference between groups on olfactory threshold, odour discrimination, cued identification, or free identification scores using a standardised smell test (the Sniffin' Sticks test). This suggests that sensory compensation in blind individuals is not pronounced in olfactory abilities when measured by standardised smell tests. Using the same test, another recent study by Majchrzak et al. (2017) compared a heterogeneous group of visually impaired participants (n = 99) with sighted controls (n = 100). They also found no significant difference in odour identification or discrimination tasks, further suggesting that blind individuals do not have an enhanced sense of smell.

General-loss hypothesis

The consequences of blindness on the remaining sensory modalities, however, is still under debate (Gurtubay-Antolin and Rodríguez-Fornells, 2017). In contrast to the literature discussed that argues that blind individuals have enhanced sensitivity of their remaining sensory modalities (compensatory hypothesis), it has also been suggested that visual deprivation leads to maladjustments in remaining modalities (general-loss hypothesis). This is particularly the case for modalities that include spatial information (e.g. audition, touch) since localisation is hypothesised to benefit from visual calibration (Gori et al., 2014a; Gori et al. 2014b). For example, research suggests that blind individuals are impaired in auditory spatial tasks such as bisection (Gori et al., 2014a), vertical localisation (Lewald, 2002; Zwiers, Van Opstal and Cruysberg, 2001) and absolute distance discrimination (Kolarik et al., 2013). Evidence also suggests blind individuals are impaired in tactile spatial tasks including haptic orientation discrimination (Postma et al., 2008), visual spatial imagination (Noordzij, Zuidhoek and Postma, 2007) and rotation of object arrays (Ungar, Blades and Spencer, 1995). Cappagli, Cocchi and Gori (2017) investigated both tactile and auditory spatial perception in the same study and found substantial spatial impairment in congenitally blind children and blind adults for auditory distance perception and proprioceptive reproduction (hand-pointing in the haptic domain) when compared to blindfolded sighted participants.

This supports the notion that visual calibration is necessary for spatial perception in auditory and haptic domains. Indeed, auditory distance accuracy and variability are improved in the presence of additional congruent visual cues in sighted individuals (Anderson and Zahorik, 2014; Calcagno et al., 2012; Finnegan, O'Neill and Proulx, 2015, 2017). Moreover, Cappagli et al. (2017) found that late blind individuals performed significantly better than sighted subjects in both auditory and tactile space perception tasks. This superior performance of late blind individuals may be due to practice effects, since after vision loss their spatial judgements must rely solely on auditory cues, for example, learned early in life, as reported by Cappagli et al. (2017). However, this assumes that during early development vision calibrates hearing in encoding spatial information (Gori et al., 2014a; Pasqualotto and Proulx, 2012). While this study only included three late blind individuals and requires further replication, these preliminary results, that congenitally blind individuals were severely impaired while late blind individuals had superior abilities compared to sighted individuals, suggest that space perception may be drastically weakened due to the lack of visual calibration over the auditory and haptic modalities during a critical period of development.

Impact of perception on higher cognition

Thus far we have reviewed the perceptual changes that occur with visual experience or the lack thereof. Given that most higher-level cognitive processing is based on inferences about the outside world that are validated with perceptual information, any initial changes in sensation or perception will have higher-order consequences (Proulx, 2013). One such example is the behaviours that are classified as aspects of spatial cognition. Spatial cognition has been tested in blind individuals for a suite of behaviours, including memory for arrays of objects lying within the manipulatory space (arm's length), environmental knowledge, wayfinding and navigation. On the one hand, some researchers have reported results suggesting that congenitally blind people do not fully develop spatial cognition, and thus perform poorer than sighted and late blind participants (Pasqualotto and Newell, 2007). On the other hand, other researchers have reported that visual experience is not necessary for the development of spatial cognition and that blind individuals can perform spatial tasks without visual experience (Landau, Gleitman and Spelke, 1981).

We hypothesised that these conflicting findings could be resolved if another factor were considered that would classify these studies by the frame of reference required for the task (Pasqualotto and Proulx, 2012). Shelton and McNamara (2001) noted that objects can be mentally represented with respect to the position of the observer (an egocentric frame of reference) or with respect to the position of the object in the environment (an allocentric frame of reference).

Earlier research with sighted participants found that people have a preference for the allocentric representation (Mou and McNamara, 2002). If the objects are lined up in rows and columns, then we remember that format rather than how they looked from the view from an angle, for example. This is also true if you blindfold the participants and walk them from one "home" location to each object in turn. Sighted participants will prefer the allocentric reference frame over the egocentric one. In our study we were curious whether having visual experience during child development is key to create the structures in the brain to support such another-centred reference frame. We therefore tested people who were congenitally blind, participants who were sighted for some period of time and then became blind later in life and sighted participants. We blindfolded everyone and walked them to the locations of objects in a large room. Later we tested them on a computer with a virtual pointing task: "Imagine you are at the cup facing the book, point to the pan."

First we found an interesting difference between the congenitally blind and sighted people: although the sighted people preferred the other-centred, or allocentric, reference frame, the congenitally blind participants preferred the self-centred or egocentric reference frame. The important piece of the puzzle, however, was whether the late blind people would perform like the congenitally blind, showing that current visual experience matters, or like the sighted, showing the role of early visual experience. The results were clear: the late blind performed the same as the sighted participants. Therefore having the experience of vision early in life lays the groundwork in the brain for the representation of locations in a different reference frame than that found in people who never had visual experience.

The crucial finding from our work on spatial cognition that resolves the prior conflicting findings is that the difference between the blind and sighted participants was a matter of kind, rather than degree. That is, all three groups performed at a similar level of accuracy, but with different techniques or strategies revealed by the reliance on different spatial frames of reference. Moreover, the reliance on egocentric versus allocentric frames of reference makes sense given the strengths of visual versus auditory and tactile perception: sensing distant (out of reach), silent objects in parallel (Proulx, Brown et al., 2014). The distal and parallel features of visual processing give rise to the utility of vision as a calibrator for multisensory spatial information (Pasqualotto and Proulx, 2012), and thus provides the neural means for mapping the relative locations of objects to one another (allocentric) rather than just in relation to the location of the perceiver (egocentric). Interestingly we found similar differences between the congenitally blind on the one hand and the sighted and late blind on the other hand in a mental number line task (Pasqualotto, Taya and Proulx, 2014) that likely draws upon similar representations of space and magnitude in the posterior parietal cortex.

In contrast, work in another area of cognition, memory, has revealed consistent advantages in working, semantic and episodic memory in those without visual experience (congenital visual impairment). Initial work examining semantic memory (remembering words) found better performance in the congenitally blind than other participants (Amedi et al., 2003). Moreover, activity in the "visual" cortex of the occipital lobe correlated with the number of words correctly remembered in the congenitally blind but not in the other participants. This neural plasticity (taking advantage of the normally visual cortex for another task) allowed for a greater number of items to be remembered; was the quality of the memory representation better as well? We later assessed this with a memory task that is sensitive to the fidelity of memory by distinguishing real and false memories. The prior finding by Amedi et al. (2003) was replicated (the congenitally blind remembered more words than the other participants), but additionally we found those without visual experience also had far lower rates of false memory compared to other participants, too (Pasqualotto, Lam and Proulx, 2013). This and other work examining short-term memory suggests that the advantage in congenitally blind participants arises from improved stimulus encoding, perhaps resulting from cross-modal recruitment of what are normally visual areas of the brain (Rokem and Ahissar, 2009).

Critical periods for visual development: evidence from sight restoration

A critical period for vision is a window of time in which there must be visual input to develop neural connections and the ability of sight (Daw, 1998). This was first proposed by Hubel and Wiesel (Hubel and Wiesel, 1964; Wiesel and Hubel, 1965a, 1965b), and their findings relating to binocular deprivation will be discussed given its relevance to human blindness. They sutured the eyelids of kittens after birth for three months. Upon sight restoration, the kittens still appeared blind – bumping into objects and losing sight of passing objects. This was also supported by neurological evidence. The lateral geniculate nucleus (LGN), the main connection between the optic nerve and the primary visual cortex (V1), was reduced in size by 40%, and many cells in V1 did not respond to visual stimulation (Daw et al., 1992; Hubel, Wiesel and LeVay, 1977). It was therefore concluded that there is a critical period for vision in cats between 3 weeks and 3 months of age, and that a lack of visual stimulation during this time means that sight cannot develop. A critical period for vision has also been supported by evidence in macaque monkeys and rodents (Fagiolini et al., 1994; Hubel et al., 1977). This suggests that different species have their own critical period for visual development. Given ethical reasons, it is of course difficult to test critical periods in humans. Despite this, it has been proposed there is a critical period between birth and 2 years when the lateral geniculate nucleus (LGN) becomes its adult size (Hickey, 1977), or up to 6 years of age when the cortical architecture becomes refined (Lewis and Maurer, 2005). Nevertheless, it is vital to establish how necessary critical periods are for visual development, since many congenitally blind individuals are not treated due to the belief that they would not develop sight upon sight restoration having missed a critical period (Kalia et al., 2017).

A unique opportunity to study critical periods in humans has emerged in the last decade from Project Prakash in India. India has the world's largest population of blind children, with 90% unable to obtain an education and fewer than 50% surviving until adulthood, yet nearly 40% of these children can be treated, for example because their blindness is from cataracts (Kalia et al., 2017). Project Prakash provides free screening and treatment for children in India and as of 2014, 42,000 children have been screened with approximately 2,000 being treated (www.projectprakash.org). Alongside providing sight and improving the quality of life of thousands of children, testing these children after sight restoration provides information about visual development in humans.

Kalia et al. (2014) tested children after sight restoration following early-onset (blind before 1 year of age) and extended blindness (blind for 8–17 years). Children were tested on contrast sensitivity, which is the ability to perceive changes in luminance between regions that are not separated by a definitive border. Contrast sensitivity improved within the first few weeks after surgery and continued to improve for two years. This development was independent of the age of sight onset, showing that the duration of blindness did not influence their contrast sensitivity development. Interestingly, contrast sensitivity no longer develops in typically developing individuals of the same age, and the rate of development exceeded those of infants in two individuals (Atkinson, Braddick and Moar, 1977; Banks and Salapatek, 1978). This first shows how the visual system can retain considerable plasticity, even when blindness extends critical periods. Furthermore, it provides evidence that a critical period may not be as critical for visual development as previously thought, because sight restoration after early-onset and extended blindness enabled sight development. This challenges the initial work by Hubel and Wiesel (1964) and suggests we should remain optimistic for sight restoration after childhood.

Further evidence of the critical period not being so critical is provided by findings in object recognition and face categorisation with sight restoration children. Held et al. (2011) presented children with a Lego-like object which the children studied by only touch (while blindfolded). They then presented this object with another distractor object and children were then asked to identify the original object by sight. Immediately after surgery, children were 58% accurate, but this rose to 80% after one week (Held et al., 2011). In a face categorisation task (Gandhi et al., 2017), children were shown images ranging from faces to randomly selected non-face images, with three intermediate stages of increasing face-like patterns between. Children were asked whether the image was a face or not. Immediately after surgery, children performed poorly (less than 50% accuracy), but this rose to approximately 90% after six months. Alongside this improvement, children's false identification of non-faces dropped, too. This further illustrates the rapid improvement in visual development after early-onset and extended blindness, challenging the notion of an essential critical period early in life.

While evidence from sight restoration studies challenges a critical period for visual development early in life being crucial for vision to later develop, it may be possible that this critical period still occurred but was delayed until their sight restoration. For example, it has been found in rats and kittens that the critical period is mediated by the neurotransmitter GABA. Dark-rearing reduces the function of GABA that delays the onset of the critical period, suggesting that later exposure to light (i.e. sight restoration) could initiate a critical period later in life thus the children may not have *missed* a critical period, but this may have been *delayed* (Hensch, 2005a, 2005b; Mower, 1991). However, research suggests that the critical period was only delayed if there was no exposure to light at all. Since light can still enter the eye even with dense cataracts, sight restoration children in the studies discussed would therefore not be raised in total darkness and thus a delayed critical period may not apply. For example, research found that exposure to light for just six hours prevented the delayed onset of the critical period in kittens as the GABA pathway was stimulated by even this brief exposure to light (Mower, Christen and Caplan, 1983). However, this exposure to light was extremely intense (from a flashlight), whereas Project Prakash children would only see dim light due to their cataracts, which may not be intense enough to stimulate the critical period. Since it is unknown how much light the children could detect, it is still an open question whether a critical period for vision was delayed or missed. Nevertheless, the rapid improvements made by the sight restoration children, despite having severe visual impairment for their first few years of life (8–17 years), suggests we should be optimistic for vision restoration later in life.

In the face categorisation task with sight restoration children by Gandhi et al. (2017), they found that the improvement in face categorisation was independent from visual acuity development because face categorisation improvement exceeded visual acuity improvement. Furthermore, they also tested age-matched controls wearing blur goggles causing them to have similar acuity to post-operative children (Gandhi et al., 2017). These controls were still highly accurate at the face categorisation task, suggesting that face categorisation does not depend on visual acuity. Given these results, it suggests there may be multiple critical periods for different visual functions (namely visual acuity and face categorisation), challenging the idea of a critical period as a unitary construct. Indeed, this is supported by animal studies. For example, Harwerth et al. (1986) found different critical periods for rods and cones, monocular spatial vision and binocular vision in macaque monkeys. Furthermore, in ferrets there is evidence that the critical period for orientation selectivity ends earlier than the critical period for ocular dominance (Chapman and Stryker, 1993).

In addition to providing evidence for two separate visual functions with different critical periods, the data from sight restoration studies also suggest face categorisation is more resilient to visual deprivation than visual acuity, given its faster development (Gandhi et al., 2017). It remains an open question, however, as to *what* makes a visual function susceptible or resilient to early deprivation. It has been suggested that earlier manifesting visual functions are more vulnerable to visual deprivation (Sengpiel, 2007). Evidence from Gandhi et al. (2017), however, challenges this notion, because face categorisation is evident in neonates (Fantz, 1965; Mondloch et al., 1999) while neonate visual acuity is still poor (Kellman and Arterberry, 2000), suggesting face categorisation is an earlier manifesting visual function than acuity. It is therefore important for future research to investigate what makes a visual function susceptible or resilient to early deprivation to further understand visual development following sight restoration. This shows us how sight restoration studies provide evidence of multiple critical periods within visual development, which may have varying degrees of resilience to visual deprivation. Moreover, the blind brain retains considerable plasticity, which may explain the rapid improvement in contrast sensitivity, face categorisation and object recognition after sight restoration.

The metamodal hypothesis of computational (non-sensory) brain organisation

The rapid improvement in object recognition and face categorisation from studies of sight restoration may be explained at a neural level by the *metamodel hypothesis*. This suggests that the organisation of specialised cortical regions in the human brain are independent from the sensory input (Pascual-Leone and Hamilton, 2001). For example, the "visual" cortex can also receive auditory and tactile stimuli but is referred to as the "visual" cortex because there is a preference for visual input since the spatial functions inherent to the striate cortex are best accomplished using visual information (Proulx, Brown et al., 2014). Crucially, visual input is not the *only* sensory input that the "visual" cortex can process (Liang et al., 2013; Liang, van Leeuwen and Proulx, 2008), as recent studies have demonstrated that other sensory information such as sound, touch and even pain evoke activity in the occipital cortex.

In this view, a congenitally blind individual may already have a representation of objects or faces in the visual cortex that have been built up from tactile or auditory input (Pietrini et al., 2004; Ricciardi et al., 2009). Thus, upon sight restoration, the new visual input may be re-routed to these already existing cortical regions for representing objects and faces, discussed in more detail later in the following section. This therefore enables rapid improvement in tasks such as object recognition since a *new* cortical representation for objects need not be created. Evidence to support the metamodal hypothesis comes from visually impaired as well as sighted individuals.

First, there is evidence from functional brain imaging studies showing activation of the visual cortex in early blind subjects during braille reading (Burton, Sinclair and Agato, 2012;

Burton et al., 2002; Sadato et al., 1996) and other forms of tactile stimulation such as during a one-back vibrotactile matching task (Burton, Sinclair and McLaren, 2004). To assess a causal link between visual cortex activation and task performance, Cohen et al. (1997) used repetitive transcranial magnetic stimulation (rTMS) to disrupt the primary visual cortex while participants were reading braille. They found there was an increase in braille reading errors when repetitive transcranial magnetic stimulation (rTMS) bursts were applied to the visual cortex, but stimulation of a control area (somatosensory cortex) produced no such effects. In contrast, when sighted participants read embossed Roman letters, TMS to the visual cortex showed no effect on tactile performance, whereas similar stimulation is known to disrupt their visual performance. This suggests that the visual cortex is necessary for braille reading even in the absence of visual input. However, a limitation of this study is that the TMS was applied during performance, and so other effects are not controlled for, such as changes in attention. Addressing this limitation, Kupers et al. (2007) tested task performance 15 minutes after repetitive transcranial magnetic stimulation (rTMS) in which the effects of TMS could still be assessed outside the stimulation period. They tested participants on three consecutive braille words as a repetition priming task. Due to the repetition priming, subjects made significantly fewer mistakes and read faster in the second and third presentation of the same word list. However, after repetitive transcranial magnetic stimulation (rTMS) to the visual cortex, this repetition priming effect was diminished and participants made significantly more reading errors. These effects were not seen after repetitive transcranial magnetic stimulation (rTMS) to a control area (the somatosensory cortex), in line with Cohen et al. (1997). These studies suggest that despite visual deprivation, the visual cortex has a functional role in blind individuals.

The visual system is classically divided into a dorsal and a ventral stream, involved in motion and object recognition respectively (Mishkin and Ungerleider, 1982). In further support of the metamodal hypothesis, there is evidence that these streams are preserved in the absence of vision, suggesting that the so-called "visual" cortex also processes information carried by non-visual sensory modalities (Kupers and Ptito, 2014; Proulx, Ptito and Amedi, 2014). For example, the lateral occipital tactile vision area (LOtv) is an object-selective area in the ventral visual pathway (Lacey et al., 2009) yet evidence suggests that this area of the ventral pathway is not specific to just visual input. For example, in both blind and sighted individuals, the lateral occipital tactile vision area (LOtv) responds to soundscapes of specific objects created by a visual to auditory sensory substitution device called the "vOICe", which translates visual shape information into an auditory stream (Amedi et al., 2007), thus showing how auditory stimuli activates the ventral stream. Similarly, evidence suggests this is also the case when perceiving objects from tactile stimuli. For example, Ptito et al. (2012) used a visual to tactile sensory substitution device that translates visual images into electro-tactile stimulation that is transmitted to the tongue via a 12 × 12 electrode array. In a shape recognition study, fMRI data showed that both blind subjects and blindfolded sighted controls activated the lateral occipital tactile vision area (LOtv). This supports the notion that the lateral occipital tactile vision area (LOtv), part of the ventral stream, subserves an abstract or supramodal representation of shape that is preserved in congenitally blind individuals. Moreover, in sighted individuals, the lateral occipital tactile vision area (LOtv) is shown to respond selectively to objects not only by vision but also by touch (Amedi et al., 2001; Amedi et al., 2007; Pietrini et al., 2004). This further suggests the ventral stream is genuinely modality dependent, and that the supramodal nature is not the result of brain reorganisation in congenital blindness.

In specific relation to a modality independent representation for faces, the fusiform face area (FFA) is an area of the ventral stream that receives input from the lateral geniculate nucleus (LGN) and projects into V1, which is associated with face processing in sighted individuals

(Haxby et al., 1999). There is evidence that congenitally blind individuals show more activation in the fusiform face area (FFA) when hearing voices, compared to late blind and sighted individuals (Gougoux et al., 2009). This suggests that the fusiform face area (FFA), part of the "visual" cortex, is also responsive to relevant auditory stimuli associated with a face (voices) and that the fusiform face area (FFA) subserves an abstract representation of faces regardless of the sensory modality (Pietrini et al., 2004).

Given the evidence that the ventral stream, in particular the lateral occipital tactile vision area (LOtv) for object recognition and the fusiform face area (FFA) for face recognition, is preserved in congenitally blind individuals, this suggests that the visually impaired may have representations for faces and objects provided by their auditory and haptic experience of the world. How, then, do these metamodel representations enable such rapid improvement in object recognition and face categorisation in sensory restoration?

Cross-modal plasticity: cortical reorganisation or unmasking?

The review of the literature above suggests that the visual cortex can be activated by other sensory modalities and is functionally active in congenitally blind individuals who lack visual experience. There are two competing hypotheses put forward to explain this cross-modal plasticity in the blind brain. On the one hand, according to the *cortical reorganisation hypothesis*, cross-modal brain responses are mediated by the formation of new pathways in the sensory-deprived brain. Animal studies suggest that when the brain is deprived of visual input at an early age, tactile and other non-visual information are re-routed to the visual cortex (Chabot et al., 2008; Karlen, Kahn and Krubitzer, 2006, 2009; Piché et al., 2007). On the other hand, according to the *unmasking hypothesis*, loss of sensory input induces unmasking and strengthening of *existing* neuronal connections. A key piece of evidence to distinguish between these hypotheses is whether cross-modal plasticity occurs slowly, consistent with cortical reorganisation through novel neuronal pathways, or quickly, consistent with an unmasking of existing neuronal connections. Given such rapid improvement in visual tasks in the sight restoration studies, this favours the unmasking hypothesis, since this time frame is too rapid for new neuronal connections to be formed. But is this sort of plasticity restricted to those with sensory impairments? It is not – other research has found that short-term sensory deprivation and training can also reveal this cross-modal plasticity in sighted adults. Merabet et al. (2008) blindfolded sighted individuals for five days while they learnt braille. After this sudden vision restriction, the visual cortex became activated with tactile information after two days, which then reversed as soon as the blindfold was removed. This provides evidence for profound and rapidly reversible neuroplastic changes, which the authors suggest is from the sudden unmasking of existing connections and a shift in connectivity. Perhaps sudden visual experience rapidly unmasks connections, potentially enabling visual input to access these existing object or face representations, resulting in rapid improvement in face categorisation and object recognition, as seen in the sight restoration children. This suggestion is further supported by evidence that the maturation of a new neuron takes four to six weeks (Brady et al., 2011). Their improvement within a week, therefore, cannot be a result of *new* neural connections between visual input and the visual cortex, but is more likely to utilise the existing neural architecture representing faces (e.g. fusiform face area (FFA)) and objects (e.g. lateral occipital tactile vision area (LOtv)) that visual input can be directed to via the unmasking of existing connections.

This suggests how visual development may be rapid in individuals, despite missing a critical period from extended blindness. However, this evidence for the unmasking of existing neurons (Merabet et al., 2008) is from sighted individuals, and so its generalisability to sight restoration children could be limited given the potential differences in brain structure between sighted and blind individuals. Research has found structurally different visual areas as well as different connections between these and tactile areas in blind individuals compared to sighted (Büchel, 1998; Ptito et al., 2008). However, other recent research in visually impaired adults who learned to interpret auditory displays of images via sensory substitution showed the same cross-modal plasticity over an even briefer time period of only two hours of training (Striem-Amit et al., 2012). Thus this finding generalises across both sighted and visually impaired people and suggests that the cortex is highly plastic and able to re-route information displayed to the other senses or via sight restoration in just a matter of hours via existing multisensory neural connections (Proulx, Ptito and Amedi, 2014).

Molyneux's question

This potential mapping of new sensory input on to existing representations draws on Molyneux's question, a nearly 400-year-old philosophical question asking whether someone born blind could distinguish between a sphere and a cube by sight alone upon sight restoration (Morgan, 1977). John Locke and other empiricists believe the answer would be "yes" because humans have an innate conception of an object that is separate from all sensory input. Sight restoration projects such as research with sensory substitution and Project Prakash offer unique opportunities to address this question. Given the initial failure to accurately identify objects (Held et al., 2011) the answer might be "no". However, given there is no data for their rapid improvement within the first week, it could be possible that this improvement and their success at this task is evident much earlier than one week, possibly within the first couple of hours or days. Given vision is a completely brand-new experience for these individuals, it is perhaps unrealistic to think their neural circuits can process visual information immediately upon sight restoration, however, this ability may occur within a short period of time, especially given the evidence of the unmasking of existing neurons occurring in just two days (Merabet et al., 2008), and some sensory substitution training can evince successful performance and neural plasticity in only two hours (Striem-Amit et al., 2012). Indeed it is even possible for naïve participants to perform well on an optician's visual acuity test without any training at all (Haigh et al., 2013). Given the possibility of rapid re-routing of information between visual input and existing representations, there is potential that Molyneux's question is more realistically answered with a "yes" if allowing a few hours until testing.

Conclusion

"We see with the brain, not the eyes" (Bach-y-Rita, Tyler and Kaczmarek, 2003). The most crucial aspect of this review is that "seeing" the world might be different for those with visual impairments compared to those with vision, but that their perception is just as rich and varied due to the compensatory effects of practising to experience the world through the other senses. This has important consequences for approaches to accessibility. Of course the visually impaired are still faced with the challenges of a world largely designed by the sighted for the sighted, and so some way of accessing visual information is often necessary. Most famously, one might think of technologies such as the white cane and braille as ways to render information normally seen as something that can be felt. New approaches are taking this even further by transforming images into a format that other senses can process, and this is called sensory substitution (Bach-y-Rita et al., 2003), a topic discussed at greater length in another contribution to this volume. The key to sensory substitution is that all perception ultimately takes place in the brain, thus turning images into sounds (Brown and Proulx, 2013, 2016; Haigh et al., 2013; Proulx et al., 2016) or something that can be touched (Bach-y-Rita et al., 1969; Chebat et al., 2007; Chebat et al., 2011) has demonstrated a fascinating potential of the brain for taking such sensory input and processing it in a metamodal framework (Proulx et al., 2014). There is still much to be learned about the "blind brain", with great potential both for a basic understanding of how all brains work and for developing new assistive technology to best tap into that potential.

References

Amedi, A., Malach, R., Hendler, T., Peled, S. and Zohary, E. 2001. Visuo-haptic object-related activation in the ventral visual pathway. *Nature Neuroscience*, 4(3), 324–330.

Amedi, A., Raz, N., Pianka, P., Malach, R. and Zohary, E. 2003. Early "visual" cortex activation correlates with superior verbal memory performance in the blind. *Nature Neuroscience*, 6(7), 758–766.

Amedi, A., Stern, W.M., Camprodon, J.A., Bermpohl, F., Merabet, L., Rotman, S., Hemond, C., Meijer, P. and Pascual-Leone, A. 2007. Shape conveyed by visual-to-auditory sensory substitution activates the lateral occipital complex. *Nature Neuroscience*, 10(6), 687–689.

Anderson, P.W. and Zahorik, P. 2014. Auditory/visual distance estimation: Accuracy and variability. *Frontiers in Psychology*, 5, 1097.

Atkinson, J., Braddick, O. and Moar, K. 1977. Development of contrast sensitivity over the first 3 months of life in the human infant. *Vision Research*, 17(9), 1037–1044.

Bach-y-Rita, P., Collins, C.C., Saunders, F.A., White, B. and Scadden, L. 1969. Vision substitution by tactile image projection. *Nature*, 221(5184), 963–964.

Bach-y-Rita, P., Tyler, M.E. and Kaczmarek, K.A. 2003. Seeing with the brain. *International Journal of Human–Computer Interaction*, 15(2), 285–295.

Banks, M.S. and Salapatek, P. 1978. Acuity and contrast sensitivity in 1-, 2-, and 3-month-old human infants. *Investigative Ophthalmology & Visual Science*, 17(4), 361–365.

Beaulieu-Lefebvre, M., Schneider, F.C., Kupers, R. and Ptito, M. 2011. Odor perception and odor awareness in congenital blindness. *Brain Research Bulletin*, 84(3), 206–209.

Brady, S., Siegel, G., Albers, R.W. and Price, D. 2011. *Basic neurochemistry: principles of molecular, cellular, and medical neurobiology*. London: Academic Press.

Brown, D.J. and Proulx, M.J. 2013. Increased signal complexity improves the breadth of generalization in auditory perceptual learning. *Neural Plasticity*, 2013(879047), 1–9.

Brown, D.J. and Proulx, M.J. 2016. Audio-vision substitution for blind individuals: Addressing human information processing capacity limitations. *IEEE Journal of Selected Topics in Signal Processing*, 10(5), 924–931.

Büchel, C. 1998. Functional neuroimaging studies of braille reading: Cross-modal reorganization and its implications. *Brain*, 121(Pt 7), 1193–1194.

Burton, H., Sinclair, R.J. and Agato, A. 2012. Recognition memory for braille or spoken words: An fMRI study in early blind. *Brain Research*, 1438, 22–34.

Burton, H., Sinclair, R.J. and McLaren, D.G. 2004. Cortical activity to vibrotactile stimulation: An fMRI study in blind and sighted individuals. *Human Brain Mapping*, 23(4), 210–228.

Burton, H., Snyder, A.Z., Conturo, T.E., Akbudak, E., Ollinger, J.M. and Raichle, M.E. 2002. Adaptive changes in early and late blind: A fMRI study of braille reading. *Journal of Neurophysiology*, 87(1), 589–607.

Calcagno, E.R., Abregú, E.L., Eguía, M.C. and Vergara, R. 2012. The role of vision in auditory distance perception. *Perception*, 41(2), 175–192.

Cappagli, G., Cocchi, E. and Gori, M. 2017. Auditory and proprioceptive spatial impairments in blind children and adults. *Developmental Science*, 20(3), e12374.

Cattaneo, Z., Fantino, M., Tinti, C., Pascual-Leone, A., Silvanto, J. and Vecchi, T. 2011. Spatial biases in peripersonal space in sighted and blind individuals revealed by a haptic line bisection paradigm. *Journal of Experimental Psychology: Human*, 37(4), 1110–1121.

Chabot, N., Charbonneau, V., Laramée, M.E., Tremblay, R., Boire, D. and Bronchti, G. 2008. Subcortical auditory input to the primary visual cortex in anophthalmic mice. *Neuroscience Letters*, 433(2), 129–134.

Chapman, B. and Stryker, M.P. 1993. Development of orientation selectivity in ferret visual cortex and effects of deprivation. *Journal of Neuroscience*, 13(12), 5251–5262.

Chebat, D.R., Rainville, C., Kupers, R. and Ptito, M. 2007. Tactile-"visual" acuity of the tongue in early blind individuals. *Neuroreport*, 18(18), 1901–1904.

Chebat, D.R., Schneider, F.C., Kupers, R. and Ptito, M. 2011. Navigation with a sensory substitution device in congenitally blind individuals. *Neuroreport*, 22(7), 342–347.

Cohen, L.G., Celnik, P., Pascual-Leone, A., Corwell, B., Falz, L., Dambrosia, J., Honda, M., Sadato, N., Gerloff, C., Catala, M.D. and Hallett, M. 1997. Functional relevance of cross-modal plasticity in blind humans. *Nature*, 389(6647), 180–183.

Cuevas, I., Plaza, P., Rombaux, P., De Volder, A.G. and Renier, L. 2009. Odour discrimination and identification are improved in early blindness. *Neuropsychologia*, 47(14), 3079–3083.

Daw, N.W. 1998. Neurobiology: Columns, slabs and pinwheels. *Nature*, 395(6697), 20–21.

Daw, N.W., Fox, K., Sato, H. and Czepita, D. 1992. Critical period for monocular deprivation in the cat visual cortex. *Journal of Neurophysiology*, 67(1), 197–202.

Fagiolini, M., Pizzorusso, T., Berardi, N., Domenici, L. and Maffei, L. 1994. Functional postnatal development of the rat primary visual cortex and the role of visual experience: Dark rearing and monocular deprivation. *Vision Research*, 34(6), 709–720.

Fantz, R.L. 1965. Visual perception from birth as shown by pattern selectivity. *Annals of the New York Academy of Sciences*, 118(21), 793–814.

Fieger, A., Roder, B., Teder-Salejarvi, W., Hillyard, S.A. and Neville, H.J. 2006. Auditory spatial tuning in late-onset blindness in humans. *Journal of Cognitive Neuroscience*, 18(2), 149–157.

Finnegan, D.J., O'Neill, E. and Proulx, M.J. 2015. Compensating for distance compression in audiovisual virtual environments using incongruence. *34th Annual Chi Conference on Human Factors in Computing Systems, Chi 2016* (pp. 200–212). San Jose, CA: ACM.

Finnegan, D.J., O'Neill, E. and Proulx, M.J. 2017. An approach to reducing distance compression in audiovisual virtual environments. *Sonic Interactions for Virtual Environments (SIVE), IEEE 3rd VR Workshop*, 1–6. doi: 10.1109/SIVE.2017.7901607

Finocchietti, S., Cappagli, G. and Gori, M. 2015. Encoding audio motion: spatial impairment in early blind individuals. *Frontiers in Psychology*, 6, 1357.

Gandhi, T.K., Singh, A.K., Swami, P., Ganesh, S. and Sinha, P. 2017. Emergence of categorical face perception after extended early-onset blindness. *Proceedings of the National Academy of Sciences USA*, 114(23), 6139–6143.

Ghazanfar, A.A. and Schroeder, C.E. 2006. Is neocortex essentially multisensory? *Trends Cognitive Science*, 10(6), 278–285.

Goldreich, D. and Kanics, I.M. 2003. Tactile acuity is enhanced in blindness. *Journal of Neuroscience*, 23(8), 3439–3445.

Gori, M., Sandini, G., Martinoli, C. and Burr, D.C. 2014a. Impairment of auditory spatial localization in congenitally blind human subjects. *Brain*, 137(Pt 1), 288–293.

Gori, M., Vercillo, T., Sandini, G. and Burr, D. 2014b. Tactile feedback improves auditory spatial localization. *Frontiers in Psychology*, 5, 1121.

Gottfried, J.A. 2006. Smell: Central nervous processing. *Advances in Otorhinolaryngol*, 63, 44–69.

Gougoux, F., Belin, P., Voss, P., Lepore, F., Lassonde, M. and Zatorre, R.J. 2009. Voice perception in blind persons: A functional magnetic resonance imaging study. *Neuropsychologia*, 47(13), 2967–2974.

Gougoux, F., Lepore, F., Lassonde, M., Voss, P., Zatorre, R.J. and Belin, P. 2004. Neuropsychology: Pitch discrimination in the early blind. *Nature*, 430(6997), 309.

Gougoux, F., Zatorre, R.J., Lassonde, M., Voss, P. and Lepore, F. 2005. A functional neuroimaging study of sound localization: Visual cortex activity predicts performance in early-blind individuals. *PLoS Biol*, 3(2), e27.

Grant, A.C., Thiagarajah, M.C. and Sathian, K. 2000. Tactile perception in blind braille readers: A psychophysical study of acuity and hyperacuity using gratings and dot patterns. *Perception & Psychophysics*, 62(2), 301–312.

Gurtubay-Antolin, A. and Rodríguez-Fornells, A. 2017. Neurophysiological evidence for enhanced tactile acuity in early blindness in some but not all haptic tasks. *Neuroimage*, 162, 23–31.

Haigh, A., Brown, D.J., Meijer, P. and Proulx, M.J. 2013. How well do you see what you hear? The acuity of visual-to-auditory sensory substitution. *Frontiers in Psychology*, 4, 330.

Harwerth, R.S., Smith, E.L., Duncan, G.C., Crawford, M.L. and von Noorden, G.K. 1986. Multiple sensitive periods in the development of the primate visual system. *Science*, 232(4747), 235–238.

Haxby, J.V., Ungerleider, L.G., Clark, V.P., Schouten, J.L., Hoffman, E.A. and Martin, A. 1999. The effect of face inversion on activity in human neural systems for face and object perception. *Neuron*, 22(1), 189–199.

Held, R., Ostrovsky, Y., de Gelder, B., deGelder, B., Gandhi, T., Ganesh, S., Mathur, U. and Sinha, P. 2011. The newly sighted fail to match seen with felt. *Nature Neuroscience*, 14(5), 551–553.

Hensch, T.K. 2005a. Critical period mechanisms in developing visual cortex. *Current Topics in Developmental Biology*, 69, 215–237.

Hensch, T.K. 2005b. Critical period plasticity in local cortical circuits. *Nature Reviews Neuroscience*, 6(11), 877–888.

Hickey, T.L. 1977. Postnatal development of the human lateral geniculate nucleus: Relationship to a critical period for the visual system. *Science*, 198(4319), 836–838.

Hubel, D.H. and Wiesel, T.N. 1964. Effects of monocular deprivation in kittens. *Naunyn-Schmiedeberg's Archives of Pharmacology*, 248, 492–497.

Hubel, D.H., Wiesel, T.N. and LeVay, S. 1977. Plasticity of ocular dominance columns in monkey striate cortex. *Philosophical Transactions of the Royal Society of London. Series B, Biological Sciences Royal Society (Great Britain)*, 278(961), 377–409.

Hugdahl, K., Ek, M., Takio, F., Rintee, T., Tuomainen, J., Haarala, C. and Hämäläinen, H. 2004. Blind individuals show enhanced perceptual and attentional sensitivity for identification of speech sounds. *Cognitive Brain Research*, 19(1), 28–32.

Kalia, A., Gandhi, T., Chatterjee, G., Swami, P., Dhillon, H., Bi, S., Chauhan, N., Gupta, S.D., Sharma, P., Sood, S., Ganesh, S., Mathur, U. and Sinha, P. 2017. Assessing the impact of a program for late surgical intervention in early-blind children. *Public Health*, 146, 15–23.

Kalia, A., Lesmes, L.A., Dorr, M., Gandhi, T., Chatterjee, G., Ganesh, S., Bex, P.J. and Sinha, P. 2014. Development of pattern vision following early and extended blindness. *Proceedings of the National Academy of Sciences*, 111(5), 2035–2039.

Karlen, S.J., Kahn, D.M. and Krubitzer, L. 2006. Early blindness results in abnormal corticocortical and thalamocortical connections. *Neuroscience*, 142(3), 843–858.

Karlen, S.J., Kahn, D.M. and Krubitzer, L. 2009. Effects of bilateral enucleation on the size of visual and nonvisual areas of the brain. *Cerebral Cortex*, 19(6), 1360–1371.

Kellman, P.J. and Arterberry, M.E. 2000. *The cradle of knowledge: Development of perception in infancy.* Cambridge, MA: MIT Press.

Kolarik, A.J., Pardhan, S., Cirstea, S. and Moore, B.C. 2013. Using acoustic information to perceive room size: Effects of blindness, room reverberation time, and stimulus. *Perception*, 42(9), 985–990.

Konishi, M. 2000. Study of sound localization by owls and its relevance to humans. *Comparative Biochemistry and Physiology. Part A, Molecular & Integrative Physiology*, 126(4), 459–469.

Kupers, R., Beaulieu-Lefebvre, M., Schneider, F.C., Kassuba, T., Paulson, O.B., Siebner, H.R. and Ptito, M. 2011. Neural correlates of olfactory processing in congenital blindness. *Neuropsychologia*, 49(7), 2037–2044.

Kupers, R., Pappens, M., de Noordhout, A.M., Schoenen, J., Ptito, M. and Fumal, A. 2007. rTMS of the occipital cortex abolishes braille reading and repetition priming in blind subjects. *Neurology*, 68(9), 691–693.

Kupers, R. and Ptito, M. 2011. Insights from darkness: What the study of blindness has taught us about brain structure and function. *Progress in Brain Research*, 192, 17–31.

Kupers, R. and Ptito, M. 2014. Compensatory plasticity and cross-modal reorganization following early visual deprivation. *Neuroscience & Biobehavioral Reviews*, 41, 36–52.

Lacey, S., Tal, N., Amedi, A. and Sathian, K. 2009. A putative model of multisensory object representation. *Brain Topography*, 21(3–4), 269–274.

Landau, B., Gleitman, H. and Spelke, E. 1981. Spatial knowledge and geometric representation in a child blind from birth. *Science*, 213(4513), 1275–1278.

Leclerc, C., Saint-Amour, D., Lavoie, M.E., Lassonde, M. and Lepore, F. 2000. Brain functional reorganization in early blind humans revealed by auditory event-related potentials. *Neuroreport*, 11(3), 545–550.

Legge, G.E., Madison, C., Vaughn, B.N., Cheong, A.M. and Miller, J.C. 2008. Retention of high tactile acuity throughout the life span in blindness. *Perception Psychophysics*, 70(8), 1471–1488.

Lessard, N., Pare, M., Lepore, F. and Lassonde, M. 1998. Early-blind human subjects localize sound sources better than sighted subjects. *Nature*, 395(6699), 278–280.

Lewald, J. 2002. Vertical sound localization in blind humans. *Neuropsychologia*, 40(12), 1868–1872.

Lewis, T.L. and Maurer, D. 2005. Multiple sensitive periods in human visual development: Evidence from visually deprived children. *Developmental Psychobiology*, 46(3), 163–183.

Li, W., Luxenberg, E., Parrish, T. and Gottfried, J.A. 2006. Learning to smell the roses: Experience-dependent neural plasticity in human piriform and orbitofrontal cortices. *Neuron*, 52(6), 1097–1108.

Liang, M., Mouraux, A., Hu, L. and Iannetti, G.D. 2013. Primary sensory cortices contain distinguishable spatial patterns of activity for each sense. *Nature Communications*, 4, 1979.

Liang, M., van Leeuwen, T.M. and Proulx, M.J. 2008. Propagation of brain activity during audiovisual integration. *Journal of Neuroscience*, 28(36), 8861–8862.

Majchrzak, D., Eberhard, J., Kalaus, B. and Wagner, K.H. 2017. Do visually impaired people develop superior smell ability? *Perception*, 46(10), 1171–1182.

Matteau, I., Kupers, R., Ricciardi, E., Pietrini, P. and Ptito, M. 2010. Beyond visual, aural and haptic movement perception: hMT+ is activated by electrotactile motion stimulation of the tongue in sighted and in congenitally blind individuals. *Brain Research Bulletin*, 82(5–6), 264–270.

Merabet, L.B., Hamilton, R., Schlaug, G., Swisher, J.D., Kiriakopoulos, E.T., Pitskel, N.B., Kauffman, T. and Pascual-Leone, A. 2008. Rapid and reversible recruitment of early visual cortex for touch. *PLoS One*, 3(8), e3046.

Merabet, L.B. and Pascual-Leone, A. 2010. Neural reorganization following sensory loss: The opportunity of change. *Nature Reviews Neuroscience*, 11(1), 44–52.

Merabet, L.B., Rizzo, J.F., Amedi, A., Somers, D.C. and Pascual-Leone, A. 2005. What blindness can tell us about seeing again: merging neuroplasticity and neuroprostheses. *Nature Reviews Neuroscience*, 6(1), 71–77.

Metatla, O., Bryan-Kinns, N., Stockman, T. and Martin, F. 2015. Designing with and for people living with visual impairments: Audio-tactile mock-ups, audio diaries and participatory prototyping. *Codesign*, 11(1), 35–48.

Metatla, O., Correia, N.N., Martin, F., Bryan-Kinns, N. and Stockman, T. 2016. Tap the ShapeTones: Exploring the effects of crossmodal congruence in an audio-visual interface. *34th Annual Chi Conference on Human Factors in Computing Systems, Chi 2016* (pp. 1055–1066). San Jose, CA: ACM.

Mishkin, M. and Ungerleider, L.G. 1982. Contribution of striate inputs to the visuospatial functions of parieto-preoccipital cortex in monkeys. *Behaviour Brain Research*, 6(1), 57–77.

Mondloch, C.J., Lewis, T.L., Budreau, D.R., Maurer, D., Dannemiller, J.L., Stephens, B.R. and Kleiner-Gathercoal, K.A. 1999. Face perception during early infancy. *Psychological Science*, 10(5), 419–422.

Morgan, M.J. 1977. *Molyneux's question: Vision, touch and the philosophy of perception.* Cambridge: Cambridge University Press.

Mou, W. and McNamara, T.P. 2002. Intrinsic frames of reference in spatial memory. *Journal of Experimental Psychology: Learning Memory, and Cognition*, 28(1), 162–170.

Mower, G.D. 1991. The effect of dark rearing on the time course of the critical period in cat visual cortex. *Brain Research: Developmental Brain Research*, 58(2), 151–158.

Mower, G.D., Christen, W.G. and Caplan, C.J. 1983. Very brief visual experience eliminates plasticity in the cat visual cortex. *Science*, 221(4606), 178–180.

Noordzij, M.L., Zuidhoek, S. and Postma, A. 2007. The influence of visual experience on visual and spatial imagery. *Perception*, 36(1), 101–112.

Pascual-Leone, A. and Hamilton, R. 2001. The metamodal organization of the brain. *Progress in Brain Research*, 134, 427–445.

Pascual-Leone, A. and Torres, F. 1993. Plasticity of the sensorimotor cortex representation of the reading finger in braille readers. *Brain*, 116(Pt 1), 39–52.

Pasqualotto, A., Lam, J.S. and Proulx, M.J. 2013. Congenital blindness improves semantic and episodic memory. *Behaviour Brain Research*, 244, 162–165.

Pasqualotto, A. and Newell, F.N. 2007. The role of visual experience on the representation and updating of novel haptic scenes. *Brain and Cognition*, 65(2), 184–194.

Pasqualotto, A. and Proulx, M.J. 2012. The role of visual experience for the neural basis of spatial cognition. *Neuroscience Biobehaviour Review*, 36(4), 1179–1187.

Pasqualotto, A., Taya, S. and Proulx, M.J. 2014. Sensory deprivation: Visual experience alters the mental number line. *Behaviour Brain Research*, 261, 110–113.

Piché, M., Chabot, N., Bronchti, G., Miceli, D., Lepore, F. and Guillemot, J.P. 2007. Auditory responses in the visual cortex of neonatally enucleated rats. *Neuroscience*, 145(3), 1144–1156.

Pietrini, P., Furey, M.L., Ricciardi, E., Gobbini, M.I., Wu, W.H., Cohen, L., Guazzelli, M. and Haxby, J.V. 2004. Beyond sensory images: Object-based representation in the human ventral pathway. *Proceedings of the National Academy of Sciences USA*, 101(15), 5658–5663.

Postma, A., Zuidhoek, S., Noordzij, M.L. and Kappers, A.M. 2008. Haptic orientation perception benefits from visual experience: Evidence from early-blind, late-blind, and sighted people. *Perception Psychophysics*, 70(7), 1197–1206.

Proulx, M. 2013. Blindness: Remapping the brain and the restoration of vision. *The Psychological Science*. Accessed 11 January 2019. www.apa.org/science/about/psa/2013/02/blindness.aspx.

Proulx, M.J., Brown, D.J., Pasqualotto, A. and Meijer, P. 2014. Multisensory perceptual learning and sensory substitution. *Neuroscience Biobehaviour Review*, 41, 16–25.

Proulx, M.J., Gwinnutt, J., Dell'Erba, S., Levy-Tzedek, S., de Sousa, A.A. and Brown, D.J. 2016. Other ways of seeing: From behavior to neural mechanisms in the online "visual" control of action with sensory substitution. *Restorative Neurology and Neuroscience*, 34(1), 29–44.

Proulx, M.J., Ptito, M. and Amedi, A. 2014. *Multisensory integration, sensory substitution and visual rehabilitation*. London: Pergamon.

Ptito, M., Matteau, I., Zhi Wang, A., Paulson, O.B., Siebner, H.R. and Kupers, R. 2012. Crossmodal recruitment of the ventral visual stream in congenital blindness. *Neural Plasticity*, 2012(304045). https://doi.org/10.1155/2012/304045

Ptito, M., Moesgaard, S.M., Gjedde, A. and Kupers, R. 2005. Cross-modal plasticity revealed by electro-tactile stimulation of the tongue in the congenitally blind. *Brain*, 128(Pt 3), 606–614.

Ptito, M., Schneider, F.C., Paulson, O.B. and Kupers, R. 2008. Alterations of the visual pathways in congenital blindness. *Experimental Brain Research*, 187(1), 41–49.

Ricciardi, E., Bonino, D., Sani, L., Vecchi, T., Guazzelli, M., Haxby, J.V., Fadiga, L. and Pietrini, P. 2009. Do we really need vision? How blind people "see" the actions of others. *Journal of Neuroscience*, 29(31), 9719–9724.

Roder, B., Teder-Salejarvi, W., Sterr, A., Rosler, F., Hillyard, S.A. and Neville, H.J. 1999. Improved auditory spatial tuning in blind humans. *Nature*, 400(6740), 162–166.

Rokem, A. and Ahissar, M. 2009. Interactions of cognitive and auditory abilities in congenitally blind individuals. *Neuropsychologia*, 47(3), 843–848.

Rombaux, P., Huart, C., De Volder, A.G., Cuevas, I., Renier, L., Duprez, T. and Grandin, C. 2010. Increased olfactory bulb volume and olfactory function in early blind subjects. *Neuroreport*, 21(17), 1069–1073.

Rosenbluth, R., Grossman, E.S. and Kaitz, M. 2000. Performance of early-blind and sighted children on olfactory tasks. *Perception*, 29(1), 101–110.

Sadato, N., Pascual-Leone, A., Grafman, J., Ibañez, V., Deiber, M.P., Dold, G. and Hallett, M. 1996. Activation of the primary visual cortex by braille reading in blind subjects. *Nature*, 380(6574), 526–528.

Sathian, K. 2000. Practice makes perfect Sharper tactile perception in the blind. *Neurology*, 54(12), 2203–2204.

Scheller, M., Petrini, K. and Proulx, M.J. 2018. Perception and interactive technology. In J.T. Wixtted (ed.), *Stevens' handbook of experimental psychology and cognitive neuroscience* (vol. 2, pp. 1–50). Hoboken, NJ: Wiley & Sons.

Sengpiel, F. 2007. The critical period. *Current Biology*, 17(17), R742–743.

Shelton, A.L. and McNamara, T.P. 2001. Systems of spatial reference in human memory. *Cognitive Psychology*, 43(4), 274–310.

Sorokowska, A. 2016. Olfactory performance in a large sample of early-blind and late-blind individuals. *Chemical Senses*, 41(8), 703–709.

Spence, C. 2011. Crossmodal correspondences: a tutorial review. *Attention, Perception and Psychophysics*, 73(4), 971–995.

Sterr, A., Green, L. and Elbert, T. 2003. Blind braille readers mislocate tactile stimuli. *Biological Psychology*, 63(2), 117–127.

Sterr, A., Muller, M.M., Elbert, T., Rockstroh, B., Pantev, C. and Taub, E. 1998. Changed perceptions in braille readers. *Nature*, 391(6663), 134–135.

Striem-Amit, E., Cohen, L., Dehaene, S. and Amedi, A. 2012. Reading with sounds: Sensory substitution selectively activates the visual word form area in the blind. *Neuron*, 76(3), 640–652.

Ungar, S., Blades, M. and Spencer, C. 1995. Mental rotation of a tactile layout by young visually impaired children. *Perception*, 24(8), 891–900.

Van Boven, R.W., Hamilton, R.H., Kauffman, T., Keenan, J.P. and Pascual-Leone, A. 2000. Tactile spatial resolution in blind braille readers. *Neurology*, 54(12), 2230–2236.

Voss, P., Lassonde, M., Gougoux, F., Fortin, M., Guillemot, J.P. and Lepore, F. 2004. Early- and late-onset blind individuals show supra-normal auditory abilities in far-space. *Current Biology*, 14(19), 1734–1738.

Wan, C.Y., Wood, A.G., Reutens, D.C. and Wilson, S.J. 2010. Early but not late-blindness leads to enhanced auditory perception. *Neuropsychologia*, 48(1), 344–348.

Wiesel, T.N. and Hubel, D.H. 1965a. Comparison of the effects of unilateral and bilateral eye closure on cortical unit responses in kittens. *Journal of Neurophysiology*, 28(6), 1029–1040.

Wiesel, T.N. and Hubel, D.H. 1965b. Extent of recovery from the effects of visual deprivation in kittens. *Journal of Neurophysiology*, 28(6), 1060–1072.

Wong, M., Gnanakumaran, V. and Goldreich, D. 2011. Tactile spatial acuity enhancement in blindness: evidence for experience-dependent mechanisms. *Journal of Neuroscience*, 31(19), 7028–7037.

Zwiers, M.P., Van Opstal, A.J. and Cruysberg, J.R. 2001. A spatial hearing deficit in early-blind humans. *Journal of Neuroscience*, 21(9), 141–145.

4

On being blind

Gaylen Kapperman

Introduction

An introduction is in order here. At this time in my life, I am totally blind. Because I inherited an eye disease, Stargardt's, I have had useable sight for several decades. When one is afflicted with Stargardt's disease, one begins life as a sighted individual with the prospect of slowly losing one's sight over a span of several decades until one is totally blind. Thus, I have lived a portion of my life as a sighted individual, a portion of my life as a low vision person and currently as a person who is totally blind. Thus, I can speak to the issues involved in all three conditions as well as the challenges involved in losing one's vision slowly over time. I will address those issues using my personal experience as examples. Many individuals who are visually impaired have experienced the same or very similar challenges to those I will address in the following pages.

My father and mother carried the gene, ABCA4, recessively, the most common gene that results in Stargardt's disease. Thus, neither one was visually impaired. They spawned five offspring, three of whom are visually disabled. I am the oldest of the five and two of my sisters are also afflicted with Stargardt's. I have a brother and a sister who are normally sighted. All of us have children and none of them are visually disabled.

Stargardt's disease involves the photoreceptor cells of the retina. The centrally located receptors, the cones, begin to deteriorate first. As a consequence, at the onset of the deterioration process, one loses one's central vision, the portion of one's visual field in which one sees most clearly. At this point, one continues to be able to see peripherally. Using one's peripheral vision only, one's visual acuity is reduced markedly. One has "side vision" remaining. As the disease progresses, the peripheral photoreceptors, the rods, become involved and deteriorate slowly. As the process continues over decades, one eventually loses all ability to see. One reaches the point of total blindness. The speed of the deterioration of vision differs in individuals one from another but if the individual lives long enough, his or her visual condition will progress to the point of complete blindness.

The degeneration of my eyesight probably began some time shortly after my birth. Over the following seven years, it decreased to the point of my being somewhat visually impaired. During those first seven years, my father and mother and grandparents did not recognise that my eyesight was decreasing. The first hint of things to come came during the first day of my elementary school days. At the beginning of the day, the teacher attempted to determine which of the children could not see what was written on the blackboard. I assume that that was a very rudimentary method for determining which children were nearsighted and needed glasses. Of course, I was the only youngster in the class who could not discern anything the teacher wrote on the blackboard. As a consequence, my parents were advised to take me to see an optometrist in order to be fitted for glasses.

My initial appointment with the optometrist resulted in his confirming that I had a severe visual condition. It was relatively easy for the optometrist using an ophthalmoscope to visualise my retinas. At that young age, my retinas had deteriorated to the point that it was extremely evident that a disease process was in progress. The optometrist indicated to my parents that I should be seen by an ophthalmologist.

At this point, one of the many challenges faced by parents of young visually impaired children came to the fore. That challenge is misinformation being given by medical authorities. I remember travelling to a then well-regarded ophthalmological clinic with my parents. After checking in and waiting some minutes, I was called into the examination room by the nurse. My parents were not allowed to accompany me. I remember the doctor putting eye drops in my eyes. Then I was escorted out of the room and sat with my parents while the eye drops took affect, increasing the diameter of my pupils. After some time, I was called back into the examination room, once again, not accompanied by my parents. I remember vividly the ophthalmologist examining my eyes after having administered a visual acuity test. He shone a bright light into both of my eyes taking his time to carefully examine my retinas. After due course, I was once again escorted out of the room and told to sit in the waiting room while my parents were called into the examining room to speak with the doctor. I sat there patiently waiting for their return. I remember seeing them come out of the room walking slowly and exhibiting physical traits that showed anguish with shoulders bowed. Of course, I could not see their facial expressions. As I write this, I can still conjure up the scene. My parents quietly told me to come with them after my father consulted with the woman who sat at the reception window. On our walk back to the car, little was said. I could sense a deep sadness on the part of both of my parents. I remember wondering what the problem was. To reiterate, I was only 7 years old. On the trip back home when we stopped for a break, I was allowed to have any kind of candy I wanted, and I was encouraged to choose as much as I wanted.

Because the clinic was some distance from my home, the trip lasted for several hours. We arrived home late. My mother prepared some food. After that, I was told to go to my room and go to bed. My bedroom adjoined the room in which my parents sat and discussed the information they had received from the doctor. The door was left open. I crawled into bed but did not fall asleep immediately. I listened to my parents discuss the situation not knowing that the doctor had given them radically false information. The doctor had told them that I would be totally blind by the age of 14 and that they should rush me through the impending eight grades to have me enter high school as soon as possible because once I lost all of my vision, my education would come to an end. Yes, that is true, I am not exaggerating! This was the first of a very long list of misinformation that my parents and I received through the years, most of which emanated from medical personnel and quacks!

As my eyesight grew worse as the years passed, my parents attempted to find possible cures. One possible remedy recommended to them was to have me "seen" by a nationally known faith healer. Fortunately, they did not act on that recommendation. In retrospect, I am certain that the faith healer's subordinates would not have allowed him to attempt to employ his "magic" on me because they would have recognised that even his "exceptional powers" would not have been sufficient to remedy my situation.

Another possible remedy recommended to my parents was to have me treated by a chiropractor who was, in fact, a quack. He was a very cunning charlatan. Unfortunately, my parents did succumb to that recommendation. In retrospect, as an adult looking back at this experience, I assume that he may not have been a licensed chiropractor. At any rate, he had developed a reputation among very naive "farm folks" that he could cure all diseases by applying his "hands-on" approach. According to him, there was no condition that he could not treat successfully.

Many individuals who have deteriorating eye conditions fall victim to charlatans from time to time. Luckily, I did not suffer any untoward effects from the "treatments" that lasted for two years until my parents finally brought it to an end.

I was 12 years old when my father sold the farm and we moved to a neighbouring small town where he purchased a business. At that point, I met two more challenges. I attended the local school there. At that age, my eye disease had progressed to the point that I was forced to hold the reading material within an inch of my nose. As my eyesight diminished, my reading speed decreased dramatically. At that point, I was unable to finish all of the assignments during school hours, so I brought my books home regularly. I studied every evening after dinner on a regular basis. I met the challenge of having to put forth much more effort than the other students to accomplish the same amount of work.

At this point, I was enrolled in seventh grade. That is when the next challenge began, bullying by the other boys. These were boys with whom I had not grown up as was the case when I attended the rural school while living on the farm. Before that point, I had never been singled out by other boys for harassment. My reaction to the challenge that the bullying presented was to fight back viciously. I recall that there were several boys who thought it was their mission to "rough me up". As each one gave it his best to give me a good beating, I fought back ferociously. I remember fights in the boys' restroom, on the playground and in the gym. Of course, all of these took place out of sight of the teachers. Each time another boy began attempting to "rough me up", I would retaliate generally by hitting them hard and fast with my fists. I never lost a fight. Generally, after I had beaten each of the bullies, they thought discretion was the better part of valour and the bullying stopped.

My next bullying challenge resulted in a near-death experience. It came my way one day during the summer between the eighth and ninth grades. I was with some boys in the park that was situated several blocks from my home. No other adults were in the vicinity. Only boys of my age and somewhat older made up the group. Suddenly one of them grabbed me and threw me to the ground. I began to fight back but this time, I was not on my feet and thus could not fight back with fists. He had grabbed me from behind around my neck and was positioned behind me on the ground with his legs wrapped tightly around my waist. He began to pull down with his legs and tightened his grip on my neck with his arms and pulled upward. I struggled mightily but could not cause him to release his grip. Because he was strangling me, I could not speak because no breath was passing over my vocal chords. Other boys stood watching as the struggle continued. The next thing I remembered was "waking up" lying face down in the grass. I was in much pain. My back was injured and there was pain emanating from my neck. Apparently, the boys had begun to run away because they thought the aggressor had killed me. As I gained consciousness, I heard one of them yell to the others, "he's moving!" Some of them came back to my location and stood there looking at me while I lay on the ground attempting to regain my composure. Some were laughing and grinning while making comments. I lay on the ground for several minutes until I gained enough strength to stagger to my feet. I walked home in excruciating pain. I never did tell my parents what had happened.

I continued to think about the incident for several days. I made a pledge to myself that that would never happen again. I would never be a victim of such an attack. I knew a boy who lived not far from me. He had never been involved in any of the bullying. One day, previous to the incident, he had shown me a switchblade that he owned. I remembered that. I walked to his house to talk to him. I made him a very generous offer for his switchblade. I paid him a considerable amount of money for the knife because I wanted to be armed at all times. I was determined never to be a victim again.

At the beginning of my high school career, starting in the ninth grade, I carried the switchblade everywhere I went. I made an effort to show it to the other boys in high school. I did this generally in the boys' restrooms where I knew the teachers would not be present. My carrying a switchblade all through my high school years was a very successful resolution to the problem of the bullies selecting me for special treatment. Attempts to bully me never took place by any of the boys in my school thereafter! My willingness to "push back" solved that immediate problem.

When I enrolled in high school, I met the challenge of participation in extra-curricular activities by getting involved in athletics. In high school, the boys were offered the opportunity to do after-school sports. During the four years of high school I played American football and participated on the track and field team. I could not participate in basketball because the ball moved too fast for me to see it.

I enjoyed playing American football. It is a very rough game in which considerable physical aggression is required. I enjoyed that aspect of the game.

When I played football during practice or during games, no special adaptations were made for me because of my being severely visually impaired. At the time, I estimate that my acuity may have been approximately 20/200 (+1.0 Log MAR) or slightly less. To the credit of the coaches, I was given no quarter. I was not in any fashion given any type of "special" consideration.

My participation in football undoubtedly helped me overcome the challenge of the absence of social acceptance by the other students that is so often experienced by severely visually disabled teenagers. During my senior year, I was given the honour of being the homecoming king. My selection took place as a result of the vote of the students in the school. I was convinced that I did not deserve the honour. In years past, it had always been bestowed on one of the best players in the senior class. I was not one of the best players. I, undoubtedly, was honoured by the students because I was the nicest senior football player. I never bullied other students as did several of my senior football team mates. I made an effort to be friendly to everyone I met. I never manhandled them in the boys' restroom. I never made malicious comments to them. As a consequence, I was forced to endure the humiliation of riding on the back of a convertible car with a crown on my head and a cape over my shoulder pads, sitting next to my queen as we were driven around the periphery of the football field basking in the applause of the assembled crowd!

Little did I know but the worst was yet to come. The homecoming dance was to be held immediately after the game, giving enough time for those attending the dance an opportunity to change into appropriate clothing. I hurried in the locker room, showered quickly, dowsed myself with sweet-smelling aftershave, put on my coat and tie and quickly exited to the parking lot. There, I had arranged with a friend to be able to stash a bottle of cheap whisky in his car. I was exceptionally nervous because I knew from previous homecoming dances that the king and queen started the celebration by dancing together in front of the entire student body and teachers. I was very unsure of my ability to dance. Thus, I began guzzling whisky and chain-smoking Winston cigarettes, remaining slumped down in the front seat of the car with my bottle of whisky in my hand sipping from it nervously. Eventually, one of my friends came to the car, opened the door and told me that the principal was looking for me. The dance was to begin, and several people had been given the task of finding me. Fortified with alcohol,

I acquiesced and exited the car. I was already somewhat inebriated but was determined to appear to be sober. I walked into the school and was met by my girlfriend who immediately began admonishing me for my disappearing act. I ignored her verbal assault and took her by the hand and we walked into the high school gym where the dance was to be held. At my entrance, applause rose up from a large, very blurry assembled crowd. I could not recognise any single individuals in the crowd that surrounded the dance floor. That inability was not due entirely to the over-consumption of alcohol!

Apparently several hundred people had been waiting for me to make my appearance while I had been hiding in the car in the parking lot getting drunk. I did not see my queen until she walked up to me and she said something to the effect, "Let's do it!" We walked on to the middle of the dance floor and the music began. I concentrated hard to stay in time. My queen, who dated an older man, commented on how good a dancer I was. That comment through me off my concentration and I remember making a misstep but managed to regain my concentration and stayed in time with the music throughout the dance. When the music ended, again we walked off the dance floor to the applause of the assembled crowd. I would have rather had been on the football field bashing heads with the largest, meanest opponent that could have gone against me!

After my initial faltering beginning to my social life during the seventh and eighth grades, my social life began to flourish in high school, starting with my freshman year. I attribute this to two factors. As previously noted, first and undoubtedly foremost, my participation in after school athletics engendered greater acceptance by the boys who held the highest esteem among the teenagers – the athletes. A second factor of perhaps lesser influence, yet perhaps contributory was my academic ability. In every class, I occupied one of the positions of highest achievement.

My not possessing a driver's licence (due to my poor vision apparently) was another challenge that I faced. My social life flourished despite my inability to drive a car. In rural Nebraska, it was absolutely necessary that every boy have a driver's licence and every boy owned his own vehicle at or before age 16. It was, then, commonly accepted among the adults in the community that teenage boys were permitted to operate vehicles of all kinds well before the commonly accepted age limit. As a consequence, I had ample opportunities to accompany my friends in travelling about the area in their vehicles.

I met the challenge of achieving at a high academic level through sheer dint of long hours of study despite my relatively busy social life. Because I had nothing but a small video projector, one of the first low vision aids, located in my bedroom at home, I brought the majority of my textbooks home each day to study during the evening after dinner. I had no other low vision aids. Reading was extremely slow and laborious. I would continue until I had completed all of my assignments. In many cases, I did not finish the task until midnight.

In school, I used very thick magnifying glasses that had been affixed in frames like regular glasses. By leaning over and placing my nose nearly on the page, I was able to read. If writing with a pencil was required, I could move away from the page sufficiently to fit the pencil between my magnifying glasses and the paper. My handwriting was larger than that of my classmates.

I did not have the advantage of having a specially trained teacher. When I reached the age of 16, personnel from the Nebraska state rehabilitation agency were allowed to advise my parents and me. I was assigned a rehabilitation counselor. I assume that he discussed my situation with the high school officials.

During my high school years, I assumed a leadership role. I held various elected positions on the student council. In addition, in one incident, I became a leading social activist.

At the beginning of my high school years, we were able to receive one TV channel. Perhaps two years later, a second TV station was established close enough for us to receive that channel also. My TV watching was not limited to the local news. To the sheer joy of my teenage friends and me, the second TV station broadcasted a programme specially designed for teenagers, American Bandstand. The programme emanated from Philadelphia and was hosted by Dick Clark. It featured rock 'n' roll artists and Philadelphia teenagers dancing to the music. The programme was extremely popular in my teenage community. Then, suddenly, one day the programme was taken off the air. All of us were extremely disappointed. I leaped into action. I called the management of the TV station to try to gather information about why the programme was removed. I was told that it was not popular enough. I knew that that probably was a false rationale for its removal. I did not know how to countermand the argument. In order to prove that it was popular among my friends, I designed a petition, one in which the undersigned demanded to have the programme reinstated. I passed the petition around in school. Everyone signed it. At the end of the day, it was given back to me with an enormous number of signatures. That evening, I wrote a cover letter and addressed an envelope to the management of the company and put it in the mail. I never received a reply. In retrospect as an adult in thinking about that situation, I am sure that it was taken off the air for religious reasons. That was my first attempt at political action and it ended in failure!

With regard to my watching TV, I would indicate that for a considerable period of years, I was able to watch TV. I do not know the very last time that I was able to view the picture on a TV screen, but I was able to watch TV until I was perhaps 50 years old. During the intervening years, I lay on the floor in front of the TV. The TV was situated near the floor. My family members who could see well were able to view the screen positioned higher than my head. That approach worked well for many decades. Now that I can no longer watch TV or see movies, it is one of many activities that I miss among the numerous activities in which I participated. Even though many movies and many TV shows are audio described for the blind, the best audio description does not fully replace being able to view the screen. Thus, I count not being able to watch TV or movies as one among many losses in my life as a result of becoming totally blind.

During my senior year in high school, the next challenge arose – the question of what I would do after graduation. In the past, from time to time, I had overheard my parents and grandparents discussing my future. No one in my extended family had attended college or any post-secondary educational programme of any sort. My father and grandparents did not hold high school diplomas. My mother was the most educated person in the extended family with a high school diploma. As a consequence, the circumstances pertaining to my life after high school was of some concern to my family members because of their very limited experience with regard to post-secondary education. When I was assigned an advisor from the state rehabilitation agency, my family was afforded information concerning possibilities for a future life. One of those possibilities was attending college.

The next challenge that I faced was providing proof that I was worthy of being supported in my pursuit of a college degree. In discussions with my advisor, it was determined that I should undergo a thorough psychological examination by a psychologist. A day was set when he was to come to our home to perform the evaluation. I remember sitting at the dining room table with the gentleman. He opened his satchel to bring out several items. These were the assessment instruments.

We began the assessment after he asked questions about my life and the types of activities in which I was involved. The two major instruments were a test of my manual dexterity and the other was an IQ test. After I completed the manual dexterity test, I felt that he thought I was not very adept at handling small bolts, washers and nuts, placing the washers on the bolt and attaching the nut to the top of the bolt and placing them in holes on a board. I believe that my ineptitude was due to the lack of fine-motor coordination and the inability to see the small holes where the bolts were to be inserted.

The second test involved many items that dealt with my mental acumen. I continued to answer the questions one after another. It required a lengthy period to complete the exam. At the conclusion, the psychologist calculated the score. Before the exam he had told me that this was an IQ test to determine how smart I was. As a consequence, after he completed the calculations, I asked him how well I did. He said I did very well. I then asked him what my IQ was. He said that it was against professional ethics for him to tell me, but he assured me that I was smarter than he was. The outcome of the assessment resulted in my being encouraged to enrol in a university.

During my senior year, arrangements were made for my taking the college admissions exam, the Scholastic Aptitude Test (SAT). I was allowed to use my low vision aid device in my small study room. The principal was responsible for overseeing the administration of the exam. I was given 1.5 times the normal amount of time to complete all sections. I worked as fast as I could in completing the various parts of the exam. At the end of the time period, the principal came to the room to collect the completed exam. I was not able to finish all of the items. Some weeks later, the principal came to one of my classes and interrupted the class to beckon me to the hallway. He excitedly announced that I had done exceptionally well on the exam. The principal's enthusiasm may have stemmed from the fact that I was severely visually impaired and, as a result, I was not expected to do well. The low expectations held by others regarding my capability has haunted me through the years.

The first time that others' low estimation of my ability first came to my notice was in English class during my freshman year in high school. During that year, the first of a very long list of incidents confirming the misplaced attitude of adults became apparent to me. One day in English class, the English teacher launched into a discussion about college. He asked us if we wanted to know who should go to college and who should not. Of course, all of us 14-year-olds in unison indicated, yes, we wanted to know. He began listing the names of the members of the class as he surveyed the class visually. I noted rather quickly that he was listing the "smart kids!" The dumb kids' names and my name were not mentioned as potential college students. After a momentary pause in my thinking, I surmised that I was not included among the supposedly college-ready students was because I was visually impaired. Very easily, I discounted his judgement as being wrong. That attitude on my part has served me well down through the decades! I can remember only one time when I took the advice of an adult or an authority figure in my life. In remembering the many pieces of advice that I have been given, welcome or not, not one was, in my mind, valid. I will note these in the following paragraphs.

I chose to attend a small liberal arts college in Nebraska against the wishes of my rehabilitation counselor and the approach taken by the state rehabilitation agency in general. It was common to encourage all of the blind and severely visually disabled college-age young people in Nebraska to attend the University of Nebraska in Lincoln. The reason for attempting to discourage me from attending the small private liberal arts college was because the cost of attending that institution of higher learning was much more than attending the University of Nebraska. That fact was explained to me directly by my counselor in a discussion with him regarding my future. I indicated that if the agency would pay the usual amount that it paid for all of those attending the University of Nebraska, I would make up the remainder of the costs with scholarships and other sources of funding. My counselor indicated that he would bring the matter to the agency head. Sometime later, he informed me that the arrangement was approved.

I had made an application for admission to the small college before having discussed the situation with my counselor. I was admitted in a relatively short period of time. I followed the notification of admission with communications in which I inquired about scholarships. I was awarded a substantial one along with the funds committed by the rehabilitation agency, but I still needed additional funding. Since my father was deceased, I was eligible for a moderate amount of money supplied monthly by the social security administration. Thus, the three sources of funding were sufficient to support my attending the most expensive school in Nebraska. This was, again, a very wise choice on my part that went counter to the advice of older individuals in my life. I received an outstanding education in the college and got considerable individual attention that would not have been afforded me at the University of Nebraska, which was much larger than my small college. There were many advantages that came my way because of my attending the school of my choice.

One major adaptation that the college authorities afforded me was that they gave me permission to study in a small room in one of the older classroom buildings. I brought several pieces of equipment to use in my studying and, as a consequence, there was not sufficient space in the very small dormitory rooms where we were housed because each room housed two boys. As a result, I had a very secure, quiet location in which to study. I needed that type of environment because I spent many more hours studying than did every other student on the campus. Without the distraction of my roommate and other boys in the dormitory, I was able to study as efficiently as I could, reading perhaps 80 words per minute and having to take frequent breaks to rest my eyes.

To begin our studies, all freshmen were asked to choose a major. I chose mathematics. I had two reason for that choice. First of all, mathematics was one of my favourite subjects in school. I was particularly adept at it. Second, assignments in math did not require a large amount of reading. A long assignment might consist of five to ten pages of material, whereas, in other areas of study, generally, throughout the semester, hundreds of pages of reading were required. During the years that I was a student in various institutions of higher education, none of the currently existing assistive technology had been invented. I was left with my thick glasses and reading with my nose on the page at a very slow pace. My choice of mathematics was my solution to that very vexing problem of reading especially slowly.

When I attended classes, I could not see what was written on the blackboard. As a consequence, I listened as closely as possible, but never took notes. Generally, I learned the content by studying the textbooks carefully and not depending on any information that may have been imparted in class. In fact, I may have been able to complete the major in mathematics without having to attend class except when tests were given.

Based on our choice of majors, we were given our class schedules listing the courses for which we were registered by our academic advisor. I, of course, was enrolled in a mathematics course along with 12 semester hours of other courses that were common to entering freshmen. I did not realise that the math course in which I was enrolled was not included in the array of required courses for majoring in mathematics. It was the generally required math course of all students who did not major in math. I came to that realisation some time later in the semester when engaged in conversation with other students some of whom had declared math as their major area of study. This was yet another example of lower expectations for me by the significant adults in my life. That error on the part of my advisor caused me to spend a fifth year working toward a bachelor's degree because I was not able to begin the sequence of requirements for a math major until my sophomore year. In retrospect, this is an example of the few times when poor advice led to a very good outcome.

The major advantage that five years as an undergraduate afforded me was that it enabled me to major in German as well as mathematics. My preparation in German resulted in several extraordinarily advantageous opportunities for me that would not have accrued to me if I had not majored in German as well as mathematics.

In summary, the major in German afforded me several advantages. First of all, after eventually having graduated with a master's degree, I was awarded a Fulbright Fellowship to study at the University of Heidelberg, Germany, for one year. Following that experience, I was employed to teach German and mathematics at a school for blind children. Later in my professional life, as a university professor, I have chosen foreign language instruction for blind students as one of my specialty areas in which I have published. Thus, not all of the advice based on low expectations for me resulted in misfortune.

Academic achievement was highly valued at the liberal arts school where I began my academic career. As a consequence, all of the students' GPAs were listed by name in a location outside of the registrar's office. With today's emphasis on confidentiality, that appears to be a gross violation. At that time, it was not considered as such. I believe that it was used by the faculty as a method to spur on the lesser-achieving students to increase their efforts. At any rate, a freshman girl and I received the two highest GPAs in the school. She and I achieved four A grades and one B plus. This was the time in higher education before grade inflation became commonplace! A grade of C was considered to be average and in almost all courses was achieved by the majority of students. Thus, our very high GPAs were noted in the school newspaper. The headline in the first issue of the spring semester announced that a freshman boy and girl had received the highest grades during the previous fall semester. Our names and pictures were displayed on the front page along with short articles about each of us. Not one mention was made that I was visually impaired! That fact about me played no part in the editor's decision to focus on me along with the high-achieving girl.

During the spring semester, the fraternities and sororities offered invitations to join them. One of the fraternities offered "bids" to only the most intellectually talented boys in the freshman class. I was offered an invitation and I chose to join it. As a consequence, I was well accepted by a very academically talented group of young men some of whom became lifelong friends. I contend that the decision on the part of the members of the fraternity to offer me an invitation was based on the fact that I could help win the annual academic trophy awarded each year to the fraternity, which demonstrated the highest commitment to scholarship based on its collective GPA. My newly adopted brotherhood had never lost the trophy since its inception decades before. Thus, I was viewed as a potential contributing member to the goal of the group. I contend that I would not have had this type of opportunity had I attended a very large university. As a consequence, my tendency to go against the advice of my elders resulted in yet another very beneficial outcome in my life.

My social life at college began very slowly. For the first year, it was nearly nonexistent. During the first semester, I did nothing but eat, sleep and study. To meet yet another challenge, developing a reasonable social life, I was determined to change my approach. At the beginning of the second semester, I determined that I could not keep up an extraordinarily rigorous work schedule. Thus, I did not spend every waking hour in my study room. I began observing the female students on campus. Because I had remaining vision at approximately 20/200 (+1.0 Log MAR) acuity, I was able to see the girls if I was in close proximity. I made very unsuccessful attempts to become acquainted with some of them. Each time, I was rebuffed in polite and not so polite terms. I am certain that I was known as the "blind kid" on campus.

Despite a series of failures, I continued my attempts to become acquainted. One particular girl struck my fancy. I had observed her in line for lunch and dinner several times. She was accompanied by several other girlfriends. She had reddish-blonde hair, a great smile, a terrific figure and seemed to be very well liked by her girlfriends. I never did see her in the company of another male. All of these factors peaked my interest. I asked about her among some of the boys in my dorm. They agreed to use their influence among the females on campus to find out information about her. Not a long while later, I found out her name and home town. She lived only about 25 miles from the college.

Now that I had as much information about her as I thought I could get, I was determined to make acquaintance with her. Luckily, one day while walking through the dining room carrying my tray of food, I happened to walk toward the table where she and her girlfriends were sitting. As I approached, I noted that there was an empty chair next to her. I asked politely if the chair was taken. And of course, it was not. I sat down with the hope of engaging her in conversation. Unfortunately, she did not want to talk with me. She turned her back to me and continued to talk with her girlfriends. They also paid no attention to me. As a matter of fact, their attitude was one that gave me the impression that I had entered a "no man is welcome" zone! After just a short while, they decided to get up and be on their way. Not one of them had acknowledged my existence. I assume that one or more of them had been in some my classes where they observed me writing notes with my head down and nose close to the paper. I did not remember having a class with the red-headed girl, but she certainly did not want to meet me. I counted that incident among the many rebuffs that I had suffered. I assumed that the females on campus did not view me as a likely dating partner because of my being severely visually impaired.

The wife of one of the professors was employed by the rehabilitation agency to be my reader. Her husband was one of the professors in the Department of Elementary Education. He, of course, knew about my situation and where I studied and the equipment I used. He invited me to speak to both sections of his introductory course in elementary education to describe in detail how a disabled youngster had made his way through the 12 grades. He was well ahead of the time in that regard. Nowadays, it is common that people who major in any aspect of professional training for teachers are exposed in some fashion to the needs of disabled children. At any rate, unknown to me, the red-headed girl who was the object of my interest attended one of the sections of the course in which I spoke. Later, I discovered that she had sat in the back row. Of course, I did not see her. Luckily, she took an interest in my story and, as a consequence, in me. One of the details that I described to the assembled students was where I studied and the arrangement of my equipment in my study room. Thus, they all knew where my study room was located.

Some of the students had gone to the dean to ask that the building I studied in be open to them also as they complained that they could not concentrate in the dorms because of the noise and disruption caused by the other less-studious students. The dean gave me the assignment of watching over the building and closing it at night and asking the students to leave after 10 pm each evening. I was in charge of the building. I agreed to that plan readily.

One evening, while I was studying, I knew there were several other students in the various classrooms. Suddenly there was a knock on the door. I looked up and there the red-headed girl was standing with a gorgeous smile on her face. She asked if she could come in and have a cigarette with me. The only rooms in the building where smoking was allowed were the professors' offices. Since my study room was formerly a professor's office that was in considerable disrepair, I smoked there. She knew this. Of course, I was more than pleased to welcome her into my space. She sat down, lit a cigarette and introduced herself. I told her that I already knew her name. She was slightly amused, and I think pleased to a certain extent. She told me that she was impressed with the "talk" that I had given in her class and she wanted to know more about me. We talked for bit and exchanged personal information about ourselves including where our home towns were located and information about our families. She and I had a regrettable fact in common in that both of our fathers had died when we were teenagers. I invited her to eat lunch with me the next day. I waited for her at the entrance of the dining room and to my delight, she approached me and we walked in together and ate lunch. That was a beginning of a wonderful romance and eventually resulted in our marriage three years later. Once again, my refusal to heed the advice of my elders resulted in yet another wonderful outcome! If I had attended the University of Nebraska, I would never have had a chance to meet the love of my life!

During our undergraduate days, we spent an enormous amount of time together. We ate lunch and dinner together every day. She came to the classroom building where I was in charge and spent time studying. We always set aside sufficient time to be with one another, shall we say, romantically. As a consequence, I undoubtedly had the most flourishing romantic life of perhaps any other man on campus! Thus, my social life moved from dismal to spectacular in a relatively short period of time.

Another misadventure with the medical profession occurred during my undergraduate days at college. I had decided that I ought to visit an ophthalmologist to have my eyes examined. I do not remember why I thought that that was a good idea. By that time, I knew that there was no cure for my eye disease. At any rate, I made an appointment with an eye specialist. I made my way by bus to the city where he was located. During the exam period, he indicated, as I knew, that there was no treatment that would cure my eye disease. He indicated to me that the disease I had, which he did not name, was inherited. He asked me if I had a girlfriend. I said yes, I did. He then asked if I planned to marry her. At that time, marriage had not been upper-most in my mind. I thought about it for a moment and said, yes perhaps! He said, well, then you need to have a vasectomy! I was somewhat uncertain what was involved in the operation. He then told me that he had a friend in the clinic who was an urologist and he might be able to "take me" right then. He called his friend on the phone and quickly explained the situation. He had a young man in his office who has an inherited eye disease and he needs to have a vasectomy. He asked his friend if he could see me right away. He then turned to me and told me that his friend could see me right then. He gave me directions to his friend's office. I was to turn left out of his office, follow the corridor and turn right and at the end of that corridor was the location of his friend's office. Well, instead of turning left out of his office, I immediately turned right, sped up to nearly a running pace, burst through the front door, ran across the front area of the clinic, saw a cab, jumped in and gave the driver orders that I wanted to be taken to the bus station immediately just as fast as he could go! He indicated that I had run by an elderly woman who was making her way to his cab. I told him that she could catch the next one and that he should start driving immediately to the bus station! I wanted to get away from the misguided doctor just as fast as I could! Once again, my refusal to take the advice of authority figures in my life came to the fore. As I write this, I have one very wonderful daughter who actually is my genetic daughter and has some of my characteristics – something I would not have, had I obeyed the doctor's orders.

The eye specialist was not the only medical professional who recommended eugenics for me. Sometime after we had been married, I visited the family doctor for a reason of which I have no recollection, but I certainly do remember the discussion with him. He was the family doctor for my then wife's family including her mother and her sisters. In my discussion, he indicated to me that my mother-in-law had indicated to him that I was afflicted with an inherited eye disease. I told him that that was true. Once again, I saw well enough that merely by observing me, one could not discern that I was visually impaired unless one saw me reading or if was very observant. The doctor was neither. He indicated that when my wife and I decided to have children, I could have a vasectomy, but we could take her to Omaha to the medical school there. Arrangements could be made for one of the young medical students to meet us there and he could donate semen that could then be placed inside her! He assured me that the medical students there were smart and were high-quality males. I told him "Hell no!" I am not going to do that! I was offended at the suggestion and made certain he knew that. I also then discovered that my mother-in-law had severe reservations about my marrying her daughter. Apparently, she had talked to the family doctor about this most unfortunate situation. Once again, my obstinate refusal to take the advice of others served me well!

The sexy redhead and I were married one year before I graduated. She graduated one year ahead of me and took a position as an elementary education teacher while I completed my studies, majoring in mathematics and German and was awarded a secondary teaching certificate. I completed student teaching in mathematics in a local high school near the college.

After I graduated, my wife and I moved to a neighbouring state where we both enrolled in graduate school. I began my training as a teacher of blind youngsters. During the year that we lived there, I applied for the Fulbright Fellowship to study special education for blind and visually impaired children in Germany. I had become acquainted with the process of applying for prestigious post-baccalaureate fellowships due to my membership in the academically oriented fraternity. The professor who was our advisor urged many of the members of the fraternity to apply for various fellowships with the intention of studying in post-baccalaureate programmes. During my years as a member of the fraternity, I attended several small celebrations in which we informally honoured our older brothers who were awarded numerous very prestigious fellowships. As a consequence, I was cognisant of the process involved in applying for those fellowships.

While I attended graduate school, one piece of advice I received from a professor resulted in an excellent outcome. While I spent an enormous amount of time completing the very rigorous application process for the Fulbright, I sought out the German professor on campus to seek his advice. During the very arduous application process, one of the items to be completed was related to at which university the applicant desired to study. I made an appointment with the German professor to pose the question as to which one he might recommend. He indicated that most Americans liked Heidelberg and that it was an excellent city in which to live. As a consequence, I noted that in my application. This is one very rare example in which the advice of an elder actually was of value to me.

I can summarise our year in Germany by indicating that it was one of the best years of our lives. We travelled widely. Once again, I would have found that to be exceptionally difficult had I not been with my sighted partner. When we reached various cities, we depended upon her ability to see and my ability to speak German. Together, we enjoyed a very exciting year in Germany.

As the year came to an end, it was time for us to return to the United States and begin work. One evening we sat together and scanned a book that I had brought with us. It was a book published by the American Foundation for the Blind in which all of the contact information for all agencies serving the blind in the United States were listed. We turned from one state to the other listed in the book to decide where we might wish to live. For those states that we agreed upon, I wrote letters of inquiry to the schools for the blind located there. The only school official from which I received a positive response was the superintendent of the Kansas School for the Blind located in Kansas City, Kansas. I went to the post office and sent a telegram back to him accepting his offer of employment as a teacher of math and German. Upon our return to the United States, once I had arrived at the school, and become acquainted with other staff members, I learned that he had fired his German teacher and his math teacher had left at the end of that school year. Then, one day, he received a letter from a young man, named Kapperman, living in Germany who was a certified teacher of math and German and who held a secondary teaching certificate as well as a certificate in teaching blind and visually impaired students. It is no wonder that I was hired sight unseen!

We moved to Kansas after arriving back in the United States. My wife obtained a teaching position in the Kansas City school district. We spent three years there with my teaching at the Kansas School for the Blind and her teaching third grade in the Kansas City schools.

During the third year in Kansas City, I applied for admission to a doctoral programme in a neighbouring state. I was accepted and at the close of the third year in Kansas City, we moved to the location where the doctoral programme was located. I was determined to become a professor. As a consequence, I worked hard to complete the requirements for the degree in record time. Once again, my wife was an invaluable aid in that she worked as a special educator teaching in one of the local schools.

Once I graduated having completed the doctoral program, I took a position as an assistant professor in the Visual Disabilities Program at Northern Illinois University. At that time, I still maintained some usable sight. Because closed-circuit television had just been developed for use by visually impaired individuals, I began using that device. That technological advance proved to be of invaluable aid to me.

My first challenge as a visually impaired university professor came about when I was awarded my first competitive grant. The major faculty member with whom I worked became extremely jealous of my accomplishment. He was fully sighted, and I was severely visually impaired and that fact, I believe, caused him to resent my accomplishment. Winning federal grants was a very highly prized activity in my department. As a consequence, I am convinced that the fact that I was able to succeed in that area when many other members of the faculty could not, led to a great amount of resentment on his part. At that point, our relationship began a downward spiral and never did recover its original level of cordiality. I was unable to find a solution to this predicament. Our relationship came to a sudden end at his very unexpected, early death.

I have continued to be one of the most successful procurers of grants in the department and in college and university through the decades. I have found that the resentment toward me as a result of my success was not limited to my original coworker. This very unfortunate attitude on the part of others has become apparent to me on numerous occasions since I began as a university professor and researcher.

The latest incident in which resentment toward me was revealed in very stark terms occurred when a new dean attempted to "encourage" me to resign my position. She made a valiant effort to arrange the circumstances of my work to such an extent that I would voluntarily quit. My situation was such that she was not allowed to fire me outright. In short, she enlisted the aid of three subordinates to accomplish the goal. These were two associate deans and a chairwoman. The details describing their unsuccessful efforts are two complex to enumerate here. Suffice it to say that they are all no longer working at Northern Illinois University and I am still employed at that institution. I believe that the fundamental reason for her resentment and subsequent attempts to get rid of me was that I was the highest paid professor in the college, and because I am blind, that fact was more than she could tolerate.

The resentment is not limited to sighted colleagues and administrators. I have sensed the same resentment on the part of some of my blind and visually impaired graduate students. Apparently, they are jealous of my success as a fellow visually impaired person. That most unfortunate attitude prevails in other cultures as well as among disabled individuals. My approach is to accept the fact that I will engender ill will from others because I am a successful individual in an area in which competition is rigorous. I have never allowed the less than admirable attitude on the part of others to deter me from my efforts to succeed. There is little that I can do to nullify their attitudes and thus I ignore it for the most part.

Another challenge that I find to be most disconcerting is the inability to negotiate social situations. When I had a bit of useful vision, I was able to participate in social gatherings nearly as competently as fully sighted individuals. Now that I am totally blind, I find social situations to be one of the most vexing problems I face. I do not have a method by which to overcome this challenge. As a consequence, down through the years, my social life has diminished considerably. I attend fewer parties and I am invited to fewer social gatherings with individuals who once were close friends. I believe that many of them feel a bit uncomfortable in my presence now that I can no longer function visually as I had in the past. My social isolation has grown commensurately as my eyesight has grown worse.

My solution to my failing social life is to not retire from my position as a professor. I maintain my position as a professor emeritus continuing to work with graduate students and to interact with them and a small number of professional colleagues. I continue to work on new projects in which I develop innovative solutions to problems faced by blind and visually impaired children and adults. A small number of professional colleagues and graduate students work with me on teams led by me. The individuals I choose to be members of my teams are those who do not harbour ill will toward me because of my success.

Another challenge that I face along with all of my totally blind brothers and sisters is the ability to negotiate the environment. I use a guide dog rather than a cane. I have several reasons for making that choice. First of all, I am an extremely poor cane traveller! Second, a dog enables me to travel much more efficiently in the environment moving quickly from point A to point B without undue delay! Third, it is my opinion that the sighted public is much more willing to accept a blind person using a guide dog than one using a white cane.

Another vexing challenge is the inability to travel by car independently. I am able to purchase expensive cars for my wife to drive. In addition, I hire private drivers. I am extremely fortunate in that I do not need to use public transport. Once again, my ability to amass a reasonable amount of personal funds has enabled me to overcome this challenge.

I have met the challenge of maintaining my home and surrounding area by employing others to do the work. I never have mowed a lawn, I have never toiled in maintaining the vegetation surrounding my home, I do not shovel snow, I never repair any type of equipment in the home, I do not clean the rooms in my home nor do I do laundry. I employ others to do all of those chores. I am absolutely certain that even if I had perfect sight, I would not do any of that work about the home! I realise that the vast majority of blind individuals do not find themselves in such an advantageous situation.

I meet the challenge of handling written work by using the very latest assistive technology. Once again, I am very fortunate in that I can afford to buy the most up-to-date equipment and software that I need. With the use of technology, I am able to manage any tasks that require my dealing in one manner or another with the written word or figures. Living as a financially secure individual has enabled me to meet many of the challenges that blindness brings with it!

Conclusion

Others have told me that they believe that I am so successful because I am extremely resilient. I just never give up. My array of personality traits includes extreme self-confidence. Also, I am given to taking risks. I believe that my high level of self-confidence engenders that approach to life. The fact that I have stated these rather socially inappropriate self-appraisals readily indicates to the reader why I am given to generating resentment in others and finally, I simply do not care if that is the result!

Part II

Cerebral visual impairment/ cerebral visual processing

5

Cerebral (cortical) visual impairment in children

A perspective

Gordon N. Dutton and Corinna M. Bauer

Introduction

The key rigorous standard for all children with cerebral (cortical) visual impairment (CVI) is to give them full access to all the information and skills they need to learn.

The authors have seen the lives of hundreds of children with CVI enhanced by successful pursuit of this aphorism.

Effective learning underpins child development, but children cannot learn from the unintelligible. When salient adaptations are made for children with CVI to render their worlds accessible and meaningful, their low expectation "learning difficulties" are transformed into high expectation "learning challenges".

CVI, its origin, nature, impact and amelioration, is a broad topic (Dutton and Bax, 2010; Lueck and Dutton, 2015; Zihl and Dutton, 2014). This chapter seeks to complement current literature with some explanatory and practical insights.

A recent systematic review has defined CVI in a child as "a verifiable visual dysfunction, which cannot be attributed to disorders of the anterior visual pathways or any potentially co-occurring ocular impairment" (Sakki et al., 2018). Unstable imagery due to associated disorders of eye-movement control can diminish vision further (Jacobson et al., 2002). CVI has many possible variables, giving every affected child their own unique pattern of visual experience, limitations and resulting behaviours. These need to be identified, characterised, profiled and regularly addressed throughout the child's life (Atkinson, 2017; Chokron and Dutton, 2016; Martín et al., 2016; Philip and Dutton, 2014; Philip et al., 2016).

Ocular visual impairment (OVI) due to bilateral eye or optic nerve disorders resembles a filter limiting visual input into an intact mental processing unit. On the other hand, it is an anomaly of intrinsic brain image processing that can interfere with looking, seeing, perceiving, recognising, interpreting, focusing in upon and moving through the visual world. CVI can range greatly in nature and degree and can influence any aspect of daily life. Moreover, other mental and motor functions can be impaired by collateral brain injury or dysfunction.

CVI has become the leading cause of visual impairment in children in high-income countries, as well as an increasingly frequent cause in low-income nations (Kong et al., 2012). OVI is becoming less common, in part due to the combined success of immunisation for rubella and improved outcomes from eye surgery. CVI on the other hand is becoming more frequent owing to effective paediatric intensive care, causing increased survival rates in infants and children who sustain brain injury (Shirley et al., 2017).

In OVI the brain cannot learn from what it does not perceive, but it can develop differently. For example, in people with no vision from early on in life, the brain parts that process incoming visual image data, the occipital lobes, can functionally reconfigure and create alternative representations of the surroundings through echolocation. This yields transient perceived imagery created through mental analysis of echoic sound (Thaler et al., 2011; Thaler and Goodale, 2016; Thaler et al., 2016). This has been called "flash sonar", owing to the transience of the imagery seen after each successive tongue click and consequent echo (Kish and Hook, 2017). Sight is thus a mental process, with echolocation, for example, giving "visual" experience from auditory input, through cross-modal neuroplasticity.

CVI can co-exist with retinopathy of prematurity (Jacobson and Dutton, 2000), or optic nerve hypoplasia (Dutton 2013; Zeki, Hollman and Dutton, 1992). Moreover, early-onset CVI can result in fewer nerve fibres in the retina and optic nerve, probably due to nerve cell death back into the eyes (by retrograde trans-synaptic degeneration), where it can be identified with optical coherence tomography (OCT) imaging of the retina (Jacobson, Ygge and Flodmark, 1998; Lennartson et al., 2017). So, the distinction between OVI and CVI is not distinct.

Sensory inputs are integrated by the mind into singular experiences. This means that one sense can compete with another for attention, especially when the capacity for processing visual information in time and/or space is diminished. For example, background noise or visual clutter can interfere with learning (Simonsen et al., 2008). Also, it is important to recognise that CVI is commonly associated with optical error, impaired focusing, or both. So, all children with CVI must be optometrically screened for these conditions and appropriate spectacles given if needed (Das et al., 2010; Saunders et al., 2010).

From early infancy, child development depends on perception to a significant degree (Leong et al., 2017). Yet, infants and children can only learn from what they are able to see, hear and appreciate. For children with CVI, applying parenting and educational approaches based on the needs of typical children cannot and does not work well. Traditional habilitation strategies for children with OVI may be ineffective or even detrimental for a child with CVI (Groenveld, Jan and Leader, 1990), and clear "inside-to-out" ways of envisioning how every affected child, each with their own unique form of CVI, are needed. This means we need to know each child's set of perceptual limits and how and why these constrain learning, to work out how each child can be parented and taught using perceptible and meaningful approaches.

A major aim of disability legislation is to afford access. To meet with the spirit of such legislation, each scenario a child needs to learn from must be accessible. This short chapter outlines some of the basic principles of what parents, carers, and professionals need to know to work out how to achieve this goal for the child with CVI under their care.

The creation of vision by the brain

Imagery of our surroundings is brought into focus on the retinae of both eyes, where it is converted into electrical signals and transferred via a pair of relay stations, the lateral geniculate bodies, to the back of the brain (the occipital lobes and the adjacent middle temporal lobes). This is where rapid initial processing of the incoming information from the whole visual fields takes place, with the brain creating our perception of light level, clarity, contrast, colour and movement.

When you place your hands over your ears, your thumbs as they point backwards overlie your occipital and middle temporal lobes. This is where static and moving image processing

Tree of vision

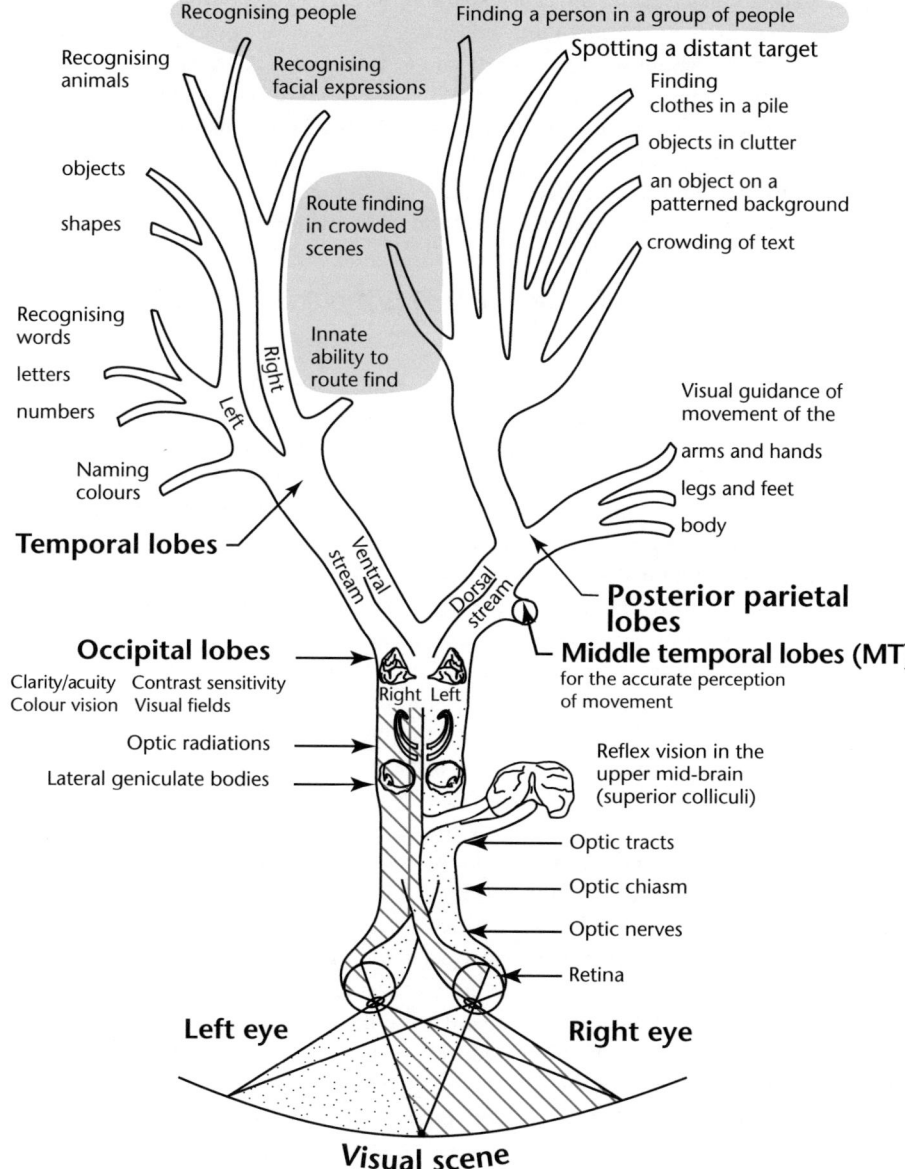

Figure 5.1 Tree of vision: stylised diagram of the visual functions of the brain depicted in the form of a tree. The roots represent the eyes taking in the imagery. The trunk and main branches represent the main visual pathways, and the small branches depict the functions served.

Source: Adapted from Lueck and Dutton (2015).

respectively, take place. Processed visual information is rapidly transferred along the ventral stream (which runs through the inferior longitudinal fasciculus) to your temporal lobes underlying your palms, and along the dorsal stream (which runs through the superior longitudinal fasciculus) to your posterior parietal lobes, underlying your fingers. This whole process comprises a complex dynamic interplay of visual information (Milner and Goodale, 2006) (see Figure 5.1).

The temporal lobes contain an ever-expanding library of everything we have learned to recognise. Comparison of the incoming information with what is stored in our visual library enables us to both recognise what we know, and to learn and remember what is new.

The posterior parietal lobes construct a 3D mapped emulation of our visible (as well as audible and tactile) environment (Pinel and Barnes, 2014). This allows us to locate ourselves in relation to our surroundings and lets us move freely and accurately. Without our knowing, this visual perceptual integration takes place (Goodale and Milner, 2013; Milner and Goodale, 2006) within a time frame of around a tenth of a second (Liu et al., 2017).

Where is the "picture" of what we see? Is it out in front of us, or is it in our minds?

Vision arose at an early stage of animal evolution to guide movement. When we watch sighted animals of all sizes negotiate 3D space by means of vision, we may be forgiven for thinking that the process is simple. Yet, it's miraculous. From moment to moment our minds compute a dynamic triple coincidence. Our mental maps of our bodies seamlessly integrate with our visual perceptual maps of our surroundings, to be matched to our actual position within the physical structure of our environment. How is this achieved?

Just as a tablecloth will make a transparent table visible, the conscious temporal lobe imagery cloaks our non-conscious 3D mapped posterior parietal construct of our surroundings and thereby lets us know not only what we are looking at (from the overlying imagery), but where it is with respect to ourselves (from the underlying 3D mental construct of the structure and locations of the elements of the visual scene). Run up a flight of stairs. Do you consciously see and locate each step? No. We can move rapidly through 3D space, non-consciously by means of vision, without realising how we are doing it. It is this moving 3D map in our posterior parietal lobes that orchestrates this miracle (Arcaro et al., 2018; Goodale and Milner, 2013).

Most of the time we are "grounded" by touch. Supplementary visual mapping of our surroundings informs us of our location. Our knowledge of the positions in space of our body and limbs (proprioception) is integrated into the mental map. Our balance system ties into this visual analysis. Inside our inner ears there are balance receptors. Minute lumps of calcium linked to nerve endings that detect gravitational forces, act as plumblines. When they are off-centre, their messages to the brain lead to automatic action to prevent falling. This fast process is controlled in the brainstem at the top of the spinal cord, and it is linked to vision. Have you ever straightened a picture on a blank wall? How did you know it was not vertical? It didn't match your inner plumb line created by your balance system, so you adjusted it to do so. This sense of balance is reciprocally corroborated by vision. When climbing on to a chair our balance systems ensure that we don't fall and are aided by our using vision to map the horizontal and vertical elements of our surroundings to reinforce our sense of stability. All this takes place non-consciously (unless we choose to think about it) (Pinel and Barnes, 2014).

The tiny disparity in timing for sound reaching each ear is processed in such a way that we can locate where sound is coming from. We can then point to its origin, showing that we can relate this both to ourselves and to our environment. Without our knowing, this information too is mapped in our posterior parietal lobes and temporal lobes (Thaler et al., 2016).

Nerves called proprioceptors in the 12 muscles that move our eyes, and the multiple neck muscles that move our heads, give immediate feedback about the direction we are looking at any one moment (Donaldson, 2000; Weir, Knox and Dutton, 2000). This is integrated with our dynamic balance systems. In this way, the 3D mental emulation of our surroundings mapped to our body position does not go off-kilter when we move our head and eyes around, and the picture is stabilised. The stable jigsaw imagery that our minds assemble as we look from one part of the scene to another is integrated into our visual mindset, as an accurately located seamless whole, matched to our 3D mental construct of our body shape, size and position, which is fed by neural feedback from our limbs, muscles and joints.

This joined-up mapping process informed by these multiple inputs, relates the position of your body to your location, by creating an internal, ever-changing in real time, accurately located multi-modal mental construct of yourself within your surroundings, allowing you to move comfortably and accurately, even through complex moving scenes (Milner and Goodale, 2006; Pinel and Barnes, 2014).

To sum up, our minds receive visual information and create from it the picture of what we are looking at. Our heads and eyes move as they survey the scene, capturing key elements, to build the imagery up. The visual brain receives this image information and "zips it up" into a very slightly delayed real-time, seamless whole, with respect to our head and eyes. Image timing systems, served by the middle temporal lobes (Zihl and Heywood, 2015) and coordinated in part by the cerebellum (Voogd et al., 2012), ensure that the timing of our image processing and eye movements closely match what we are seeing and doing, to what is happening around us. The posterior parietal lobes non-consciously map this dynamic virtual scene with respect to our bodies, while the temporal lobes consciously identify the salient elements in the scene and, if previously unknown, learn from them. The frontal lobes intimately connect with this process and enable us to make choices about, for example, where to look, where to go and how to get there. In this way the continuous ever-changing flow of our vision, consolidated by balance, touch, hearing and knowledge of self, becomes a creation of mind, informed by our prior knowledge and experiences, that we co-locate with the geometry of our apparently ever-changing surroundings as we elect to move through them. Ongoing anticipation of the outcome of our forthcoming movement through our surroundings and our forward planning of this process are informed by visual, haptic and higher-memory functions.

CVI results from disturbance of this complex process, leading to an atypical visual construct in mind that becomes the affected person's normal framework of perception. By recognising that dysfunction of the visual brain can affect any of the many elements of the mental process of vision outlined above, it becomes clear that there must be any number of patterns of "alternative normal vision" among those with CVI, each with its own unique impact.

Children's fascination, exploration and play in the 3D world drive early development, but they can only learn from what they are able to perceive, interpret and understand. In a sense, we as parents and professionals are outside our children's minds, attempting to look in. So, the best estimates that we can make of what they can and cannot see are informed by a detailed analysis of their visual behaviours and measurement of their vision and visual performances, interpreted in the light of our understanding of how the brain sees and what happens if the process is disturbed. These estimates can then be used to make each salient element of their surroundings (and every salient element of what we want them to access and learn from) easily accessible, perceptible, understandable and learnable for as much of their active lives as possible. As parents we do this intuitively, founded in part upon our memories of how our parents and teachers looked after us, but for the child with alternative vision, knowledge of how the child sees is needed in order to modify our parenting strategies accordingly, so it is imperative that parents are taught about their child's vision, its nature and its impact.

Successful learning is motivational, self-driven and underpinned by optimal neuroplastic brain growth and development (Kish and Hook, 2017). To enhance this process during each stage of their development, we need to come to understand and know each child's unique profiles of perceptual, motor and intellectual capabilities and limitations. In this way, we can work within this window of opportunity as we strive to accord accessible and attractive meaning to their worlds, crafting the keys to match their locks and opening their mental doors to what were hitherto inaccessible opportunities.

Children with CVI respond to their visual worlds in three principal ways: they may adapt their approaches, they may react to what they are unable to deal with or they may not respond or react (to what they do not see). The consequences of CVI in children need to be profiled, as they not only give clues to the nature of their vision, but they also give inspiration for how we can alter their circumstances to enable them to learn and function most effectively (see Hyvärinen, Chapter 7 this volume; Lueck and Goodrich, Chapter 8 this volume).

What is going on inside the brain of the child with CVI?

Recent brain imaging studies have shown that those with OVI neuroplastically develop different compensatory or alternative brain pathways while those with CVI manifest significantly narrower visual tracts in the brain, which could underlie impairment in visual search, by limiting visual parallel processing capacity (Martín et al., 2016).

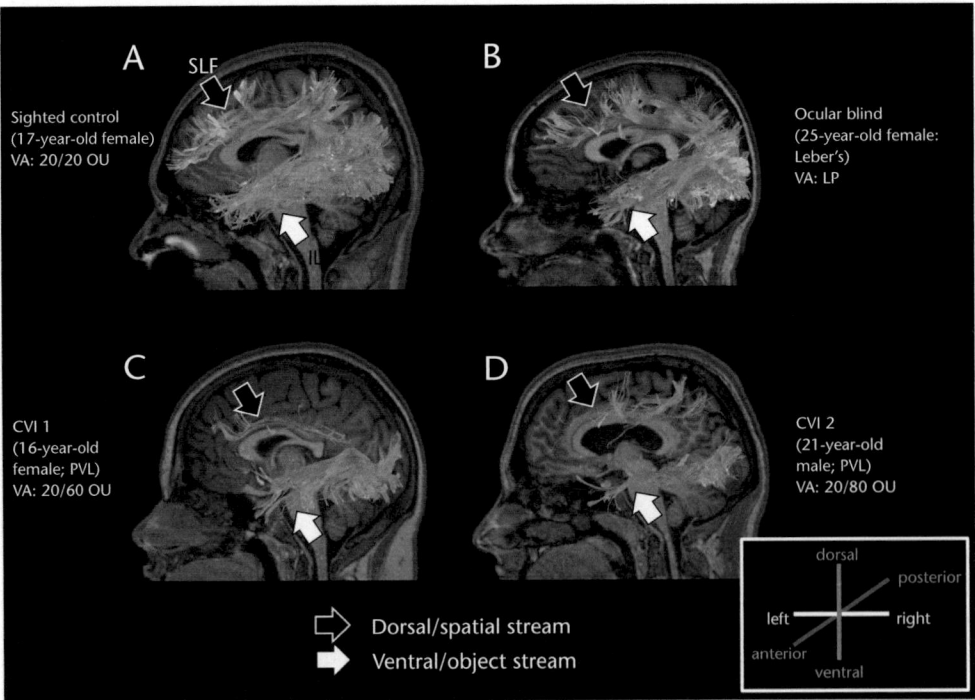

Figure 5.2 Reconstruction of the white matter pathways of the dorsal stream and the ventral stream.

Source: Adapted from Martín et al. (2016).

Figure 5.2 shows reconstructions of the white matter pathways of the dorsal stream, called the superior longitudinal fasciculus (SLF, black arrow) and the ventral stream, called the inferior longitudinal fasciculus (ILF, white arrow), in (A) a sighted control, (B) OVI and (C and D) CVI participants. Both pathways show robust connections in the individual with OVI, despite his only ever having had no more vision than light perception. Both individuals with CVI (C and D), however, demonstrate reduced white matter connections of the dorsal stream (black arrow), but only the individual with inability to recognise faces (or prosopagnosia) and other characteristic ventral stream impairments, shows a reduction in size of the ILF. This is not surprising given the high prevalence of dorsal stream dysfunction among individuals with CVI, while ventral stream impairments tend to be less common (Dutton, 2009).

Ten ways in which children can be visually affected by CVI

Any element of the way the brain processes visual information can be affected in almost any combination and degree. For every child with CVI, all of the following issues must be probed. This can be done by first taking a structured history from parents or carers (Zihl and Dutton, 2014) and by measuring functional vision (Hyvärinen et al., 2012). This also needs to become the role of visual impairment assessment teams including teachers, who need to observe the child's performances with salient tests, recognising that diagnostic vision testing by the medical profession is not functional.

It is only through taking a history and assessing visual performance in day-to-day life oneself that one can truly understand what the child is seeing and ensure that all materials and methods being used to teach the child are accessible. In education this entails diagnostic teaching (Lueck and Dutton, 2015). A move towards this policy is essential if children with CVI are not to be disadvantaged by inaccessible teaching materials and methods (Martín et al., 2016).

The limitations that need to be sought, documented and worked within for every child with CVI include the following:

1   Impaired central visual functions of acuity, contrast perception and colour perception.
2   Visual field impairment, and/or impaired visual attention to one side or down below.
3   Impaired perception of movement.
4   Difficulty handling the complexity of a visual scene, manifesting as inability to find an object among other objects or against a patterned background or to find a person in a group (dorsal stream dysfunction).
5   Impairment of visually guided movement of the body (dorsal stream dysfunction) and further evidence of associated lower visual field impairment.
6   Impaired visual attention due to underlying dorsal stream dysfunction.
7   Behavioural difficulties or distress associated with crowded environments or people approaching unexpectedly (because they pop out from a non-sighted area of the visual field, or because of impaired visual parallel processing and mapping of the scene).
8   Impaired ability to recognise what is being looked at and to navigate by means of visual recognition (ventral stream dysfunction).
9   Illusions such as persisting vision (called palinopsia in which the image of what was last seen persists and is superimposed upon the image of the next visual scene). This can only be subjectively described by those affected.
10 Hallucinations. These can be formed or unformed and can in some children relate to visual brain seizure activity. Again, hallucinations can only be subjectively described by those who are affected.

A "thinking in threes" approach to the subject of CVI

While disorders of the eyes and optic nerves disrupt visual input into an intact brain, disorders of data processing by the brain affecting mental image creation, are more complex, because any of the brain's myriad functional interconnections can be impacted. The subject of CVI is big and can appear overwhelming, so it helps if it can be broken down into bite-sized chunks to create a memorable mental checklist (Gawande, 2011). Thinking in threes provides a useful way of doing this (Backman, 2005).

Three overlapping categories of affected children are described (Lueck and Dutton, 2015), these comprise the following:

1   *Children with profound visual impairment due to CVI*, who need alternative approaches to substitute for lack of vision. Some functional vision is commonly present.
2   *Children with CVI who have functionally useful vision and cognitive challenges*, who show widespread brain dysfunction affecting vision, intellect and often mobility.
3   *Children with CVI with functionally useful vision, who perform at or near the typical academic level for age*, who are the least affected. They may show minor impairment of intellectual function and mobility. Disorders of visual perception and/or visual guidance of limb and body movement may be present, often with typical or slightly reduced primary visual functions. (*Infants with CVI whose low vision has an unknowable destiny* comprise an important supplementary group).

The brain and vision

Considering the whole brain, simplistically it has three principal parts:

1   The front, which thinks, plans and behaves.
2   The middle, which feels and moves the body and processes language.
3   The visual brain at the back, which sees.

When all three are affected, multiple disabilities result, with vision often being profoundly affected. When the middle and back are affected, cerebral palsy is frequently accompanied by CVI, often with typical intellect, and when only the back is affected, CVI alone is likely to be present. CVI can occur in a wide variety of ways in any of these three common scenarios.

Within the visual brain, there are also three principal elements:

1   The combined "occipital and middle-temporal lobes", which receive and process visual information about these key elements:

   (a) The whole visual field.
   (b) Central vision with respect to (i) clarity (acuity), (ii) contrast/light brightness and (iii) colour.
   (c) Movement of the imagery (processed by the middle temporal lobes).

2   The temporal lobes provide the image library against which the processed information from the occipital lobes is compared to bring about learning and recognition of the appearance of:

   (a) People.
   (b) Shapes and objects.
   (c) Routes and locations (i) out and about, (ii) within buildings and (iii) within storage spaces.

3   The posterior parietal lobes parallel process and map the 3D scene:

(a)   To guide movement of the hands, feet, limbs and body in any environment.
(b)   To appraise the whole scene, enabling visual search.
(c)   To provide the material for the frontal lobes to choose to give visual attention to.

The three principal cross-referenced senses that are integrated into what we "know" to be our singular overall mode of perception at any one time are (1) vision, (2) hearing and (3) touch. Hearing and touch can likewise be impaired in children with CVI and should also be considered.

The three additional mainly non-conscious senses related to vision comprise (1) our knowledge of position in space or proprioception, (2) our balance and (3) our mental timing centres that deal with the speed and passage of events. These too can be impaired.

Impaired vision interferes with three key needs, each with three elements, comprising:

1   Access to information, whether (i) distant, (ii) at intermediate distance such as in a room or (iii) nearby.
2   Mobility through 3D space, of (i) our upper limbs, (ii) our lower limbs and (iii) our bodies.
3   Social interaction that needs (i) visual search to find friends, (ii) visual recognition of people and (iii) recognition and understanding of the language of facial expression and gesture.

Each of these "threes" outlined above is important to examine in children with CVI.

By routinely applying this prior knowledge to in-depth history taking and assessment, to actively seek out difficulties the child may have, a comprehensive profile of the child's functional capacities and their limits emerges. This in turn guides habilitation and education by ensuring that those parenting and working with the affected child can capitalise upon their new-found in-depth understanding of their child's abilities and behaviours, aiming to make everything being used to teach the child entirely accessible, and knowing the origin of behavioural difficulties and how to deal with them.

Applying this knowledge to habilitation/rehabilitation comprises three approaches:

1   Compensation for the lack of function, for example enlargement of print for low visual acuity, or increased spacing of print for impaired visual parallel processing.
2   Alternative approaches, for example listening to the spoken word instead of reading.
3   Training the child in all salient strategies within the child's capabilities.

The above method of thinking is of course not comprehensive, but it provides a useful and effective mental tool to guide assessment and to plan how to help children with CVI. The identification of specific issues using these tools can lead to further salient approaches. This rationale needs to be integrated with an overall evaluation seeking to determine:

1   The child's prior knowledge, strengths and abilities.
2   Other disabilities and their impact, including the child's mental capacity.
3   The child's mental status considering whether the child affected is (i) fearful, (ii) anxious or (iii) depressed for any reason, and determining what assessments and interventions may need to be taken if any of these three states of mind are evident (Dutton and Bax, 2010).

Once one has addressed these issues, a set of three profiles often emerge:

1. The profile of anxieties and fears

Fear and anxiety may negatively impact a child's ability to learn (National Scientific Council on the Developing Child, 2010). CVI can be a cause of fear or anxiety for a range of reasons. For example, low vision can cause accident and injury. Impaired mapping of the visual scene can cause imagery to be mislocated, and so moving imagery has been described as appearing to loom into view. Visual field deficits can have the same effect. Impaired recognition of people and mislocation of sound (commonly described by the parents of children with CVI, but yet to be researched) can cause anxiety in social situations. Imagine a kiss on your right cheek, if you have inability to see to your right due to right hemianopia, and you cannot detect the approaching face (see Chapter 6). Emerging recognition by the child with CVI that they lack skills that others have, can lead to social isolation owing to appearing different to others, while bullying can lead to discomfiture, lack of confidence and anxiety. All reasons for anxiety need to be sought, identified if present and addressed in order to foster a mental and emotional profile conducive for learning.

2. The profile of abilities

Abilities are the child's strengths and can serve as gateways to learning. Thus, if we first and foremost identify what the child can do and enjoys doing, then these activities can act as the building blocks to develop further strengths and skills. In essence, this approach provides the guide to how to parent and teach the child using wholly accessible, interesting and meaningful child-centred and child-focused motivational activities and experiences. Happy and motivated children learn well when pathways to attainment are identified, developed and applied.

Thinking in threes once more, one can consider abilities under the categories of *emotional and social skills* (Goleman, 1996), *intellectual skills* and *practical and motor skills and abilities*.

1   *Emotional and social skills* include (i) the ability to master communication and language, (ii) the facility to develop theory of mind or the capacity to understand the feelings of others and (iii) the ability to master and control emotion.
2   *Intellectual skills* underpin the ability to (i) learn, to (ii) imagine and to (iii) plan.
3   *Practical, sporting and musical skills* include (i) mobility in all its guises, (ii) hand–eye coordination and dexterity and (iii) the higher-order skills to imagine, plan and carry out meaningful sets of actions.

Music is an important element to consider, where (i) listening, (ii) creating and (iii) performing can all be inspiring and motivational, and in our experience has the capacity to kick-start development of other skills.

3. The profile of visual and perceptual limitations

Each and every visual function outlined above needs to be evaluated functionally in terms of what needs to be done, to ensure that all materials and approaches to play and learning are made accessible for each child with CVI. This information is configured and presented in terms of the adaptations and alternative approaches needed to give the child access to all salient elements of their world. For example, felt-tip pens with a line width known to make all lines visible, are used to render eyes and facial features in storybooks visible.

Aspects of cerebral auditory impairment that can compound the difficulties of CVI

Children with CVI may have additional hearing disabilities that need to be actively sought out. Not only can there be impairment of hearing due to ear disorders, but mental processing of sound can also be affected.

The cerebral auditory impairments that we have encountered are analogous to the visual disabilities. Dorsal stream dysfunctions can lead to difficulty extracting the sound of voices in noisy places and inability to know where sounds are coming from, while ventral stream difficulties can relate to impaired voice recognition (Rauschecker, 2011), but this is less common in our experience.

Empowering affected children, their parents and carers by skilled teaching about the specific effects of CVI and how to deal with them

In an ideal scenario, (i) medical diagnosis, (ii) characterisation of functional skills and limitations and (iii) training of the child (when apposite) by parents and those supporting the child need to be seamless. This requires well-organised teamwork with good communication. In our experience the medical approach needs to be relinquished soon after diagnosis (except for the ongoing care of associated conditions such as seizure disorders), in the context of a well-informed, loving, positive, supportive model of care matched to the child's needs. This approach intuitively guides optimal management and habilitation by (i) parents, (ii) teachers and (iii) mobility specialists, in decluttered home and school environments. (At home, school and out and about, plain bedsheets that can hide any muddle, or a pop-up tent for the child to go inside, can instantly create a calm working space for those with impaired visual parallel processing.)

Thumbnail sketches of a range of CVI case studies

A coloured tent helps vision emerge and be retained by eliminating clutter

Ali, aged 9, has profound quadriplegic cerebral palsy. She had light perception only, even in a multisensory room. Crowds or noise caused distress.

Surrounded by an orange tent to eliminate clutter and mute ambient sound, her response was immediate. For the first time in her life she gazed around smiling. A few subsequent months of short daily periods in the tent, enabled Ali to change from shouting, to making gentle sounds with turn-taking and looking around, giving attention even when outside the tent. This suggests that Ali has impaired visual and auditory parallel processing and that the quiet, and elimination of clutter throughout her visual field, was the catalyst for the new development of her improved quality of life (Little and Dutton, 2015).

Eliminating clutter helped an infant to reach out and explore for the first time

Ben was 11 months old. He had sustained brain injury due to lack of blood supply during birth. This affected both posterior parietal lobes. Despite intact motor function, he had never reached out to grasp anything.

His cot was lined with a white sheet and all clutter was removed, bar one toy at the far end. Within 20 minutes he had moved toward the toy and picked it up (Zihl and Dutton, 2014). Following able parenting, he is now doing well at mainstream school, confounding his initial prognosis. His persisting lower visual field impairment corroborates the site of his neonatal brain injury: his posterior parietal lobes.

Impaired visual search and poor visual guidance in a 10-year-old boy

A 10-year-old boy had had a heart infection when aged 3 (Gillen and Dutton, 2003). This caused indirect damage from bleeding into both posterior parietal lobes. He recovered well, but at age 10 could not read long words, follow text, write words in a line or copy, as print matched to his age had, for him, become too small and crowded. He was losing confidence. He often walked into people as if they were not there, or did not see moving objects like cars and impaired visual scanning was evident. Going down stairs and stepping off kerbs were difficult. Yet his optics, visual acuities, 3D and colour vision were normal. His visual fields could not be plotted because he could not simultaneously see the central and peripheral targets. He could not look at specified targets, but his eye movements to instructions like "look up", were normal. He took a long time to find an item of clothing in a pile or on a patterned bed spread, or a pencil on a cluttered desk. His behaviours, symptoms, signs and brain imaging were consistent with the diagnosis of a variant of Balint syndrome, comprising inability to see more than one or two items at once at any moment, inaccurate visual guidance of reach and inability to move his eyes to a nominated target. Apparent impairment of his lower visual field, and inability to see fast-moving targets are typical accompaniments.

An approach using his strengths and abilities was encouraged. He learned to scan the ground ahead. His environment was de-cluttered. Well-spaced text and masking of the text above what he was reading (rather than below, which interferes with accessing the next line) was adopted. Auditory and verbal strategies of listening and dictating to a scribe were implemented. He learned to employ his visual scanning, hearing, touch and proprioception to locate and reach for objects to better effect, gaining greater independence and self-esteem. His prior behavioural outbursts due to frustration also became infrequent.

"Baby talk" language training leads to understanding in a 7-year-old child with CVI

Ben aged 7 had profound CVI and no understanding of language. He bit, pinched, scratched and hair pulled, with terrified outbursts of screaming. His congenital brain disorder gave him a visual acuity of 6/200 (by preferential looking). He would focus on a single item, walk toward it with arms extended, grasping it on collision with it. This item was shortly relinquished in favour of another one discovered at random. He had bilateral occipito–parietal brain changes, and no evidence of vision in his lower visual field. The combination of these features fitted well with the hypothesis that he had profoundly impaired visual parallel processing with profound impairment of visual guidance of movement (Balint syndrome) (Dutton, 2018).

Progressively decluttering his world, using a tent for him to retire to regularly, while lovingly employing consistent, repeated, single, salient, prolonged word utterances, matched contemporaneously to each singular experience, as described by Sally Ward in her book *Baby Talk* (Ward, 2004) has led to progressive receptive and expressive language development, and has ameliorated his frustration and fear. He is now a happy boy and his behavioural outbursts have all but abated.

Baby talk puts simple words to the infant's experience. The same approach is of course needed for simultanagnosia because words applied to what the child is not focusing on have no meaning, and so cannot be learned from.

The girl whose upward, but not downward, reach and grasp are accurate

An 18-year-old girl who was born at 24 weeks gestation approached one of the authors at a meeting where they were both contributing. She asked why she was clumsy.

She was found for the first time to have no detectable visual function below 30 degrees from the horizontal. When asked to reach out for objects in her intact lower visual field she consistently did so inaccurately, with a wide gap between fingers and thumb as she did so. However, her reach in her upper visual field was accurate, with a normal in-flight gap between fingers and thumb as her hand reached out for the proffered objects. This is at the time of writing, a hitherto unpublished observation. She now stores many of her key possessions above eye level, where they are much easier to find and reach for.

Blindsight in a child, and how it can be used to train reading by "imagined pantomiming"

A 5-year-old girl needed brain surgery to stop bleeding inside her head after she fell out of a window. Despite this, the blood vessels to her occipital lobes became blocked by being kinked, and she lost her vision. Vision recovered sufficiently to allow her to move around, but she was unable to recognise anything. However, it was found that she could recognise shapes by moving her finger along the lines she felt unable to see (Lueck and Dutton, 2015). She was later taught to do this by imagining she was moving her finger around the images of shapes (Goodale and Milner, 2013), and through this method she has even learned to read large print, as well as learning to read braille.

Persisting perception of movement in those with loss of the occipital lobes is called the Riddoch phenomenon (Riddoch, 1917), and can accurately guide movement despite lack of measurable sight. This case shows that this phenomenon in a child can be capitalised upon to good effect. The following YouTube recording describes the same condition in an adult seen by one of the authors: www.youtube.com/watch?v=9ABQ-U6V0tY.

Is sound localisation difficult for children with CVI, as well as the visual issues?

John was a 10-year-old boy attending mainstream primary school. He had sustained superior posterior periventricular white matter injury related to premature birth and had lower visual field impairment. He showed difficulty finding items in his bedroom or his mother in a group and could not work out where someone was calling from. He rarely if ever looked at the face of anyone talking to him. He explained he could not locate the origin of sounds and could not listen while looking at a face. He was given a mobile phone to find family members who phone him rather than calling out. He has learned how to glance, then turn and smile at his mother's face once she has finished speaking. This has helped build their relationship.

For soccer he chooses to play in goal. When asked what a ball looks like when kicked, he answered, "It disappears for about a metre of course, then comes back when it slows down". On assessment he could not count fingers on a quickly moving hand, differentiating them only when the hand moved slowly.

Once his visual difficulties had been recognised, understood and explained, John became much happier, and able to adapt to his own normality. Foremost for John, he was no longer criticised for bad performance, but instead praised for doing so well in the light of the new knowledge.

Additional visual difficulties described by those affected and by parents

CVI is a developing subject. The development of an evidence base for all new topics starts with observation and hypothesis. Each of the following scenarios has been commonly witnessed by, and described to the authors, but are not well recognised.

Could light gazing be a sign of simultanagnosia vision?

Children who gaze at lights need to have their attention broken to look at something else. Those who are older and able to communicate say they are unable to look away from lights, and this is uncomfortable. The majority of such children appear to only be able to focus on one item at a time. This suggests that they may have simultanagnostic vision. In young affected children without language, the baby talk strategy outlined above (Ward, 2004) can be rewarded by language developing for the first time.

Is flinching in response to a distant movement due to impaired 3D and temporal mapping of space?

Children with CVI who flinch in response to a non-threatening movement, often have inaccurate guidance of their movements, or optic ataxia. Does this mean that impaired mapping of external space leads to inability to locate the position of such movements, which are thus seen as threatening or even frightening?

Can cerebral visual impairment be masked?

It has been argued that around 40% of the brain serves vision. It is therefore highly likely that children with cerebral palsy or major developmental dysfunctions, may have additional hidden visual difficulties, because affected children cannot describe them, or because the evident motor impairments have taken precedence. The default condition for all such children needs to be that they may have CVI, until proved otherwise, rather than the other way round.

Can CVI present with features of an alternative diagnosis?

Features of CVI can be seen in children with developmental coordination disorder (DCD) (Chokron and Dutton, 2016), autistic spectrum disorder (ASD) and attention deficit hyperactivity disorder (ADHD) (Lueck and Dutton, 2015), and ideally needs to be sought out and identified in all affected children, because their management can be altered to good effect when the origin and profile of the behavioural features of these conditions has been identified.

Conclusion

We need to appreciate how the child with CVI is experiencing the world, not just seeing it. Only then can we start to recognise and empathise with their experiences and how they feel.

Only then can we appreciate their limitations and strengths, and ensure they are comfortable and happy, avoiding or preventing scenarios that cause anxiety and fear. This philosophical approach consistently helps the child with CVI to learn, because salient information can then be made to fall within the child's capacity to access and understand it, at his or her level of development. With full knowledge of what the child already knows, the provision of intuitively micro-stepped, progressive, fully accessible, small, repeated, consistent, meaningful and motivational enhancements immediately following each successive experience (both planned and unplanned) progressively leads from the known into the just knowable unknown, resulting in exciting ongoing progressive developmental strides in children with CVI, if not all children.

The unique functional profile of every child with CVI necessitates an approach that identifies and capitalises upon the child's skills and abilities, while ensuring that they are each taught with entirely accessible methods that motivate and excite them. It is now well known that one cannot make a child learn, they have to do it themselves, but they can only do so when the world is accessible, meaningful and interesting. Learning is then exciting and motivational.

The key to bringing out the very best in children with CVI is to learn and to master the requisite skill set. The best outcomes we have seen have come when parents have been well taught about their child, have taken up the challenge and have been the prime movers.

Parental in-depth education and empowerment are axiomatic to a successful outcome (CVI Scotland, 2017).

We must never use our own perceptions, to guide our educational approach to children with CVI, we must always use theirs.

References

Arcaro, M.J., Thaler, L., Quinlan, D.J., Monaco, S., Khan, S., Valyear, K.F., Goebel, R., Dutton, G.N., Goodale, M.A., Kastner, S. and Culham, J.C. 2018. Psychophysical and neuroimaging responses to moving stimuli in a patient with the Riddoch phenomenon due to bilateral visual cortex lesions. *Neuropsychologia*, S0028–3932(18), 30204–30205.

Atkinson, J. 2017. The Davida Teller Award lecture, 2016: Visual brain development: A review of "dorsal stream vulnerability" motion, mathematics, amblyopia, actions, and attention. *Journal of Vision*, 17(3), 26.

Backman, B. 2005. *Thinking in threes: The power of three in writing.* Fort Collins, CO: Cottonwood Press.

Chokron, S. and Dutton, G.N. 2016. Impact of cerebral visual impairments on motor skills: Implications for developmental coordination disorders. *Frontiers of Psychology*, 7, 1471.

CVI Scotland. 2017. *CVI Scotland* [e-resource]. Accessed June 2018. https://cviscotland.org.

Das, M., Spowart, K., Crossley, S. and Dutton, G.N. 2010. Evidence that children with special needs all require visual assessment. *Archives of Disease in Childhood*, 95(11), 888–892.

Donaldson, I.M. 2000. The functions of the proprioceptors of the eye muscles. *Philosophical Transactions of the Royal Society of London B Biological Sciences*, 355(1404), 1685–1754.

Dutton, G.N. 2009. "Dorsal stream dysfunction" and "dorsal stream dysfunction plus": A potential classification for perceptual visual impairment in the context of cerebral visual impairment? *Developmental Medicine and Child Neurology*, 51(3), 170–172.

Dutton, G.N. 2013. The spectrum of cerebral visual impairment as a sequel to premature birth: An overview. *Documenta Ophthalmologica*, 127(1), 69–78.

Dutton, G.N. 2018. Parallel processing [blog]. CVI Scotland. Accessed 21 December 2018. https://cviscotland.org/news/gordon-duttons-blog-18-12-01-2018.

Dutton, G.N. and Bax, M. 2010. *Visual impairment in children due to damage to the brain: Clinics in developmental medicine No 186.* London: MacKeith Press.

Gawande, A. 2011. *The checklist manifesto: How to get things right.* London: Profile Books.

Gillen, J.A. and Dutton, G.N. 2003. Balint's syndrome in a 10-year-old male. *Developmental Medicine and Child Neurology*, 45(5), 349–352.

Goleman, D. 1996. *Emotional intelligence: Why it can matter more than IQ.* London: Bloomsbury.

Goodale, M.A. and Milner, D.A. (2013). *Sight unseen* (2nd ed.). Oxford: Oxford University Press.

Groenveld, M., Jan, J.E. and Leader, P. 1990. Observations on the habilitation of children with cortical visual impairment. *Journal of Visual Impairment and Blindness*, 84, 11–15.

Hyvärinen, L., Walthes, R., Freitag, C. and Petz, V. 2012. Profile of visual functioning as a bridge between education and medicine in the assessment of impaired vision. *Strabismus*, 20(2), 63–68.

Jacobson, L.K. and Dutton, G.N. 2000. Periventricular leukomalacia: An important cause of visual and ocular motility dysfunction in children. *Survey of Ophthalmology*, 45(1), 1–13.

Jacobson, L.K, Ygge, J. and Flodmark, O. 1998. Nystagmus in periventricular leucomalacia. *British Journal of Ophthalmology*, 82(9), 1026–1032.

Jacobson, L.K, Ygge, J., Flodmark, O. and Ek, U. 2002. Visual and perceptual characteristics, ocular motility and strabismus in children with periventricular leukomalacia. *Strabismus*, 10(2), 179–183.

Kish, D. and Hook, J. 2017. *Echolocation and flash sonar*. Louisville, KY: APH.

Kong, L., Fry, M., Al-Samarraie, M., Gilbert, C. and Steinkuller, P.G. 2012. An update on progress and the changing epidemiology of causes of childhood blindness worldwide. *Journal of the American Association of Pediatric Ophthalmology and Strabismus*, 16(6), 501–507.

Lennartsson, F., Nilsson, M., Flodmark, O. and Jacobson, L. 2017. Damage to the immature optic radiation causes severe reduction of the retinal nerve fiber layer, resulting in predictable visual field defects. *Investigative Ophthalmology and Visual Science*, 55(12), 8278–8288.

Leong, V., Byrne, E., Clackson, K., Georgieva, S., Lam, S. and Wass, S. 2017. Speaker gaze increases information coupling between infant and adult brains. *Proceedings of the National Academy of Sciences of the United States of America*, 114(50), 13290–13295.

Little, S. and Dutton, G.N. 2015. Some children with multiple disabilities and cerebral visual impairment can engage when enclosed by a "tent": Is this due to Balint syndrome? *British Journal of Visual Impairment*, 33(1), 66–73.

Liu, L., Wang, F., Zhou, K., Ding, N. and Luo, H. 2017. Perceptual integration rapidly activates dorsal visual pathway to guide local processing in early visual areas. *PLoS Biology*, 15(11), e2003646.

Lueck, A. and Dutton, G.N. 2015. *Impairment of vision due to disorders of the visual brain in childhood: A practical approach*. New York: AFB Press.

Martín, M.B., Santos-Lozano, A., Martín-Hernández, J., López-Miguel, A., Maldonado, M., Baladrón, C., Bauer, C.M. and Merabet, L.B. 2016. Cerebral versus ocular visual impairment: The impact on developmental neuroplasticity. *Frontiers of Psychology*, 7(7), 1958.

Milner, D.A. and Goodale, M.A. 2006. *The visual brain in action* (2nd ed.). Oxford: Oxford University Press.

National Scientific Council on the Developing Child. 2010. *Persistent fear and anxiety can affect young children's learning and development*. Working Paper No. 9 [e-publication]. Accessed February 2018. www.developingchild.net.

Philip, S.S. and Dutton, G.N. (2014). Identifying and characterising cerebral visual impairment in children: A review. *Clinical and Experimental Optometry*, 97, 196–208.

Philip, S.S., Tsherlinga, S., Thomas, M.M., Dutton, G.N. and Bowman, R. 2016. A validation of an examination protocol for cerebral visual impairment among children in a clinical population in India. *Journal of Clinical Diagnostic Research*, 10(12), NC01–NC04.

Pinel, J.P.J. and Barnes, S.J. 2014. *Introduction to biopsychology* (9th ed.). London: Pearson Education.

Rauschecker, J.P. 2011. An expanded role for the dorsal auditory pathway in sensorimotor control and integration. *Hearing Research*, 271(1–2), 16–25.

Riddoch, G. 1917. On the relative perceptions of movement and a stationary object in certain visual disturbances due to occipital injuries. *Proceedings of the Royal Society of Medicine*, 10(Neurological Section), 13–34.

Sakki, H.E.A., Dale, N.J., Sargent, J., Perez-Roche, T. and Bowman, R. 2018. Is there consensus in defining childhood cerebral visual impairment? A systematic review of terminology and definitions. *British Journal of Ophthalmology*, 102(4), 424–432.

Saunders, K.J., Little, J.A., McClelland, J.F. and Jackson, A.J. 2010. Profile of refractive errors in cerebral palsy: Impact of severity of motor impairment (GMFCS) and CP subtype on refractive outcome. *Investigative Ophthalmology and Visual Science*, 51(6), 2885–2890.

Shirley, K., Chamney, S., Satkurunathan, P., McLoone, S. and McLoone, E. 2017. Medscape: Impact of healthcare strategies on patterns of paediatric sight impairment in a developed population 1984–2011. *Eye (London)*, 31(11), 1537–1545.

Simonsen, B., Fairbanks, S., Briesch, A., Myers, D. and Sugai, G. 2008. Evidence-based practice in classroom management: Considerations for research to practice. *Education and Treatment of Children*, 31(3), 351–380.

Thaler, L., Arnott, S.R. and Goodale, M.A. 2011. Neural correlates of natural human echolocation in early and late blind echolocation experts. *PLoS One*, 6(5), e20162.

Thaler, L. and Goodale, M.A. 2016. Echolocation in humans: An overview. *Wiley Interdisciplinary Review of Cognitive Science*, 7(6), 382–393.

Thaler, L., Paciocco, J., Daley, M., Lesniak, G.D., Purcell, D.W. Fraser, J.A., Dutton, G.N., Rossit, S., Goodale, M.A. and Culham, J.C. 2016. A selective impairment of perception of sound motion direction in peripheral space: A case study. *Neuropsychologia*, 80, 79–89.

Voogd, J., Schraa-Tam, C.K., van der Geest, J.N. and De Zeeuw, C.I. 2012. Visuomotor cerebellum in human and nonhuman primates. *Cerebellum*, 11(2), 392–410.

Ward, S. 2004. *Baby talk*. London: Random House.

Weir, C.R., Knox, P.C. and Dutton, G.N. 2000. Does extraocular muscle proprioception influence oculomotor control? *British Journal of Ophthalmology*, 84(9), 1071–1074.

Zeki, S.M., Hollman, A.S. and Dutton, G.N. 1992. Neuroradiological features of patients with optic nerve hypoplasia. *Journal of Pediatric Ophthalmology and Strabismus*, 29(2), 107–112.

Zihl, J. and Dutton, G.N. 2014. *Cerebral visual impairment in children*. New York: Springer Verlag.

Zihl, J. and Heywood, C.A. 2015. The contribution of LM to the neuroscience of movement vision. *Frontiers in Integrative Neuroscience*, 9, 6.

6

A personal perspective on CVI

Nicola McDowell

Introduction

Imagine living in a world of visual uncertainty. A world that at times seems to shimmer and shake and there is nothing you can do to make the image you are seeing stay still. A world where you can suddenly be surrounded by unknown faces, even when you are in a room full of your family and friends. A world where personal possessions, such as clothing, books and jewellery can suddenly disappear into a black hole, seemingly never to be found again, no matter how hard you try to find them. A world that in the blink of an eye, can become so frightening and overwhelming you feel as if your life is in danger and the resulting panic you feel makes it hard for you to breathe. A world that at times makes you start to doubt your own sanity and ability to mix with your peers. Now imagine that this world of visual uncertainty is actually a common, yet often undiagnosed, invisible disability. A disability that is not only invisible to everyone around you, but also invisible to you. Now imagine living with this disability and in this world for years, without realising that your brain is actually not correctly interpreting the image your eyes are seeing. I don't have to imagine what this world would be like, I live with this uncertainty every day.

A CVI journey

I have a disability called cerebral visual impairment (CVI) (see Chapter 5) and although it is now the most common cause of vision impairment affecting children (who grow up to be affected adults) in the developed world (Fazzi et al., 2007), it is a very poorly understood impairment, which is an issue I can relate to. I have lived with CVI for over 20 years now, as a result of a brain injury when I was a teenager. However, for 17 of those years, I was completely unaware I even had this condition! Although it seems hard to imagine now, for most of these years, I did not even realise that the many challenges I faced in everyday life, such as having difficulty mixing in a large group of people, struggling to get through a family meal without knocking over a glass and not being able to navigate my way around an unfamiliar environment, actually had anything to do with my vision at all.

As a result of my impairment not being identified, I adopted certain adaptive behaviours that were often misinterpreted as anti-social, controlling and being obsessed about routines and organisation. Thinking about it now, it is very easy to understand why these kinds of behaviours developed. The main CVI issues I am affected by, including simultanagnosia (an inability to see more than one object at a time), optic ataxia (difficulties with visually guided movement) and apraxia of gaze (difficulty with directing one's gaze to different visual objects) (Dutton, 2015; Goodale, 2013; Pawletko, Chokron and Dutton, 2015), caused me to start to doubt my ability to participate in society. Over time, I simply lost all confidence in doing activities that most people take for granted and as an adult I struggled with tasks such as doing the weekly grocery shop for my family, getting money out of an unfamiliar cash machine or taking my children to the playground by myself.

I therefore see myself as fortunate to have finally received the correct diagnosis of CVI. This happened as a result of a chance meeting with an expert on the subject, at a conference for professionals working in the field of educating children with visual impairments. For someone who understands this condition, my visual behaviours were easy to recognise and attribute to CVI. For me, finally getting a reason for my difficulties, was life-changing, as it explained why I find the world so different to those around me. Getting the right diagnosis, therefore, helped me to understand myself again, which allowed me to start developing strategies to help alleviate the effects of my visual difficulties. This in turn, resulted in me slowly rebuilding my confidence in my ability to participate in society again. However, as I have learnt the hard way, simply getting a diagnosis of CVI does not make it obvious to the general public or even to the people close to you, including family and friends, what your specific needs are.

The reason for this is that I am an independent, professional adult and CVI is my only impairment, so I do not look any different to the next person. I can walk down the street and blend in with the crowd, as I do not use a mobility cane (out of pure stubbornness and possible denial of the potential benefits), or have a guide dog, which are often seen as the symbols of blindness and low vision. This means, that to the outside world, I look just the same as everyone else going about their daily business and therefore everyone just assumes that I do not require any assistance – which is exactly how I want it to be, most of the time.

Unfortunately, however, this also means that people do not see the intense emotional struggle that occurs every time I walk in a busy, crowded environment. People do not see the constant battle of trying to fight the vision issues, which cause strangers to loom unexpectedly at me from all angles, which at times can be very frightening. People do not see my confusion, knowing that often things are not where my eyes seem to tell me they are, and I know I will embarrass myself by either grasping at thin air or knocking things over. People do not see the constant game of roulette that I face, while trying not to barge into unsuspecting pedestrians because I have misjudged their movement and inaccurately mapped the environment around me. People do not understand the unconscious emotional reactions I have developed from past negative experiences that cause me to feel anxious without really understanding why. These emotions exacerbate the exhausting impact of being constantly on the alert, with my brain's primitive fight or flight response ready to trigger at any moment and cause me to completely panic. People do not see that at the same time as all of this, I am trying to achieve the almost impossible task of attempting to look normal and totally in control. If the people around me were aware that I was constantly battling this internal turmoil, they would realise that at times I am not actually a capable adult at all, and I would be exposed as a fraud; an exposure that I am constantly fighting against.

However, there is a problem with keeping this inner turmoil hidden. When my CVI causes me to do something that seems unacceptable to the general public, such as knocking over a small child, whose unpredictable movement is impossible for me to follow, or stepping out in front of a car or a bike on the road that I just did not see, I do not get the special considerations someone with a disability might receive. Instead, when these kinds of encounters have occurred, I have been yelled at and abused for being careless, self-absorbed and not watching where I am going. Most people can brush off an experience like this as simply a moment of inattention and an accident, but not me. I have experienced humiliating encounters such as this on so many occasions in the last 20 years that it has slowly eroded my confidence in being in society, and on many occasions has resulted in my doubting my ability to even leave the safety of my own home.

At other times, forcing myself to cope in challenging environments has led to a state of being in which I am so incapacitated by the overwhelming amount of sensory information swamping my already reduced cognitive processing abilities, that I am unable to function in any normal way. This state has been referred to as a "CVI meltdown" (CVI Scotland, 2017a). When I am subject to a CVI meltdown, I am functionally blind and cannot move independently, I also lose all of my cognitive abilities and cannot even string a sentence together or understand what people are saying to me. Being in this state is incredibly emotionally overwhelming and I often panic that I am not going to be able to save myself from the situation. A good example of experiencing a CVI meltdown in a public arena was the time I decided that I would try and walk up the main shopping area of Melbourne by myself, while visiting the city for a conference. After having spent three days in this unfamiliar environment, I was already physically and emotionally exhausted from the extra exertion it took just to map my new surroundings. Therefore, this seemingly simple feat of walking up town by myself may have already been outside my capabilities at the time and it was probably extremely foolish of me to even try. However, I was urged on by a strong sense of determination and just a small touch of stubbornness to carry on with this activity, which I had been planning for a couple of days. As the storm clouds of a CVI meltdown started to gather, I became increasingly more terrified that I would get lost and be unable to find my way back to anywhere that was remotely familiar. Although I am quite capable of looking after myself when in a cognitively conscious and functioning state, and know what to do if I feel that I need help, this all changes when I am completely overwhelmed by my visual disabilities. When experiencing a CVI meltdown, I am powerless and unable to implement any strategies that will help me to get through this. In most situations, I also do not really know what I perceive to be the terrifying monster I am facing and fighting to get away from. I cannot articulate the terror I am feeling in any way and I understand, that to anyone else, it just seems incomprehensible that I could be so frightened by the world around me. During my walk in Melbourne, the full impact of my CVI meltdown saw me cowering in a corner between a shopfront and a building column, trying desperately to find enough oxygen in the air to stop myself from passing out.

The very nature of my CVI means that I am constantly walking a tightrope between the able-bodied and disabled worlds. A tightrope that I often have no control over when I am going to fall. At times, however, the disparity of living between these two worlds – going from being totally independent and fully capable one moment, to being completely overwhelmed by my visual issues and requiring assistance the next – is soul destroying. Each morning I wake up wondering how much my visual impairment is going to impact on me over the course of the day. Depending on the environment I am in and my emotional state at any given time, I can move from being almost fully sighted and fully functional, to having low vision and needing some assistance to move around, to being functionally blind and struggling to make decisions for myself, all in a matter of minutes. I constantly have to weigh up the relative benefits of declaring my disability in different situations and trying to explain to the people around me how I am affected (which is no easy task, as CVI doesn't just have a simple explanation one can spout out to people and expect them to understand straight away), or keeping my situation to myself and maintaining the fierce independence my personality mostly demands of me.

But as I have learnt the hard way, desperately holding on to a level of independence out of pure stubbornness can actually do more harm than good, especially in this fast-paced, modern world we live in. Take, for example, a challenging situation I experienced when trying to fly domestically after a work trip away. As anyone who does this regularly can appreciate, the irritating announcement over the loud speaker that your flight has been cancelled and that you need to retrieve your luggage from the baggage-claim area and re-check in for alternative flights, is something we all dread. For most people, although frustrating, completing the required steps would be relatively straightforward. However, this may not be the case for someone who is in an unfamiliar airport and who went through the initial check-in with a colleague, so did not take any notice of where the desks were, but is now by themselves and most importantly, they have CVI. This is the situation I found myself in, and the debilitating effects of anxiety and panic kicked in before the announcement had even been completed. For me it was like the perfect storm. I was already tired from a mentally draining couple of days of intense new learning and now the thought of not getting home to my family that night was enough to send me into a downward spiral. I'm sure most people can understand the emotional upheaval of disrupted travel plans, but it's the impact of these emotional behaviours on one's already impaired visual functioning skills that is often the final nail in the coffin for someone with CVI. As I panicked, the world started to visually crumble around me. I was unable to read signs and I did not feel that I could move safely among the throngs of other travellers, as I couldn't work out whether the tiles on the ground in front of me were flat or actually steps. I also had difficulty hearing any further announcements and instructions over the loud speaker, and I could not establish where I was and where I needed to go. All I wanted to do was slump to the floor and cry. Imagine that! A grown woman, professionally dressed and clutching a laptop bag, collapsed on the floor sobbing! Although I had enough cognitive ability left to realise that this wasn't going to help, I did not have enough functioning to do much else. So, I did something that I find extremely difficult – I asked for help. However, again, my hidden disability fooled the general public and the airport assistant simply started spouting off directions for where I needed to be. Another CVI-related issue is that I am unable to mentally picture or map a verbal image or directions, so after his first "turn left at" I was more lost than ever. This nightmare threatened to continue unabated, as I stumbled around the airport, fighting the tears from rolling down my cheeks. Luckily, I was saved from this nightmare, when I was rung by an assistant from the airline to inform me of the cancelled flight (something I obviously already knew). To this hero on the phone, I simply said that I was visually impaired, that I was lost in the airport and that I did not know where to get my bag from. She straight away detected the emotion and panic in my voice, and simply told me to stay where I was and that she would send someone to find me and help. My faith in humankind's support of people with disabilities was completely reaffirmed that day, as a kind and compassionate airline assistant located me after I had given a couple of landmarks as to where I was, took care of getting my bag and checking me into an alternative flight home. She then personally guided me to the gate lounge where I could wait and recover in relative peace.

Having the flawed character trait (for someone in my situation) of always fighting to be independent, the thought of needing to be rescued was something that I thought I would struggle to deal with. However, this experience actually taught me an important life lesson. I have a disability that most of society is not even aware of, and consequently, does not really understand. It is therefore up to me to make my disability known and understood. Not only is it important for me to do so, it is also my responsibility as a disabled person, especially for everyone else that also lives with CVI. People in general are very willing to help those in need, which is something we see on a daily basis all over the world. However, to do so, people need to be given the opportunity to understand what one is dealing with. No one can possibly help if they do not understand what the world is like for someone with CVI.

With this enlightened awareness, I have been able to develop simple strategies to help make these situations somewhat easier to cope with. For instance, while in crowded and cluttered environments, I make sure I give myself regular breaks away from the noise and visual clutter, to give my brain a chance to unwind and reset, before it has to wind up again and interpret the chaos around me. This is an extremely important strategy and has saved me in situations similar to the Melbourne shopping expedition, and stopped the CVI storm clouds from rolling in on a number of occasions. Implementing this approach can be as easy as finding a quiet spot where I am away from crowds. If I cannot find somewhere to remove myself to, I simply shut my eyes and use mindfulness breathing techniques to block out the other sensory information, such as noises and smells. I also better understand the limits of my capabilities and do not venture into environments that I know will be difficult for me, such as a hectic shopping mall on Christmas Eve. I now take more notice of my emotional state and fatigue levels, and make sensible decisions about whether I will be able to handle different situations and events, such as going out for dinner at a busy restaurant after a stressful day at work. I have also recognised the importance of having "safe places" (CVI Scotland, 2017b) that are clutter free, quiet and peaceful for me to be in. A safe place is somewhere that I can regularly retreat to when I am feeling overwhelmed by the events of everyday life, even when I am away on holiday. The most obvious safe place is my home environment, however, I have also learnt to turn hotel rooms and outdoor environments, such as the beach, into safe places as well. Probably the most important strategy I have implemented, and the one that was the hardest for me to develop, was being open and honest with the people around me, and explaining my visual needs to them. This has made it easier to ask for help when needed, as people then understand what I need and why.

However, this has only become possible because I have been granted the gift of awareness and an in-depth understanding of my disability. I now understand the basic science of how the brain processes vision and how the different visual issues associated with CVI impact visual processing. I have also explored this further and have a clear understanding of how this impacts me specifically. For instance, because of my simultanagnostic visual dysfunction, I am aware that I am never going to be able to locate someone in a crowd of people. When meeting people, I therefore, ask them to find me, and so I plant myself in a certain location until they have spotted me, instead of my trying to search for them. I know this will be a fruitless search that will result in my becoming highly anxious and stressed and dealing with even further reduced visual function. Another example, is around my mobility in a crowded moving environment. As a result of my difficulty with creating an effective 3D map of the environment around me, especially when there are lots of visual and auditory distractions, I know I am going to miss obstacles, possible hazards and sometimes even people. If possible, I therefore ask to be sight guided by family, friends and colleagues.

Having the awareness that my disability can impact upon me more on some days than others, due to both external and internal factors, is also very important. As I have already explained, external factors such as the nature of the environment I am in, the number of distractions around me, issues with glare and lighting and internal factors such as my emotional state and fatigue levels, are elements I have to take into consideration every time I prepare myself to leave the house. Unfortunately, disasters can happen when I do not consider these factors. Recently on a whim, I decided to venture out on what should have been a straightforward trip to my local shops to purchase a birthday present for my niece. On this day, I was quite fatigued and stressed after a busy morning at work. It was also very windy and bright outside, and the glare was making it difficult to see clearly. Not long after leaving the office,

I noticed someone had left a stack of papers on the roof of their car while unlocking their car door across the street to my left. In an instant, I became completely engrossed in watching this person desperately trying to catch each page as they all started to flutter away down the street. I continued walking while watching this comical scene on my left, quietly chuckling to myself at their misfortune, when suddenly out of nowhere something attacked me on my right. I was instantly knocked to the ground and my heart started to pound as I struggled to get to my feet ready to run away from this daring midday attacker. Imagine my horror, when instead of turning to face this unknown assailant, I was greeted with a peaceful, sturdy parking meter that had always been there. It hadn't moved, it hadn't sprung up out of nowhere, it had just been completely invisible to me on my right-hand side. The distraction of someone else's misfortune had inadvertently caused my own visual inattention to kick in and I had forgotten all my rules of safe travel. Some might say it was justice served for laughing at someone else's expense, but the impact of the sudden collision severely jolted my head, causing a painful headache that lasted a couple of days, cracked a back tooth, injured my knee and severely bruised my pride. A lesson learnt in the most brutal of ways.

This incident served to remind me that it is difficult for me to be spontaneous and attempt to do something without fully considering the different aspects of a specific situation first. On this day, I did not think about how I was feeling, or whether I had enough energy to be able to maintain full concentration and visual attention while navigating my way through the unseen hazards and people on the busy city streets. The distraction caused me to turn my focus from the footpath in front of me and the resulting lack of visual attention had a disastrous effect. Although this was one of my worst vision-related accidents, there have been many others like this, which have caused me to adopt certain behaviours in order to try and keep myself safe. Most of the time, I am now a very cautious person. I also feel like I have to be in control of what is happening around me and what activities my family and I are going to participate in so that I am able to prepare myself beforehand for every potential issue that may arise during the activity. I find it hard to enjoy activities that have been sprung upon me when I do not have any time to prepare myself, especially when they are in unfamiliar environments. I also need to know if there is going to be a safe place for me to escape to whenever I am away from home, which can make holidays difficult. Unfortunately, these behaviours make me look like a very controlling and demanding person. But as I have just highlighted, at times it is necessary to be like this, in order to function in a world where my visual issues make it hard to understand the scene in front of me.

In some situations, however, I have been able to make changes to the way I go about living my life, to ensure that I am able to alleviate some of the more disabling effects of my visual condition in certain situations. An example of this is when I am participating in the enjoyable social activity of eating out at a café or restaurant. Before I understood my visual needs, I would blindly enter different eating establishments, sit somewhere at random and struggle to cope for a period of time, before I would inevitably have to leave, as a result of experiencing another CVI meltdown. This occurred because I never thought of trying to make the situation better for my specific needs. I never thought about what the actual venue would be like, whether it would be cluttered and crowded with lots of tables and chairs that would make it difficult to move through, whether the lighting would be bright enough for me to see easily or whether it might be so dim that I would struggle to even read the menu. I never used to think about where I sat at the table or what I was viewing in front of me from that position. The reason for this is that I never considered that these factors could actually impact on how well I was able to function in these environments or how long I was able to stay there (most of the time, it was only about an hour at the most). Having to leave early all the time, as a result of challenging visual environments making me feel physically ill and triggering a severe headache, is something that I find incredibly frustrating.

But once I did start taking my visual needs into consideration, I was able to engage in this kind of activity more easily and I found that I also enjoyed these social outings a lot more. If possible, I now preview different environments to make sure they are "CVI friendly". In my hometown, I have a number of different locations that I like to go, as I know I will not be so affected by my visual difficulties in these spaces. So, whenever possible, I organise it so that these are the venues we go to for different events, such as birthday dinners and nights out with friends. Specific requirements of these venues are that they are well lit and that any hazards are easily identifiable. For instance, the edges of steps and any trip hazards are painted a contrasting colour so that they stand out and easily grab my visual attention. I also ensure that all signage is clear and easy for me to read, especially bathrooms, which reduces the risk of an embarrassing incident, such as walking into the men's toilet (it is surprising how many men's and women's toilet signs are incomprehensible when one is highly stressed and visually not functioning well). I also think carefully about where I am going to sit within the restaurant and try to be the first person to sit at the table so that I get the most optimal spot before others join me. It is important for me to be facing into as blank a scene as possible, as this will reduce the visual distraction and allow me to converse with others more easily. Now that family, friends and colleagues understand this need, they have no issue with letting me pick my seat first.

For me, another important aspect of suitable eating places is that they do not have loud music playing in the background and that the space does not create an echo. Other people with CVI have described the difficulty of being able to concentrate on visual information in front of them when there is competing auditory information and vice versa. I know that for me, I find it impossible to hear what someone is saying if there is competing noise and an overload of visual information. I generally have to choose between listening to what my friends are saying and shutting out all the visual imagery, or viewing the visual scene and switching off to what they are saying. Of course, this also means that sometimes I have to be a bit ruthless about who I am going to be sitting next to. If I do not make a wise decision about my dinner companion, I can spend the entire night completely disengaged from everyone else, because I am unable to block out the one loud person sitting next to me.

However, as we all know, it is not possible for one to always pick the particular destination of a social gathering or work-related function or pick who you are going to sit next to. For this reason, I often find myself having to deal with challenging situations in unfamiliar environments, most of which I am unable to preview prior to the event. From experience, I know that after only a short period of time, I will struggle to function both visually and cognitively in these environments and this has led to changes in my social interactions and the development of specific, sometimes even anti-social, behaviours. A good example of this is the creative strategies I have developed to avoid being greeted by an acquaintance or friend with a kiss on the cheek. One of my main CVI-related issues is that I have a right-sided hemianopia as well as right-sided hemi inattention, and I quite often forget that I even have a right side at all and walk around oblivious to anything happening to the right of me (one day I left the house only brushing the left side of my hair and I sometimes leave half the washing on the line!). This means that when someone is coming into kiss me on the cheek on my right side, I often do not even know they are there until I feel their warm breath and gentle touch of their lips on the side of my face. As one can imagine, I find this sudden invasion of my personal space very frightening and the physical reaction of jerking my head away in surprise and panic has resulted in many a comical accident, including kisses on the neck, head butts and even for one unsuspecting greeter, a kiss on the lips. Not only do these incidents humiliate me (and often the person who was simply trying to greet me), they also cause me a great deal of anxiety leading up to different events, as I spend hours trying to establish how I can avoid the whole greeting experience. However, the tactics that I use, such as standing at the back of the group and not making eye contact with people, or not responding to their greeting advances, just make me look rude and unfriendly.

There are many other situations that cause others to view me in this light – as someone that is impolite, aloof and who does not actually enjoy spending time with others. Most of the time, I can understand why I may be viewed like this. I often do not respond to people waving at me or calling out to me from a distance, which people assume is because I do not want to talk to them. When in fact, it's because I haven't even seen or heard them. I sometimes struggle to make eye contact with people while talking to them, because of any visual distractions in the environment behind them, which my gaze gets constantly drawn to. So I avoid large group discussions to reduce the chances of coming across as bad mannered and inattentive. I often pull out of social activities at the last minute, because on the day I have realised that I am actually just too exhausted to attend, which means people have stopped asking me to join them at different events. I am always the first person to leave any large social gathering to ensure that I avoid the stress and embarrassment of suffering another CVI meltdown in public, which again makes me look anti-social. The knowledge that I am autobiographically portraying this social outcast persona, is something that upsets me greatly, because this is not who I really am. I would love to be the last person to leave a party for once. I would love to feel comfortable and confident mixing and mingling in different social settings, and to initiate the kissing on the cheek of an old friend I have not seen in a while. And I would love to be known as a social, easy going and relaxed person.

I used to think this was the price that I had to pay for being able to continue walking the tightrope between the able-bodied and disabled worlds. But as I continue down this journey to CVI enlightenment, I am beginning to see the world a little bit differently. I have, therefore, realised that this might not be the best way forward. After only recently being empowered through the correct diagnosis for my difficulties, for the first time in over 20 years, I have now started to embrace the uniqueness of my life with CVI. For a long time, my impairments have been a big part of who I am and have, at times, restricted me from participating in different activities. However, I now know that these impairments do not define me. I am a person first and foremost and it just so happens that I have a "different normal" brain, which has created a very complex visual world for me. When I am open and honest about what it is like to live in this world, people are quick to accept the way I behave and the actions I take – no matter how strange it might seem!

When I sit back and think about this, I have also come to realise that it is important for me, as the disabled person, to have more faith in the way that society perceives me and my abilities. This is a message that I would like others affected by CVI to embrace. Fortunately, as a professional working in the field of education and rehabilitation of children who are blind or who have low vision, I am in the position to be able to pass on this positive belief in humankind to the children I work with, their families and support teams. I have finally learnt that when armed with an effective CVI toolbox full of diverse strategies and approaches for dealing with different challenging situations, and combining it with the knowledge that if I explain what support I need from the people around me, I do not have to continue through life worrying about which side of the tightrope I am going to fall on any given day. In fact, I do not have to worry about walking the tightrope at all. I can continue on, not living in two worlds, just living in one. A world that accepts me for who I am. And hopefully, by sharing this insight, children with CVI will grow up never experiencing what it is like to live life walking on a tightrope.

Conclusion

But I need help to make this happen. Society as a whole needs to understand what the world is like for those of us living with CVI and learn to interpret our behaviours and emotional responses. Especially when it relates to children. Teachers need to understand that the tantrums, aggression, crying and refusal to participate in different activities, might not actually be the child being defiant, not being interested in learning or not being able to participate in a formal educational setting. The child may simply be terrified by the frightening visual scene he or she cannot understand and is constantly on high alert, waiting for the CVI meltdown clouds to roll in once again, but is unable to articulate to anyone what they are experiencing. The adults around these children also need to realise that there is a reason for the child's controlling and demanding behaviour and it's not simply a way of getting more attention. Family and friends need to understand that the anti-social behaviours that both children and adults display, is not by choice. These behaviours are a necessity to be able to continue functioning in what can be a very confusing and exhausting world at times. People also need to realise, that often, we need help to feel safe in different environments, even when they are familiar to us. We need people to understand that clutter and crowds seem like terrifying monsters and make us feel that our lives are constantly being threatened. We also need to know that our emotional reactions in different situations will not be misinterpreted or trivialised. But most importantly, all of us with CVI, including both children and adults, need to know that it is acceptable for us to use whatever behaviours, strategies or methods we need to get through each day – even when they do not make sense to anyone else. With global acceptance of this, over time, we will learn to trust the world around us and be at peace with who we are.

References

CVI Scotland. 2017a. *CVI Scotland* [e-publication]. Accessed 14 October 2017. http://cviscotland.org/documents.php?did=1&sid=55.

CVI Scotland. 2017b. *CVI Scotland* [e-publication]. Accessed 22 October 2017. http://cviscotland.org/documents.php?did=1&sid=68.

Dutton, G.N. 2015. Eye movement disorders in children with cerebral visual impairment In A. Lueck and G.N. Dutton (eds), *Vision and the brain: Understanding cerebral visual impairment in children* (pp. 177–188). New York: AFB press.

Fazzi, E., Signorini, S.G., Bova, S.M., La Piana, R., Ondei, P., Bertone, C., Misferari, W. and Bianchi, P.E. 2007. Spectrum of visual disorders in children with cerebral visual impairment. *Journal of Child Neurology*, 22(3), 294–301.

Goodale, M.A. 2013. Separate visual systems for perception and action: A framework for understanding cortical visual impairment. *Developmental Medicine & Child Neurology*, 55(Suppl. 4), 9–12.

Pawletko, T., Chokron, S. and Dutton, G.N. 2015. Considerations in the behavioural diagnosis of CVI: Issues, cautions, and potential outcomes. In A. Lueck and G.N. Dutton (eds), *Vision and the brain: Understanding cerebral visual impairment in children* (pp. 145–176). New York: AFB Press.

7

Assessment of visual processing functions and disorders

Lea Hyvärinen

Introduction

This chapter describes assessments and clinical examinations of school children with visual processing disorders using transdisciplinary assessment based on observations and testing by teachers, parents, caregivers and therapists and observations and examinations by all medical specialists and psychologists in the care of the child/student. This chapter also discusses important clinical test situations repeated at school, where the educational vision team benefits from a new view on testing. To measure functions that have not yet been possible to assess, may require a visiting specialist to examine students at the school or to allow a teacher or therapist to accompany a student in clinical test situations. The latter function is routine in many hospitals in assessment of students with multiple disorders. This also improves ergonomics during testing.

Infants and children with visual processing disorders are a heterogeneous cohort, the largest and growing group of infants and children with visual disorders. Teachers' and therapists' role is important; their observations and questions to medical specialists on students' strategies guide doctors in choosing clinical tests for in-depth examination. Refraction and correction of refractive errors, eye movements and accommodation should be repeated before testing sensory functions:

- Visual acuity (VA) as optotype acuity at near, also with tightly crowded optotypes to reveal increased crowding effect
- VA at distance with 100% spacing in line test; if this is difficult, then with single optotypes
- Grating actuity (GRA)
- Low contrast VA and GrA
- Visual adaptation, colour vision, motion perception and visual fields.

Many schools have lists of functions that should be observed and discussed with vision rehabilitation specialists (see Figure 7.1)

This overview begins with three case histories to depict some clinical examinations and assessment of visual processing functions in transdisciplinary examinations of educational and medical vision teams. These students taught us important details about their visual problems and education.

Case 1

In 1976, the first Vision Rehabilitation Centre in Helsinki, Finland, started to function in collaboration with the Finnish and Swedish Schools for the Blind and Visually Impaired. In 1977, a 6-year-old boy was referred for consultation because no one was able to measure his visual acuity. The boy saw well enough for almost normal looking orientation and moving. He had large angle, horizontal nystagmus and his test results were surprising: the measurement had to be made at an unusually short distance, 30 cm from the boy's eyes. At that distance he could with difficulty recognise the LEA symbols on the uppermost, 30M line; thus his visual acuity was 0.01 (6/600). His grating acuity was surprising, at 4cpd, which did not match his VA value. Therefore contrast sensitivity measurement was made at the Department of Psychology when the boy came for his next visit.

The contrast sensitivity curve showed normal values at the lowest grating acuity values until value 1 cpd, after which the curve bends down reaching the X-axis at 4 cpd. The CS curve depicts how much visual information is transferred (moved) from the eyes to the brain at different grating frequencies (X-axis) and contrast levels (Y-axis); the X just above the X-axis depicts the information transferred by the high-contrast visual acuity measurement (Hyvärinen and Jacob, in press). This was our first experience of a cortical lesion that had caused "cortical blindness", with visual acuity barely 0.01 (6/600, 20/2000), yet the boy was *not* blind.

This boy's occipital cortex was found severely atrophic. This explained the nearly total loss of recognition functions, except *visual information in motion, also at low contrast,* possibly arriving via the *tectopulvinar pathway* and via V5 to the remaining atrophic occipital lobe and temporal and parietal functions.

Case 1 was our first dramatic experience on how visual acuity does *not* depict a child's visual functioning. His grating acuity value seemed to be closer to his functional vision: he moved freely, played with a soccer ball in the corridor as long as it moved. If the ball was not moving, he seemed not to notice it. This group of children is often classified as "blind with blind sight" but they may have *motion perception that is not measured.*

In the 1970s several leading laboratories were studying pathways for visual information into the brain other than the well-known retinocalcarine pathway. After a monkey, Helen, was blind after surgical removal of the calcarine cortex (now known as the area V1) but later in her retirement learned to use vision, it was apparent that there must be another pathway.

Miller, Pasik and Pasik (1980) reported on measurements of responses to gratings in superior colliculus: "Monkeys with total bilateral ablation of the striate cortex, however, retain a residual capacity for pattern discrimination and also can differentiate between a vertical and an oblique luminous bar" (p. 1510). This confirmed our guesses. Monkeys responded to gratings up to 4 cpd as did the boy with visual acuity 0.01. Apparently, humans also had this newly discovered pathway. Later it was called the tectopulvinar pathway going via superior colliculus in tectum and pulvinar nucleus in thalamus to MT/V5 (middle temporal visual area/visual area 5) and further into occipital and parietal lobes.

This bright boy studied in a local school in his hometown with occasional support periods on the elementary level (one week in a year) provided by the School for the Blind. At the university he completed a postgraduate degree (PhLic). In his studies and his work he did not use an assisting person, which each "visually impaired" (by VA-value) university student and later adult was eligible for in Finland. His main interests in his undergraduate and postgraduate studies were conflict and terrorism, and he has continued his research further in this field. He lives independently and uses public transport, although he is eligible to use a taxi and to have a personal assistant in daily tasks, both services he does not use, because he functions well. Grating acuity

4 cpd means useful information for many tasks, especially for orientation and moving. Texts must be enlarged and for longer texts, scanning and speech synthesiser are used.

This case showed us that much more should be learned about brain functions before we could correctly measure visual functioning of all children.

Case 2

Among hundreds of youngsters with brain damage-related cerebral palsy and visual field loss, there is one documented case of an individual whose visual fields during a long treatment with baclofen intrathecally and orthopaedic manual therapy (OMT) quite unexpectedly could be measured with normal size. This young man described his story at a conference in Dortmund 2010 and I use parts of his talk (that we wrote together) in this report:

> I was born in 1984 with brain damage, which was due to placenta ablation. My eye movements did not differentiate from my head movements, yet I learned to read at age 3 using head movements. I saw facial expressions and had normal visual acuity. I grew up with no visual or motor memory. I have always had good corrected visual acuity and no problems in reading.
>
> When I was 11 years old, my family bought me Microsoft's Flight simulator. Training with this programme started my slow visuospatial development, as it helped me experience movement and viewpoints in a new way.
>
> At 14 years of age, my right hand had developed well enough to allow use of an electric wheelchair outdoors but I had no knowledge of the route to home. Dr Lea made a video of the route from school to my home walking in front or behind my wheelchair to document the route, with my therapist and my classroom assistant. I watched the video every evening and after a month I had learned the route. However, the route from home to school was a new route. I could not reverse the route from school to home because I had no concepts for directions and no visual imagination where to handle the information. I had good visual acuity and large enough visual field for orientation but *could not move my attention into the left lower part of the visual field during testing*. After 34 months of intensive training my visual fields could be recorded of normal size. I had seen the visual field in the same size during all years so the test results were wrong. This is a common finding in children and adults with cerebral palsy.
>
> At school, I used auditory learning strategies in mathematics, which was very challenging. Math is a strongly spatial subject and I did not have spatial awareness. At 17 years of age I started to use a computer program called MathCAD, designed for working with symbolic mathematics. It acted as a replacement for spatial memory. I had some spatial awareness but was mostly *a talking head without body awareness*.
>
> Before intrathecal baclofen was started in January 2004, I had rigid joints and weak circulation particularly in the limbs and trunk, which added to my stiffness. My head control and speech were fairly good for a spastic person. I had *no virtual visual world*. I could not form a lasting memory of how objects such as flowers looked like. I was unable to extrapolate features of visual scenes and remember them. I had no sensory imagination, was unable to create virtual environments described in fictional novels and poems. I was dependent on immediate visual information. Control of visual attention was inflexible. *I had to move my head to consciously shift visual attention*.
>
> Many of the effects of the baclofen treatment could be felt immediately after the pump was installed when I was 19 years old in January 2004. During the first night after the operation, when I woke up I wondered what was in the foot end of my bed. I felt my toes

for the first time. In October 2004, ten months after the pump was installed I perceived two lines going up diagonally when Dr Lea drew them but when the pencil did not move, the diagonal lines did not have any direction, their position continuously changed as if they were "vibrating". The horizontal line did not move. This indicated that the perception of some line directions was unstable.

In 2006, my visual fields started to improve during each orthopaedic manual therapy (OMT) session and could be recorded of normal size 34 months after intrathecal baclofen was started. *Although I had experienced the size of my visual field always of normal size, I could not move my attention down and left during the perimetric testing.* Next, spasticity decreased, motor functions improved, I experienced "depth", and working memory improved.

During the third year (2006) movements became smoother and the inhibition of immediate movements developed. During the fourth year I learned to use hands together. I have since learned a variety of motor skills like pouring fluid in glass, which I had trained since I was 4 years old.

My awareness of body height improved in 2006, as soon as I was able to transfer weight on to the pelvis. In 2007 to 2008, the fourth and fifth year, I started to develop a virtual visual space in which to manipulate objects. In 2008, I realised that my body image had developed to the point where I could actually enjoy shopping for clothes. In November 2009 I did not notice myself that I started to use a spoon to take a piece of cake while saying a sentence – two demanding functions simultaneously. This year's (2010) highlight was when I learned to manipulate shirts, something my therapist and I thought to be impossible.

To me it looks like that perception of distances and directions must work well before perception of space is possible. It has been a slow development. First, I was able to model the concepts of "from me" and "toward me"; then development continued steadily from there on. (These concepts could be trained in infancy from the beginning of early intervention.) It seems that virtual visual scenes and the capability to analyse "real" visual scene develop together. The emergence of virtual visual space happened in tandem with the improvements in understanding real space.

Another important area of improvement is the subjective experience and perception of emotions (development of *mirroring*). Social interaction is much easier now because I can better model the motives and intentions of others. This area of experiences is very hard to explain. Somehow also seeing, looking at objects is more enjoyable. Objects also have a multidimensional, emotional content. Depth perception and episodic memory improve due to visual input. In summary, I feel like I was born again as a more flexible, emotionally richer, more social person.

I believe that my case is a good example of how the compound effect of medication and intensive physiotherapy and occupational therapy has transformed my life. The effect of *baclofen* can be felt in the decrease of spasticity and disappearance of painful spasms. The effect of OMT can be felt during the therapy as the decrease of the joint rigidity and pain, and as improvement in the body image. I experienced an obvious enlargement of the visual fields several times immediately after the 60 min OMT sessions before the enlargement became permanent. The final improvement occurred at a time when the continuous *neural white noise from the spastic muscles decreased* and sensory functions in general improved.

Case 3

Face blindness is a poorly known visual processing problem. It can be an inherited disorder but more often it is a part of brain damage during birth or soon after birth due to a motor disorder (often cerebral palsy) and is often accompanied by difficulties in learning route-based orientation, due to loss of recognition of landmarks on routes. Since the child may have several other "hidden" weak areas of functioning, therapists and teachers are instrumental in interdisciplinary working with a rehabilitation ophthalmologist and several other medical specialists. I could not examine Eva each year, but I could activate help, usually from the School for Vision Impaired Children when problems occurred. Many details are included with the hope that they will be helpful in assessments of other children with similar problems.

Eva was born 15 weeks premature as a very small infant. She survived with several disorders typical to prematurity: mild motor problems of legs and hands and *weak accommodation*, structural and functional changes in lungs and mouth functions, motor problems in swallowing (she could swallow only fluids), and difficulties in the perception and awareness of environmental structures, especially stairs and surface qualities, and problems in sensory integration.

Group training in warm water at the age of 2 years and 9 months caused a panic reaction that was found to be due to fear when not recognising her mother among five mothers wearing the same colour swimming suit and cap. This situation was treated by using a headband around her mother's thigh. Her family observed Eva further and reported that Eva *did not recognise family members by faces but by clothing and voice.*

When assessed a week later, Eva had alternating esotropia corrected with +2.50/+2.75 spectacles for distance. She did not have near correction, the angle was larger at near so she needed new glasses. Her visual acuity was 0.63 (6/10) with single LEA symbols at 40 cm distance (Playing Cards test) and 0.2 (6/30) with the standard line test with LEA symbols in each eye. The difference between these two values was outside the range of normal and meant difficulty in keeping details apart, i.e. *increased crowding effect.* Distance visual acuity was 1.0 (6/6) with single symbols; line test was not yet possible. The low-contrast Hiding Heidi picture at 2.5% contrast was noticed at 2 m (6') distance; this measures maximum visual communication distance (in populations with low contrasts on their very fair or very dark faces) and meant that for visual communication we should be at about half the distance or closer, in order to be seen comfortably by Eva. Detection grating acuity with the LEA gratings was 25 cpd, i.e. she responded to the difference between the grey surface and stripes. How she saw the lines was impossible to know. Visual fields measured with confrontation were of normal size. Her eyes were structurally normal, with no retinal or optic nerve changes. Discussion Eva's activities and behaviours with her mother revealed that she had problems in several visual functions.

Visual symptoms typical to brain damage-related vision loss

All answers to the following questions were "Yes": variation in visual functioning; early development of speech; prefers talking with adults to playing with children; crowded places problematic; problems with shadows and thresholds; walks over toys and falls; uses siblings and adults as helpers in visual tasks; difficulties in finding toys on patterned surfaces; difficulties in noticing fast moving objects; in playground does not play like other children. Eva had also poor recognition of body forms (Gestalt); she had not seen the difference between her grandmother and a school child with a rucksack on the street.

Eva was eligible for a twice-yearly repeated two-day long neuropsychological evaluation for two years. The functions assessed and reported during developmental evaluations were: tests WPPSI-R, NEPSY; concentration and endurance in solving tasks, eye–hand coordination; interpretation of pictures; scanning and the size of the observational field, *left lower field weak*; recognition of faces in pictures and during communication; visual deductions and interpretations; use of visual information: missing parts, blurry pictures; constructing a new picture of parts of a picture; copying of geometric forms; building a picture of its parts; drawing free hand; finding objects in a new room. The evaluation report described Eva as friendly, determined and pertinent. If she did not understand an expression or word, she asked what the word meant; she played with other children, accepted invitations to play and invited other children to play with her.

When clinical tests for visual processing were used at the age of 4½ years the differences in the recognition functions were apparent: in the tasks of *early processing* in the occipital lobe, Eva grasped the LEA rectangles correctly (eye–hand coordination) and placed them on rectangles of the same length without difficulty (pure visual comparison of size). Similarly, the LEA mailbox game showed normal perception of orientation of the slot. The test was held in *horizontal* direction because Eva had *limited rotation of her wrist* (a common problem in children with cerebral palsy). Training of the observed weak functions was included in the early intervention programme. She could use simultaneous recognition of form and colour in the Colorama game. She could not perceive the difference between a smiling and a sad face in well-drawn, simple pictures (a recognition task at full contrast of non-moving forms) although she could respond to the low contrast Hiding Heidi test in motion. Her binocular line acuity (100% spacing between symbols) at distance was 0.8 (6/9) at full contrast; 0.3, (6/18) RE and 0.25, (6/24) LE at 2.5% contrast at a distance of 3 m, and binocular near line acuity 0.5 (6/12) at full contrast, i.e. lower than distance VA, slightly improved with new near add but still lower than at at distance. This depicts *increased crowding effect*, i.e. difficulties in keeping details apart. Copying of lines at the age of 5 years showed that orientation of lines was difficult to perceive and to use for copying, especially in angles. The difficulties in spatial orientation persisted both in egocentric small space and in the environmental orientation. Her weak motion perception was noticed later also in larger spaces: she did not perceive bicycles and cars in motion. Her uneven profile of visual functioning was a warning sign on visual processing disorders. The university hospital arranged an MRI. It showed *periventricular leukomalasia*.

Occupational therapy by an imaginative therapist started and was instrumental in developing basic understanding of structure of her body, directions and distances, gross and fine motor functions, facial expressions and better tolerance to tactile information. Since Eva did not seem to perceive surface structures, training of long cane techniques using a Pathfinder cane was started. When using the cane for the first time on a cobblestone street Eva asked, "How can a street be so bumpy?" which clearly revealed her difficulties in perceiving surfaces. A part of occupational therapy was later used for riding to entice Eva to use her hands to touch animals, brushes and pieces of apples and carrots at the same time as it was training of balance. She did not learn to recognise her horse, which was not a problem because the horse recognised Eva at distance. The supporting activities were regularly reported to the day care personnel. The first few months went well; the teachers and children always wore something easily recognisable. When Eva moved to the group of older children her face blindness was no more considered.

Problems in day care at the age of 5 years

When Eva was included in a small day care group of eight children with special needs, the day care personnel felt that the girl recognised them and did not use individual details as distinctive marks. Therefore, Eva's ability to recognise her peers was tested using pictures of faces. She did not recognise anybody. When she was told that the pictures were pictures of her day care group, she said: "This is my picture because I am the only child with glasses". She recognised spectacles, not her face. She did not recognise even her best friend, the only dark child in the group but could correctly match the pictures, i.e. her picture perception was good enough for correct matching, but she did not recognise the facial features of her peers – these are two different functions. The result of the test did not change the opinion of the staff at the kindergarten; they considered Eva to be "a spoiled child with autistic behaviours". The teachers felt that her atypical visual communication, "avoiding eye contact" was a sign of autism. They did not believe that Eva did not perceive eyes and was looking for details that she could see, like hair, ear rings, etc. That time it was still common that kindergarten teachers did not know the differences in behaviours of children with visual processing problems from those of children with autism spectrum disorders.

Second preschool year at the kindergarten

Because of Eva's developmental and growth delay, a decision was made to give her an extra preschool year in the same kindergarten. She was now seen as a big girl and was asked to eat warm lunch, which she could not do. Therefore, chewing and tongue functions were observed and her swallowing reflex was found to be abnormal in a video fluorographic recording. Eva had learned to let fluids run down into the oesophagus by tilting her head backwards (nobody had noticed that as a sign of problematic swallowing; it was considered "one of her odd behaviours"). First tube feeding and after a few months, feeding directly into her very small stomach through the "button" took six hours during the day and seven hours during the night.

Orientation in space remained problematic at the age of 5 years; she did not find the way from the yard to her home door in a three-story apartment house, which her younger brother (by two years) noticed before adults did and spontaneously started to function as Eva's personal guide. Eva did not see the difference between the pavement and the street and she didn't see cars coming. She was taught to stay on the lawn close to the house when she heard a car coming.

Grade 1 at the School for Visually Impaired Children

There had been marked development in compensating strategies in most areas of functioning, but so much special teaching was still needed that the first school year at the School for Visually Impaired Children was considered advisable. The teaching programme was a combination of that of a regular school and a special school. Eva had physiotherapy once a week and speech therapy twice a week at the school. Tube feeding through the "button" was no problem at the special school where she could have the meals while sitting in the classroom. When the gastrostomy was operated, Eva was 14 kg (31 lb) and looked like a tiny waif. Two years later at the Special School Resource Center she was 25 kg (55 lb) and looked like a regular schoolgirl.

Daily training of routes helped Eva to learn a few routes within the school building starting from a certain door as the origin; no map-based orientation developed. When she was asked to explore a model and find out where on the school compound the place depicted by the model might be, she did not know. Her O&M teacher asked her to "enter the space with your hand through the door and walk further". After a few seconds Eva said, "This place is not at school, this is my dorm; my room is this one." She could describe all the rooms. *Her hand was more skilled in exploration of space than her sight.*

Eva had learned to observe her visual functions and could describe that small spots like full stops and commas disappeared sometimes and after a while reappeared. People's faces disappeared also, especially eyes and mouth for longer times than dots. There were holes in her attention, which few children report. Before coming to school her vision had been examined in an ophthalmologist's office where the LEA near test with 25% spacing between the symbols could be used for the first time and the VA value with that test was 0.8 (6/9) while with 100% spacing it was 1.0 (6/6) and at 2.5% contrast 0.5 (6/12), i.e. all visual acuity values had become typical normal findings. At school half a year later, VA at distance with the line test was 1.0 (6/6) and near vision acuity was 1.0 with 100%, 50% and 25% spacing with LEA symbols. Thus, in this test situation with the LEA symbols, increased crowding was no more measurable. However, tight spacing of letters in words made reading impossible for more than 15 minutes and pictures with many details could not be interpreted.

Processing functions of pictures of concrete objects (LEA symbols, used in early examinations) and letters are processed in different networks and thus VA values can be different if these networks are differently damaged. Visual acuity should be measured with both types of tests with abstract optotypes: letter and number optotypes, as soon as the child learns them. This is now possible with the visual acuity test: "FOUR tests in ONE" with tests based on the four Sloan letters, the four LEA numbers, and the four LEA symbols and the international reference optotype, four Landolt-Cs.

Using a pencil caused spasms and pain in the hands. Pain was apparently limiting Eva's participation in sports, but she said that she was tired. Often her "tiredness" disappeared after a short while so she was apparently not aware of pain in the legs or had no words to describe what she felt. A few months later Eva started to complain about pain in the legs after walking a kilometre. She was *becoming aware of her body and spasms in the legs*.

At the resource centre Eva saw other children using closed-circuit television magnification systems (CCTV) for reading and wanted to try it. She found reading with magnification easy and asked whether she could have a CCTV at her local school. In the home town the decision was "No" but a long letter from the resource centre managed to change the decision, although we could not explain *why* reading was easier with a CCTV. Eva's fixation and saccades were carefully measured in a basic science laboratory and found to be perfect. Eva could read 12-point text for about 15 minutes, whereas she could read with the CCTV as long as she wanted. The video magnifier made Eva able to read her Harry Potter books.

The resource centre reported a detailed description of Eva's school situation, devices and needs for special attention at the local school, but unfortunately grades 2, 3 and 4 in the local school were a severe disappointment to Eva, her family and the resource centre. Eva received for her new school a CCTV with blackboard camera, a slanting board, lamp, telescope and a magnifier. During the winters of second and third grade both of her classroom teachers stayed only one year and did not have time to learn about Eva's special situation. Therefore, teaching was in the hands of Eva's assistant who had not wanted to participate in the training at the resource centre and whose experience was in assisting older boys with behavioural problems. When she saw Eva, a small, friendly, quiet girl she made her own diagnosis that Eva had "no real problems" and did not follow most of the recommendations by the resource centre. Auditory books and other materials were ordered late, in the third grade so late that they had not arrived before the Christmas vacation. This classroom assistant told the other children in the classroom that *they did not need to talk to the disabled girl*. Eva was also left alone by other children in the school playground.

Eva should have started typing lessons and should have received a small computer in 2010 but nothing happened for two years. Eva "saw too well" and "was only mildly spastic". The "mild" spasticity of the hands allowed the use of one hand for about 15 minutes, after which the hand was so spastic and aching that the pencil had to be moved to the other hand for the next 15 minutes. Even if Eva's handwriting slowly improved, she could not read it after a few days, so her mother had to read it aloud for examinations. Special teachers from the resource centre visited Eva's school to discuss the advice but no changes happened. Finally, Eva received a small computer donated by someone outside of the school.

During the ophthalmological examinations, visual acuity and contrast sensitivity values remained as before. Eva could see slow-moving pictures (Pepi test) and biological motion (Walking Man test) but did not properly perceive and copy movements in gymnastics or perceive moving or distance of bicycles and cars on the street. Loss of high-speed motion made lip-reading difficult.

Grades 5 and 6 at the local school

With her own computer and PleXtalk Eva had become faster in homework and had more time for reading for pleasure and writing her fantasy novels. She used first 40-point font, later 28 or 20-point Arial when typing, enlarging it on the screen. At school, spatial problems in maths had decreased and the number line was stable. Eva does not recognise fish and wrote the names of the fish correctly in a test by using unrelated details in the pictures to remember the names; in most pictures she used plants to help her recognise the fish. Eva's mother did not inform the teacher because Eva had trained herself to remember the names of the fish by using visual information available to her.

During the measurement of visual fields on the fifth grade at the age of 10½ years Eva's visual fields were again measured using a technique where the child is asked to "look through the black hole in the direction of the tester's *voice*" (not *at* the hole, i.e. no visual motor task) and "let the eye jump on the white dot when it appears somewhere". With this technique her visual fields were full whereas in the standard measurement visual fields were in different meridians 20–40 degrees smaller. Eva and many other children with cerebral palsy cannot divide their attention between several tasks (simultan agnosia), which makes the measurement of visual fields difficult.

Eva had a new teacher in fifth grade, who had interest in and the opportunity to observe Eva's functioning. She noticed the ineffective work of the assistant but could not get her to be moved or to improve. The teacher suggested to Eva's family that together they could start working for the move to another school with the help of the resource centre. The usual planning meeting for special education was held at the new school with the head master, the special teacher from the resource centre, Eva's classroom teacher and mother. *The classroom assistant was not present at the meeting but was asked to order the books for the next year. She did not do that.* Eva's mother learned about the delay in ordering the books in May, but the Library for the Blind was able to arrange all books and other materials during the summer.

Grades 7, 8 and 9 in the new local school

Before she started at her new school Eva had intensive training in orientation. This included exploring the new school. Eva took her cane with her because "it would teach her where there are stairs". *Perception of surfaces and recognition of their structures had improved a little* but to move comfortably Eva must remember structures of surfaces and routes based on few landmarks. Eva's special teacher at the resource centre arranged also a meeting with the teachers of the new school to decide on details: for example, a part of materials would be on a USB. Eva needed much less time for homework in the same subjects she had in her previous school even if home assignments were now longer.

In Eva's class in seventh grade, three girls of immigrant families started to ask Eva when they did not understand some words. These girls and Eva spent much time together even when language difficulties were overcome. Eva told them about her difficulties in looking at faces and the girls were never bothered by it. It was as if, "being different" from other students, Evan and her friends became a close group, her first group of friends at school.

At the new school, Eva had "one task on the paper" in the first math examination; she received B+. In her old school her math exams *had several tasks crowded on each page and resulted in D– to C*. After this exam in her new school all her math exams resulted in A–.

In the yearly follow-up of her vision, in the left lower visual field there was a patchy area where the isopter showed some defects in repeated measurement. This weakness in the lower left visual field had been noticed in the first two-day long neuropsychological assessment but not in the clinical examinations: this I/4 isopter was smaller in the previous measurement and thus did not go through the weak area. This suggests that repetition of clinical tests is important.

Eva had regular school books, the same books as her peers but as talking books, and electronic books with workbooks where the answers could be written on the page. She used her dictaphone to dictate her notes on the next day's homework. Eva's devices were a laptop with several programmes, e.g. ZOOM-text, a large extra screen, wireless keyboard and mouse and a printer and scanner at home. She also had devices for auditory materials, such as the small PleXtalk that can be carried and the PleXtalk 2 for copying books from the Library of the Blind and the digital dictaphone. Eva had electronic books in maths and three languages. At school there was a video projector in almost all classrooms. Other devices were her canes, spectacles, magnifier and several cardboard pieces with "windows" to cover information around the task material, enlarged printed materials at school and most of the printed materials on her USB, also examination materials, which Eva could enlarge on her computer. She had learned to use her devices so well that she had more time than before to read other books.

Eva's orientation in terms of space had not shown significant improvement. She did not dare to move alone for the fear of getting lost. She would yield bicycles in the wrong direction and did not notice the curbs or cars. Perception of surface qualities had not improved so in new areas she had to use a cane to be aware of the surface structure. Despite good training in orientation and moving she had either to move with a group, or use a human guide in orientation, so she mostly stayed at home reading.

The dog guide

During the fall term of the seventh grade, the owner of an 8-year-old guide dog passed away. The dog could not be given to a blind adult so close to its retirement age, so the School for Guide Dogs contacted Eva's family asking whether they would consider having the dog. This big black dog became Eva's best friend. It required long walks, which decreased the dog's weight by 9 lb in 12 months and added to Eva's weight nearly as much. Eva's sports teacher trained her for the competitions that were in September 2011 at the resource centre. Eva won the triathlon: shot-putting (6.6 lb), throwing ball and the 66-yard dash and to her surprise also the 440-yard sprint.

When I tested Eva's vision before her profile was written, the LEA Grating Acuity test was available for the first time. Eva saw the broad (1 cm) black lines with sharp edges at 60 cm distance but a few centimetres farther away the edges became jagged. Eva's grating acuity was thus 0.5 cpd while her optotype acuity was 1.0 (6/6) when measured with line tests and 2.0 (6/3) with single optotypes. Finer grating lines were seen at the edge of the test; the centre was "empty" with a few colourful spots floating in it. The grating size was 6.5 degrees at the distance of 2 metres, so the 4cpm/cm lines were seen at approximately 15 cpd at the edges of this 6.5 degree central area. Resolving of fine lines was best in the ambient vision, not in the central, focal vision in the fovea, Because the fine lines were not seen in the centre, it was easy to understand the great need of magnification required for reading.

The Profile of Visual Functioning (2011) (Figure 7.1) recorded Eva's functions as:

- normal/typical (N) and number 1;
- impaired but useful (I) and number 2;
- profoundly impaired (P) and number 3.

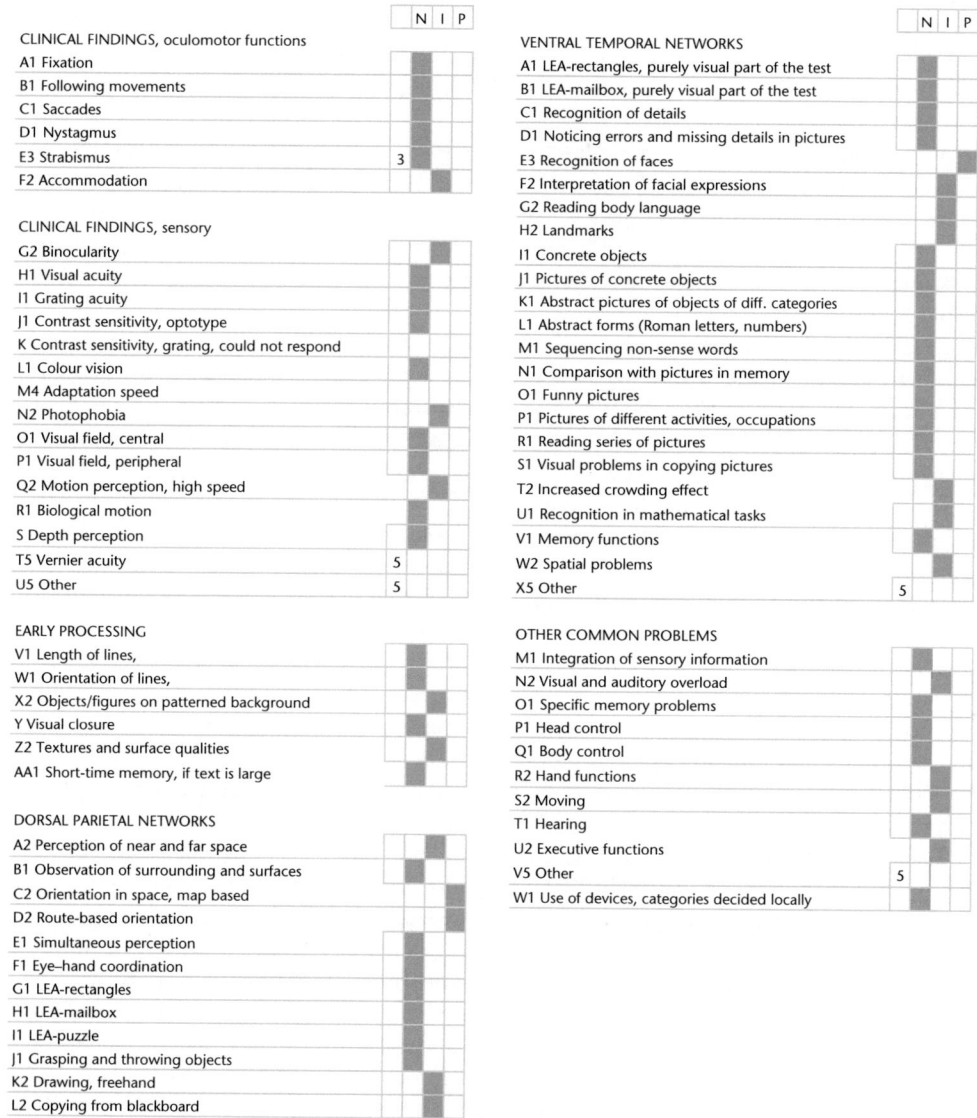

Figure 7.1   Profile of a child's (Eva) visual functioning.

Note: Both map-based and route-based orientation are marked "profoundly affected". Eva had a dog guide.

This disturbance in the centre of the grating depicts loss of visual field and has been known since the 1970s in measurements of contrast sensitivity using gratings. The first person with this kind of strange central field was an amblyopic laboratory technician who answered correctly also with his amblyopic eye because he could see the straight lines at the edges. In his case, the lines were a tangled net in the centre (Hyvärinen and Jacob, in press).

Fine lines are details in letters. If they are not seen, then magnification need in the central, focal area is unusually great (CCTV), even if in the ambient area fine lines can be seen. During measurement of grating acuity, remember to ask how the grating lines look like (for details of the measurement see Hyvärinen and Jacob, 2019).

In recognition functions Eva had her greatest problems in face recognition and interpretation of facial expressions, where loss of information in high-speed motion complicates communication situations.

As we experience in Eva's case, children with brain damage-related loss of several visual processing functions and other functional problems may have a bumpy road through early intervention and education. Fortunately, with the supporting strategies and devices it is often possible to train children to cope with their functional situation. If we can train and support early intervention teams, families and schools, the future of these children will be much brighter than it is now.

Eva did not tell her mother or the medical professionals details about her first classroom assistant, but made the decision to discuss the problems with her special teacher at the School for the Visually Impaired. At the School for the Visually Impaired, children were accepted as they were; everyone was different in one way or other. This is crucial for the functioning of children at schools that are not fully inclusive.

I met Eva after she finished her school with fine marks and she now studies archaeology and history of cultures at university. I shortened old reports to show especially my medical colleagues how little we often know about the difficulties that our patients may have at school, in terms of participation and environment but also not getting the devices or special materials that they need (to secure these much-needed resources, doctors' statements are usually accepted).

What can we learn from these three case histories? These intelligent students with visual impairments could discuss their strengths and weaknesses, and despite special needs, cause no problems in their classrooms because they use compensatory techniques. They have impaired vision but function like typical students when using their devices and special learning strategies. They are a gift to the rehabilitation services opening new windows into atypical visual functioning.

These three students also demonstrate that visual acuity does *not* alone depict visual functioning: the first student had visual acuity 0.01, used and uses techniques typical to blind students in demanding near tasks, had typical vision for orientation and moving and functioned well in daily tasks based on low but sufficient visual transfer function, contrast sensitivity. The second student had normal visual acuity but very slow development of directions and distances, spatial awareness and attention, which required years of training. The third student had visual acuity 2.0 (6/3) with single optotypes and 1.0 (6/6) with line test at distance but used CCTV and later scanned texts to read because fine grating lines could not be seen. She is a user of a dog guide because her awareness of space and recognition of landmarks did not develop. These children could describe their functions and problems clearly, which is not common in the large cohorts of children with multiple disorders affecting also use of vision. They require specific observation and testing. Young children with communication problems must be assessed using observations in clinical test situations and all functions during the day, to observe what they notice and are interested in and how they reach for objects.

Transdisciplinary assessment based on the information and questions from schools has not been earlier evaluated comparing routines from several countries. During the CVRS Conference in June 2017, the Dutch research group (Boot et al., 2017) reported their systematic review on visual dysfunctions in children with brain damage. Their conclusion was that the present status of research in the field of cerebral visual impairment (CVI) does not allow correlation between aetiology, location and perceptive visual dysfunctions in children with brain damage or a brain development disorder. A limiting factor was the small number of objective tests performed in children experiencing problems in visual processing. Based on recent insights in visual information processing, the research group recommended an alternative approach for the definition of CVI that is based on visual processing, rather than anatomical landmarks.

Clinical assessment of atypical visual functioning for education and rehabilitation

In structuring the assessment, we should keep in mind that visual disability can be due to the following:

1   *Damage to the eyes and visual pathways* that alter the quality of the visual information entering the brain. This requires many tests.
2   Children with visual processing disorders usually do not have total loss of visual processing in their hemi- or quadrant-anopias of the visual field. The damage is in the pathway between LGN, lateral geniculate nucleus and V1 area and may not affect the tectopulvinar pathway; there can be normal motion perception that normally sighted individuals depend on in their peripheral vision (Jan et al., 1987). Ophthalmology has had limited interest in motion perception when diagnosing individuals with "hemianopia" (blind in half of their Goldmann visual fields although flicker perimetry can show near normal function and these persons can have normal functioning in traffic, based on motion vision).
3   Damage to the *ocular motor functions* and *accommodation* (because near VA and glasses should be checked).
4   *Changes in the processing of visual information* in the brain, both the early processing in the occipital lobe and higher processing should be covered.

All these changes need to be considered in the assessment of visual functioning and remembered also when we discuss processing disorders because all three problems may simultaneously affect a child's functioning. Additional disorders and developmental delays can also limit use of vision.

Assessment of visual functioning of the majority of children/students with atypical vision is best based on transdisciplinary or interdisciplinary working between parents, people in care and therapies of these children and teachers and other school personnel at the local schools, the special schools' resource centres, and rehabilitation departments of hospitals where children may spend extended periods for treatment of their other disorders.

In Finland and a few German-speaking areas in Europe, we have good experiences of examinations and assessments of complex cases at special schools where teachers and therapists can arrange the time of the testing when the student is functioning well (or unusually poorly) and testing does not disturb classroom work, because the student does not travel to be tested. Ergonomics of these students are often complex and can be well arranged at schools and some homes, but seldom in hospitals. Teachers and therapists can support the student during tests, learning details about each student's examination. If videos are made, they can help to improve the later repetition of the measurements at school, so only purely medical tests are performed at the hospitals. This helps to reduce expenses, the travelling of students and improves the quality of testing. It is seldom possible to arrange calm and successful test situations in hospitals, compared to those at special schools. The information from individual test situations remains at the school and benefits all future students.

Children with motor problems, especially cerebral palsy, are one of the largest cohorts of students with visual processing disorders. It is possible that some of them can use vision well only if they stand or sit quietly, some of them cannot speak, so answering involves pointing at the correct answer. This is a technique we use in visual acuity tests systematically, although answering by naming test optotypes is still commonly used. Answering by naming adds several other functions in the test situation: remembering, knowing the correct name of the optotype, being able to say and pronounce it. Pointing must be used also in colour vision testing, which is one of the problematic tests, because the colour surfaces must not be touched. The hand/arm movements of the student may not be accurate so the student must be supported to keep the pointing safe, yet at the same time the adult must not interfere with answering. The end of the stick is covered with soft cloth and even then should not touch the colour surfaces. This type of testing has been possible only at special schools and has been presented in some training courses as a possibility for Farnsworth's colour vision test using the large test caps (Panel 16 colour vision test, Good Lite). If a student is seen to bring colourful objects close to the eye, colour information on a large area of the retina it is also tested.

Another possibility of answering in Farnsworth's test is having two sets of the test and have the row of caps in front of the student in the correct order and show the student one of the test caps at a time moving it along the test row and asking the student to say "stop" or anything he can say or give a sign to answer that the test cap is the same as a cap in the correct order line. This test situation has seen several variations at different schools.

PROCESSING OF VISUAL INFORMATION
EARLY PROCESSING
Length of lines, orientation of lines,
Perception of objects/figures against background
Visual closure, crowding effect
Stereopsis, figures in motion
Short-term memory

VENTRAL NETWORKS*
Details in pictures, noticing errors and missing details in pictures
Textures and surface qualities
Recognition of familiar and unfamiliar faces
Facial expressions, body language
Landmarks, concrete objects, pictures of concrete objects
Abstract pictures of objects of different categories
Abstract forms (Roman letters, other characters, numbers)
"Reading" series of pictures, visual problems in copying pictures
Scanning lines of text
READING uses both recognition functions and awareness of spatial structures
MATHEMATICS, recognition, memory and spatial problems in the abstract
Mathematical space (number line, pictures of three-dimensional structures)

DORSAL NETWORKS*
Perception of near and far space
Orientation in space, map-based, memorising routes
Motion perception, depth perception
Simultaneous perception and simultanagnosia
Eye–hand coordination, grasping and throwing objects
Drawing, free-hand
Copying from near/from blackboard

MIRROR NEURON SYSTEM
Early visual communication
Intuitively understanding other people's emotions and intentions
Learning movements by copying

*Ventral and dorsal networks have been called "streams", but in a stream, flow is in one direction whereas in the huge visual networks the flow is in two opposite directions. Understanding this two-way moving makes the complex visual system easier to understand: information coming from the eyes is "filtered" by the visual information coming down from the specific cortical areas. If the cortical function is atypical, even normal visual information coming from the eyes gets an unusual structure at the LGN and the child's functioning is atypical.

Schools in different countries stress observation and assessment of different visual processing functions mentioned in the lists like those in Figure 7.1. The list should cover all functions that are atypical as well as the normal functions during the observations. It is important to repeat the clinical vision tests (same tests as at the hospital) at schools to find whether the values are the same as at the hospital. If the findings are different, they should be discussed in detail, including oculomotor functions, accommodation, spectacles for distance and near testing, and ergonomics; also, the time of the day and possible effect of medications. Further, *attentional control* that selectively modulates visual information processing should be assessed (see Cases 2 and 3). Attention to information in the visual field may have small "holes" or loss of large parts of the field where attention cannot be shifted.

Clinical measurements are usually at the beginning of the Profile of Visual Functioning list (see Figure 7.1) and are explained to therapists, teachers, parents, medical specialists and their teams and psychologists. Observations on functions of ventral and dorsal networks and mirror neuron network functions, "mirroring", are agreed upon and each function is marked as "typical", "impaired but useful" or "profoundly damaged".

Young children (1–3 years) should be trained for testing, sometimes also examined for visual functioning as a part of activities in the nursery school because they often need a long time to develop the concepts required in testing at different levels. For example, when playing with the LEA Puzzle, the concept "same colour" is used in the beginning of training, then the black-and-white side and "same form". Testing visual acuity as a matching game is the only purely visual test situation. Naming adds language, vocabulary and pronunciation in the test situation and thus decreases the use of vision.

The type and role of vision loss in a child's functioning can be in part assessed by medical services, but in order to meet the needs of early intervention and education, numerous activities and tasks should be observed during therapies, early intervention activities and at local and special schools. Findings during all activities and test situations are summarised in a list. These lists are planned together with all observers and testers and final lists are unique to each child/student based on what can be tested and observed. The slots for names of functions that cannot be tested are left empty because in the future assessments they may be used. Empty slots in the profile lists are also used for unusual functions. This kind of summary list of functions shows how many more normal functions there are than impaired functions, which is important information to parents and teachers in the beginning of early intervention and a school year.

Infants and young children cannot be tested with the same tests as well-functioning school children. For them there are easier tests that do not require advanced skills in answering. Instead of usual line tests with 100% spacing, miniature line tests (LEA Symbols Crowded Symbol Book) with only three symbols on a horizontal and a vertical line, the middle optotype has the same crowding as the optotypes in a standard line test. The child must have learned the concept "centre" or "middle" for this test.

Single optotype tests like the LEA Symbols Single Symbol Book are most often used; the LEA Flash Cards are used if several types of answering must be tried and the Playing Cards and Domino Cards for near. The LEA Puzzle can be used in therapies and nursery schools as well at home and in hospitals to help young children to develop the concept "same" so that they can be tested with visual acuity tests. Names can be used when the child spontaneously has used names for the forms; these names should not be laughed at or criticised. Children should never experience failing in a test situation. For more details and basic rules on visual acuity tests, visit www.lea-test.fi.

We also need to assess nearly blind infants and children with almost no clinically measurable visual functions, except "awareness/weak response to light" and with a few motor or other disorders. We should discuss interventions to develop functions of blind infants/children and at the same time to support the use of the very limited vision. Many vision therapists use illuminated and fluorescent toys that can be used first in darkened rooms or in "black light" to increase contrast. Toys should have interesting forms and surface qualities because these infants and children depend on the tactile and haptic information of their hands. Bright colours flashing and moving as "stimulation" may startle and awaken an infant for a moment but contain nothing that could be remembered and connected to something real.

Some infants and children are likely to have visual processing disorders as a part of their severe brain damage that has caused such a delay in development that often only observations by experienced therapists and teachers can register improvement in weak visual responses. These children are blind in clinical examinations, but they may have useful vision, often visual information in motion. Observations by teachers, therapists and parents are important in the assessment of these children. Therefore, all workers need training in early intervention for blind infants as well as exposure to pleasant visual information. Infants with multiple problems should be in kangaroo care (skin- to-skin contact) when they are small infants and close to another person if they are so big that they can be on an adult's lap for only short times. To develop their awareness of social connections and skills is as important as in the care of typically developing children. Joy and warm relationships are the most important "medications" for the development of their brain and emotions. Many students at early developmental level may have nearly normal functions in a limited area.

It took Dr James Jan years to activate medical doctors to examine and assess children with other cortical processing functions than amblyopia because these problems were not included in the basic training of medical students and residents. Presently we have similar problems in the assessment of visual processing because there are misunderstandings in words. "Low vision" was introduced by Eleanor Faye, Gerard Fonda and their co-workers as the "grey area between blindness and sightedness" for adults and students whose special needs should be understood. "Low vision" contained all atypical visual functions that limited participation and learning at school. It was used in the guidelines *Management of Low Vision in Children* written in Bangkok in 1992 by the task group chosen by ICEVI and WHO and published in 1993 as guidelines for assessment of visual functioning at schools (WHO, 1993).

As we have seen in the three case histories and assessment of children with motor problems, clinical assessments should be thorough. Assessments are now often limited and misleading, visual acuity has a dominant position and grating acuity is seldom measured. Form perception at low contrast levels, i.e. contrast sensitivity, and motion perception are important functions in communication and in perceiving and recognising environment but are not measured even for traffic vision of teenage students. Visual field measurements do not test motion perception, although flicker sensitivity would be an easy test and would be especially important in hemi- and quadrantanopia that are used to limit functioning in traffic and several occupations.

Conclusion

The clinical examinations and assessments of vision should be based on information from observations of parents, care givers, therapists and teachers to help them and medical and rehabilitation specialists and ophthalmologists and optometrists to understand the child's visual functioning and to use all standard tests, including tests for early visual processing as well as higher-processing functions.

Visual acuity values should *not* be used to limit educational or medical services for students with visual processing disorders, as it is now done in many countries. Visual acuity alone does not depict quality of visual functioning. Each student's functioning, participation and environment should be thoroughly assessed to find the strengths and weaknesses of functions and available compensatory strategies.

References

Boot, F.H., Pel., J.J.M, van der Steen, J. and Evenhuis, H.M. 2017. Cerebral visual impairment: Which perceptive visual dysfunctions can be expected in children with brain damage? A systematic review. Abstract, presented at the CVRS Conference, June.

Hyvärinen, L. In press. Instructions. Accessed 15 May 2018. www.lea-test.fi.

Hyvärinen, L. and Jacob, N. 2019. *WHAT and HOW does this child see?* (2nd ed.). Helsinki, Finland: MacKeith Press.

Jan, J.E., Groenveld, M., Sykanda, A.M. and Hoyt, C.S., 1987. Behavioural characteristics of children with permanent cortical visual impairment. *Developmental Medicine & Child Neurology*, 29(5), 571–576.

Miller, M., Pasik, P. and Pasik, T. 1980. Extrageniculo-striate vision in the monkey. VII. Contrast sensitivity functions. *Journal of Neurophysiology*, 43, 1510–1526.

World Health Organization. 1993. *Management of low vision in children.* Report of a WHO consultation, Bangkok, 23–24 July 1992. Accessed 12 December. http://apps.who.int/iris/handle/10665/61105

Part III
Education

8

Trends in low vision education

Learning from the past, looking to the future

Amanda Hall Lueck and Gregory L. Goodrich

Introduction

Methods in the education of children who have low vision have changed over time. An understanding of past influences that have led to current practices in low vision education can assist in identifying essential elements that have shaped current education practices and provide insight and direction as services continue to evolve.

Definitions of terms

Definitions for low vision and partial sight have changed over time and can be different in different countries or regions.

Low vision, as used in this chapter, is a functional definition, and refers to a vision impairment that is severe enough to impede an individual's ability to learn or perform usual tasks of daily life, given that individual's level of maturity and cultural environment, but still allows some functionally useful visual discrimination. Low vision cannot be corrected to normal by regular eyeglasses or contact lenses and covers a range from mild to severe vision deficit but excludes full impairment of functional vision. The majority of persons who are legally blind are included within the low vision classification (Bailey and Hall, 1990; Lueck, 2004a; Lueck et al., 2008).

Although partial sight is synonymous with low vision in some countries or organisations (e.g. EBU, 2003; Department of Health, 2013), the terms will be differentiated in this chapter. Early educational programmes for children with "partial sight" who had sufficient functional vision to access educational materials were designed for those with milder degrees of low vision, although the precise visual acuity cut-off is not clear. Later in the twentieth century, in education settings in the United States, children with partial sight were noted to have visual acuities from 20/70 (6/21 or .54 logMAR) to better than legal blindness, which is 20/200 (6/60 or 1.00 logMAR) in the better eye with best correction in the United States. The term partial sight is no longer clearly defined in US federal education legislation although the term is mentioned within the federal regulations under the Individuals with Disabilities Education Act) (IDEA, 2004 P.L. 108–446, 34 C.F.R §300.8). As Spungin and Huebner have noted (2017), the term is no longer in general use, although, when used, it is often assumed to refer to children who are not legally blind but have limited visual acuity in the better eye with best correction.

As used in this chapter, partial sight refers to children with visual impairments who do not fall within the legal blindness category, while low vision refers to children with visual impairments who encompass the full array of functional vision including those who are legally blind with functional vision (i.e. the ability to use vision in planning and performing a task; Lueck, 2004a). This is important because many educational practices related to functional vision assessment and intervention apply to all children with low vision, including those who are legally blind with some functionally useful visual discrimination (e.g. American Printing House for the Blind, 2015; Spungin and Huebner, 2017). Children who were legally blind were not routinely provided vision instruction during the first part of the twentieth century.

A brief history of early low vision education services in the United States

Schools for the blind in the United States were initially modelled after those in Europe. Earliest schools were first established during the late 1700s and included the National Institute for Blind Youth in France c.1786 and the Liverpool School for the Indigent Blind, c.1785 in England (AFB, 2009; Historic England, 1975; Pritchard, 1963) with schools formed in Edinburgh and Bristol in 1793 and London in 1800 (Pritchard, 1963). Classes for children with functional vision came later. According to Hathaway (1932), the first European class for children with "partial sight" began in 1802 by Frans Gahels but no further details were provided. Later, recognition of the need for special schooling for children with partial sight in England (many of whom had high myopia and were enrolled in schools for the blind) led to establishment of what were called "Schools for Myopes" by James Kerr and Bishop Harman around 1908 (Pritchard, 1963). A special school was established in Germany for children with partial sight in 1907 and in Strasbourg in 1909 (Hathaway, 1932).

Special schools for children who were blind began in the United States in the 1800s. In these schools, children who were considered blind but who had available vision were taught braille. Some children with partial sight may have entered special schools where they were also taught braille but the use of vision for reading was discouraged. It is likely some of these children were visually reading the braille dots since it is reported that they were required to wear aprons and eye collars to prevent this practice (Goodrich and Huebner, 2010).

The school for "myopes" in London was visited by an American, Edwin Allen, then director of the Perkins Institute in Massachusetts. He was looking for ways to educate the children who had low vision under his care. He went on to start the first "Conservation of Vision" class in the United States in 1913 in Roxbury, Massachusetts. Another class, started by Robert Irwin in Cleveland, Ohio, followed that same year (Roberts, 1986). These programmes spread throughout the United States and Canada.

The initial classes for children with functional vision in the United States were called "Classes for Partially Seeing Children". The term "Conservation of Vision Classes" was then adopted and subsequently shortened to "Sight-Saving Classes". It was thought, at the time, that using vision would lead to further deterioration of sight, thus conservation of available vision was considered a hallmark of these classes with curricula designed to limit the use of vision while promoting auditory and tactile methods (Hatlen, 2000). Sight-saving emphasised the need to conserve vision and, according to Hathaway (1932), avoided any negative connotations associated with the term "partially seeing". Children with low vision who had learned braille were discouraged from reading the braille dots visually (Irwin, 1920).

Table 8.1 Children enrolled in sight-conservation classes in Cleveland: degree of vision of 181 children c.1920.

Degree of vision		N	%
6/9	20/30	4 (myopes)	2.2
6/12	20/40	7 (myopes)	3.8
6/15	20/50	17	9.4
6/18	20/60	14	7.7
6/21	20/70	25	13.8
6/24	20/80	24	13.2
6/30	20/100	25	13.8
6/36	20/120	26	14.3
6/60	20/200	32	17.6
5/60	20/240	6	3.3
4/60	20/300	1	.5

Source: Adapted from Irwin (1920).

In sight-saving classes, children read large print for short periods of time to "conserve" their vision. Children were either in segregated sight-saving classes or integrated primarily for oral work with typically sighted peers. Children with additional disabilities were not generally enrolled in these classes. Hathaway (1932) reports that one condition for entry was "average normal mentality".

Students enrolled in the sight-saving classes in the Cleveland Public Schools, (numbering 1 per 1,000 students) were two to three times the number of pupils who were blind in the 1920s (Irwin, 1920). Hathaway (1932), however, noted that in cities with fully developed programmes by the 1930s, the number would more likely be 1 per 500 pupils. Table 8.1 presents data provided by Irwin (1920) on the degree of vision of 181 children enrolled in early sight-conservation classes in Cleveland.

One concern for these early sight-saving classes was whether or not a child with myopia should be enrolled. That decision was thought to rest with the child's ophthalmologist who was called upon to weigh several factors that also required approval by the child's education agency: (1) the child's visual acuity – 20/70 (6/21 or .54 LogMAR) in the better eye with correction; (2) 4 or more diopters of myopia; (3) the progressive nature of the visual condition; (4) the likelihood to benefit from the sight-saving class curriculum. It was recommended that children with a visual acuity of 20/200 (6/60 or 1.00 logMAR) or less would not be able to use the equipment in a sight-saving class (Hathaway, 1932, 1933). Table 8.1, however, shows that about 20% of the children in early sight-saving classes in Cleveland had vision of 20/200 (6/60 or 1.00 logMAR) or lower, and almost a quarter of the children (23%) had visual acuities from 20/30 (6/9 or .18 logMAR) to 20/60 (6/18 or .48 logMAR).

Hathaway (1933, p. 15) states:

> It was current opinion that because of the seriously defective vision by which pupils in sight-saving classes were handicapped, they should not be educated beyond what the elementary school had to offer. For some time, so tacit was the acceptance of this opinion, that higher education for these children was not even a moot question, except to the individual teacher who saw the need for some action, especially in the case of myopic children.

Hathaway goes on to say that as individual teachers of sight-saving classes began to offer services to post-elementary school students, more formal methods were instituted to provide support for these children at higher grades. By 1933, 14 of the 48 states committed funds to the education of partially sighted children.

Curricula in the sight-saving classes, where the environment was structured to encourage ease of vision use with limited strain on the eyes, later expanded to include the teaching of reading, writing and mathematics requiring the "close use of the eyes" (Hathaway, 1932, p. 13), as well as, handwork and typewriting (which was treated as a special subject). Subjects such as geography, history, natural sciences and appreciation of music, were taken within regular education classes along with typically sighted peers, with the preparation done by a sight-saving class teacher. Aylesworth (1932) notes that lighting levels and materials were adapted to reduce strain on the eyes, and close visual work was kept to short durations of 5 to 20 minutes. Children who were legally blind with low vision were expected to learn braille and use tactile and auditory learning modes (Hatlen, 2000).

In the 1920s special university programmes with a curriculum outlined by the National Society for the Prevention of Blindness were made available for the training of teachers for children with low vision (Goodrich and Huebner, 2010). In reference to teachers in sight-saving classes, Hathaway (1933, p. 337) states that, "Above all, she should possess excellent sight, because she will be required to spend this most generously to save that of her pupils."

Throughout the first half of the twentieth century in the United States, most children with very severe visual impairments attended residential schools for the blind for their education. Children with partial sight were to be provided services in local school programmes. Hathaway, in 1932, indicated that 14 states provided financial support for these classes based upon each state's education regulations. It is unclear how extensive and consistent the curricula were for these local sight-saving classes. Moreover, children with multiple disabilities or intellectual disabilities were not enrolled in either residential schools for the blind or in local sight-saving classes.

All of this changed with several key developments, spurred by scientific findings and events surrounding two major eye diseases: retinopathy of prematurity and congenital rubella. In the 1930s, ophthalmologists reported no scientific support for the belief that the use of vision would lead to further damage to eyesight (Goodrich et al., 2008). That belief, however, persisted in the sight-saving literature. Still, the finding of no harm from using vision did lead to an increase in the use and production of large print material for children with functional vision. In the late 1940s and early 1950s, retrolental fibroplasia (RLF) (now called retinopathy of prematurity or ROP) became a major cause of visual impairment in children in the United States. The large number of children with severe visual impairment due to RLF required special education services (Silverman, 1980), but many parents did not want to send their children away from home to residential schools for the blind. This parent movement became the driving force for the development of more local school programmes to address the needs of children with severe visual impairments. However, the expansion of local school programmes did not alter the educational options for children with low vision who were legally blind. They were still expected to learn braille. Additionally, children with partial sight often received minimal specialised instruction and services, primarily through the provision of large print books and lessons in typewriting (Hatlen, 2000) even though the number of local school programmes increased.

The visual qualifications for services for children with partial sight was an issue discussed in the literature of the day. For example, one suggestion for the provision of educational services for children with partial sight was offered by Hathaway et al. (1959, p. 16) and included children who have:

- 20/70 (6/20 or 0.54 logMAR) or less visual acuity in better eye with all necessary medical and surgical treatment plus necessary lenses. "These children must have a residue of sight that makes it possible to use this as the chief avenue of approach to the brain."
- "[A] visual deviation from normal, who, in the opinion of the eye specialist, can benefit from the special education facilities provided for the partially seeing."

In addition, according to Hathaway et al. (1959, p. 16), temporary special education may be advisable for children who have:

- undergone eye operations, especially enucleation of an eye and need re-adaptation in use and psychological adjustments;
- muscle anomalies, especially strabismus, in cases in which re-education of the deviating eye and psychological adjustments are necessary.

It is worth noting that these criteria went beyond the use of visual acuity alone and did not include a definitive cut-off level for partial sight as a determinant for the need for special education related to vision when other factors indicated such services would be of benefit. It also included children who were legally blind but use vision as a primary avenue for learning. Furthermore, Winifred Hathaway, a pioneer in the education of children with low vision, noted that the legal definition of blindness in the United States is "not a useful definition of blindness from the educational viewpoint" (Hathaway et al., 1959, p. 17). She believed that many children who were legally blind should be identified as partially seeing (i.e. "low vision" in current terminology). Hathaway emphasised the importance of considering the needs of each child, along with the need to determine educational procedures by medical advisers in cooperation with educational authorities.

Into the 1960s and later, many teachers still held the belief that the use of vision for near tasks would damage eyes (Goodrich and Huebner, 2010; Hatlen, 2000). These sight-conservation beliefs were successfully challenged by the landmark work on vision utilisation by Natalie Barraga (1964), a major breakthrough in the education of children with low vision. Barraga's research showed that a period of systematic teaching of vision use (30 hours of instruction over 3 months) for children aged 6 to 13 years with low vision (20/200 [6/60 or logMAR 1.00]) to object perception in either eye) increased visual behaviours as measured by a visual discrimination scale that she created. These findings called into question the basic premise of sight-saving classes that dominated education for children with low vision in the first third of the twentieth century and continued beyond the mid-century despite medical evidence to the contrary. By presenting the opportunity to learn to use their vision, students who had no previous instruction in vision use for near work showed an increase in functional vision. Barraga's vision utilisation programme was adopted in many classrooms across the country for children with low vision (Barraga and Morris, 1980). As a secondary consequence to Barraga's work, there was renewed emphasis in the use of print of various sizes for reading for children with functional vision (Roberts, 1986).

Another key development centred on the composition of the low vision population in the 1960s due to an epidemic of congenital rubella. This led to an increase in the number of children who were deafblind due to congenital rubella syndrome. While this influx of children required special education services, available teachers of students with visual impairments were not prepared to address the special needs of these children with visual, hearing and other disabilities.

By the mid-twentieth century, the ways in which children with low vision were educated shifted due to advances in medical understanding, changes in the population of children with low vision, general education legislation that required all children to receive an education through high school (Spungin and Huebner, 2017) and advances in educational practice related to vision utilisation. Increased demands were being placed upon local school programmes, and available teachers began to add to their skills to address the intervention needs of children with low vision and children with visual impairments and multiple disabilities. Personnel preparation programmes started to address these issues in their teacher training programmes by adding new methods to deliver relevant curricula in more inclusive settings. These programmes coincided with the emergence of orientation and mobility programmes propelled, in large part, by the increasing population of adult veterans served by the government's veterans administration facilities (Goodrich and Huebner, 2010).

History of access to print enlargement systems: from standardisation to individualised options

A review of the history of print enlargement systems for children who have low vision provides some perspective into ways in which different factors have aligned to influence education practice. In the early 1900s through the 1960s, students requiring large print materials were limited to standardised print sizes used by book publishers. The most appropriate print sizes recommended for children have changed over time. Eakin and McFarland (1960), in a short history of the selection of type for early large print books, indicate that the initial large print books were created by Robert Irwin for students in the Cleveland schools in 36 point Clearface type. This type, however, was found to be too large for most students. Studies directed by Irwin from 1919 to 1920 analysed performance with 18, 24, 30 and 36 point type sizes along with tests of various spacing between letters and between lines. From the results of these studies, it was concluded that Caslon Bold 24 point type was the most effective print for production purposes for the Cleartype Series books, the most widespread large print books of their time. These books were produced for 25 years, ending in 1942.

Interest in print size standards for large print materials was renewed in the 1940s when offset lithography allowed greater ability to adjust print sizes. While the Cleartype Series books were produced with a letterpress system (i.e. typeset print) with constant type size, Stanwix House publishers, producers of a major line of large print books in the United States, began its production of Large Type Editions in 1946 using offset lithography (i.e. photographic enlargement of pages). This method was more economical, but presented a need to standardise the measurement of type that was optically enlarged. To do this, Stanwix House used the height of capital letters as the measurement base for type size determination (Eakin and McFarland, 1960).

Funded by the Act to Promote Education of the Blind of 1946 (APH, n.d.), large print books were provided free of charge to children who were legally blind in the residential schools thereby increasing the distribution and use of large print. In 1948, the American Printing House for the Blind (APH) also began producing these large print books. These became available to students enrolled in public institutions throughout the United States including local school programmes in 1956 (Hudson, personal communication, 2017; Scholl, Mulholland and Loergan, 1986). Since 2001, books produced by APH have used digital technology from electronic files, making it more feasible to produce texts in a variety of print sizes. Large print books are now available from a variety of commercial sources that also use digital technology.

Over the years, print size standards for large print production have varied. In 1965, the National Society for the Prevention of Blindness in the United States recommended 18 to 24 point type for the production of large type materials for individuals with partial sight, and in 1970, the National Accreditation Council for Agencies Serving the Blind and Visually Handicapped recommended a minimum size of 16 point for enlarged type as well as the use of 18, 20 and 24 point when appropriate (Carroll, Trautman and Collingwood, 1970). For working-age adults, Sutton (2002), in a guide developed for the American Council for the Blind, recommended that documents be enlarged to 18 point type to make them accessible to a larger number of individuals, although 14 point type was said to conform to some regulations for large type.

For schoolchildren, the American Printing House for the Blind initially printed books in 18 point, and until recently their large print books, reproduced photographically, were enlarged to 14 point type. When APH shifted to digital layout using electronically accessible textbooks, the usual type size in large print books changed back to 18 point type, although special requests for other type sizes are now accommodated (Kitchel, personal communication, 2006). In its recommendations for optimal readability, APH recommends at least 18 point type (Kitchel, n.d.), along with specifications for line and letter spacing as well as font style. Initially large print books were oversized, bulky and cumbersome (Barraga, 1983), but today's popular large print titles from major publishers often come with lighter weight paper and use of white space (i.e. reduced margins) on a page is maximised so that they more closely match the size of their regular print counterparts (GALE, 2016; Hitchner, 2016).

The need to provide enlarged type has also varied across grades in the school system. In primary grades in the United States, print size in standard textbooks is usually 16 to 18 point type and sometimes 20 point type. Enlargement, therefore, may not be needed for these materials. By the third grade in elementary school, however, the print usually gets smaller – 12 to 14 points in size. By sophomore year in high school, usual textbook print in the main sections of books is 10 to 12 point type. Therefore, the need to enlarge material becomes more common in the later grades as standard print size declines.

Standards for type size in large print textbooks have been established by many states. In California, 20 point type is considered the minimum size for the main text of state adopted textbooks for students with visual impairments from kindergarten through eighth grade (California Department of Education, 2016). Other factors besides print size were found to affect the ability to read print and ensure that students with visual impairments would be able read print optimally and to follow class assignments. Many of these are also included in the *California Guidelines for Large Print Instructional Materials* (California Department of Education, 2016) such as:

- retention of the integrity, pagination and format of every page in the original;
- removal of background material;
- use of dark, black print having good contrast;
- reversal of white text on a dark background to black on white;
- provision of headings of sufficient contrast;
- maintaining navigation cues given by headers; and
- ensuring that headings are prominent and of good contrast if they have not been converted to black.

The introduction of optical and electronic devices for reading have reduced students' reliance on standardised large print in hard copy, allowing print size to be individualised to meet the needs of each child and revolutionising reading for children who have low vision.

According to Goodrich and Sowell (1996), the increased use of low vision optical devices in the United States in the mid-twentieth century was promoted by the work of two men. William Feinbloom created a variety of low vision devices to meet the needs of his patients. Alfred Kestenbaum designed the small-diameter high-plus lens for reading for low vision patients. Around the time that low vision devices became more varied and accessible in the mid-1950s (Goodrich and Sowell, 1996), the first low vision clinics opened at the New York Lighthouse and the Industrial Home for the Blind in 1953 (Scholl et al., 1986).

Low vision optical devices were prescribed and used with schoolchildren around the same time that low vision services for adults were increasing. The use of low vision optical devices in the schools, however, was often overshadowed by the use of large print materials and, later, by newly developed closed-circuit television magnification systems (CCTVs), the first type of electronic magnification device. The initial CCTV was developed by Samuel Genensky in 1969 (Goodrich and Sowell, 1996). Since these electronic "reading machines" were able to provide very high levels of magnification, they made reading possible for many schoolchildren when available large print materials were too small for the children to decipher. They also enabled the students to read materials typically available in the classroom without the need for school staff to prepare "hard copy" enlargements ahead of time, which could be time-consuming and costly. CCTVs also allowed children to enlarge photos, diagrams and other objects thus providing access to materials beyond print and reading. The advent of the CCTV launched an era of increased print accessibility through electronic magnification for persons with visual impairments.

It is ironic that, early in the twentieth century, all students who were legally blind were encouraged to read braille, even when they had significant useful vision, while later in the century, students with low vision were encouraged to read print that was so enlarged using CCTVs that it was not possible for them to develop efficient literacy skills. As use of CCTVs spread, some children with extremely limited vision were taught to read with a CCTV system by greatly enlarging the letters on the viewing screen, thereby limiting the image on the viewing screen to one word or even only a few letters at a time. Concurrently, braille literacy was not encouraged for these students, and as a consequence, reading, for these children, was a slow and laborious process. The slow, laboured print reading speed that resulted often did not allow these students with very limited vision to develop sufficient literacy skills to maintain adequate progress in school.

The use of large print rather than braille for children with low vision was called into question in the 1990s, most notably by a major consumer organisation advocating for individuals who were blind (e.g. National Federation of the Blind, 2009) as well as education experts who concluded that access options to appropriate literacy media was lacking at that time (Committee to Develop Guidelines for Literarcy, 1991). This ignited a resurgence in instruction in braille literacy skills for students who could not read well enough to acquire effective literacy skills using regular print, large print, optical magnification or electronic magnification alone. Determination of appropriate reading media for students based upon individualised assessments is now a critical component of education programmes for students with low vision (Koenig et al., 2000). The teaching of braille literacy skills in schools has increased with renewed vigour.

The limited use of low vision optical devices in schools has also been a cause for discussion (Corn and Ryser, 1989). Efforts to encourage the use of optical devices by children with low vision in schools accelerated in the middle to late 1980s. Studies were conducted that demonstrated that the use of these devices, rather than hard copy large print, did not adversely affect reading performance and in some cases, could ultimately improve it (Lussenhop and Corn, 2002). These studies articulated advantages in the use of low vision optical devices compared to the use of large print and CCTVs for students with low vision. These included (1) cost-saving compared to the expensive CCTVs and the cost of producing large print books; (2) portability across many environments unlike standard CCTVs and bulky large print material; (3) individualised prescription of devices to meet each student's specific print size requirements as opposed to the use of hard copy large print materials produced only at pre-determined sizes for adopted textbooks and other materials; (4) greater ability to utilise typical reading material in the schools, worksite, and community and, therefore, greater ability to participate in usual activities in these varied environments; and (5) increased reading speeds with optical devices compared to large print over time for many students (Corn et al., 2003; Corn and Ryser, 1989). Methods to promote effective multidisciplinary assessments, instruction and follow-up in the use of optical devices were developed and shown to be effective (Corn et al., 2003; Cowan and Shepler, 2000a, 2000b; Kitchel, Hotta and Scott 2001; Koenig, Layton and Ross, 1992; Smith, 2004; Smith and Erin, 2002). The use of optical devices as primary modes to promote reading literacy declined with the introduction of more sophisticated and portable electronic methods of print enlargement. Children with low vision who use electronic devices such as smartphones, tablets and small portable electronic magnification devices do not stand out from their sighted peers as they did with specialised optical devices or bulky large print materials. They have also made it possible for these children to easily integrate into online social networks with peers. While the primary uses for optical devices have likely changed with the advent of e-books and portable electronic devices that provide advantages previously limited to optical reading devices, optical devices remain less expensive, less prone to breakdowns and play a major role for successful completion of specific visual tasks.

Recent methods to produce large print materials using electronic files have made it possible to produce customised large print in varying sizes, fonts and formats for standardised textbooks and individualised printed matter. Low vision optical devices have improved optics and lighting systems. New portable, handheld electronic devices for reading have been created that are lighter in weight and increasingly affordable. Improved desktop CCTV systems with simpler controls, better screen resolution, line marking systems and improved ability to vary colour and contrast, with the ability to upload electronic content are also on the market. Computer software systems used with digital textbooks have the capability to vary the characteristics of print and give consumers the means to customise print (e.g. size, colour, contrast, polarity, line spacing) and text presentation methods (e.g. a word at a time, a line at a time, continuously scrolled text or words). Portable computing tablets have been developed that enlarge and manipulate print features of electronic files or print from web pages on the Internet. Additionally, electronic devices with programmes that pair print reading with voice output are available and can assist both skilled and struggling readers who have low vision (Kamei-Hannan, Brostek Lee and Presley, 2017; Presley and D'Andrea, 2009).

Results from investigations on methods to improve reading effectiveness with respect to print size, optical device use, electronic magnification and training effects on reading performance with optical and electronic devices are being integrated into education curricula (e.g. Bailey et al., 2003; Corn, Wall and Bell, 2002; Goodrich and Kirby, 2001; Goodrich et al., 2000a, 2000b; Lovie-Kitchin et al., 1994; Lueck et al., 2003). Methods to assess print characteristics that promote optimal reading performance on an individualised basis (e.g. Ahn and Legge, 1995; Calabrese et al., 2016; Kran and Mayer, 2015; Legge et al., 1989; Lueck and Bailey, 2018; Presley and D'Andrea, 2009) have contributed to educators' ability to determine the best reading medium or media to address children's individual reading needs as part of a comprehensive learning media assessment (Koenig and Holbrook, 2005). Media alternatives may include a single medium or a combination of large print, optical magnification, electronic magnification, tactile or auditory presentations. When matching students' print reading requirements to reading mode alternatives, the selection of the optimum method for the delivery of reading material must also take into account students' cognitive and physical abilities as well as their visual capabilities and personal preferences (Lueck et al., 2001). Most importantly, the use of braille is mandated in current federal legislation for students who are blind or visually impaired unless it is determined that the use of braille or instruction in braille is not appropriate for the child now or in the future through an assessment completed by the student's instructional team (Individuals with Disabilities Education Act, 2004; Section 614 (d)(3)(B)(iii)). Thus, braille literacy skills must be promoted when it is clear that visual reading media may not adequately support the acquisition or use of literacy skills for all students with low vision.

Complex interplay of factors affecting current and future service provision

The brief historical review of educational programmes for children with low vision along with the evolution of print enlargement systems highlights a number of interconnected influences that continue to contribute to the development of services for children who have low vision. Major influences are listed in the sections that follow.

Legislative mandates

In the first three-quarters of the twentieth century, the quality and availability of programmes for children with low vision varied between individual states and in school districts within them, but this changed as federal legislation mandated more consistent and equal services across the United States (Smith, Geruschact and Huebner, 2004). In 1975, the basic right to a free, appropriate public education for all children with disabilities, along with procedural safeguards to protect these rights, were mandated with the passage of the Education for All Handicapped Children Act of 1975 (PL94–142). This led to more consistency in education programmes for children with visual impairments across the country. Additional legislation has mandated procedural safeguards to protect the right of all children to receive an education in the least restrictive environment (e.g. Individuals with Disabilities Education Act; IDEA 2004, P.L. 108–446). The make-up of the least restrictive environment has received attention from the field of visual impairment in the United States. Rather than expecting all children who have visual impairments to be fully included in general education classrooms at all times, it is currently recommended that a variety of educational setting options be made available to best address the changing needs of children with visual impairments, including those with low vision. This has led to the model that offers a continuum of service delivery alternatives in settings that range from specialised schools for the visually impaired to fully inclusive programmes with typical peers in local schools. Within this model, the type of programme required by a particular student is not fixed and can be modified as the student's identified needs change over time (California Department of Education, 2014). The visual impairment community in the United States now advocates a flexible approach to programming from least to most intensive, with no one placement more desirable than another, but determined on an individual basis (Lewis and Allman, 2017).

Curriculum guidelines

Curricular areas available to children cover a range of instructional topics. The Core Curriculum (i.e. what a student must learn by graduation from high school) is addressed as needed, but a disability-specific curriculum called the expanded core curriculum (ECC) (Hatlen, 1996) has been introduced as a critical educational component for all children with visual impairments including those with low vision. The ECC is a framework for disability-specific instruction required by students who are blind or visually impaired that was designed to address the unique disability-specific needs of each child not covered in the Core Curriculum. Areas include compensatory access (including communication), sensory efficiency, assistive technology, orientation and mobility, independent living, social interaction, recreation and leisure, career education and self-determination (Allman and Lewis, 2014a). For teachers of students with visual impairments, ways to combine the full range of disability-specific instruction with other daily programming for children with visual impairments has been encouraged (Allman and Lewis, 2014b). While the ECC presents an ideal for services, it has been noted that not all ECC areas have been routinely covered in school programmes for children with all degrees of visual impairments (Lohmeier, 2005; Wolffe et al., 2002). For children with low vision, for example, orientation and mobility instructional methods have been highly refined since this specialty was first introduced in the schools, but it has been documented that children with low vision are underserved in this area compared to students who are blind (Corn, 2007; Fazzi and Naimy, 2010; Smith et al., 2004; Wall, Emerson and Corn, 2006). Finally, functional vision assessments conducted by teachers of students with visual impairments and orientation and mobility instructors are now implemented in school programmes. Teachers have added this skill to their toolkit so that they may better understand the way students use their vision in school, home and community environments. Coupled with a comprehensive eye examination and clinical low vision evaluation, the functional vision examination provides a basis for determining appropriate programming for students who have low vision (Erin and Corn, 2010; Lueck, 2004b).

Composition of the population of children with low vision

The majority of students classified with visual impairments in schools in the United States have low vision. In addition, most children with visual impairments have multiple disabilities (Hatton, Ivy and Boyer, 2013; Kirchner and Diamant, 1999). As educators have adjusted to these population shifts, another one has occurred in recent years with the increase in children with visual impairments due to disorders of the visual brain (called cerebral/cortical visual impairment or CVI). This increase has been related to the increased survival rate of very low birth weight premature infants and improved medical care of newborns with life-threatening conditions (Dutton and Lueck, 2015). CVI is now the major cause of visual impairments in children in high-income countries and is increasing in low-income countries (Dutton and Lueck, 2015). New methods for identification, assessment and interventions are required for children with this complex condition (Lueck and Dutton, 2015; Lueck, Dutton and Chokron, in press), and these must be introduced in basic professional training programmes for a variety of service providers and in ongoing professional development programmes.

Criteria for entitlement to education services

Since the 1930s, legal blindness in the United States has been defined as 20/200 (6/60 or 1.00 logMAR) in the better eye with best correction or a visual field with a diameter not exceeding 20 degrees stemming from the American Medical Association's definition and the US federal government's social security administration regulations (Goodrich, 2015; Goodrich and Huebner, 2010). With the advent of CVI, a new category, "function at the definition of blindness", has been added to a major US federal entitlement programme that maintains a national registry for children with legal blindness. This category refers to children whose visual performance is affected by brain injury or dysfunction when visual function meets the definition of blindness (i.e. the children function at a level equivalent to those who are legally blind) as determined by an eye care specialist or neurologist (American Printing House for the Blind, 2017). Moreover, the definition of the term visual impairment for entitlement to services, based on measures of visual acuity and visual field is being questioned with respect to entitlement to education and rehabilitation services in the United States (Goodrich, 2015). Entitlement to educational services at the federal level has been based on function, without discrete visual acuity requirements as stated in the Individuals with Disabilities Education Act (IDEA, 2004 P.L. 108–446, 34 C.F.R §300.8).

In 2017, a directive from the US Office of Education (Ryder, 2017) further clarifies this functional definition of visual impairment as, "*any* impairment in vision that, *even with correction*, adversely affects a child's educational performance" (p. 2), ensuring that children with any type of uncorrectable visual condition that affects a child's performance in the education setting can receive special education. This clarification means that states in the United States who currently have entitlement programmes guidelines based on visual acuity will be required to alter these guidelines for special education related to visual impairment.

This clarification for service provision might propel yet another shift in the population of children who are determined to have visual impairments as well as the types of programmes offered in the schools. Since many of these children may have visual issues that were previously addressed by eye doctors or their support staff through vision therapy, their issues have not been addressed in traditional teacher training programmes, and they are not currently served by teachers of children with visual impairments (Lawson et al., 2017). This new directive also does not differentiate vision impairment due to ocular vs brain-based conditions. This opens the door for services for all children with CVI who cannot access educational materials through the use of vision. It remains to be seen how services for all children with visual impairments will move forward based upon this more expansive understanding of the definition of visual impairments within educational services. At this point it is unclear how programmes in the schools will be operationalised to address this directive or which specialists will be assigned as primary case managers for children with these additional medical conditions that lead to visual impairments under the expansive interpretation. School staff will require additional training to understand these conditions and the educational needs of these children in order to serve them appropriately. It is possible that current medical/educational partnerships will be reconfigured as new service paradigms are formed.

Advances in educational research related to low vision education

Intervention approaches for children with low vision have become more refined over time as new research outcomes have emerged (Erin and Corn, 2010; Lueck, 2004b). Training in visual skills, for example, has become more varied and more interwoven into real-world tasks following the original vision utilisation programme developed by Barraga in the 1960s (Barraga, 1964) and in early "visual stimulation" programmes. Vision stimulation programmes were meant for children with very severely impaired vision and involved the presentation of high-intensity visual targets to stimulate or improve sight (Bell, 1986). These were largely replaced by the introduction of more systematic programming that includes stepwise visual development goals with measurable outcomes, predominantly taught within real-world tasks (e.g. Barraga and Morris, 1980; Goetz and Gee, 1987a, 1987b; Hall and Bailey, 1989; Harrell and Akeson, 1987; Lundervald, Lewin and Irvin, 1987). Vision intervention techniques now include an array of options that can be combined to promote use of vision and access to learning such as instruction involving vision skills and behaviours, visual environmental adaptations, sensory substitutions, assistive devices and the integration of vision with other senses (Lueck, 2004b). With the proliferation of new and effective vision intervention strategies for children with low vision, both teachers of students who have visual impairments and orientation mobility specialists have had to augment their skill sets as new methods have been developed.

Technological advances and low vision education practice

Technology to improve performance outcomes and access to the general and special education curriculum has revolutionised education programming for children with low vision as it has for all children with disabilities (Presley, 2010). Rapid advances in technology have led to remarkable strides in access to instruction and social networking for students with visual impairments. To implement new technological solutions, it has been incumbent upon educators to maintain a high level of technological expertise through pre-service and in-service training approaches. As with all major changes, initial reluctance to alter accepted practice can be a factor when new skills must be acquired and the advantages of new methods are not well understood. On the other hand, technology can be very alluring, resulting in the enthusiastic adoption of technological methods without consideration of potentially negative consequences. It is, therefore, important to delineate advantages and disadvantages of technological innovations to ensure their judicial use in ways that do not disregard needed instruction in basic skills that are the backbone for learning. This was a lesson learned with the adoption of CCTV systems for reading for children with severely impaired vision that led to a decrease in critical instruction in braille literacy.

Availability of qualified teachers

Teacher availability depends upon existing funds for hiring teachers, legislation that mandates teacher qualification requirements, and the number of qualified teachers in the employment pool. Areas of instruction for children with low vision have increased over time, and education programmes have been stretched to provide sufficient support to students in schools. This has been due in large part to funding levels that have not increased to address identified curricular needs of this population, as well as the overall shortage of well-qualified teachers of students with visual impairments. Teacher shortages can be attributed, in part, to reduced funding for university personnel preparation programmes (Spungin and Huebner, 2017). In addition, qualified teachers need continuing education to have up-to-date knowledge and skills. Curricula in personnel preparation programmes for pre-service teachers and continuing education for veteran teachers require regular updates to incorporate new developments emerging from education research, medical advances, population changes and legislative mandates. Furthermore, it often takes time for new methods, ideas and policies to be adopted or implemented within the education community when they call into question earlier beliefs, methods or principles. This was seen, for example, with the long period of time it took to fully institute instructional methods that moved from sight conservation to vision utilisation. New methods or ideas require teachers to re-examine existing methods and learn new techniques that may require time and effort.

With the explosion of research in medicine, education, general special education and visual impairment education, teachers are being asked to upgrade their skills as never before. The breadth of material that teachers of children with visual impairments, including those with low vision, must cover is astounding. They must (1) provide support for the core curriculum as well as specialised instruction related to the expanded core curriculum, (2) work with a broad age range of children from birth to 22 years and (3) address the myriad concerns of diverse populations that include children with intellectual and other disabilities as well as children whose only disability is a visual one. It has become increasingly difficult for teachers to maintain and update a full repository of skills that address all the needs of the children with low vision that they serve. A chronic shortage of teachers of students with visual impairments and orientation and mobility specialists (Cross, 2016) has led to increased caseloads, creating limited time to provide services to individual children. Rather than provide direct service to many children under their care, teachers of the visually impaired often can only provide consultation service for school staff or families along with specialised materials for children. This approach is often seen as the only way to realistically meet the needs of all children on their caseload due to limited time or administrative directives. Additionally, some teachers find it necessary to pass on portions of their work to a para-educator who may not have sufficient training to effectively implement teaching strategies (Holbrook and Blankenship, 2017).

The critical and continually expanding knowledge base of educational strategies for students with low vision can improve the quality and extent of their instructional options. However, the reduced contact time available for students in many local school programmes presents a disheartening dilemma between the vast and expanding knowledge base and the limited time to implement that knowledge. Specialised programmes designed to provide intensive training related to low vision, through special master's, certificate or endorsement programmes for a variety of professionals (Goodrich and Huebner, 2010), do not generally meet licensing requirements for teachers in the schools, and therefore have not be able to add to the available pool of teachers of the visually impaired, orientation and mobility specialists or other specialised staff such as occupational therapists who work on visual skills in educational settings. While the overall needs of children with low vision are becoming more defined and detailed, due to an increasingly sophisticated practice and evidence-base, the support to address these recognised needs has not been forthcoming. This has occurred despite efforts to address the teacher shortage, expand the curricula in personnel preparation programmes and provide funding opportunities for low vision services and education (Goodrich and Huebner, 2010). In 2004, it was found that elementary school children with low vision in the United States generally did not have access to the full general education curriculum equal to their fully sighted peers nor did they receive support in the least restrictive environment, even though these principles were mandated by law and supported by national initiatives and guidelines. Much of the known information about service provision for students with low vision had not been absorbed into the knowledge base of the administrators and teachers surveyed (Smith et al., 2004). And since 2004, the amount of information teachers of the visually impaired require has skyrocketed. The trend toward limited services for students with low vision in the schools has yet to be overcome, requiring more research, funding, education of service personnel, and clarifications of guidelines for service that reach those in the field.

Conclusion

Past practices in the education of children with low vision demonstrate how methods and principles were tied to the social and scientific fabric of their time. Major breakthroughs at various junctures, derived from medical and educational discoveries, population changes, technological innovations and pioneering ideas served to propel the field beyond conventional paradigms that were accepted practice at the time. The integration of new methods into practice have been supported through additional legislation, funding for implementation, restructuring of service delivery models and policies and additions or modifications to professional training programmes. Many of the significant themes that were evident in the first part of the twentieth century also emerged in subsequent years with the specific issues within them linked to the tenor of the times. Topics in these overall themes related to the education of children with low vision have included:

- determination of the roles played by new technologies;
- considerations related to the breadth and depth of disability-specific curricula;
- availability and structure of educational placement options;
- decisions about criteria for entitlement to government and agency education services;
- changing population dynamics that necessitate revisions to education practices and existing service models;
- need for collaborative methods of assessment and intervention across key professions; and
- provision of professional training to keep up with emerging recommended practices.

Insights into the operation of forces that have driven contemporary practice through an examination of past trends can help to provide perspective and direction for the development of new systems that will lead to optimum education services for children who have low vision.

References

Ahn, S.J. and Legge, G.E. 1995. Printed cards for measuring low-vision reading speed. *Vision Research*, 35(13), 1939–1944.

Allman, C.B. and Lewis, S. 2014a. A strong foundation: The importance of the expanded core curriculum. In C.B. Allman and S. Lewis (eds), *ECC essentials: Teaching the expanded core curriculum to students with visual impairments* (pp. 15–30). New York: AFB Press.

Allman, C.B. and S. Lewis, S. (eds). 2014b. *ECC essentials: Teaching the expanded core curriculum to students with visual impairments*. New York: AFB Press.

American Foundation for the Blind. 2009. *200 years the life and legacy of Louis Braille* [e-publication]. Accessed June 2017. www.afb.org/LouisBrailleMuseum/braillegallery.asp?GalleryID=46.

American Printing House for the Blind. 2015. *Annual report 2015: Distribution of eligible students based on the federal quota census of January 4, 2014 (fiscal year 2015)* [e-publication]. Accessed July 2017. www.aph.org/federal-quota/distribution-2015.

American Printing House for the Blind. 2017. *An overview of federal quota* [e-publication]. Accessed July 2017. www.aph.org/federal-quota.

American Printing House for the Blind. n.d. *The history of the American Printing House for the Blind: A chronology* [e-publication]. Accessed August 2017. www.aph.org/about/chronology.

Aylesworth, F.A. 1932. Sight-saving classes in Toronto. *Canadian Medical Association Journal*, 27(4), 407–409.

Bailey, I.L. and Hall, A. 1990. *Visual impairment: An overview*. New York: American Foundation for the Blind.

Bailey, I.L., Lueck, A.H., Greer, R., Tuan, K.M., Bailey, V. and Dornbusch, H. 2003. Understanding the relationships between print size and reading in low vision. *Journal of Visual Impairment and Blindness*, 97(6), 325–334.

Barraga, N.C. 1964. *Increased visual behavior in low vision children*. New York: American Foundation for the Blind.

Barraga, N.C 1983. *Visual handicaps and learning*. Austin, TX: Exceptional Learning.

Barraga, N.C. and Morris, J.E. 1980. *Program to develop efficiency in visual functioning*. Louisville, KY: American Printing House for the Blind.

Bell, J. 1986. An approach to the stimulation of vision in the profoundly handicapped visually handicapped child. *British Journal of Visual Impairment*, 4(2), 46–48.

Calabrèse, A., Owsley, C., McGwin, G. and Legge, G.E. 2016. Development of a reading accessibility index using the MNREAD acuity chart. *JAMA Ophthalmology*, 134(4), 398–405.

California Department of Education. 2014. *Guidelines for programs serving students with visual impairments 2014, revised edition* [e-publication]. Sacramento, CA: author. Accessed July 2017. www.csbcde.ca.gov/Documents/VI%20Guidelines/VI_Guidelines_110314.pdf.

California Department of Education. 2016. *Guidelines for large print materials* [e-publication]. Sacramento, CA: author. Accessed July 2017. www.cde.ca.gov/re/pn/sm/lpguidelines.asp.

Carroll, T.J., Trautman, R.L. and Collingwood, H. 1970. *Standards for production of reading materials for the blind and visually handicapped*. New York: National Accreditation Council for Agencies Serving the Blind and Visually Handicapped.

Committee to Develop Guidelines for Literacy. 1991. Selecting appropriate learning media for visually handicapped students. *RE: view*, 23(2), 64–66.

Corn, A.L. 2007. On the future of the field of education of students with visual impairments. *Journal of Visual Impairment and Blindness*, 101(12), 741–743.

Corn, A.L., Bell, J.K., Andersen, E., Bachofer, C., Jose, R.T. and Perez, A.M. (2003). Providing access to the visual environment: A model of low vision services for children. *Journal of Visual Impairment and Blindness*, 97(5), 261–272.

Corn, A. and Ryser, G. 1989. Access to print for students with low vision. *Journal of Visual Impairment and Blindness*, 83(7), 340–349.

Corn, A., Wall, R. and Bell, J. 2002. Impact of optical devices on reading rates and expectations for school-age children and youth with low vision. *Visual Impairment Research*, 2(1), 33–41.

Corn, A.L., Wall, R.S., Jose, R.T., Bell, J.K., Wilcox, K. and Perez, A. 2002. An initial study of reading and comprehension rates for students receiving optical devices. *Journal of Visual Impairment and Blindness*, 96(5), 322–324.

Cowan, C. and Shepler, R. 2000a. Activities and games for teaching children to use magnifiers. In F.M. D'Andrea and C. Farrenkopf (eds), *Looking to learn: Promoting literacy for students with low vision* (pp. 167–188). New York: AFB Press.

Cowan, C. and Shepler, R. 2000b. Activities and games for teaching children to use monocular telescopes. In F.M. D'Andrea and C. Farrenkopf (eds), *Looking to learn: Promoting literacy for students with low vision* (pp. 137–166). New York: AFB Press.

Cross, F. 2016. Teacher shortage areas nationwide listing 1990–1991 through 2016–2017. US Department of Education, Office of Postsecondary Education. Accessed 23 July 2017. www2.ed.gov/about/offices/list/ope/pol/tsa.pdf.

Department of Health. 2013. *Certificate of vision impairment: Explanatory notes for consultant ophthalmologists and hospital eye clinic staff* [e-publication]. Accessed July 2017. www.gov.uk/government/publications/guidance-published-on-registering-a-vision-impairment-as-a-disability.

Dutton, G.N. and Lueck, A.H. 2015. Introduction. In A.H. Lueck and G.N. Dutton (eds), *Vision and the brain: Understanding cerebral visual impairment in children* (pp. xvii–xxi). New York: AFB Press.

Eakin, W.M. and Mcfarland, T.L. 1960. *Type, printing, and the partially seeing child*. Pittsburgh, PA: Stanwix House.

Erin, J.N. and Corn, A.E. (eds). 2010. *Foundations of low vision: Clinical and functional perspectives* (2nd ed.). New York: AFB Press.

European Blind Union Commission on Activities of Partially Sighted People. 2003. *EBU policy statement on low vision* [e-publication]. European Blind Union. Accessed July 2017. http://euroblindstatic.eplica.is/fichiersGB/pspolicy.html#32.

Fazzi, D.L. and Naimy, B.J. 2010. Orientation and mobility services for children and youths with low vision. In A.L. Corn and J.N. Erin (eds), *Foundations of low vision* (2nd ed., pp. 655–721). New York: AFB Press.

GALE. 2016. The biggest large print myths busted! [e-publication]. Accessed July 2017. http://blog.gale.com/lpmyths.

Goetz, L. and Gee, L. 1987a. Functional vision programming: A model for teaching visual behavior in natural contexts. In L. Goetz, D. Guess and K. Stremmel-Campbell (eds), *Innovative program design for individuals with dual sensory impairments* (pp. 76–97). Baltimore, MD: Paul Brookes.

Goetz, L. and Gee, K. 1987b. Teaching visual attention in functional contexts: Acquisition and generalization of complex motor skills. *Journal of Visual Impairment and Blindness*, 81(3), 115–117.

Goodrich, G.L. 2015. The evolution of the definition of legal blindness. In A.H. Lueck and G.N. Dutton (eds), *Vision and the brain: Understanding cerebral visual impairment in children* (p. 7–8). New York: AFB Press.

Goodrich, G.L., Arditi, A., Rubin, G., Keefe, J. and Legge, G.E. 2008. The low vision timeline: An inter-active history. *Visual Impairment Research*, 10(2–3), 67–75.

Goodrich, G.L. and Huebner, K.M. 2010. Low vision: A history in progress. In A.L. Corn and J.N. Erin (eds), *Foundations of low vision: Clinical and functional perspectives* (pp. 35–66). New York: AFB Press.

Goodrich, G.L. and Kirby, J. 2001. A comparison of patient reading performance and preference: Optical devices, handheld CCTV (Innoventions Magni-Cam), or stand-mounted CCTV (Optelec Clearview or TSI Genie). *Optometry*, 72(8), 519–28.

Goodrich, G.L., Kirby, J., Keswick, C., Oros, T., Wagstaff, P., Donald, B., Hazan, J. and Peters, L. 2000a. Reading, reading devices, and the low vision patient: Quantifying benefits of CCTV versus optical aids. In C.S. Stuen, A. Arditi, A. Horowitz, M.A. Lang, B. Rosenthal and K. Seidman (eds), *Vision rehabilitation: Assessment, intervention, and outcomes* (pp. 333–337). Lisse, Netherlands: Swets & Zeitlinger.

Goodrich, G.L., Kirby, J., Keswick, C., Oros, T., Wagstaff, P., Donald, B., Hazan, J. and Peters, L. 2000b. Training the patient with low vision to read: Does it significantly improve function? In C.S. Stuen, A. Arditi, A. Horowitz, M.A. Lang, B. Rosenthal and K. Seidman (eds), *Vision rehabilitation: Assessment, intervention, and outcomes* (pp. 230–236). Lise, Netherlands: Swets & Zeitlinger.

Goodrich, G.L. and Sowell, V.M. 1996. Low vision: A history. In A.L. Corn and A.J. Koenig (eds), *Foundations of low vision: Clinical and functional perspectives*. New York: AFB Press.

Hall, A. and Bailey, I.L. 1989. A model for training vision functioning. *Journal of Visual Impairment and Blindness*, 83(8) 390–396.

Harrell, L. and Akeson, N. 1987. *Preschool vision stimulation: It's more than a flashlight: Developmental perspective for visually and multiply impaired infants and preschoolers*. New York: American Foundation for the Blind.

Hathaway, W. 1932. *History and development of sight-saving classes in the United States*. Paper presented at the third annual meeting of the International Association for Prevention of Blindness, 19 November, Paris, France.

Hathaway, W. 1933. Educational opportunities in the United States for partially seeing children. *Journal of Educational Sociology*, 6(6), 331–338.

Hathaway, W., Foote, F.F., Bryan, D. and Gibbons, H. 1959. *Education and health of the partially seeing child*. New York: Columbia University Press for National Society for the Prevention of Blindness.

Hatlen, P. 1996. The core curriculum for blind and visually impaired students, including those with additional disabilities. *RE: view*, 28(1) 25–32.

Hatlen, P. 2000. Historical perspectives. In M.C. Holbrook and A.J. Koenig (eds), *Foundations of education. Volume 1: History and theory of teaching children with visual impairments* (pp. 1–54). New York: AFB Press.

Hatton, D.D., Ivy, S.E. and Boyer, C. 2013. Severe visual impairments in infants and toddlers in the United States. *Journal of Visual Impairment and Blindness*, 107(5), 325–336.

Historic England. 1975. *When was the first school for blind pupils established in Britain?* [e-publication]. Accessed July 2017. https://historicengland.org.uk/listing/what-is-designation/heritage-highlights/when-was-the-first-school-for-blind-pupils-established-in-britain.

Hitchner, A. 2016. *Spotlight on sharing: Rethinking large print*. Colorado Virtual Library [e-book]. Accessed July 2017. www.coloradovirtuallibrary.org/resourcesharing/spotlightonsharing/rethinking-large-print.

Holbrook, M.C. and Blankenship, K.E. 2017. Professional practice. In M.C. Holbrook, T. McCarthy and C. Kamei-Hannan (eds), *Foundations of education. Third edition, volume 1: History and theory of teaching children and youths with visual impairments* (pp. 322–346). New York: AFB Press.

Irwin, R.B. 1920. *Sight-saving classes in the public schools*. Harvard Bulletin VII. Cambridge, MA: Harvard University Press.

Kamei-Hannan, C., Brostek Lee, D. and Presley, I. 2017. Assistive technology. In M.C. Holbrook, T. McCarthy and C. Kamei-Hannan (eds), *Foundations of education. Third edition, volume 1: History and theory of teaching children and youths with visual impairments* (pp. 611–653). New York: AFB Press.

Kirchner, C. and Diamant, S. 1999. Estimate of number of visually impaired students, their teachers, and orientation and mobility specialists: Part 1. *Journal of Visual Impairment and Blindness*, 93(9), 600–606.

Kitchel, J.E. (n.d.). *APH guidelines for print document Design* [e-publication]. Accessed July 2017. www.aph.org/research/design-guidelines.

Kitchel, J.E., Hotta, C. and Scott, C. 2001. *Envision program*. Louisville, KY: American Printing House for the Blind.

Koenig, A.J. and Holbrook, M.C. 2005. *Leaning media assessment: A resource guide for teachers* (2nd ed.). Austin, TX: Texas School for the Blind.

Koenig, A.J., Holbrook, M.C., Corn, A.L., Depriest, L.B., Erin, J.N. and Presley, I. 2000. Specialized assessments for students with visual impairments. In A.J. Koenig and M.C. Holbrook (eds), *Foundations of education. Second edition, volume II: Instructional strategies for teaching children and youths with visual impairments* (pp. 103–153). New York: AFB Press.

Koenig, A.J., Layton, C.A. and Ross, D.B. 1992. The relative effectiveness of reading in large print and with low vision devices for students with low vision. *Journal of Visual Impairment and Blindness*, 86(1), 48–53.

Kran, B.S. and Mayer, D.L. 2015. Assessment of functional vision: Clinical assessment and suggested methods for educators. In A.H. Lueck and G.N. Dutton (eds), *Vision and the brain: Understanding cerebral visual impairment in children* (pp. 277–342). New York: AFB Press.

Lawson, H., Lueck, A.H., Moon, M. and Topor, I. 2017. *The role and training of teachers of students with visual impairment (TSVIs) as a special educator and why TSVIs do not provide vision therapy services. Low Vision Position Paper #4.* Association for the Education and Rehabilitation of the Blind and Visually Impaired [e-publication]. Accessed July 2017. https://aerbvi.org/resources/publications/position-papers.

Legge, G.E., Ross, J.A., Luebker, A. and Lamay, J.M. 1989. Psychophysics of reading VIII: The Minnesota low-vision reading test. *Optometry and Vision Science*, 66(12), 843–853.

Lewis, S. and Allman, C.B. 2017. Educational programming. In M.C. Holdbrook, T. McCarthy and C. Kamei-Hannan (eds), *Foundations of education. Third edition volume 1: History and theory of teaching children and youths with visual impairments* (pp. 280–321). New York: AFB Press.

Lohmeier, K.L. 2005. Implementing the expanded core curriculum in specialized schools for the blind. *RE: view*, 37(3), 126–133.

Lovie-Kitchin, J.E., Oliver, N.J., Bruce, A., Leighton, M.S. and Leighton, W.S. 1994. The effect of print size on reading rate for adults and children. *Clinical and Experimental Optometry*, 77(1), 2–7.

Lueck, A.H. 2004a. Comprehensive low vision care. In A.H. Lueck (ed.), *Functional vision: A practitioner's guide to evaluation and intervention* (pp. 3–24). New York: AFB Press.

Lueck, A.H. 2004b. *Functional vision: A practitioner's guide to evaluation and intervention.* New York: AFB Press.

Lueck, A. and Bailey, I.L. 2018. *Decision making guide to print size selection.* Louisville, KY: American Printing House for the Blind.

Lueck, A.H., Bailey, I.L., Greer, R., Tuan, K.M., Bailey, V. and Dornbusch, H. 2003. Exploring print-size requirements and reading for students with low vision. *Journal of Visual Impairment and Blindness*, 97(6), 335–354.

Lueck A.H., Chen, D., Kekelis L.S. and Hartmann, E. 2008. *Developmental Guidelines for infants with visual impairment: A manual for early intervention* (2nd ed.). Louisville, KY: American Printing House for the Blind.

Lueck, A.H., Dote-Kwan, J., Senge, J. and Clark, L. 2001. Selecting assistive technology for greater independence. *RE: view*, 33(1), 21–33.

Lueck, A.H. and Dutton, G.N. (eds). 2015. *Vision and the brain: Understanding cerebral visual impairment in children.* New York: AFB Press.

Lueck, A. H., Dutton, G.N. and Chokron, S. In press. Profiling children with cerebral visual impairment using multiple methods of assessment to aid in differential diagnosis. *Seminars in Pediatric Opthalmology*.

Lundervald, D., Lewin, L. and Irvin, L. 1987. Rehabilitation of visual impairments: A critical review. *Clinical Psychology Review*, 7(2), 169–185.

Lussenhop, K. and Corn, A. L. 2002. Comparative studies of the reading performance of students with low vision. *RE: view*, 34(2), 57–69.

National Federation of the Blind. 2009. *The braille literacy crisis in America: Facing the truth, reversing the trend, empowering the blind. A report to the nation by the National Federation of the Blind* [e-publication]. Accessed July 2017. https://nfb.org/images/nfb/documents/pdf/braille_literacy_report_web.pdf.

Presley, I. 2010. The impact of assistive technology assessment and instruction for children and youths with low vision. In J.N. Erin and A.E. Corn (eds), *Foundations of low vision: Clinical and functional perspectives* (2nd ed., pp. 589–654). New York: AFB Press.

Presley, I. and D'Andrea, F.M. 2009. *Assistive technology for students who are blind or visually impaired: A guide to assessment.* New York: AFB Press.

Pritchard, D.G. 1963. *Education and the handicapped child 1760–1960.* London: Routledge and Kegan Paul.

Roberts, F.K. 1986. Education for the visually handicapped: A social and educational history. In G.T. Scholl (ed.), *Foundations of education for blind and visually handicapped children and youth* (pp. 1–17). New York: AFB Press.

Ryder, R.E. 2017. *Memorandum on the eligibility determinations for children suspected of having a visual impairment including blindness under the Individuals with Disabilities Education Act.* Washington, DC: Office of Special Education Programs OSEP 17–05.

Scholl, G.T., Mulholland, M.E. and Loergan, A. 1986. Education of the visually handicapped: A selective timeline. In G.T. Scholl (ed.), *Foundations of education for blind and visually handicapped children and youth* (pp. 1–17). New York: AFB Press.

Silverman, W.A. 1980. *Retrolental fibroplasia: A modern parable.* New York: Grune & Stratton [e-publication]. Accessed July 2017. www.neonatology.org/classics/parable.

Smith, A.J., Gerushact, D. and Huebner, K.M. 2004 Policy to practice: Teachers and administrators views on curricular access by students with low vision. *Journal of Visual Impairment and Blindness*, 98(10), 612–628.

Smith, J. 2004. Teaching telescope use for school-age students, In A.H. Lueck (ed.), *Functional vision: A practitioner's guide to evaluation and intervention* [Appendix 9.2]. New York: AFB Press.

Smith, J.K. and Erin, J.N. 2002. The effects of practice with prescribed reading glasses on students with low vision. *Journal of Visual Impairment and Blindness*, 96(11), 765–782.

Spungin, S.J. and Huebner, K.M. 2017. Historic perspectives, In M.C. Holbrook, T. McCarthy and C. Kamei-Hannan (eds), *Foundations of education. Third edition volume 1: History and theory of teaching children and youths with visual impairments* (pp. 3–49). New York: AFB Press.

Sutton, J. 2002. *A guide to making documents accessible to people who are blind or visually impaired, American Council for the Blind.* Individuals with Disabilities Education Act, 20 U.S.C. § 1400 (2004) [e-publication]. Accessed July 2017. www.sabeusa.org/wp-content/uploads/2014/02/A-Guide-to-Making-Documents-Accessible-to-People-Who-are-Blind-or-Visually-Impaired.pdf.

Wall Emerson, R.S. and Corn, A.L. 2006. Orientation and mobility content for children and youths: A Delphi approach pilot study. *Journal of Visual Impairment and Blindness*, 100(6), 331–342.

Wolffe, K.E., Sacks, S.Z., Corn, A.L., Erin, J.N., Huebner, K.M. and Lewis, S. 2002. Teachers of students with visual impairments: What are they teaching? *Journal of Visual Impairment and Blindness*, 96(5), 293–304.

9

Formal and non-formal education for individuals with vision impairment or multiple disabilities and vision impairment

Current trends and challenges

Vassilios Argyropoulos and Frances Gentle

Introduction

It is evident that almost 15%, or more than 1 billion of the global population, has some type of disability or a combined set of disabilities such as physical, sensory, mental and/or developmental (WHO, 2018a). In line with the increasing number of disabilities – or at least the detected number of disabilities – several models of disability have been developed, including the medical and social-anthropological models of disability. The medical model presents and "interprets" disability as an individual "tragedy" or "bad luck"; whereas the social-anthropological model identifies disability as a social phenomenon caused by social oppression or prejudice. These models differ in terms of their respective disciplines and origins of interpretations that have led to the medicalisation or socialisation of disability respectively (Anastasiou and Kauffman, 2003; Barnes, Mercer and Shakespeare, 1999; Finkelstein, 1980; Oliver, 1990).

The disability models and their interpretations have a significant impact on ideological content and practice. However, educators and other professionals are generally less concerned about conceptual disagreements regarding the ontology of disability, and more concerned with the care and development of children and young people with disabilities who are under their care. Beaudry (2016), for example, discusses the option of a neutral concept of disability, an open-ended concept "broad enough to encompass the examination of various ethical issues (such as oppression, minority rights, or physical discomfort)" (p. 210). This type of a disability model may be the case for many professionals and practitioners because it has the potential to incorporate all contemporary trends and changes that take place in all aspects of life.

The dynamic appearance and influence of other variables that were not as evident in previous decades – such as the global humanitarian consequences of regional conflicts, natural disasters and mass human migration – are reshaping the nature of educational service delivery (Allman and Slavin, 2018). The United Nations, for example, is working with the international community to develop guidelines on inclusion of persons with disability in humanitarian action, including guidelines for education in emergencies and disaster readiness programmes in schools

(Inter-Agency Standing Committee, n.d.). New orientations and interpretations in education and values are emerging that are responsive to the diversity of cultural, religious and social backgrounds and beliefs. The emergence of formal and non-formal governmental and civil society services for persons with disabilities, the increased emphasis on bioethics, the incredible evolution of assistive technology and the updated WHO international classification of functioning, disability and health (ICF) with incorporated elements of biopsychosocial theories, will have strong impact on conceptual considerations regarding disability and inclusion (Argyropoulos and Kanari, 2015; Ouellette, 2011; Tudge et al., 2009; WHO, 2001, 2018b). It is noteworthy that within these complex social, cultural and political changes and transformations, the phenomenon of inclusion of students with disabilities in mainstream educational settings has been prioritised in many education systems across the world and is considered by policy makers as a requirement for social inclusion and cohesion. The prioritisation of disability-inclusive education is proclaimed in the United Nations Convention on the Rights of Persons with Disabilities (United Nations, 2006), and in the Education 2030 Agenda and Sustainable Development Goals (UNESCO, 2015) addressing the goal of "inclusive and equitable quality education and promoting lifelong learning opportunities for all". The United Nations and global community have established a broad range of targets and indicators to measure national progress in achieving free, equitable and quality education at all levels (primary, secondary or tertiary), including those who are considered vulnerable or at risk (e.g. persons with disabilities) by the year 2030 (UNESCO, 2015).

Individuals with vision impairment: trends, formal and non-formal education

The World Health Organization (WHO) (2018a) estimates that 285 million people are visually impaired worldwide, consisting of 39 million people who are blind and 246 million people with low vision. Although vision impairment and blindness belong to the domain of the low-incidence disabilities, WHO's estimate is substantial. The needs of the global population of people with vision impairment may fall under common categories and needs (such as the need to develop social skills and establish relationships, the usage of assistive technology, the desire for normalcy and/or the need to confront successfully all type of barriers) (Johnson-Jones, 2017), but at the same time, people with vision impairments and blindness comprise a highly heterogeneous group with a wide range of educational, developmental and physical abilities and needs, which require specialised support and services (Best, 1992; Candlin, 2003; Huebner, 2000; Scholl, 1986).

During the past three decades, there has been a dramatic increase in the number of individuals with vision impairments and additional disabilities (MDVI) within the general population of people with vision impairments. Global measures of the number of children with MDVI vary between 30% and 70% of the overall population of individuals with vision impairments (Kyriacou, Pronay and Hathazi, 2015) However, despite the growing numbers of people who are diagnosed with MDVI, there are limited case studies or projects available regarding this population.

In addition to blindness or vision impairment, a child may have such additional disabilities as cognitive, developmental, hearing, physical or mobility impairments (Hatton et al., 1997; Kyriacou et al., 2015). Every student with MDVI presents a unique educational challenge. The group of people with MDVI constitutes a distinct, diverse and heterogeneous one with a unique set of needs that are mainly associated with each individual's combination and severity of disabilities (Holbrook and Koenig, 2000).

Despite these growing numbers, a review of literature suggests there are limited published case studies or projects regarding this population. The changing distribution within the population of people with vision impairment entails different approaches to the notion of disability in terms of designing and implementing educational models with a "more inclusive character". Stangvik (2014) asserts that global polices and local values regarding persons with disabilities are "struggling" to find a balance, as global trends are increasingly having an impact on local populations. Educational settings are recognised by the global education community as places offering equal opportunities for all students to participate and learn. Current educational trends are shaped by previous trends, with consequences for students and educators alike. Changes regarding global policies, societal norms and inclusive thinking, together with technological advances in information access, have brought about corresponding changes in curricula, instructional materials, as well as in assessment and teaching methods (Nilholm, 2006; Norwich, 2002, 2008).

All the above trends and changes brought to the fore active agents of cultural and social life that contribute significantly to the process of learning through non-formal educational contexts (see Grajcevci and Shala, 2016). Examples of non-formal educational contexts include museums, cultural and environmental settings, community-based learning centres, hospitals and health clinics, whereas formal educational settings refer to structured context, such as schools, or training organisations (Norqvist and Leffler, 2017; Romi and Schmida, 2009). Learners in the broad range of non-formal educational contexts cannot be considered as a "general" or homogeneous group, but rather persons with differing needs, abilities, interests, expectations and ages; with differing social, educational, religious or ethnic backgrounds (Black, 2005; Hooper-Greenhill, 1999). The need of museums, for example, to address and develop new audiences – including audiences who are traditionally excluded, such as people with vision impairment – together with the need to build sustainable relationships with their audiences, has led museums to investigate the nature of access and existing barriers that limit access. In some museums, such as the Smithsonian Accessibility Programme in the United States, steps have been made toward a wider accessibility for people with disabilities. These steps include guidelines for an accessible environment within the framework of universal design, and the introduction of anti-discrimination legislation in different countries, for example US and UK legislation in 1990 and 1995 respectively (National Archives UK, 1995; US Congress, 1990). Legislative reforms and related research have resulted in the application of universal design principles to improve accessibility for people with disabilities (also see Australian Government AusAID, 2013).

In recent years, many non-formal educational service providers have been engaged in the process of developing a wide range of services, activities and practices, including educational programmes for school-age children, people with disabilities and other groups (e.g. elderly people), and workshops, seminars, educational material, publications, outreach programmes and loan services (UNESCO, 2016). Recognition of the heterogeneous nature of non-formal education recipients has led many non-formal education providers to redefine their relationships with their visitors and their social and educational roles in order to respond to the needs of the population and contemporary social changes (Hooper-Greenhill, 2006; Hooper-Greenhill et al., 2000).

Non-formal and formal education are conceptualised as collaborative, organised actions that shape learning networking (Colardyn and Bjornavold, 2004; Grajcevci and Shala, 2016; Romi and Schmida, 2009). However, they differ in the following two basic components:

(a) *Assessment*: formal education includes exams, tests, ongoing evaluations, whereas this is not the case for non-formal educational contexts.
(b) *Participation*: formal education generally requires compulsory attendance for a specified number of years, whereas non-formal educational activities are generally provided on an informal or voluntarily basis.

In essence, non-formal education can be considered as a complement to formal education, and both types of education aim to build fertile links between childhood and lifelong learning (Eshach, 2007; Grajcevci and Shala, 2016; Norqvist and Leffler, 2017; Romi and Schmida, 2009; UNESCO, 2015).

Hence, it appears that the notion of education has expanded in response to current technological, cultural, societal and political changes and challenges that are taking place globally.

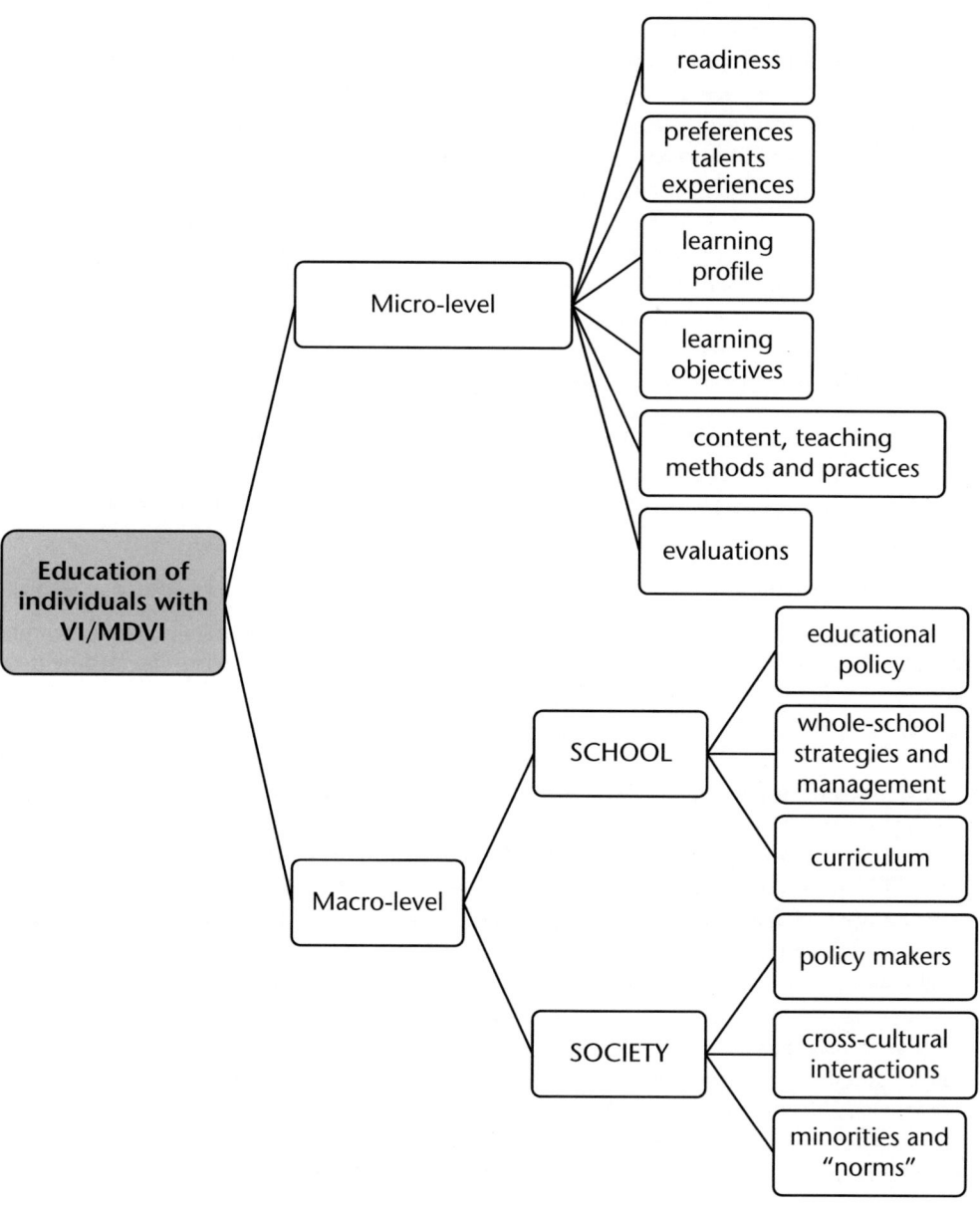

Figure 9.1 Components of micro- and macro-level approaches to formal and non-formal education of people with VI or MDVI.

These changes usually shake the edifice of educational systems, teaching methods and practices. Inclusive education is at the forefront of such global challenges as humanitarian conflict and human migration; with the United Nations and global education community working to respond to the needs of people who are confronted with discrimination or are at risk of social exclusion (UNESCO, 2015). Educational and social imbalances, lead to new directions – to new balances – such as: (a) development of new educational schemes and methods under the umbrella of formal and non-formal education (Colardyn and Bjornavold, 2004; Romi and Schmida, 2009); (b) development of collaborative networking between government, civil society and formal and non-formal education providers, such as schools and museums (Romi and Schmida, 2009; Sandell, 2003); and (c) development of new instructional and teachers' training models through bio-ecological models for human development and ethics in educational and psychological research (McLinden et al., 2016; McLinden et al., 2017; Swenson, 2007).

In this chapter, the authors explore the dimensions and qualities of education for people with vision impairment and MDVI within the contemporary scheme of formal and non-formal education. Discussion will include Rourke's (2005) stages of micro-level and macro-level approach of analysis. The micro-level approach includes actions and interactions that take place within a unit. It refers to the individual or small group of individuals (in our case persons with VI or MDVI) in a particular context (e.g. school or museum). The micro-level approach will include roles and identities under the scope of differentiated instruction (DI) and universal design for learning (UDL). The macro-level approach and analysis refers to the "global" level of interactions that take place in broader contexts and have an impact on the population being studied, for example persons with VI or MDIV. Figure 9.1 depicts roughly the components of micro- and macro-level approaches to formal and non-formal education that will be addressed in this chapter in relation to education of individuals with VI or MDVI (see Figure 9.1 on p. 121).

Micro-level approach

Formal and non-formal educational settings seem to have a pivotal role in implementing inclusive responses to the diversity of learners who have VI or MDVI. The development of collaboration and partnerships between formal and non-formal education service providers is considered significant for the evaluation and improvement of related activities, the growth in inclusive practices and the provision of opportunities for quality, equitable educational and cultural outcomes for all. In this chapter, micro-level analysis of educational services for people with VI and MDVI will be shaped by the concept of differentiated instruction (DI) and universal design for learning (UDL) principles (McGuire, Scott and Shaw, 2006; Rose and Meyer, 2006). UDL principles include the planning of instruction and accessibility options to maximise the capacity of learners to access and engage with the curriculum and teaching/learning activities (Van Garderen and Whittaker, 2006; Wehmeyer, 2006).

The spectrum of activities that are conducted by formal and non-formal education service providers resemble the qualities of differentiation and universal design for learning. Formal and non-formal approaches are closely related and depend on each other for an educational system's success (Hall, Strangman and Meyer, 2013). Research by Tomlinson and colleagues (Tomlinson, 2000; Tomlinson and Eidson, 2003; Tomlinson and Strickland, 2005), highlighted that educators and other professionals have the option to differentiate at least four elements that are based on a learner's readiness, interest and/or learning profile:

- *Content*: what the learner needs to learn or how the learner will gain access to the information.
- *Process*: activities in which the learner engages in order to make sense of the content.

- *Product*: the ways that the learner responds, rehearses, applies or extends what he or she has learned during the process.
- *Learning environment*: the way the classroom works and how teachers and students collaborate and respond to all interactions that take place during the learning activities.

All the above elements of differentiation can be incorporated in the broader concept of universal design. Implementation of the principles of universal design requires assessment and evaluation of each student's learning needs and strengths, irrespective of the environment (e.g. learning, technical, cultural, entertaining, etc.). Implementation of universal design principles in curriculum, pedagogy and teaching and learning strategies, enables educators and other professionals to respond to the widest possible audience using the minimum possible number of adaptations and with the highest possible learner access and engagement (Stephanidis et al., 1998; Tokar, 2004). Furthermore, implementation of universal design principles in terms of the learning environment and learning procedures, leads to the notion of "universal design for learning" (UDL) (Heacox, 2009). According to Heacox (2009), universal design for learning involves establishing a learner profile through formal and informal assessment, and includes evaluation of the readiness and interest of each learner. By using the principles of UDL, educators and trainers can plan a "Differentiated Learning Programme", consisting of successive stages of differentiated content, process, product and learning environment. Process and product differentiation is discussed in more detail later in this chapter. The more organised the teacher training processes are in terms of UDL, the more effective they can be in addressing participant readiness, interest and learning profile (Broderick, Mehta-Parekh and Reid, 2005; Voltz et al., 2005).

A final consideration is the research emphasis on UDL in conjunction with assistive technology and self-esteem. Such studies suggest drawing linkages with UDL when establishing syllabus frameworks and educational interventions (Murray et al., 2004; Terwel, 2005).

Differentiating the content

Touch and hearing are the primary senses that people with VI and MDVI use to access print or digital information and to acquire knowledge about attributes of the environment within which they live and interact. Recent developments in technology, including in-build accessibility options in iOS and android devices, offer the possibility of converting printed materials into such modalities as aural-audio, tactile, visual, audio-tactile and visual-audio-tactile (Brock and Jouffrais, 2015). Technology has become an enabler of "multi-sensory" learning environments through which the person is exposed to differentiated, interactive content and contexts that can be operational and functional on a stimulus-response basis. Interactivity and differentiation are predicated on systematic functional vision assessment that results in well-documented learning profiles of students' preferred sensory channels and literacy media.

Visual modalities

When content differentiation is based on visual adaptations, then a series of tasks take place in which technology has undoubtedly a pivotal role to play. Visual adaptations may be grouped into print enlargements (e.g. computer generated or photocopy enlargement) and magnification devices. Magnification devices may also be discerned in optical low vision devices and video magnifiers (e.g. closed–circuit television [CCTV]). Optical low vision devices in turn are categorised into near vision devices (e.g. illuminated and non–illuminated handheld and stand magnifiers and spectacle-mounted magnifiers) and distance vision devices (e.g. handheld monoculars, binoculars and bi-optic telescope systems or telescopes). The baseline of these devices is usually twofold; lighting improvement and contrast (Byrne et al., 2016; Corn, DePriest and Erin, 2000). Video magnifiers, such as CCTVs, constitute a special type of magnification device that can be distinguished into desktop magnifiers and portable magnifiers (Bennett, 1997; Markowitz, 2006). These devices generally render the visual content in all colours and saturations in order to produce a great variety of contrast settings (Bennett, 1997; Markowitz, 2006). In essence, content visual differentiation is based on amplification of visual information through appropriate magnification and includes degrees of flexibility in order to meet the unique visual needs and preferences of each person.

People with vision impairment will generally select the technology and optical aides that maximise the use of their vision. Eye conditions that are variable, likely to change or progressive, require careful consideration of the person's current and future needs and capabilities. Similarly, persons with fluctuating or low visual stamina may prefer to use a combination of magnification and voice output, together with braille as an additional literacy option. Presley and D'Andrea (2009) emphasise the following two major factors when assessing visual access to printed information:

1   The person's preferred working distance, that is, the distance between the reading material and the person's eyes.
2   The person's working duration, that is, the amount of time the person can read before experiencing significant visual or postural fatigue.

Presley and D'Andrea (2009) recommend measuring the person's preferred reading distances, reading speed and fluency and any physical behaviours that may result in postural or visual fatigue. Approximate oral reading rates for spot reading tasks and extended reading (e.g. 3–5 minutes of oral reading), should be measured using the person's preferred font size, font type and reading distance. The authors recommend including a broad range of print materials in the assessment process, such as newspapers and magazines, clothing tags, mathematical and prose texts.

When assessing non-readers, visual images (e.g. photographs), black and white line drawings and (if appropriate), individual letters and numbers may provide a more accurate measurement of visual abilities for reading and viewing.

Aural modalities

Another way to convert learning materials for students with VI or MDVI is to create auditory formats. Auditory adaptations make feasible the blind person's access to a vast amount and range of information. The provision of appropriate auditory materials, based on assessment of the individual's preferred learning media and use of sensory channels, is an effective method of developing listening skills and abilities. These skills serve as an additional (or alternative in case of total blindness) literacy, enabling students with VI or MDVI to keep up with their peers in the classroom (Rose and Dalton, 2006).

Auditory adaptations are feasible through the provision of auditory devices or contemporary implementations of assistive technology. The effort to provide access to aural learning material has revolved over time around the following four major approaches:

(a)   *Recording devices*, such as tape recorders, CD players, MP3 players, iPads and iPhones, which allow students to record instructional lessons and to review pre-recorded information and texts.
(b)   *Talking devices*, such as talking calculators, watches, blood measure meters and reading machines. These devices may be used in cultural centres, and include talking three-dimensional maps

that provide descriptive information for orientation. Audio information may be scripted into tactile exhibit elements in museums and art centres, which is activated according to the user's will. Hands-free auditory devices enable tactile exploration using both hands (Ziebarth, 2010).

(c) *Auditory books or digital talking books (DTBs)* are an important component of the assistive technology repertoire, and constitute the evolution from analogue cassettes to digital online formats. A very good example is the case of DAISY digital talking books. DAISY (digital accessible information system) is the published standard for formatting and converting paper-based books into the digital talking books format (Chaisanit and Suksakulchai, 2011). In addition, another example is the ePub formats (electronic publication), which constitutes a general-purpose format and can be used for many kinds of publications because it enables conversion to a range of formats. They are designed to be compatible with any e-reader that supports open formats (Junus, 2012).

(d) *Screen readers* are software that can be installed in personal computers, tablets, phones etc., and reads aloud the text that appears on the screen. In essence, screen readers transform the text on the screen into an audio modality through synthetic speech (Ashok et al., 2017; Postello and Barclay, 2012).

It is not uncommon for professionals to hear the recommendation from general educators and employers that listening to human or synthetic speech is a sufficient literacy medium for people with low vision or blindness. Such a perspective does not take into consideration the pleasure gained from immersion in the printed (or brailled) word, from reading and re-reading favourite passages from treasured novels and poetry and from exploring the visual and physical layout features of scientific, mathematical or geographical information. There is no doubt that in contemporary classrooms, boardrooms and workplaces, people with vision impairment and other print disabilities must possess the necessary knowledge and skills to listen, comprehend and respond to human, recorded or synthetic speech. Educators and other professionals play an important role in empowering people with vision impairment to effectively use their sense of hearing to access information that has not been rendered in appropriate accessible formats in education, employment and social situations.

Tactile modalities

There is currently ongoing research regarding the key functions of the sense of touch and the links between touch and patterns of conception and cognition (Argyropoulos and Chamonikolaou, 2016; Lederman and Klatzky, 2009; Robles-De-La-Torre and Hayward, 2011). In recent years, there have been dramatic developments in haptic interfaces and differentiated tactile material, and as a result, differing perspectives and theories are emerging. Several researchers, for example, have approached the study of touch and blindness from the perspective of cognitive psychological methodology (Millar, 2006, 2008), whereas others consider touch as a substitute for vision, which functions through non-visual modalities. This approach is called the sensory substitution approach (SenSub approach) and according to Renier and De Volder (2005), the substituting modalities for vision are touch and hearing (see also Zilbershtain-Kra, Arieli and Ahissar, 2015). Research has highlighted the importance of braille literacy as a pathway to higher education and employment (Wolffe and Kelly, 2011). In the United States for example, the rate of unemployment for braille literate people is 6%, as compared with an unemployment rate of 75% for people with severe vision impairment who cannot read braille (Strobel et al., 2006). Similarly, analysis of the results of a US longitudinal study of 11,270 youths with disabilities found a significant relationship between braille literacy skills during secondary schooling and post-school paid employment and higher education (Wolffe and Kelly, 2011). Tactile adaptations are common in educational settings and comprise one of the most interesting themes in research and educational practice because they trigger perceptual and cognitive mechanisms and processes (Argyropoulos and Chamonikolaou, 2016; Millar, 2006, 2008). Tactile material may be categorised as follows:

(a) *Three-dimensional objects that can be explored from all angles.* These objects can be real or products created from three-dimensional printers, for example, miniatures, replicas and molecular models (Argyropoulos and Kanari, 2015; Holbrook and Koenig, 2000).

(b) *Three-dimensional tactile models with corresponding types of topographic reliefs, for example tactile maps and sculptures* (Teshima, 2010). Fixed position maps may constitute a good example. These maps have the advantage that they can be affixed in the environment where they can be found by persons with vision loss who can then position themselves in the correct orientation. Placement on a horizontal surface provides the map reader with a real-world orientation. Maps should be large enough to provide sufficient scale for detail, but not so large that the map readers have to change their position or reorient themselves (Ziebarth, 2010).

(c) *Two-dimensional tactile figures,* for example raised-line shapes, surfaces, diagrams and graphs, including raised-line bar graphs, line graphs and pie charts that are produced using a variety of material such as swell, plastic or regular paper (Edman, 1992; Fernandes and Albuquerque, 2012).

(d) *Tactile information, including tactile books and posters.* A synthesis of tactile materials may constitute scenario or story and together support literacy instruction (Wright, 2008).

(e) *Hard copy braille* produced by braillers (i.e., braille typewriters) or by braille embossers (printers that render print text as tactile braille cells) (Best, 1992; Holbrook and Koenig, 2000. Also braille can be rendered in soft copy (digital) format by advanced technological means and read, for example, using a refreshable braille display. Such displays consist of a series of six- or eight-dot braille cells made up of small metal or plastic pins arranged in a rectangular context and in essence converts the content into braille and displays it through the pins (Quick, 2010).

All the aforementioned different types of tactile material aim at the same target; to develop tactile skills to people with VI/MDVI and thus excel their tactual perception and cognition. Individuals with vision impairment generally use a range of technology and literacy formats to access and communicate information. The choice of format and device used for any particular activity is often associated with the nature and level of complexity of the task, the presence or absence of symbols (e.g. mathematics, computing and science), the task location, time of day and the nature and severity of vision loss. McNear and Farrenkopf (2014, p. 192) recommended the use of technology devices that maximise reading and writing tactile information, with reinforcement through auditory information. The authors noted the critical importance of technology with braille input and output, with the provision of daily opportunities to read and write with braille technology in order to develop and maintain high levels of braille literacy proficiency.

Perception by touch requires many factors to be considered; and this is because there are many sources of sensation that provide information. Tactual perception is a complex process that does not encompass only touch. Instead, it has to be considered as a kind of multi-factor processing, in which touch, posture and movement are the main complementary sources. The relative balance between these sources formulates the presuppositions for spatial coding and in turn, de-coding and interpretation (i.e. apprehension) (Millar, 1997).

The multi-factor process of touch has been studied by such researchers as Katz (1989), who asserted that touch is a complex conglomeration of functions that operate in a converging manner. According to Katz, touch is not a single sense modality and it is therefore inappropriate to refer to touch as simply a skin sensation. Katz (1989) roughly divided touch into three kinds: surface, immersed and volume touch (pp. 50–52). He stressed that numerous inputs can arise from vibrations (spaced pulses), pressure (hardness or softness) or skin sensations (impressions of roughness or smoothness, wetness or dryness, hot or cold surfaces, etc.). These various qualities and attributes of touch have been explored by contemporary researchers, including Kim, Israr and Poupyrev (2013), who asserted that "Touch and gesture interactions have rapidly proliferated in recent years and have become a de facto standard in mobile phones, tablet and desktop computers" (p. 531).

Technological advances

Technological devices and applications are increasingly playing a pivotal role in education access and communication. Advances in technology are opening new avenues for research and clinical applications, and in the process, removing barriers to communication and information access for people with VI and MDVI. The development of wearable and mobile technological devices are examples of recent breakthrough technologies that have the potential to convey and transform information through accessible and complementary formats. Audio and tactile tablets are increasingly used as sources of spatial and acoustic information, while at the same time enabling users explore tactile maps with their hands (Hakobyan et al., 2013; Velázquez, 2010).

Listed below are examples of applications that assist people with VI with navigation and real-time information:

(a) *Navigation*: sonar sensors for avoiding obstacles; radio frequency for indoor localisation global system for mobile communications in order to send alerting messages to appropriate services; and global positioning systems to provide persons with vision impairment with auditory instructions to locate outdoor reference points, such as streets, intersections, addresses and public transportation (Chandana and Hemantha, 2014; Golestanian, Siva and Poellabauer, 2017; Ramadhan, 2018; Shahu and Shinko, 2017).

(b) *Obtaining real-time, audible or visual information*: radio-frequency identification (RFID) tags for identifying the colour of clothes, tracking objects, currency denominations or products in supermarkets; text readers and audible barcode scanners for reading aloud labels, documents, banknotes and images, including faces; and enhanced images by wearable electronic eyeglasses. This group of technologies enable people with VI to quickly and efficiently convert inaccessible information into their preferred visual and/or auditory formats (Hild and Cheng, 2014; Hwang and Peli, 2014; Rotolo, Hick and Martin, 2015; Sangami et al., 2015; Stinson, 2015).

Appropriate provision of differentiated material facilitates access to the curriculum and teaching/learning activities for students with vision impairments, making them more independent, engaged and included in the learning process. Equitable access for people with disabilities to the common resources of the community, including facilities, services and products relating to housing, health, rehabilitation, education, culture, vocational training, work, politics and sports), represents the essence of an open society. The ultimate objective of differentiation and universal design is to increase the quality of life of people with and without disabilities, with respect to their independence, security and dignity, decision-making and personal responsibility.

Differentiating process and product

Differentiating process

Educators and other professionals play a significant role in the process of differentiation. By providing varied options at different levels of difficulty, they respond to each student's needs, likes and dislikes and learning readiness (Tomlinson and Allan, 2000). Educators must therefore apply a plethora of processes in order to involve their students in the process of learning. Differentiated procedures may be categorised into the following two types of strategies:

(a) *Organisational*, for example, separating students into small groups, creating flexible grouping and re-grouping, providing interest centres and establishing areas/stations for inquiry-based and independent activities (Hart, 1992; Tomlinson and Allan, 2000; Tomlinson and Eidson, 2003).
(b) *Teaching or instructional*, for example, matching students' readiness, preferences, likes and dislikes to the differentiated content; using tiered activities; offering hands-on supports for those who have difficulties or disabilities; varying the length of time a student may take to complete a task; developing activities that correspond to all types of learning; and using all differentiated learning material (Hart, 1992; Tomlinson and Allan, 2000).

Differentiated procedures may seem easy to apply or to conduct when, for example, a student with blindness is enrolled in a class or participates in a museum visit. However, appearances can be deceiving. Broderick et al. (2005, p. 198) made the following interesting comment when trying to shed light on the "tricky side" of differentiated processes:

> Flexible grouping, too, encourages students to build personal connections by working with different members of the community. It also prohibits the differentiated classroom from becoming nothing more than within-class homogeneous grouping. Teachers must be certain, however, that these groupings allow disabled students to act as helper as often as they act as helpee.

Educators may find it daunting to differentiate the learning process for classes that include students with vision impairment because visual information dominates the school day. The differentiation options, described above, have to be appropriately adapted to enable the student with VI to be actively involved and engaged in the learning process. Listed below are examples of teacher actions that facilitate differentiation in formal or non-formal educational contexts when a learner with VI is enrolled:

(a) *Verbal description and modelling movements*: these actions may be extremely useful for demonstrations, lectures, board-work, and content displayed on overhead or data projectors. Verbal description, combined with appropriate movement, such as in dramatic plays or when learning songs, will help the learner who is blind to engage with the teaching and learning activities in the classroom.
(b) *Organisational and ergonomic arrangements* that maximise the student's independent access to his or her seating, materials and storage area.

(c) *Differentiation of curriculum content* and provision of appropriate alternative formats.
(d) *Provision of hands-on opportunities* that enable students with vision impairments to confidently and equitably participate in all teaching/learning processes that take place in any formal or non-formal educational contexts. Student actions to promote independence in the learning process, such as responding quickly to instructions; learning to raise his or her hand to answer aloud; moving independently in the classroom; and independently moving from the classroom to the wider school environment (Broderick et al., 2005; Castellano, 1996; Holbrook and Koenig, 2000; Tomlinson and Strickland, 2005).

Differentiating product

Product refers to the phase where students have the chance to reflect on their understanding and express required learning in their own way, for example, responses to specific stimuli or performances, speeches, or completion of reports, tests or brochures (Tomlinson and Allan, 2000). Product differentiation is of great importance because it depends heavily on the teacher's design skills and real-time management of multiple classroom activities, combined with systematic assessment that is based on students' learning profiles and interactions within educational contexts (Dillenbourg and Fischer, 2007; Tomlinson, 2014).

Since the product constitutes learners' reflections on their understanding, it is vital to offer them a broad range of possible means to present their acquired knowledge. According to Tomlinson and Allan (2003), teachers and professionals may facilitate and encourage their learners to:

(a) express what they have learned in varied ways through differentiated content, for example, oral presentations, reliefs, models, collage, tactile posters, braille texts or even through a poem or a song individually or collaboratively, puppet show, a letter or a diagram);
(b) select their own working arrangements, for example, alone, with a group, in the lab, in the classroom, in the playground or in a multi-sensory environment; and
(c) participate in a variety of assessments at varying degrees of difficulty in order to address each learner's readiness, skill levels and preferences.

Tomlinson and Eidson (2003) highlighted that products should have clearly stated, specified criteria for success, based both on students' needs and readiness. For this to be achieved, it is essential that teachers provide a flexible range of products that are responsive to learners' talents and preferences. Product differentiation should include student use of assistive technological devices and applications that enable seamless participation in education. Teachers and professionals should therefore create learning environments where all students are expected to achieve and be successful, and where students with VI can use their preferred assistive technology to show what they have learned during classes. Product selection should facilitate students' expression of their acquired knowledge and strengths, and in so doing, promote quality, inclusive and equitable learning environments (Van de Water and Rainwater, 2001).

In the case of learners with MDVI, teachers need specialised training in order to develop the required skills and understanding to develop these students' experience and interaction with the world. Learners with MDVI represent a population that requires focused education and rehabilitation assessment and services (Chen, 2006; Chen et al., 2009; Dammeyer, 2016; Rogow, 2005). Usually the products in the field of MDVI are relevant to individualised communication and literacy modes that reflect each person's level of visual function and skills in orientation and mobility, social-emotional expression, daily living and self-determination (Chen, 2006; Chen and Haney, 1995; Dammeyer and Larsen, 2016; Dietz and Ferrell, 1993; Michael and Paul, 1991; Rowland, Stillman and Mar, 2010).

In concluding this section on process and product differentiation, it is worthwhile deferring to Broderick et al. (2005), who noted that "it is not appropriate to have only one opportunity per unit to demonstrate one's knowledge. Students need many and varied smaller opportunities throughout the course of study, and having multiple opportunities for rehearsal and practice of assessment activities" (pp. 199–200).

Differentiating the learning environment

The learning environment constitutes the fourth "pillar" of differentiation. In general, learning environment components, such as rules and norms, furniture and seat arrangement, lighting, context procedures and processes, are of great importance because they constitute the determinants of functional or non-functional learning environments. The components of learning environments mould the "climate" of the educational setting, influencing such human variables as mood, attitudes, standards and tone. George (2005) and Murray et al. (2004), highlighted the following features of positive differentiation of learning environments:

(a) Availability of areas that enable learners to work quietly and without distraction, or to work in groups (e.g. teamwork or peer tutoring). Such areas may be situated in any part of the educational setting, for example, in a science lab, the library, classroom and/or playground.
(b) Clear guidelines for independent work that are based on assessment of individual learners' needs, preferences, talents and learning profiles.
(c) Flexibility in seating arrangements and use of differentiated content.
(d) Acceptance and understanding that all students must learn to work at an appropriate pace.

According to researchers and education practitioners, school and classroom environments may require minor to major adaptations to meet the learning and visual needs of students with VI or MDVI (Holbrook and Koenig, 2000). The idea of differentiating the learning environment, as was briefly described above, has nothing to do with the notion of an over-protected or sheltered environment. On the contrary, one of the basic principles of universal design refers to each person's engagement in the learning process (Arter, 1999; McGuire, Scott and Shaw, 2006). In other words, learners should not be hampered by environmental barriers or unsuitable learning environments that result in inequitable access and participation, isolation or exclusion from the learning experience of their peers. Such examples may be found in both formal and non-formal educational settings (Argyropoulos and Kanari, 2015; Arter, 1999; Barnes et al., 1999; Lewis and Taylor, 1997; Oliver, 1990; Moussouri, 2007).

When considering formal education, the following two main aspects of the learning environment of schools can be enriched through adaptations that provide students with VI or MDVI with stimulating, safe and engaging places to move and study.

Wider school environment

Usually, the wider school environment consists of many critical reference points. Students with VI or MDVI must learn the layout of the whole school environment in order to effectively apply their orientation and mobility skills. Adjustments may include highlighting reference points, for example, skirting boards that contrast with floor and wall surfaces, tactile surface indicators on the floor for use as guiding lines. Internal support columns should be painted with bright colours, for example yellow, to alert students with low vision, and floors should be carpeted or painted with different colours to separate internal spaces. Of great importance is the avoidance of overhangs and any type of protrusion, particularly on staircases and floors when these obstacles are at head height. The edges of the staircases should be highlighted using textures or bright contrasting colours (e.g. yellow) to alert the students to potential dangers. Carpeted areas also help students with orientation and mobility, however it is important to ensure that carpets remain unbroken and uncurled at the edges (Lewis and Taylor, 1997).

Lighting and noise control can be challenging issues in school environments. All areas of the school should be well illuminated and glare-free, including stairwells and corridors. Measures for keeping the noise down include the use of carpeting and soundproofing of walls. Such measures help students to develop their listening skills by using sound cues to track the location of the teacher and their schoolmates, and to make sense of what is going on around them.

Other useful cues in school environments include environmental information in clear and enlarged print and/or braille, tactile labels and audio/tactile interactive maps that can be activated by wearable or mobile technological devices. Audio/tactile cues provide the students with spatial and acoustic information while at the same time enabling them to tactually explore the interactive maps with their hands. These maps are usually made of swell paper and represent an area or a location, which can be explored by touch. In addition, these maps can also render audio output such as verbal descriptions or soundscapes of the school environment converting the whole construction into an audio/tactile map.

Finally, an appropriate general layout of the school environment is also of importance because it enables students with VI to build mental maps for efficient orientation. Lewis and Taylor (1997, p. 197) stated that

> primary schools might be arranged with a natural progression of classes according to age down a corridor or around a reception/hall area . . . [and later on] . . . in secondary schools, specialist teaching areas are easier to locate and access if they are arranged in subject clusters e.g. science/humanities/arts.

Classroom environment

Differentiation in classroom environments is often more focused on the mobility needs of students with VI, such as seating and working positions, storage of material, display of work and adaptations for such specific activities as laboratory work.

According to researchers and practitioners (Best, 1992; Lewis and Taylor, 1997), there are fundamental considerations regarding the seating and working position of a student who has vision restrictions. Addressing such issues as lighting and location can have a positive impact on class participation and content understanding of students with VI. Hence, depending on the eye condition, a student with VI may need to sit facing the front of the classroom, near the teacher's desk or close to the window or other major light source. It is important that teachers do not stand in front of windows when speaking, as bright light or glare may prevent students with VI from attending. Hence, it is vital to review clinical and functional vision assessments in order to determine each student's visual requirements.

When considering the physical work environment in the classroom, it is important that desk and work surfaces are large enough to accommodate devices such as laptops, notetakers, braillers or portable video magnifiers and also bulky braille or large-print textbooks and resources. The student's desk and chair should be at an optimum height and preferably with an adjustable top to offer the student a comfortable and adaptable seating position throughout the day. Specialist and mainstream teachers and school principals must also consider the environmental needs of students with VI and additional disabilities, for example, the need for extra space for wheeling chairs and standing frames (Salend, 2004).

Environmental adaptations may be required for science and other practical subjects. Equitable access to science laboratories for students with VI may require electrical plugs with safety handles, secure spaces for experiments with lab sinks, switches and sockets that contrast with the walls, and labelling of chemicals, etc. in the student's preferred format (large print, braille). Physical education areas and gymnasiums should be well marked and the potential for hazards minimised (e.g. isolated seats or gym equipment).

Students who have multiple disabilities may benefit from multisensory classrooms that offer a range of multisensory stimulus, for example, bubble lamps, spotlights, star panels, fibre optics, ultra-violet lights, mirror balls, nature or animal sounds, rhythmical music and stimulating textures. The aims of multisensory classrooms include orchestrating a relaxing or stimulating atmosphere, conducting assessments of sensory or cognitive functioning or motivating students according to their needs (Ferrell, Bruce and Luckner, 2014).

A differentiated learning environment is, by definition, an environment that is responsive to learners' needs (Bently et al., 2005). Furthermore, a differentiated learning environment "acts" as the means to communicate and acquire knowledge and develop skills. Research by Bently et al. (2005), emphasised the heterogeneity of learners with MDVI, and that these learners require individualised educational approaches that promote expressive and receptive communication and literacy development. Individualised approaches may include adapted materials, assistive technologies, individualised instructional strategies and multisensory approaches (Bruce, Janssen and Bashinski, 2016; Ferrell et al., 2014). Through provision of differentiated learning environments, educators and other professionals may observe, assess and create individualised communicative profiles that serve as a starting point for planning, selecting and adapting educational materials, learning environments and play activities (Pizzo and Bruce, 2010). It has been observed that when such interactions take place within responsive learning environments, learners with MDVI may develop spatiotemporal concepts and communicative representations that are associated with tactual experiences and meaning (Martens et al., 2014; Miles, 2005).

Macro-level approach

The education of students with VI or MDVI has hitherto been described and analysed through the lens of micro-level perspectives, taking into account direct instruction and universal design for learning (UDL) principles as theoretical underpinnings. The macro-level perspective, which takes into account societal and cultural contexts, contributes to a fuller, richer picture of the educational trends of students with VI or MDVI.

Two main components of the macro-level perspective are as follows:

(a) The *formal or non-formal education system* (e.g. school, museum), which may be referred to as an autonomous organisation (system) with its own values and policies. The dynamic factors, which shape the function of a school and influence its interactions with other similar systems (e.g. other schools), include its educational policy, applied strategies, school management and curriculum (see Figure 9.1). According to Druckman (2003), these dynamic school factors have a great impact on (i) the mindset of the principal and teachers; (ii) levels of collaboration within the school and with other schools; (iii) the teaching pedagogy (e.g. child-centred or teacher-centred); and (iv) the will and capacity of the school to deliver meaningful authority (e.g. school rules, policies).

From the above components, it may be conjectured that differentiated instruction, which takes place at the micro-level of the classroom, might be difficult to apply if the "school mindset" is opposite to this approach. Such factors as school policy, level of collaboration among the principal and teachers, school mindset (e.g. inclusive or segregative thinking), level of collaboration with other educational providers (formal or non-formal), are mutually dependent, macro-level components. The nature of interactions between macro-level components will have a strong impact on teaching methods and practices that take place at the micro-level level (e.g. in the classroom).

(b) *Society*: formal and non-formal education systems operate under the influence of political, economic and cultural structures and processes. For example, adoption of the social model of disability, in contrast to the individual or medical model of disability, has had a significant impact on school policies and practices with regard to children with disabilities. The medical model of disability imposes the notion of disability as an individual matter and has a great influence on the types of educational service (e.g. inclusive or segregated), and teaching practices provided to these children and their families. The medical model of disability contributes to the perpetuation of discrimination and negative stereotyping of people with disabilities, while ignoring the role of the societal beliefs in creating and perpetuating barriers that affect and shape the experience of disability. The social model of disability highlights such issues as the failure of society to respond to the needs of people with disabilities and the discriminatory barriers and impediments that limit, isolate or exclude people with disabilities from equitable participation in all aspects of society (Anastasiou and Kauffman, 2013). In the macro-level perspective, schools are addressing different facets of inclusion as they try to balance the pros and cons of the "inclusive process". Differentiation seems to constitute one of the bright avenues for accomplishing "successful inclusion" for students with disabilities, simply because it is not a static procedure. Differentiation requires active responses to the "here" and "now" and the incorporation of new or innovative elements of societal change.

Providers of non-formal educational services, for example, educational programmes in community centres or museums, have recognised that their learners (participants, audiences) are not homogeneous or "general" groups, but rather a collection of people with diverse social, educational, religious and ethnic backgrounds and diverse interests, expectations and needs (Black, 2005; Hooper-Greenhill, 1999). Museums, for example, have developed a wide range of services, activities and practices, including educational programmes for schoolchildren and community groups, workshops, seminars, educational material and publications, outreach programmes and loan services. Recognition of the heterogeneous nature of audiences, in combination with the finding that museums have for centuries addressed the needs of marginalised social groups, has led museums to redefining their relationships with their audiences and their social and educational role (Ramey-Gassert, Walberg and Walberg, 1994). As a result, museums are well positioned to contact different people and groups, and to respond to contemporary social changes. In other words, the notion of differentiation operates within the context of cultural interactions and has led museums, and other non-formal educational service providers, to build up their own networks. In so doing, museums have increased their community outreach and strengthened their ability to influence societal values and knowledge.

Finally, the macro-level perspective regarding differentiation depends on the advantages and challenges of ethnically diverse populations, and the socio-economic and political influences that shape formal and non-formal education provision. Human migration across national borders may change the status quo within a country. Minority populations bring with them different cultures and different quality-of-life perspectives about work, education, relationships and lifestyle choices. In Europe for example, great changes have taken place in social and educational service provision as a result of recent population migration. The notion of differentiation is occupying a major role in acquiring new balance in contemporary formal and non-formal educational settings (Council of Europe, 2003).

A case study

The following case study highlights the connections between micro-level processes in schools and museums and macro-levels of analysis of schools' and museums' interactions and impact on community. This example is drawn from the three-year project entitled "Bridging the Gap between Museums and Individuals with Visual Impairments" (BaGMIVI, http://bagmivi-project.eu) (Argyropoulos, Nikolaraizi, Chamonikolaou and Kanari, 2016). All project partners were involved in the field of vision disability with different occupations and duties. Specifically, 16 partners composed the consortium of this project. Four of the 12 formal partners were universities (University of Thessaly in Greece, University Babes Bolyai in Romania, University of Sofia in Bulgaria and Eotvos Lorand University in Hungary); three were non-governmental organisations (the International Council for Education and Rehabilitation of people with Visual Impairment/ICEVI-Europe, the Bulgarian Association for Education of Visually Impaired Children and the European Blind Union-EBU); four were museums and galleries (Rakursi Art Gallery in Bulgaria, Transylvanian Museum of Ethnography in Romania, Szent István Király Múseum in Hungary and Nicholas and Dolly Goulandris Foundation Museum of Cycladic Art in Greece); and one was an IT company. The last four partners were special schools for the blind and were located in Greece, Bulgaria, Romania and Hungary respectively.

The aim of this project was to support museums to develop various practices in order to enhance the access of people with vision impairments into the museums' context and content. In order to meet the objectives of the project, the researchers realised that actions had to be taken within (micro-level) and between (macro-level) the participating museums, schools and universities. Hence, it was decided to strengthen and consolidate the existing partnerships between museums (i.e. non-formal educational context) and the universities and schools that were enrolling students with VI (i.e. formal educational settings). The BaGMIVI project included the following groups of actions, which followed a chronological order:

(a) Intensive training events for museum staff members in each participating museum. The purpose of the training events was to update museum members' on the different access practices, including access differentiation and universal design approaches. The training addressed such topics as accessible cultural content, differentiated instructional approaches and educational-museum programmes (micro-level activity).

(b) Multi-level collaboration was shaped among the university faculty members (who were experts in the field of VI or MDVI), the museum members and the school-level special educators of students with VI/MDVI (macro-level activity).

(c) Teachers provided information to the museum staff regarding the characteristics of their students who had VI/MDVI, including the type of visual disability, level of cognitive skills, additional disabilities and interests (macro-level activity).

(d) The museums and special schools for the blind started to collaborate on a regular basis in order to develop the museums' differentiated educational programmes and educational materials (macro-level activity).

(e)   Development of interdisciplinary work groups, consisting of experts, artists and other professionals, who joined the network of museum members and educators, and to consult with them about the museums' educational materials (macro-level activity).

(f)   The museums and schools started to collaborate on a regular basis to organise the "when" and the "how" of museum visits for the students with VI or MDVI (macro-level activity).

(g)   The teachers "prepared the ground" with their students for the museum visits by conducting workshops and interactive games (micro-level activity).

(h)   The researchers collected reflections and feedback from the special education teachers and students with VI/MDVI about the museums' educational programmes and learning material (micro-level activity).

(i)   Ongoing contact was established between the participating museum members and the special education teachers as well as between museum staff members and the university faculty members in order to further develop the museums' educational programmes or/and undertake repeated visits (macro-level activity).

> (Argyropoulos, Nikolaraizi, Chamonikolaou and Kanari, 2016; Argyropoulos, Nikolaraizi, Kanari and Chamonikolaou, 2016; Argyropoulos, Nikolaraizi, Kanari and Chamonikolaou, 2017; Argyropoulos, Nikolaraizi, Kanari and Chamonikolaou, Plati et al., 2017)

The above case study provides evidence that the existence of a solid, collaborative network constitutes a fertile source for converging micro- and macro-level actions and outcomes. The study focused on development of networks between different systems such as schools, museums and universities. Specifically, the networks that were established led to interdisciplinary approaches, interdisciplinary working teams and collaboration between the museums and schools, resulting in the development, delivery and review of the museums' differentiated educational programmes and materials. Small-group processes that took place at a micro-level may influence the macro-level context and vice versa (Druckman, 2003). It seems that the two perspectives (micro and macro) compose an interdependent state that reflects the networked nature of our world having at its core the cause-and-effect reasoning (collaboration or conflict) among systems (Castells, 2000; Hillman, Withers and Collins, 2009; Rethemeyer and Hatmaker, 2008).

Conclusion

Exponential growth of technological innovation has raised substantially the focus on research into the impact of educational technology on information access and participation of persons with disabilities. As a result, research and innovation have influenced traditional schemes and designs for enriching and differentiating school and classroom environments and instructional practices (Ross, Morrison and Lowther, 2010). Smart devices have the potential to bridge all the gaps between users with disabilities and their needs in home, school or work settings (Frontoni et al., 2017).

It is estimated that by 2020 there will be more than 5 billion Internet users and 80 billion connected devices worldwide will be under the service of people all over the world (Statistica, n.d.). We are entering the era of smart cars, smart homes and smart schools, which will require new approaches to macro- and micro-level differentiation in employment, education and community environments.

In this chapter, the authors have explored the models of differentiated instruction (DI) and universal design for learning (UDL). These models are complementary, interrelated and theoretical foundations for analysis of formal and non-formal education systems for learners with VI or MDVI that have much in common and support one another (Hall et al., 2013). The UDL principles, in combination with DI, are increasingly used by researchers and education practitioners to design and evaluate (i) the multitude of processes that are applied during educational and social activities, and (ii) disability-inclusive pedagogy and learning materials that promote and support educational access and engagement with the learning process (Rose and Meyer, 2006). According to Tomlinson and Strickland (2005), "we are moving from one size-fits-all classrooms to classrooms that are far more personalized to address the diversity reflected in the classrooms" (p. 184). Tomlinson proposes an overarching vision about DI with UDL qualities as flexible learning environments that are "equipped" with enriched content and a plethora of teaching and instructional processes that promote learner engagement and teacher evaluation of learning (Dodge, 2005; Roe and Egbert, 2011). We are witnessing a period of educational technological transformation, which, in combination with major global societal, cultural and political forces – the so-called "mega trends" according to Singh (2012) – will have an enormous impact on inclusive education and instruction, not only for students with VI and MDVI, but for all students.

References

Allman, K.R. and Slavin, R.E. 2018. Immigration in 2018: What is a teacher educator to do? *The Teacher Educator*, 53(3), 236–243.

Anastasiou, D. and Kauffman, M. 2013. The social model of disability: Dichotomy between impairment and disability. *Journal of Medicine and Philosophy*, 38, 441–459.

Argyropoulos, V. and Chamonikolaou, S. 2016. Investigating key functions of hand movements by individuals with visual impairment: Improving instructional practices in special education through research. *Contemporary Educational Researches Journal*, 6(1), 2–10.

Argyropoulos, V. and Kanari, C. 2015. Re-imaging the museums through "touch": Reflections of individuals with visual disability on their experience of museum-visiting in Greece. *ALTER, European Journal of Disability Research*, 9, 130–143.

Argyropoulos, V., Nikolaraizi, M., Chamonikolaou, S. and Kanari, C. 2016. Museums and people with visual disability: An exploration and implementation through an Erasmus+ project. In *Proceedings of EDULEARN16 Conference* (pp. 4509–4516). Barcelona, Spain: IATED.

Argyropoulos, V., Nikolaraizi, M., Kanari, C. and Chamonikolaou, S. 2016. Education and access of students with visual disabilities to culture: Re-defining the role of museums. In M. Carmo (ed.), *Proceedings of END International Conference on Education and New Developments* (pp. 374–378). Ljubljana, Slovenia: WIARS.

Argyropoulos, V., Nikolaraizi, M., Kanari, C. and Chamonikolaou, S. 2017. Current and future trends in museums regarding visitors with disabilities: The case of visitors with visual impairments. In *Proceedings of the 9th ICEVI Europe Conference, "Empowered by Dialogue"* (pp. 32–33). ICEVI: Bruges, Belgium.

Argyropoulos, V., Nikolaraizi, M., Kanari, C., Chamonikolaou, S., Plati, M., Markou, E. and Leotsakou, B. 2017. Bridging theory and practice in developing inclusive practices in museum: The Greek case. In *Proceedings of the 9th ICEVI Europe Conference, "Empowered by Dialogue"* (pp. 40–41). ICEVI: Bruges, Belgium.

Arter, C. 1999. Environmental issues. In C. Arter, H.L. Mason, S. McCall, M. McLinden and J. Stone (eds), *Children with visual impairment in mainstream settings* (pp. 19–28). London: David Fulton.

Ashok, V., Puzis, Y., Borodin, Y. and Ramakrishnan, I. V. 2017. Web screen reading automation assistance using semantic abstraction. In *Proceedings of the 22nd International Conference on Intelligent User Interfaces, ACM IUI 17* (pp. 407–418). ACM: Limassol, Cyprus.

Australian Government AusAID. 2013, January. Accessibility design guide: Universal design principles for Australia's aid program, Registration Number 13. Accessed 7 September 2018. www.ausaid.gov.au/publications.

Barnes, C., Mercer, G. and Shakespeare, T. 1999. *Exploring disability: A sociological introduction*. Cambridge: Policy Press.

Beaudry, J.-S. 2016. Beyond (models of) disability? *Journal of Medicine and Philosophy*, 41(2), 210–228.

Bennett, D. 1997. Low vision devices for children and young people with visual impairment. In H. Mason and S. McCall (eds), *Visual impairment: Access to education for children and young people* (pp. 64–75). London: David Fulton.

Bently, I., Alcock, A., Murrain, P., McGlynn, S. and Smith, G. 2005. *Responsive environments*. Oxford: Elsevier.

Best, B.A. 1992. *Teaching children with visual impairments*. Milton Keynes, UK: Open University Press.

Black, G. 2005. *The engaging museum: Developing museums for visitor involvement*. London and New York: Routledge.

Brock, A. and Jouffrais, C. 2015. Interactive audio-tactile maps for visually impaired people. *ACM SIGACCESS Accessibility and Computing*, 113, 3–12.

Broderick, A., Mehta-Parekh, H. and Reid, D.K. 2005. Differentiating instruction for disabled students in inclusive classrooms. *Theory Into Practice*, 44(3), 194–202.

Bruce, S., Janssen, M. and Bashinski, M. 2016. Individualizing and personalizing communication and literacy instruction for children who are deafblind. *Journal of Deafblind Studies on Communication*, 2, 73–87.

Byrne, A., Corrigan, M., Knight, M. and Wright, R. 2016. A framework for introducing access technology and optical devices to students with vision impairment. In S. Silveira, F. Gentle and D. Gallimore (eds), *Vision impairment, educational principles and practice: Some fundamentals* (pp. 51–69). RIDBC Renwick Centre Monograph No. 1. New South Wales, Australia: North Rocks Press.

Candlin, F. 2003. Blindness, art and exclusion in museums and galleries. *International Journal of Art and Design Education*, 22(1), 100–110.

Castellano, C. 1996. The blind child in the regular elementary classroom. *The National Federation of the Blind Magazine for Parents and Teachers of Blind Children*, 15(3). Accessed 7 September 2018. https://nfb.org/Images/nfb/Publications/fr/fr15/Issue3/f1503tc.html.

Castells, M. 2000. *The rise of the network society* (2nd ed.). Chichester: Wiley-Blackwell.

Chaisanit, S. and Suksakulchai, S. 2011. The online participatory DAISY talking book production system (OPDAISYS): A shared information and knowledge system for print disabled students. *Journal of Engineering and Applied Sciences*, 6, 242–249.

Chandana, K. and Hemantha, G.R. 2014. Navigation for the blind using GPS along with portable camera based real time monitoring. *SSRG International Journal of Electronics and Communication Engineering*, 1, 46–50

Chen, D. 2006. *Essential elements in early intervention: Visual impairment and multiple disabilities*. New York: AFB Press.

Chen, D. and Haney, M. 1995. An early intervention model for infants who are deaf-blind. *Journal of Visual Impairment and Blindness*, 89, 213–221.

Chen, D., Rowland, C., Stillman, R. and Mar, H. 2009. Authentic practices for assessing skills of young children with sensory impairments and multiple disabilities. *Early Childhood Services*, 3(4), 323–338.

Colardyn, D. and Bjornavold, J. 2004. Validation of formal, non formal and informal learning: Policy and practices in EU member States. *European Journal of Education*, 39(1), 69–89.

Corn, A.L., DePriest, L.B. and Erin, J.N. 2000. Visual efficiency. In A.J. Koenig and M.C. Holbrook (eds), *Foundations of education* (vol. II, pp. 464–491). New York: AFB Press.

Council of Europe. 2003. Cultural diversity and minorities. Accessed 7 September 2018. https://pjp-eu.coe.int/documents/1017981/1667911/2.7.pdf/5a6e8423-45da-4f93-b7bc-514022851a16.

Dammeyer, J. 2016. Challenges and praxis in assessment of congenital deafblindness. *Journal of Deafblind Studies on Communication*, 2(1), 63–72.

Dammeyer, J. and Larsen, F.A. 2016. Communication and language profiles of children with congenital deafblindness. *British Journal of Visual Impairment*, 34(3), 214–224.

Dietz, S. and Ferrell, K.A. 1993. Early services for young children with visual impairment: From diagnosis to comprehensive services. *Infants and Young Children*, 6(1), 68–76.

Dillenbourg, P. and Fischer, F. 2007. Basics of computer-supported collaborative learning. *Zeitschrift für Berufs und Wirtschaftspädagogik*, 21, 111–130.

Dodge, J. 2005. *Differentiation in action*. New York: Scholastic.

Druckman, D. 2003. Linking micro- and macro-level processes: Interaction analysis in context. *International Journal of Conflict Management*, 14(3–4), 177–190.

Edman, P. 1992. *Tactile graphics*. New York: American Foundation for the Blind.

Eshach, H. 2007. Bridging in-school and out-of-school learning: formal, non-formal, and informal education. *Journal of Science Education and Technology*, 16(2), 171–190.

Fernandes A.M. and Albuquerque P.B. 2012. Tactual perception: A review of experimental variables and procedures. *Cognitive Processing*, 13(4), 285–301.

Ferrell, K.A., Bruce, S. and Luckner, J.L. 2014. *Evidence-based practices for students with sensory impairments.* (Document No. IC-4). Gainsville, FL: University of Florida, Collaboration for Effective Educator, Development, Accountability and Reform Center (CEEDAR).

Finkelstein, V. 1980. *Attitudes and disabled people.* New York: World Rehabilitation Fund.

Frontoni, E., Pollini, R., Russo, P., Zingaretti, P. and Cerri, G. 2017. HDOMO: Smart sensor integration for an active and independent longevity of the elderly. *Sensors*, 17(11). Accessed 7 September 2018. www.ncbi.nlm.nih.gov/pmc/articles/PMC5713030.

George, P.S. 2005. A rationale for differentiating instruction in the regular classroom. *Theory Into Practice*, 44(3), 185–193.

Golestanian, M., Siva, J. and Poellabauer, C. 2017. Radio frequency-based indoor localization. In J.H. Ortiz and A.P. De la Cruz (eds), *Ad-hoc networks* (pp. 115–136). London: IntechOpen.

Grajcevci, A. and Shala, A. 2016. Formal and non-Formal education in the new era. *Action Researcher in Education*, 7, 119–130.

Hakobyan, L., Lumsden, J., O' Sullivan, D. and Bartlett, H. 2013. Mobile assistive technologies for the visually impaired. *Survey of Ophthalmology*, 58(6), 513–528.

Hall, T., Strangman, N. and Meyer, A. 2013. *Differentiated instruction and implications for UDL implementation.* Washington, DC: National Center on Accessing the General Curriculum, US Department of Education, Office of Special Education Programs.

Hart, S. 1992. Differentiation: Way forward or retreat? *British Journal of Special Education*, 19(1), 10–12.

Hatton, D.D., Bailey, D.B., Burchinal, M.R. and Ferrell, K.A. 1997. Developmental growth curves of preschool children with visual impairments. *Child Development*, 68, 788–806.

Heacox, D. 2009. *Making differentiation a habit: How to ensure success in academically diverse classrooms.* Minneapolis, MN: Free Spirit Publishing.

Hild, M. and Cheng, F. 2014. Grasping guidance for visually impaired persons based on computed visual-auditory feedback. In *Proceedings of the 9th International Conference on Computer Vision Theory and Applications* (VISAPP-2014) (pp. 75–78). Setúbal, Portugal: Science and Technology Publications.

Hillman, A.J., Withers, M.C. and Collins, B.J. 2009. Resource dependence theory: A review. *Journal of Management*, 35(6), 1404–1427.

Holbrook, M.C. and Koenig, A.J. 2000. Basic techniques for modifying instruction. In A.J. Koenig and M.C. Holbrook (eds), *Foundations of education. Vol. II: Instructional strategies for teaching children and youths with visual impairments* (pp. 173–193). New York: AFB Press.

Hooper-Greenhill, E. 1999. Education, communication and interpretation: Towards a critical pedagogy in museums. In E. Hooper-Greenhill (ed.), *The educational role of the museum* (pp. 3–27). London: Routledge.

Hooper-Greenhill, E. 2006. The power of museum pedagogy. In H.H. Genoways (ed.), *Museum philosophy for the twenty-first century* (pp. 235–245). Lanham, MD: Altamira Press.

Hooper-Greenhill, E., Sandell, R., Moussouri, T. and O' Riain, H. 2000. *Museums and social inclusion: The GLLAM report.* Leicester: Research Centre for Museums and Galleries, Department of Museum Studies, University of Leicester. Accessed 7 September 2018. www2.le.ac.uk/departments/museumstudies/rcmg/projects/museums-and-social-inclusion-the-gllam-report/GLLAM%20Interior.pdf.

Huebner, K.M. 2000. Visual impairment. In M.C. Holbrook and A.J. Koenig (eds), *Foundations of education* (vol. I, pp. 55–76). New York: AFB Press.

Hwang, A. and Peli, E. 2014. An augmented-reality edge enhancement application for Google Glass. *Optometry and Vision Science*, 91, 1021–1030.

Inter-Agency Standing Committee. (n.d.). IASC task team on inclusion of persons with disabilities in humanitarian action. Accessed 7 September 2018. https://interagencystandingcommittee.org/iasc-task-team-inclusion-persons-disabilities-humanitarian-action.

Johnson-Jones, K.J. 2017. Educating students with visual impairments in the general education setting. Dissertation. University of Southern Mississippi. Accessed 12 January 2019. https://aquila.usm.edu/dissertations/1337.

Junus, S.G.R. 2012. E-books and e-readers for users with print disabilities. In C. Booth (ed.), *Making libraries accessible: Adaptive design and assistive technology* (pp. 22–28). Chicago, IL: ALA TechSource.

Katz, D. 1989. *The world of touch.* L.E. Krueger (ed.). Hillsdale, NJ: Lawrence Erlbaum.

Kim, S.-C, Israr, A. and Poupyrev, I. 2013. Tactile rendering of 3D features on touch surfaces. *Proceedings of the 26th ACM UIST symposium: Haptics* (pp. 531–538). St. Andrews, UK: ACM.

Kyriacou, M., Pronay, B. and Hathazi, A. 2015. *Report of the mapping exercise carried out by the commission of persons with visual impairment and additional disabilities.* EBU document. Accessed 7 September 2018. www.icevi-europe.org/files/2015/additional-disabilities.pdf.

Lederman, S. and Klatzky, R. 2009. Haptic perception: A tutorial. *Attention, Perception and Psychophysics,* 71(7), 1439–1459.

Lewis, C. and Taylor, H. 1997. The learning environment. In H. Mason and S. McCall (eds), *Visual impairment: Access to education for children and young people* (pp. 196–204). London: David Fulton.

McGuire, J.M., Scott, S.S. and Shaw, S.F. 2006. Universal design and its applications in educational environments. *Remedial and Special Education,* 27(3), 166–175.

McNear, D. and Farrenkopf, C. 2014. Assistive technology. In C.B. Allman and S. Lewis (eds), *ECC essentials: Teaching the expanded core curriculum to students with visual impairments* (pp. 187–247). New York: AFB Press.

McLinden, M., Douglas, G., Cobb, R., Hewett, R. and Ravenscroft, J. 2016. "Access to learning" and "learning to access": Analysing the distinctive role of specialist teachers of children and young people with vision impairments in facilitating curriculum access through an ecological systems theory. *British Journal of Visual Impairment,* 34(2), 177–195.

McLinden, M., Ravenscroft, J., Cobb, R., Douglas, G. and Hewitt, R. 2017. The significance of specialist teachers of learners with visual impairments as agents of change: Examining personnel preparation in the United Kingdom through a bioecological systems theory. *Journal of Visual Impairment and Blindness,* 111(6), 569–584.

Markowitz, S.N. 2006. Principles of modern low vision rehabilitation. *Canadian Journal of Ophthalmology,* 41, 289–312.

Martens, M.A.W., Janssen, M.J., Ruijssenaars, W.A.J.J.M., Huisman, M. and Riksen-Walraven, J.M. 2014. Intervening on affective involvement and expression of emotions in an adult with congenital deafblindness. *Communication Disorders Quarterly,* 36, 12–20.

Michael, M. and Paul, P. 1991. Early interventions for infants with deaf-blindness. *Exceptional Children,* 57, 200–210.

Miles, B. 2005. Literacy for persons who are deaf-blind. Accessed 10 January 2019. https://nationaldb.org/library/page/1935.

Millar, S. 1997. *Reading by touch.* London: Routledge.

Millar, S. 2006. Processing spatial information from touch and movement: implications from and for neuroscience. In M.A. Heller and S. Ballesteros (eds), *Touch and blindness* (pp. 25–48). Princeton, NJ: Lawrence Erlbaum Associates.

Millar, S. 2008. *Space and sense.* Hove, UK: Psychology Press.

Moussouri, T. 2007. Implications of the social model of disability for visitor research. *Visitor Studies,* 10(1), 90–106.

Murray, R., Shea, M., Shea, B. and Harlin, R. 2004. Issues in education: Avoiding the one-size-fits-all curriculum: Textsets, inquiry, and differentiating instruction. *Childhood Education,* 81(1), 33–35.

National Archives UK. 1995. Disability Discrimination Act (DDA). Accessed 7 September 2018. www.legislation.gov.uk/ukpga/1995/50/contents.

Nilholm, C. 2006. Special education, inclusion and democracy. *European Journal of Special Needs Education,* 21(4), 431–445.

Norqvist, L. and Leffler, E. 2017. Learning in non formal education: Is it "youthful" for youth in action? *International Review of Education, Journal of Lifelong Learning,* 63, 235–256.

Norwich, B. 2002. Education, inclusion and individual differences: Recognising and resolving dilemmas. *British Journal of Educational Studies,* 50(4), 482–502.

Norwich, B. 2008. What future for special schools and inclusion? Conceptual and professional perspectives. *British Journal of Educational Studies,* 35(3), 136–143.

Oliver, M. 1990. *The politics of disablement.* London: Palgrave Macmillan.

Ouellette, A. 2011. Toward a disability-conscious bioethics. In *Bioethics and disability: Toward a disability-conscious bioethics.* Cambridge Disability Law and Policy Series (pp. 315–366). Cambridge: Cambridge University Press.

Pizzo, L. and Bruce, S. 2010. Language and play in students with multiple disabilities and visual impairments or deaf-blindness. *Journal of Visual Impairment and Blindness,* 104(5), 287–297.

Postello, T. and Barclay, L.A. 2012. Elementary school: Developing and refining listening skills. In L. A. Barclay (ed.), *Learning to listen, listening to learn: Teaching listening skills to students with visual impairments* (pp. 104–152). New York: AFB Press.

Presley, I. and D'Andrea, F.M. 2009. *Assistive technology for students who are blind or visually impaired: A guide to assessment.* New York: AFB Press

Quick, D. 2010. Research points to full-screen braille reading possibilities. Accessed 7 September 2018. https://newatlas.com/full-screen-braille-display/14664.

Ramadhan, A.J. 2018. Wearable smart system for visually impaired people. *Sensors*, 18, 843. doi:10.3390/s18030843

Ramey-Gassert, L., Walberg, H.J. III and Walberg, H.J. 1994. Reexamining connections: Museums as science learning environments. *Science Education*, 78(4), 345–363.

Renier, L. and De Volder, A.G. 2005. Cognitive and brain mechanisms in sensory substitution of vision: A contribution to the study of human perception. *Journal of Integrative Neuroscience*, 4, 489–503.

Rethemeyer, R.K and Hatmaker, D.M. 2008. Network management reconsidered: An inquiry into management of network structures in public sector service. *Journal of Public Administration Research and Theory*, 18(4), 617–646.

Robles-De-La-Torre, G. and Hayward, V. 2011. Force can overcome object geometry in the perception of shape through active touch. *Nature*, 412, 445–448.

Roe, M.F. and Egbert, J. 2011. Four faces of differentiation: Their attributes and potential. *Childhood Education*, 87(2), 94–97.

Rogow, S. 2005, A developmental model of disabilities. *International Journal of Special Education*, 20(2), 132–135.

Romi, S. and Schmida, M. 2009. Non formal education: A major educational force in the postmodern era. *Cambridge Journal of Education*, 39(2), 257–273.

Rose, D.H. and Dalton, B. 2006. *Plato revisited: Learning through listening in the digital world.* Washington, DC: National Center on Universal Design for Learning. Accessed 7 September 2018. www.udlcenter.org/sites/udlcenter.org/files/Plato_Revisited.pdf.

Rose, D.H. and Meyer, A. (eds). 2006. *A practical reader in universal design for learning.* Cambridge, MA: Harvard Education Press.

Ross, S.M., Morrison, G.R. and Lowther, D.L. 2010. Educational technology research past and present: Balancing rigor and relevance to impact school learning. *Contemporary Educational Technology*, 1(1), 17–35.

Rotolo, D., Hick, D. and Martin, B. 2015. What is an emerging technology? *Research Policy*, 44(10), 1827–1843.

Rourke, J.T. 2005. Levels of analysis. *International politics on the world stage* (10th ed.). New York: McGraw-Hill Higher Education.

Rowland, C., Stillman, R. and Mar, H. 2010. Current assessment practices for young children who are deaf-blind. *Research and Practice in Visual Impairment and Blindness*, 3, 63–69.

Salend, S.J. 2004. *Creating inclusive classrooms: Effective and reflective practices for all students* (5th ed.). Upper Saddle River, NJ: Pearson-Prentice Hall.

Sandell, R. 2003. Social inclusion, the museum and the dynamics of sectoral change. *Museum and Society*, 1(1), 45–62.

Sangami, A., Kavithra, M., Rubina, K. and Sivaprakasam, S. 2015. Obstacle detection and location finding for blind people. *International Journal of Innovative Research in Computer and Communication Engineering*, 3, 119–123.

Scholl, G.T. 1986. What does it mean to be blind? Definitions, terminology and prevalence. In G.T. Scholl (ed.), *Foundations of education for blind and visually handicapped children and youth* (pp. 23–33). New York: American Foundation for Blind.

Shahu, D. and Shinko, I. 2017. A low-cost mobility monitoring system for visually impaired users. In *Proceedings of the International Conference on Smart Systems and Technologies* (pp. 235–238). Osijek, Croatia: IEEE.

Singh, S. 2012. *New mega trends: Implications for our future lives.* Basingstoke: Palgrave Macmillan.

Stangvik, G. 2014. Progressive special education in the neoliberal context. *European Journal of Special Needs Education*, 29(1), 91–104.

Statistica. (n.d.). *Internet of things (IoT) connected devices installed base worldwide from 2015 to 2015* (in billions). Accessed 7 September 2018. www.statista.com/statistics/471264/iot-number-of-connected-devices-worldwide.

Stephanidis, C., Salvendy, G., Akoumianakis, D., Bevan, N., Brewer, J., Emiliani, P.L., Galetsas, A., Haataja, S., Iakovidis, I., Jacko, J., Jenkins, P., Karshmer, A., Korn, P., Marcus, A., Murphy, H., Stary, C., Vanderheiden, G., Weber, G. and Ziegler, J. 1998. Toward an information society for all: An international research and development agenda. *International Journal of Human–Computer Interaction*, 10(2), 107–134.

Stinson, L. 2015. *Guiding the blind through London's subway with estimote beacons.* Accessed 7 September 2018. www.wired.com/2015/03/blind-will-soon-navigate-london-tube-beacons.

Strobel, W., Fossa, J., Arthanat, S. and Brace, J. 2006. Technology for access to text and graphics for people with visual impairments and blindness in vocational settings. *Journal of Vocational Rehabilitation*, 24, 87–95.

Swenson, E.V. 2007. Ethics of psychological research. In S.F. Davis and W. Buskist (eds), *21st century psychology: A reference handbook* (pp. 103–114). Thousand Oaks, CA: Sage.

Terwel, J. 2005. Curriculum differentiation: Multiple perspectives and developments in education. *Journal of Curriculum Studies*, 37(6), 653–670.

Teshima, Y. 2010. Three-dimensional tactile models for blind people and recognition of 3D objects by touch: Introduction to the special thematic Session. In K. Miesenberger, J. Klaus, W. Zagler and A. Karshmer (eds), *Computers helping people with special needs* (pp. 513–514). ICCHP 2010 Lecture Notes in Computer Science, 6180. Berlin, Heidelberg: Springer.

Tokar, S. 2004. Universal design in North American museums with hands-on science exhibits: A survey. *Visitor Studies Today*, 7(3), 6–10.

Tomlinson, C.A. 2000. Differentiation of instruction in the elementary grades. Eric Digest. Accessed 7 September 2018. http://ceep.crc.uiuc.edu/eecearchive/digests/2000/tomlin00.pdf.

Tomlinson, C.A. 2014. *The differentiated classroom: Responding to the needs of all learners.* Alexandria, VA: Association for Supervision and Curriculum Development.

Tomlinson, C.A. and Allan, S.D. 2000. *Leadership for differentiating schools and classrooms.* Alexandria, VA: Association for Supervision & Curriculum Development.

Tomlinson, C.A. and Eidson, C.C. 2003. *Differentiation in practice: A resource guide for differentiating curriculum, grades 5–9.* Alexandria, VA: ASCD.

Tomlinson, C.A. and Strickland, C.A. 2005. *Differentiation in practice: A resource guide for differentiating curriculum, grades 9–12.* Alexandria, VA: ASCD.

Tudge, J.R.H., Mokrova, I., Hatfield, B.E. and Karnik, R.B. 2009. Uses and misuses of Bronfenbrenner's Bioecological Theory of Human Development. *Journal of Family Theory and Review*, 1(4), 198–210.

United Nations. 2006. *Convention on the rights of persons with disabilities* (CRPD). Accessed 7 September 2018. www.un.org/development/desa/disabilities/convention-on-the-rights-of-persons-with-disabilities.html.

United Nations Educational, Scientific and Cultural Organization (UNESCO). 2015. *Education 2030: Incheon declaration and framework for action for the implementation of sustainable development goal 4.* Accessed 7 September 2018. http://uis.unesco.org/sites/default/files/documents/education-2030-incheon-framework-for-action-implementation-of-sdg4-2016-en_2.pdf.

United Nations Educational, Scientific and Cultural Organization (UNESCO). 2016. *Building knowledge societies* (pp. 84–93). Accessed 7 September 2018. http://unesdoc.unesco.org/images/0024/002448/244834e.pdf.

United States Congress. 1990. *Americans with Disabilities Act.* Accessed 7 September 2018. www.ada.gov/ada_intro.htm.

Van de Water, G.S. and Rainwater, T. 2001. *What is P–16 education? A primer for 46 legislators.* Denver, CO: Education Commission of the States.

Van Garderen, D. and Whittaker, C. 2006. Planning differentiated, multicultural instruction for secondary inclusive classrooms. *Teaching Exceptional Children*, 38, 12–20.

Velázquez, R. 2010. Wearable assistive devices for the blind. In A. Lay-Ekuakille and S.C. Mukhopadhyay (eds.), *Wearable and autonomous biomedical devices and systems for smart environment: Issues and characterization.* LNEE 75 (pp 331–349). Berlin, Heidelberg: Springer.

Voltz, D.L., Sims, M.J., Nelson, B. and Bivens, C. 2005. A framework for inclusion in the context of standards-based reform. *Teaching Exceptional Children*, 37(5), 14–19.

Wehmeyer, M.L. 2006. Universal design for learning, access to the general education curriculum, and students with mild mental retardation. *Exceptionality*, 14, 225–235.

Wolffe, K. and Kelly, S.M. 2011. Instruction in areas of the expanded core curriculum linked to transition outcomes for students with visual impairments. *Journal of Visual Impairment and Blindness*, 105(6), 340–349.

World Health Organization. 2001. *The international classification of functioning, disability and health (ICF)*. Geneva: WHO. Accessed 12 January 2019. www.who.int/classifications/icf/en.

World Health Organization. 2018a. *Disability and health*. Media Center. Accessed 7 September 2018. www.who.int/mediacentre/factsheets/fs352/en.

World Health Organization. 2018b. *International classification of functioning, disability and health*. Accessed 7 September 2018. www.who.int/classifications/icf/en.

Wright, S. 2008. *Guide to designing tactile illustrations for children's books*. Accessed 7 September 2018. www.aph.org/files/research/illustrations/illustration.pdf.

Ziebarth, B. 2010. *What visitors with vision loss want museums and parks to know about effective communication* (White paper) (pp. 1–14). Bloomington, IN: Indiana University. Accessed 7 September 2018. www.ncaonline.org/docs/effective_communication-ziebarth.pdf.

Zilbershtain-Kra, Y., Arieli, A. and Ahissar, E. 2015. Tactile substitution for vision. *Scholarpedia*, 10(4), 32457. Accessed 7 September 2018. www.scholarpedia.org/article/Tactile_Substitution_for_Vision.

10

Transition from school to higher education
Research evidence and best practice

Graeme Douglas, Rachel Hewett and Mike McLinden

Introduction

In this chapter we focus upon the transition from school for young people with vision impairment. This transition is often seen as symbolic because it reflects a step into adulthood – leaving school and entering the labour market or university (or both). It is also practically challenging because young people are moving from one context to another. Not only will physical environments change, but expectations, support and even legal rights and responsibilities will be different. For some students, it might also coincide with leaving home for the first time.

In the first section of the chapter we outline what *transition* is and why it is considered to be so important. We argue that crucial to an understanding of transition is recognising that at its core is a developing young person – before, during and after transition. Schools, communities and families play important roles in preparing young people *for* transition by developing academic and independence skills. However, it is important to recognise that as a process, learning and development will continue *after* transition too. In this section we also outline an overview of some of the challenges of the labour market and university life. This is most obviously illustrated by the poor employment outcomes for people with vision impairment observed in most industrialised countries. It is this challenging environment that heightens the importance of adequate preparation for transition.

In the next section we outline a broad framework for thinking about education with transition in mind. A broad distinction is made between "*access to learning*" and "*learning to access*". the former focuses upon inclusive practice and environmental adjustments, while the latter focuses upon developing a young person's agency and independence. It is argued that if we attend to both these educational strategies in a balanced yet *progressive* manner then transition from school into new settings can be smooth and positive. We argue that of key importance here is that education should focus upon a "balanced curriculum" throughout the school career of young people to ensure they have the educational outcomes needed to succeed in life. To ensure there is such a balance, curriculum design should acknowledge that while progress in "core" curriculum areas is important (e.g. science, maths, English, etc.), consideration also needs to be given to areas of an "expanded core curriculum" that includes independence skills (e.g. skills in mobility, self-advocacy and technology) and career education opportunities.

While the longer-term role of education in preparing young people for life after school is central to smooth and positive transition, we recognise that the process of transition from school needs specific planning and actions. In the final sections we consider some of the research evidence and specific strategies that are associated with successful transition from school. In particular we draw upon the findings of a longitudinal transitions study that has worked with young people with vision impairment in the UK. (We provide a focused example of transition to university in the UK. Other chapters in this volume provide additional information about employment, for example see Chapter 11).

Transition from school: why is it so important?

"Transition" is the term commonly used to describe the life changes that children and young people experience as they move from one educational setting to another. This may include early years to primary/elementary school, primary to secondary/high school and secondary school to work, college or university (Nasen, 2014). In this chapter we focus mainly upon the transition from secondary school. This is a particularly important transition because in many countries this phase of education signals the end of compulsory education and a shift into adulthood, including potentially having the rights and responsibilities associated with adulthood. It can therefore be a profound transition in a young person's life given that the new context in which the young person must now function will have different expectations and will assume certain skills are in place.

In order to understand transition from school, it is useful to first consider the context to which the transition is taking place. The most obvious one is employment. Labour market statistics have consistently shown that people with vision impairment have poor employment outcomes, even in comparison to other disability groups. For example, Table 10.1 presents figures from two UK studies that show that employment rates for those with vision impairment are considerably lower than those for their sighted peers. More specifically, in relation to younger people with vision impairment, Hewett and Keil (2015) estimated that 42.8% aged 16–25 are not in employment, education or training (NEET) compared to 21.7% of 16–25-year-olds from the general population. Similar patterns have been found in other countries (e.g. Capella McDonnall, 2011).

More positively, when analysing the employment outcomes of over 1,000 people with vision impairment, Pavey, Douglas and Corcoran (2008) found that employment rates were slightly higher for people who had experienced vision impairment in childhood. This suggests an education effect; that the interventions made when young people with vision impairment are in school can have a positive impact on their outcomes in adulthood. Table 10.1 illustrates that while there is considerable disparity in employment rates between those with vision impairment and the general population, this disparity narrows as an individual's level of education increases – in fact Clements, Douglas and Pavey (2011) found that educational attainment (i.e. as measured by formal academic qualifications) was the single most significant predictor of employment in their sample of people with vision impairment.

The significance of educational attainment highlights the importance of young people with vision impairment maximising their academic qualifications, including progressing into higher education if they should wish to do so. Nevertheless, there is a range of other factors that will enable successful transition.

An important starting point in considering transition from school will therefore involve an analysis of the *resources* and *enablers* that are available to young people to help them succeed in

Table 10.1 Comparison of UK employment rates between people registered as having a vision impairment, who identify as long-term disabled with a seeing difficulty and the whole population by education level (various sources).

Group (source)	Degree or above (%)	A-level and below degree level (%)	GCSE level and other (%)	No qualification (%)	Total weighted (%)
Registered as having a vision impairment (Clements et al., 2011)	59	40	27	16	33
Self-identified as long-term disabled with a seeing difficulty (Hewett and Keil, 2016)	64	58	44	14	45
Employment for whole population (Hewett and Keil, 2016)	84	76	69	40	72

a given educational context. The challenge of ensuring there is a successful transition is that the expectations and availability of these resources is different in schools, higher education and work. Focusing upon the UK as an illustrative case, Table 10.2 presents examples of these differences for the three different contexts. The analysis makes a distinction between four types of resource that can enable people with vision impairment:

- *Human support*, i.e. people who support with tasks such as reading or technical work in a science lab.
- *Adjustments and inclusive practice*, i.e. modified materials, inclusive teaching strategies, available accessible resources.
- *Support for teaching or training*, i.e. people who will teach and train vision impaired people independence skills, e.g. mobility, technology, low vision strategies.
- *Independence and personal agency*, i.e. the skills and knowledge a young person with vision impairment might possess, e.g. topic knowledge and qualifications, mobility skills, skills with technology, braille reading, self-advocacy skills.

The differences in how school, higher education and employment (including seeking employment) operate will seem all too obvious to those who have experienced these systems: differences in expectations of self-advocacy in describing what your needs and requirements might be; different ways of interacting with a teacher, a university tutor or a line manager; even the use of different language (e.g. in England the term "special educational needs" tends to be used within schools, while "disability" is more commonly used in the adult context including within higher education). As young people may be less knowledgeable about these differences, an important role of compulsory education will be to prepare them for these changes, including supporting them in gaining relevant experience.

In the final row of Table 10.2 we also note "policy and practical tensions". An example of this is the legal duty to make "reasonable adjustments" in the UK Equality Act (2010). Reasonable adjustments refer to the positive steps organisations must take to remove the barriers associated with disability (similar legislation exists in other countries, e.g. "reasonable accommodations" in the US Americans with Disabilities Act, 1990). It is important to recognise that policies in a given country may be ambiguous, in conflict with other policy or practical pressures or simply not be implemented.

Table 10.2 Examples of enabling resources and expectations when at school, in higher education and employment (UK).

Enabling resource	Secondary school	Higher education	Employment
Levels of human support	*High levels of additional human support to aid curriculum access* (e.g. teaching assistants, specialist teachers)	*Low levels of additional human support to aid curriculum access* (some can be provided through disability support office). In some countries government schemes also offer targeted funding to individuals (e.g. Disabled Students' Allowance (DSA) in the UK)	*Low levels of additional human support to facilitate independent work.* In some countries government schemes also offer targeted funding and support to individuals (e.g. provided through occupational health and Access to Work in the UK)
Levels of adjustments and expectations of inclusive practice	*Adjustment and inclusive practice are required and expected to* ensure that the curriculum is accessible (e.g. inclusive teaching techniques, modified assessment, environmental audits)	*Adjustment and inclusive practice are required and expected to ensure that the curriculum is accessible* (e.g. accessible online resources, teaching and assessment practice). Adjustments should be anticipatory. Universities commonly fail to do this	*Adjustment and inclusive practice are required and expected to ensure that workers with disabilities are not put at a disadvantage.* While adjustments are required, these do not need to be anticipatory
Additional available support for teaching or training	*Additional educational input should be in place to teach additional curriculum* (as conceptualised by the expanded core curriculum), e.g. independence skills, mobility, use of technology	*Some additional support and equipment are available through student support services and DSA*	*Some additional support and equipment is available through Access to Work and occupational health, with the expectation that the worker would be equipped to use it*
Independence and personal agency	*Independence skills should be progressively developed during the school career.* This should be a central part of individual education plans	*Independence skills are assumed to be in place,* although some limited support to develop these skills may be available through student support services and DSA	*Independence skills should be in place,* although there may be some limited support available through Access to Work and the employer to overcome some barriers such as transport
Notable policy tensions (based upon UK)	*Policy tension*: schools are judged upon academic performance; young people require good academic grades to progress in many areas; outcomes in relation to independence may be neglected	*Policy tension*: universities assume student independence, which is not always in place. Reasonable adjustment and inclusive practice is assumed to solve most curriculum access issues – this is not the case, and these are not implemented consistently anyway. DSA is under reform, and reduction of resource and change in emphasis may make universities less inclusive	*Policy tension*: employers are expected to make appropriate reasonable adjustments for workers with disabilities, but may not have the resources or expertise to do so. The funding available for Access to Work, which can pay for support in the workplace has been reduced by the UK government

The different types of enabling resources presented in Table 10.2 inevitably overlap with one another and will shift and change over time. Most obviously, teaching and training of particular independence skills (e.g. mobility) will lead to a young person developing greater confidence and personal agency to undertake these activities independently (in this case, independent travel).

Education and transitions: "access to learning" and "learning to access"

Given that compulsory education serves a developmental and preparatory role for what comes afterwards, the idea of transition cannot be limited to a focus upon the actual *moment* when young people change settings. Rather, it is a more significant endeavour and as such is better thought of as an ongoing process over a longer time frame. It is important to conceptualise an education system that attends to preparing all young people to be included and take part in society throughout life. Education must attend to this bigger picture as well as the immediate imperative of including the young person in the learning on a given day at school. This is challenging but vital. In discussing the role of distinctive curriculum areas in the education of children and young people with vision impairment, Allman and Lewis (2014, pp. 14–15) succinctly sum this point up in arguing that education should begin "with the end in mind [. . .] focusing on the potential adult".

Common in the field of vision impairment education is the helpful distinction between different areas of the curriculum – the "core" curriculum and an "additional" or "expanded" curriculum (e.g. McLinden and Douglas, 2013). The latter is used in the UK as a term to include areas that would not typically be taught in schools as part of the core curriculum, such as mobility, low vision training and information access and social skills (e.g. having friendship groups and self-advocacy skills). In many other countries the term "expanded core curriculum" (ECC) is used (e.g. Hatlen, 1996; Holbrook and Koenig, 2000), and in the United States the ECC has been defined in detail (e.g. Sapp and Hatlen, 2010).

The ECC is clearly linked with the broad notion of promoting longer-term independence. As an example, in their article Sapp and Hatlen (2010) present two case studies of 20-year-old young men who have similar academic achievements but very contrasting levels of independence. It is argued that one had benefitted from sustained ECC intervention *throughout* his school career that the other had not (rather, the specialist teaching intervention solely focused upon material preparation, support for *academic* teaching and explaining his special needs to classroom teachers and other pupils).

The balance and dynamic between access to the core curriculum and access to the ECC can be succinctly captured through a "dual model of access":

- *Access to learning*: inclusive practice and differentiation ensuring that the child's environment is structured and modified to promote inclusion and learning and access to the core curriculum.
- *Learning to access*: learning provision supporting the child to learn independence skills in order to afford more independent learning. This is commonly conceptualised as the ECC.

In practice, the broad approaches within this dual model of access are not considered to be mutually exclusive and each will be required at different stages in the child's educational career depending on the particular curriculum context (see for example, McLinden and Douglas, 2013; McLinden et al., 2016). Nevertheless, there is a significant change over time as young people

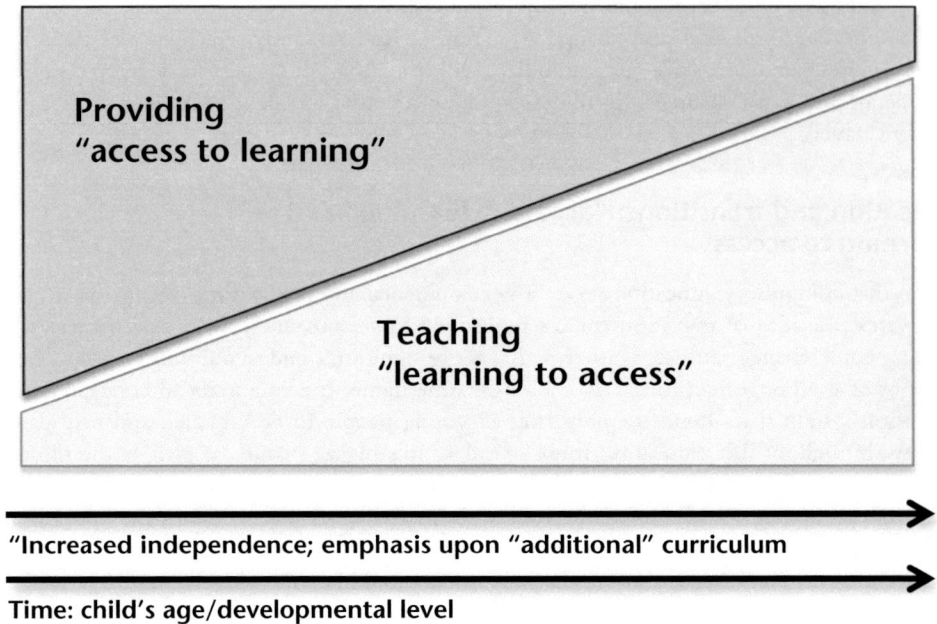

Figure 10.1   Balancing "access to learning" and "learning to access" through a young person's educational career.

develop and take greater responsibility for their learning and their lives in general. This change is most explicitly revealed at times of transition (for example, from one school to another, or when leaving school), but the dynamic between the approaches should be constant and inform the focus of educational planning at every stage not just when a key transition is approaching.

Figure 10.1 captures this dynamic relationship over a developmental timeline. Teaching young and developmentally young pupils will involve the teacher emphasising "access to learn" strategies, e.g. enlarged text books, use of teaching assistants for curriculum access tasks, sighted guide when moving around the school and specialist accessible teaching resources. "Learning to access" strategies will be emphasised in order to encourage independence. This emphasis on promoting independence access skills will increase as the child gets older and they will be encouraged to take greater responsibility for aspects of their education and life, e.g. low vision aids, touch typing, use of computers/laptops, provision of electronic files rather than hard copy material, independent mobility and self-advocacy.

Bioecological development and progressive mutual accommodations

The dual model of access highlights the careful balance required in ensuring children and young people have fair and optimised access to the core curriculum as well as structured opportunities to develop their independence over a given developmental timeframe. A bioecological perspective has been drawn upon to examine the proximal (i.e. close to the learner) and distal (i.e. at a distance from the learner) influences on promoting curriculum access within particular educational contexts (e.g. McLinden et al., 2016).

Through a bioecological perspective the nature of intervention has been highlighted as seeking to promote "progressive, mutual accommodation" (Bronfenbrenner, 2005, p. 107) between the growing individual and the changing properties of the immediate settings in which the young person with vision impairment lives (e.g. McLinden et al., 2016). As such the framework offers scope to examine the dynamic of transition "through", and "from" school, in which different strategies must work together to promote greater inclusion (see Figure 10.2):

1   *Inclusive practice*, i.e. how these barriers are addressed through inclusive design and delivery of the curriculum.
2   *Adjustments*, i.e. where it is necessary for the school, university or employer to make adjustments to meet individual needs (sometimes called "accommodations").
3   *Personal agency*, i.e. where the individual is able to make their own adjustments, drawing upon (and developing with support) their independence skills.

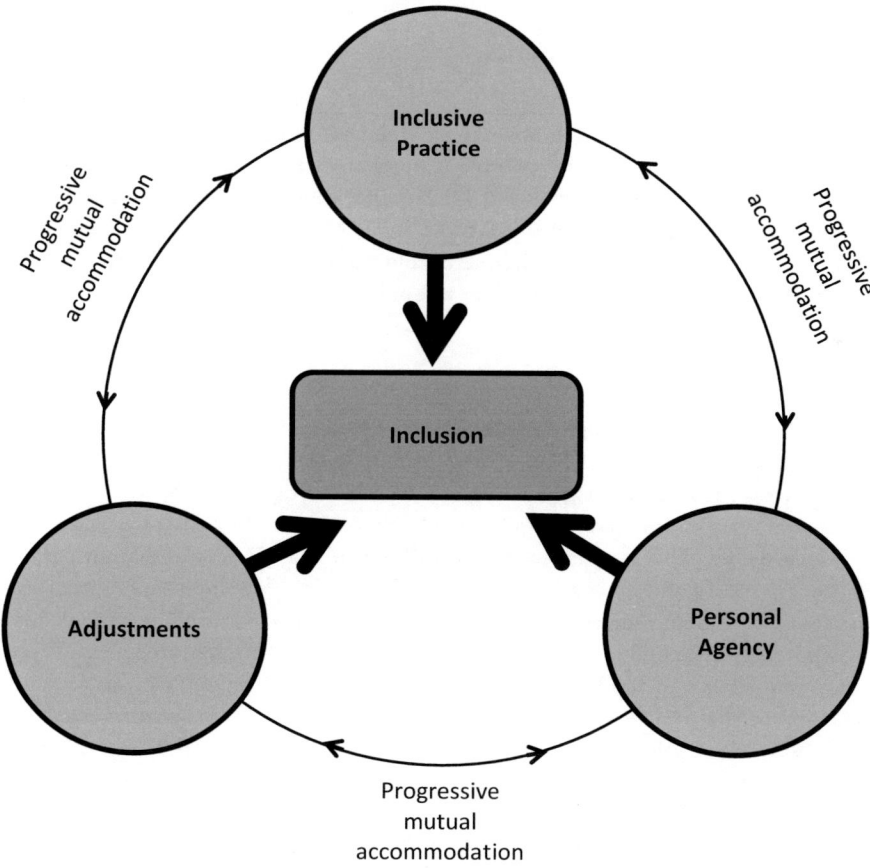

Figure 10.2 Progressive mutual accommodation through education and beyond.

Individual agency

Importantly, there is evidence that the presence of independence skills that are afforded by the ECC are associated with positive employment outcomes for people with vision impairment (e.g. Capella McDonnall, 2011; Wolffe and Kelly, 2011). Further, the importance of independence is reflected in the design of vision impairment employment services for adults. For example, Wolffe and colleagues (e.g. Wolffe 2000, 2010; Wolffe and Kelly, 2011; Wolffe and Spungin, 2002) have developed a "career education model" that emphasises that job seekers should have independence skills in place, such as daily living skills, mobility, computer/ low vision access skills, work experience (voluntary and paid) and high expectations (including role models). Employment services in the UK (e.g. Saunders, Douglas and Lynch, 2013) typically emphasise many of these independence skills in their assessments and interventions. As an example, a series of analyses of the National Longitudinal Transitions Study-2, a national study of young people in the United States, has identified a number of significant factors that impacted upon employment outcomes. These include work experience opportunities, completion of postsecondary education, mobility skills, social skills, technology skills, braille skills and careers counselling (e.g. Capella McDonnall, 2011; Cmar, 2015; Wolffe and Kelly, 2011).

Inclusive practice and adjustments

The focus upon outcomes is clearly helpful, but it is only a partial analysis. First, there is a need to ensure that compulsory education systems are designed to maximise these broader educational outcomes as part of the school system. A number of the chapters in this book explore this further (for example see Chapters 9 and 11). Second, there is a need to ensure that systems beyond compulsory education (for example, those linked to employment and higher education) are inclusive and make appropriate adjustments and accommodations and also have support mechanisms to enable continued individual development and growth.

Planning successful transition

We now turn our attention to applying the principles outlined above to consider the specifics of achieving a successful transition from school. We draw upon the "Longitudinal Transitions Study", which has recorded the experiences of a cohort of young people with vision impairment for several years as they have left school. The project started in 2010 when we recruited over 80 young people with vision impairment in England and Wales. At that time they were between the ages of 14 and 16 years (i.e. just at the end of their compulsory education). The study has followed a longitudinal qualitative design with participants being surveyed twice a year through semi-structured interviews. Some have also been involved in case study work in which they and other stakeholders have provided very detailed accounts of particular transitions. The aim of the project was to allow young people with vision impairment to give an insight into their experience of transition from school – what has worked and what has not worked (see Douglas and Hewett, 2014; Hewett, Douglas and Keil, 2017; Hewlett, Douglas, McLinden and Keil, 2017).

The participants are now all over the age of 20 years, and at the time of writing three-quarters are still actively in the project providing valuable updates on their situations, circumstances and reflections upon their transition from school. We have gathered evidence about the support they received for making transitions, levels of independence, attitudes towards independence and work experience.

In the following sections we present six important transition strategies. The strategies are of relevance to transition from school generally, but in the case of (3), (4) and (5) we present examples of young people in higher education. The final section (6) provides specific guidance on going to university:

1   Transition reviewing and planning
2   Work experience
3   Accessing information
4   Getting around independently
5   Self-advocacy
6   Specific preparation for higher education transition.

1. Transition reviewing and planning

Having completed compulsory education, which at the time in the UK was at age 16, the participants followed a number of pathways. For the majority (over 90%), this included further study in a sixth form or further education college as a first step, and about half of these participants continued on to higher education. Just four participants went straight from school at 16 years of age into apprenticeships or employment.

While the majority of participants continued studying, these transitions were not always positive ones. Over the course of the research, we have identified evidence of "churning", where the young people have repeated years in college, or repeatedly taken courses at the same level (or even lower levels) and appeared not to make positive progression. Similar findings were noted by researchers in other disciplines.

Transition from compulsory education is clearly varied and complex, but of importance is *planning* at key points in young people's education. Appropriate planning allows individuals and services to organise and prepare for the next phase (e.g. college or apprenticeship). A formal process for young people with special educational needs in England and Wales is the "transition review" (and associated "transition plan"). This is an annual meeting at school that is held to talk about the young person's future. At various stages of the study, the participants were asked to reflect upon the support that they had received during their time in education for preparing to make key decisions and transitions at age 16. Initially the participants provided predominately neutral evaluations of the support received. However, as they have got older and experienced more transitions, their analysis has become more negative. Common problems identified included the process not being "person-centred" and there being insufficient opportunity to explore their individual aspirations for the future. Challenges they faced for planning for the future included not being aware of the full range of options available, not being confident about what course(s) to study and not having the required support in place.

2. Work experience

Several studies (e.g. Capella McDonnall, 2011; Giesen and Cavenaugh, 2012) have identified previous work experience opportunities as an important factor for young people with vision impairment to be able to successfully make the transition into paid employment. It can be challenging for young people with vision impairment to find such work experience opportunities. Not only does this reduce their experience of the workplace, but it also reduces opportunities to apply and develop some of the important independence skills described elsewhere (e.g. travelling to the workplace).

The majority of the participants in the Longitudinal Transitions Study had undertaken some form of work experience through the school they attended. When reflecting back, most participants viewed work experience as having been helpful to them, particularly as it gave them experiences that they could draw upon when seeking paid employment in the future. Less positive accounts came from participants who had undertaken placements that did not align with their interests. This largely seemed to stem from schools finding it difficult to identify organisations that would be prepared to support a young person with a severe vision impairment.

Different countries have different policies and traditions in relation to work experience. Indeed, in recent years the requirement for English schools to arrange work experience placements has been dropped. Irrespective of local policies, an important role of educators of young people with vision impairment is to encourage, organise and facilitate such work placement opportunities while still at school.

3. Accessing information

Being able to access information is a key barrier faced by people with vision impairment. Referring to the dual model of access presented above, educational services are required to ensure that written material is prepared and available in an accessible format (e.g. available as braille, electronic format and large print). However, as the child develops, educational services should provide appropriate equipment and teaching to encourage efficient and independent access to information (e.g. access technology and teaching in the use of that technology). At the age at which the young person prepares to make the transition from compulsory education, we would expect that individual to be equipped with the skills required to be able to work independently in their next setting, whether that is higher education or the workplace.

Low vision aids (LVAs) offers a useful example here. LVAs are an important tool for people with low vision as they can help maximise the vision that an individual has. Despite this, less than half of the participants who had used LVAs when in school anticipated using them as they got older. Several of the participants in the study spoke negatively about using LVAs. While they attributed this partly to feeling self-conscious when using them, there were also indications that the participants had been given LVAs by staff who were unqualified to do so, which led to them being dismissive of the advantages of using LVAs in the future. However, it should be noted that some of the young people who have transitioned into employment, despite being initially reluctant to use LVAs, have since identified situations where it was helpful to use them. Several of the participants who previously used LVAs are instead choosing to use mainstream technology, such as apps on their mobile phones. While all the participants reported using a computer to access information, relatively few of them used specialist software to use the computer, preferring to make some basic adjustments such as changing the resolution or font size. Throughout the longitudinal study, we have noted many positive examples of participants using "mainstream technology" as an assistive tool; well over half of the participants described using mainstream technology in this way to help them access information independently, in the same way they would use specialist assistive tools such as LVAs.

Early introduction of braille appears to be an indicator of whether participants were likely to continue using braille into the future. Those who had the greatest opportunity to use braille once they left school were the young people using refreshable braille displays. While none of the participants used braille exclusively, most identified certain tasks that they prefer to do in braille such as for reading notes when giving a presentations or proofreading an essay.

This highlights the importance of teaching young people with vision impairment to maximise their information access skills to enable them to work as independently as possible in their next setting. Box 10.1 presents contrasting experiences of young people in higher education.

Box 10.1   Information access in higher education

One participant with severe vision impairment described herself as feeling very confident about being able to access the content of her course when she made the transition to higher education. She reported having various strategies for accessing information, primarily electronic and refreshable braille according to the task in hand and, importantly, being able to explain to others the different mediums that she would like to use. She attributed this to being able to explore different strategies when she was in school and having made her own decisions about what suited her best:

> One good thing about being in mainstream [school] was I kind of started figuring out what was necessary and what support I had as a matter of course . . . When I then transitioned to college afterwards, I went there, and I was like "I need this, and I need this, I need this format" and I knew what I needed.

In contrast, one of the participants who is sight impaired and prefers to read using large print, found it extremely difficult when she started in higher education. The institution provided her with electronic material, but as she had not used this medium when in school or college, she found it very difficult to access her course material this way: "I am just annoyed that all my stuff had to go through electronically, they don't listen that I can't work electronically. It's like trying to talk to a brick wall." It is debatable as to what a reasonable adjustment/accommodation should be in this particular case – the expectation of large print in some circumstances seems reasonable, but not in all situations. While it is important to hold a given institute to account, being able to efficiently work with electronic files is clearly a crucial skill in higher education.

(Longitudinal Transitions Study)

---

4. Getting around independently

Being able to get around independently can be a key challenge for many people with vision impairment, but one that can be overcome with appropriate environmental design and modification as well as mobility teaching (see Chapters 23 and 24). Referring to the dual model of access presented above, during their time in school young people with vision impairment should receive appropriate mobility training to ensure that they are able to move around environments safely and independently. As the young person progresses closer towards making the transition from compulsory education, we would expect an individual to have maximised their skills to be able to travel and move around independently in their next setting.

The participants' confidence in getting around independently has been a theme explored at regular points during the longitudinal transitions study. Initially the participants spoke very confidently about their ability to get around, with many noting that it was not a challenge to them having grown up in their local area. However, the overall confidence of the participants dropped as they moved into new settings, with around half saying that they did not feel prepared for getting around in new environments or for using public transport. Positively, participants who received an extensive programme of mobility support during their time in compulsory education have demonstrated confidence in getting around independently and applying their skills to new settings. Some participants who have found independent travel a challenge reported not receiving mobility support when in school, indicating that providers had focused on their immediate needs, rather than considering the broader skills that they would require as they moved into adulthood. Box 10.2 presents contrasting experiences of young people in higher education.

Box 10.2   Getting around independently in higher education

One participant had a challenging time during compulsory education in accessing specialist support to develop his mobility and orientation skills. As a result, he changed to a different school where he was able to receive a regular and structured programme to develop these skills. As a result, he felt far better prepared for making the transition to higher education and to be able to learn the necessary routes around his new environment:

> Yeah, at secondary school there was only one session every two months or something, really inconsistent. . .I wasn't independent at all at that point, I knew a tiny bit of my local area, but I just wasn't confident enough to travel on my own.

However, having had the opportunity to develop his mobility skills before leaving school he was able to use this when he went to university:

> So, I learnt so much in such a short space of time. Like I learnt the majority of the campus because I started and my routes from accommodation, all the places I needed to be within a few days and the shops within the area, and we are still working together to branch out into train stations and stuff now.

A second participant described finding getting around independently more difficult than he expected once in higher education. He had hoped to live with friends in the second year of his course, but in the end decided to stay in university halls of residence as he was concerned about living too far away from the campus:

> *Researcher*: I think before you were saying that you wanted to stay on in [university] halls. Would it have been nice to move out with your friends?

> *Participant*: It makes it more difficult. Halls is really the only option because of how close it is. Having a house just makes it . . . travelling across roads and stuff, more difficult.

Prior to leaving home he described himself as confident in getting around independently as he was very familiar with his local area. However, once in a new environment he discovered that he was not as well prepared as he anticipated.

(Longitudinal Transitions Study)

---

5. Self-advocacy

Research has identified self-advocacy as an important skill for young people with vision impairment as they transition into employment and adulthood (e.g. Hutto and Hare, 1997). Referring to the dual model of access presented above, teachers and parents will commonly advocate for children by making adjustments on their behalf and helping them manage their learning. Nevertheless, they will also encourage young people to manage their own learning and articulate their own needs. The longitudinal transitions study has identified several ways in which it is necessary for the participants to self-advocate, such as explaining their vision impairment, requesting and explaining required adjustments and addressing problems.

Several ways of developing self-advocacy skills were identified by the participants. These include having had opportunities to self-advocate when younger (for example explaining adjustments to class teachers in school or college), having a good understanding of their vision impairment and how it affects them and having a good knowledge and understanding of available specialist equipment and support to be able to explain adjustments to others. The research findings have also highlighted how important it is for young people with vision impairment to feel empowered to self-advocate, for example, through support and encouragement by parents and specialist teachers. However, the findings also illustrated how important it is for the young person to be confident about what they need to say in different situations. Lack of opportunity to self-advocate seemed to be a key explanation for this lack of confidence. Box 10.3 presents contrasting experiences of young people in higher education.

Box 10.3   Self-advocating in higher education

Higher education staff commonly rely upon students explaining their support needs and raising issues at relevant times. For students who receive specialist support packages, they are commonly required to self-advocate for the type of support they need (e.g. during a needs assessment) or communicating this support to others.

Many of the participants reported experiencing problems during their time in higher education, but some were more prepared than others in addressing these. For example, one participant shared that they had problems with their exam access arrangements, but that they challenged these as soon as they occurred, leading to more positive outcomes in the future: "When I did my exams, I didn't get all the adjustments that I needed, but I spoke to someone and they ensured I got them." In contrast, another participant experienced consistent problems in accessing course material as her department did not adhere to the reasonable adjustment plan that had been developed on her behalf. However, she did not feel confident to address these challenges, and instead graduated at the end of the course with what she felt to be a disappointing degree classification: "I don't think I was prepared at all for that one . . . I think if maybe I had been told of subtle ways . . . If I couldn't tell a teacher outright, maybe being told other methods to use."

As noted elsewhere, the conduct of some universities might be questioned in relation to their duty to make reasonable adjustments/accommodations, and this failure to follow their duty could lead to a complaint. Nevertheless, it is important (and pragmatic) that young people can articulate their own situations and requirements to ensure all stakeholders are clear about their responsibilities.

(Longitudinal Transitions Study)

---

6. Specific preparation for higher education transition

Up to this point in the chapter we have made important general observations about transition from school – issues of planning, work experience and development of independence.

Nevertheless, there are also very specific preparations that can be made in relation to transition to higher education and this will be partly linked to the systems that operate in particular countries. Even so, it is useful to consider three important aspects of preparation: choosing a higher education provider, applying for additional relevant funding and negotiating support while in higher education. In many ways, navigating these steps will involve the young person with vision impairment applying and developing their personal agency as discussed in this chapter. Box 10.4 presents some strategies based upon experiences of young people in higher education in the UK.

Box 10.4   Key preparations for HE transition in the UK

As with all people choosing a university, the main driver should be the course and subject being studied. Nevertheless, there are other issues to consider that are linked to vision impairment, including: declaring disability at the point of application; discussing the requirements of the course and access issues; consideration of the geography, living accommodation and transport; and consideration of the student support that is available. Some of these issues can be explored by the young person visiting a university in advance, and as one participant noted:

> I managed to arrange a meeting with the disability department beforehand, and that's how I knew they were so good.
>
> [They] had a good disability department, one of the best that I have seen. From my experience so far, it's been absolutely brilliant. . .they really do seem to know what they are doing, so that's good. And I had a friend who is also visually impaired who came up here and had a really positive time with the disability department and the course.

The Disabled Student Allowance (DSA) is a non-means-tested scheme available to UK-based students. DSA funds specialist equipment, non-medical support (e.g. note-takers, mobility support) and general expenses associated with a student's disability (e.g. Hewett, Douglas, McLinden and Keil, 2017). Such funding requires an application and associated assessment. It is very important for young people to understand the process and to be able to articulate their likely needs. This might involve getting support from others.

> There's a lot of things that I wasn't aware of at the time. I was very surprised with what they can actually provide, and the detail they actually go into, I had no idea there was a software programme that can read out stuff to you, if you highlighted things.

All universities in the UK, and many in other countries, will have some kind of department that oversees and arranges support for students with disability (often called a "disability support office"). Students with vision impairment should make contact with the disability support office as early as possible in their university career. They can carry out assessments of need, make arrangements and communicate with relevant staff and advise upon the available support and accommodations available (e.g. examination arrangements). Again, young people are expected to advocate for themselves in such circumstances (including how to appeal if they think support is not as it should be), as noted by a university Disability Support Officer:

> I think you have got to be aware that they are now 18, and they are coming to university, they are independent adults, we are going to treat them as an adult, and that works both ways, in that they have to let us know if things aren't right.
>
> *(RNIB, 2018; Longitudinal Transitions Study)*

Conclusion

In this chapter we have explored the process of transition from school with a particular focus on higher education. Central to our analysis has been a consideration of how education systems prepare young people with vision impairment, and the need for a broad and balanced view of curriculum and associated educational outcomes. Our analysis has drawn upon findings from the Longitudinal Transitions Study in the UK that has tracked young people as they leave compulsory education.

There are many challenges faced by young people with vision impairment as they leave school, not least the difficulties of securing paid employment and succeeding in higher education. Undoubtedly, many of the difficulties are social and physical barriers that must be challenged through campaigns and legal action: inaccessible buildings, libraries and websites and poor attitude and practice of employers and universities who fail to be inclusive and make necessary accommodations. Nevertheless, while it is clear that successful transition is linked to good support structures and an inclusive environment, it is also linked to young people developing and being able to draw on personal agency – including their ability to communicate their requirements, navigate physical and social environments, and make effective use of technology. Therefore, successful transition *from* school relies upon long-term planning and attention being given *within* school, through the development of independence skills.

References

Allman, C.B. and Lewis, S. 2014. *ECC essentials: Teaching the expanded core curriculum to students with visual impairments*. New York: AFB Press.

Bronfenbrenner, U. 2005. *Making human beings human: Bioecological perspectives on human development*. Thousand Oaks, CA: Sage.

Capella McDonnal, M. 2011. Predictors of employment for youths with visual impairments: Findings from the second national longitudinal transitions study. *Journal of Visual Impairment and Blindness*, 105(8), 453–466.

Clements, B., Douglas, G. and Pavey, S. 2011. Which factors affect the chances of paid employment for individuals with visual impairment in Britain? *WORK: A Journal of Prevention, Assessment, and Rehabilitation*, 39(1), 21–30.

Cmar, J.L. 2015. Orientation and mobility skills and outcome expectations as predictors of employment for young adults with visual impairments. *Journal of Visual Impairment & Blindness*, 109(2), 95–106.

Douglas, G. and Hewett, R. 2014. Views of independence and readiness for employment amongst young people with visual impairments in the UK. *Australian Journal of Rehabilitation Counselling*, 20(2), 81–99.

Giesen, J.M. and Cavenaugh, B.S. 2012. Transition-age youths with visual impairments in vocational rehabilitation: A new look at competitive outcomes and services. *Journal of Visual Impairment & Blindness*, 106(8), 475–487.

Hatlen, P. 1996. The core curriculum for blind and visually impaired students, including those with additional disabilities. *RE:view*, 28, 25–32.

Hewett, R., Douglas, G. and Keil, S. 2017. *Reflections of transition experiences by young people with visual impairments aged 19–22: Technical report of findings to April 2016.* Birmingham: VICTAR, University of Birmingham.

Hewett, R., Douglas, G., McLinden, M. and Keil, S. 2017. Developing an inclusive learning environment for students with visual impairment in higher education: Progressive mutual accommodation and learner experiences in the United Kingdom. *European Journal of Special Needs Education,* 32(1), 89–109. doi: 10.1080/08856257.2016.1254971

Hewett, R. and Keil, S. 2015. *Investigation of data relating to blind and partially sighted people in the Quarterly Labour Force Survey: October 2011–September 2014.* Birmingham: VICTAR, University of Birmingham.

Hewett, R. and Keil, S. 2016. *Investigation of data relating to blind and partially sighted people in the Quarterly Labour Force Survey: October 2012–September 2015.* Birmingham: Visual Impairment Centre for Teaching and Research, University of Birmingham.

Hutto, M.D. and Hare, D. 1997. Career advancement for young women with visual impairments. *Journal of Visual Impairment & Blindness,* 91, 280-295.

Holbrook, M.C. and Koenig, A.J. (eds). 2000. *Foundations of education: Instructional strategies for teaching children and youths with visual impairments* (Vol. 2). New York: American Foundation for the Blind.

McLinden, M. and Douglas, G. 2013. *Education of children with sensory needs: Reducing barriers to learning for children with visual impairment.* In A. Holliman (ed.), *Educational psychology: An international perspective* (pp. 246–255). London: Routledge.

McLinden, M., Douglas, G., Cobb, R., Hewett, R. and Ravenscroft, J. 2016. "Access to learning" and "learning to access": Analysing the distinctive role of specialist teachers of children and young people with vision impairments in facilitating curriculum access through an ecological systems theory. *British Journal of Visual Impairment,* 34(2), 177-195.

Nasen. 2014. *Transition: A quick guide to supporting the needs of pupils and their families when moving between educational settings.* Tamworth, UK: Nasen. Accessed 11 January 2019. www.nasen.org.uk/resources/resources.transition.html.

Pavey, S., Douglas, G. and Corcoran, C. 2008. Transition into adulthood and work: Findings from Network 1000. *British Journal of Visual Impairment,* 26(2), 202-216.

RNIB. 2018. Starting university [e-resource]. Accessed 1 February 2018. www.rnib.org.uk/young-people/starting-university.

Sapp, W. and Hatlen, P. 2010. The expanded core curriculum: Where we have been, where we are going, and how we can get there. *Journal of Visual Impairment & Blindness,* 104, 338–348.

Saunders, A., Douglas, G. and Lynch, P. 2013. Tackling unemployment for blind and partially sighted people Summary findings from a three-year research project. RNIB. Accessed 11 January 2019. www.rnib.org.uk/services-we-offer-advice-professionals-employment-professionals/employment-assessment-toolkit.

Wolffe, K.E. 2000. Growth and development of youths with visual impairments. In C. Holbrook and A. Koenig (eds), *Foundations of education* (vol. 1, pp. 135–160). New York: American Foundation for the Blind.

Wolffe, K.E. 2010. Rehabilitation services for adults with low vision: Personal, social and independent living needs. In A.L. Corn and J.N. Erin (eds), *Foundations of low vision* (2nd ed., pp. 729–759). New York: AFB Press.

Wolffe, K.E. and Kelly, S. 2011. Instruction in areas of the expanded core curriculum linked to transition outcomes for students with visual impairments. *Journal of Visual Impairment & Blindness,* 105, 340-349.

Wolffe, K.E. and Spungin, S.J. 2002. A glance at worldwide employment of people with visual impairments. *Journal of Visual Impairment and Blindness,* 96(4), 245–253.

11

Career education for students with visual impairments

Karen E. Wolffe

Introduction

The efficacy of infusing career education into the lives of children and youth who are disabled has been documented in special education literature since the term's formal introduction by then-US Commissioner of Education, Sydney Marland in 1971 (Brolin, 1995; Brolin and Kokaska, 1995; Kokaska and Brolin, 1985) and the culmination of these early special educators' efforts is the career education curriculum published by the Council for Exceptional Children (CEC), *Life-Centered Education* (CEC, 2012) based on their work. In the field of blindness, a body of literature has been produced that promotes the inclusion of career education in the core curriculum for students with visual impairments (Allman and Lewis, 2014; Hatlen, 1996; Holbrook, Kamei-Hannan and McCarthy, 2017; Wolffe, 1996, 1999, 2014, 2017).

Researchers have had access to detailed outcome data for students receiving special education services in the United States, including those with vision impairment. Between 2000 and 2010, longitudinal data were compiled and reported on by SRI International under the auspices of the US Department of Education's Institute of Education Sciences (IES) National Center for Special Education Research and have been made public. Secondary analyses of these data have been performed by researchers in the field of vision impairment (Capella-McDonnall, 2011; Conners et al., 2014; Kelly and Wolffe, 2012; Wolffe and Kelly, 2011) and they shed further light on the importance of career education in the lives of children with vision impairment as a primary diagnosis and those with vision impairment and additional disabilities.

The career development model

The stages of the career development model are developmental and span the life of an individual from birth to death. The stages and related content are described in the sections that follow (Wolffe 1996, 2014, 2017). Career education encompasses the first four stages of the career development model, which occur in childhood and adolescence. These stages are: career awareness, career exploration, career preparation and career placement. The final stages of the career development model, career maintenance and career mentoring, occur in adulthood and are outside the purview of educators.

Career awareness

Career awareness begins at birth when young children bond with their parents and begin to formulate ideas about who they are and how they fit into their family structure. Career awareness extends from birth through elementary school as children learn about the world around them and their roles within that world: at home, in preschool or day care settings and finally in school. Ideally, they learn organisational skills, how to follow directions, gather information about work, develop positive work habits and accrue incidental information about the world and how it operates. Children in the career awareness stage need to learn about work and about contributing to their families and society.

Career exploration

Career exploration begins in elementary school and becomes more intense during middle school or grades 6–8 and early secondary or grades 9 and 10. In this stage, children become more focused on investigating various careers and the jobs that those careers encompass while continuing to refine their work habits, knowledge, techniques used in advanced studies and skills for adult life. They refine their time and money management skills as well, and apply those skills in their daily activities. They can articulate their vocational interests, abilities, skills, values, work personalities and employment liabilities.

Career preparation

Career preparation takes places primarily in high school for most students, but often extends into postsecondary preparation if the career of choice requires advanced training. This stage typically involves the acquisition of employability skills specific to applying for first jobs and in preparation for vocational careers following the completion of prerequisite training and credentialing. The knowledge, skills and abilities that secondary students need to acquire to move successfully into placements during and following high school include: application of learned knowledge and skills in daily activities; demonstrable life and career values; avocational and vocational goals; an understanding of available jobs and resources for success in life; well-determined interpersonal skills; the ability to select, use and maintain equipment and tools; and well-developed self-esteem and self-reliance.

Career placement

While career placement begins in high school, when youth typically secure their first jobs, this stage extends for most individuals into early adulthood. This stage is where individuals secure their early work experience through entry-level, part-time and temporary jobs and build upon those experiences to find the work they want to do and are best able to do to establish their careers as adults. Skill refinement and application of learned work habits are important components of this stage.

Career maintenance

The career maintenance stage includes career stabilisation and advancement, as anticipated and if possible. Adults must apply the vocational skills, knowledge and work habits (soft skills) acquired through their work experiences to be successful. An understanding of employer expectations and how those expectations change over time is required to successfully maintain and advance a career. This stage is typically experienced by adults during their working years.

Career mentoring

Career mentoring is the final stage of the career development model and this is the stage in which more mature, experienced workers teach and guide younger workers in their fields of interest. Career mentors help younger, less experienced workers understand the nuances of the work environment, the skills and knowledge required to be successful in a chosen career and provide encouragement and insights.

Barriers and challenges

Environmental barriers

The world is designed for the majority of people living in it and they are sighted people. Although in many parts of the world there have been conscious improvements in accessibility for people without and those with reduced sight; for example, braille signage is in evidence in many public buildings and audio output on devices and tools is becoming common, there is still considerable information about the environment and what's going on within the environment that is only available through vision. In addition, accessibility is not universal; in many parts of the world, it's minimal. It's not pervasive. An individual without sight is at a disadvantage in a world where buildings don't talk to tell what they are and how to enter or exit them, what and who to find within, if it's safe to enter or prohibited and so forth. Therefore, for many blind people, the environment is still a huge barrier. Progress has been made, only to sometimes revert back to situations in which inaccessibility rules. Even the things that we laud – wonderful technological advances – continue to evolve into more graphically oriented devices with limited accessibility to those who cannot see the icons or graphics. Devices are also getting smaller and smaller, which makes them harder for people with low vision to see and use efficiently. Finally, while there is some great technology with built-in accessibility, an individual has to know how to use it and be able to afford it.

Attitudinal barriers

Other external barriers faced by children, youth and adults with vision impairment are often attitudinal. An almost universal misunderstanding about differences between people with vision loss and those who are fully sighted exists and is demonstrated when sighted people speak to others with vision accompanying blind individuals rather than to them or automatically assume that someone without sight must also have a hearing or cognitive impairment. People who know blind and partially sighted people through living or working with them, who are friends or relatives, understand that they are the same as others – that they have the same wants and desires, dreams and ambitions, fears and insecurities. Understanding and accepting people with vision impairment is not a problem for those who know them, but for those that do not it may be difficult because their understanding of blindness and its limitations or challenges is based on what they've read, seen in movies or on television and/or heard through their community. Unfortunately, the general sense among the sighted population is that blindness and severe vision loss radically restrict what someone can do and this lack of knowledge leads to attitudes of pity or compassion for many. In some cases, if a blind or partially sighted person demonstrates the ability to perform tasks of daily living, sighted people who don't know the person may attribute the performance of these skills to superhuman abilities and rather than feel compassion or pity, feel awed instead. Either attitude – pity and compassion or awe and wonderment – is troublesome because the attitude is assumed without a thorough knowledge of the individual with sight impairment and negatively influences any relationship between the parties.

Solutions

In order to resolve these challenges that young people with impaired sight face, caring adults in their lives need to do the following: convey their high expectations of children who are blind or partially sighted; encourage social engagement with sighted and visually impaired children and adults; develop children's disability-specific skills or alternatives to using vision such as reading and writing with braille or using optical devices and technology, orientation and mobility skills and adapted daily living skills; provide them with realistic feedback on their performance; and promote work opportunities. Each of these needs is further developed in the following sections.

High expectations

Significant others in the lives of children with vision impairment (service providers, parents, caregivers, siblings, extended family members, neighbours and others in the community) are encouraged to convey their high expectations of children and adolescents who are blind or have low vision both in what they say and what they do with them. Their high expectations are conveyed when they speak directly to the child with a visual impairment without condescension and about the same kinds of things they would discuss with a typically sighted child. For example, what the child is doing in school, for fun, in the community and with whom, as well as what the child dreams of becoming as an adult. Significant others need to expect the same kind of behaviour and actions from a child with a vision impairment that they would expect from a same-aged child without disabilities. They should not do for the child anything that the child is likely to be able to do for himself or herself.

Social skills

Children and youth with vision impairment may need to be taught social skills and encouraged to socialise with both other children who are visually impaired and those who are not disabled. The reason these children need structured teaching in the area of social interaction skills is that these skills are typically learned incidentally – through the casual observation of others and how they handle or respond to social engagement situations. Developmental milestones such as a smile are reinforced and maintained visually: a baby smiles and adults respond with smiles and encouragement (cooing, tickling, crooning) to elicit another smile. Without visual feedback, a smile may not be reinforced by significant others and maintained. Likewise, many of the social engagement cues, such as gesturing, facial expressions and body language, are visual in nature and difficult or impossible to interpret without good eyesight or without reporting from sighted people to a blind or partially sighted person. To assist youngsters in the acquisition of social skills, significant others must explain these nonverbal indicators and describe how they are used in social situations. They must also teach children how to reciprocate when sighted friends and acquaintances do things for them or gift them in ways that may not be obvious to the child without good vision.

Blindness-specific skills

Blindness-specific or compensatory skills are those techniques that blind and partially sighted individuals must develop to live life independently (reading Braille, using optical devices or assistive technology to access information, mastering orientation and mobility techniques and modifying the environment and tools to make them understandable without or with only limited sight). These alternatives to using sight to perform tasks are learned in addition to learning the core curriculum (language, science, mathematics, geography, history, etc.) learned by all children and youth to be successful in life. The importance of children and adolescents with vision impairment developing compensatory skills has been documented in research looking at factors that contribute to their success in life (Wolffe and Kelly, 2011).

Realistic feedback

To understand how their performance on tasks compares to the efforts of others, young people without good vision need realistic feedback from others who can observe the performances of same-aged peers. Significant others need to share with children who are visually impaired specifics about what is working well for them and where improvement is needed. This is information that typically sighted children pick up by watching others perform and seeing examples of their efforts. For example, sighted students will compare their written assignments or test results with one another or look at others' work to see how theirs compares. Children without good vision cannot surreptitiously evaluate and compare their work with the work of others – they need input from those who can see the products, compare them and report back on the similarities and differences between them. Ultimately, individuals are evaluated for positions in training and work situations based on the performance of others their age and with similar credentials. Young people with vision impairment must be able to produce as much work and sustain the same quality standards as their peers to compete with them successfully.

Opportunities to work

Significant others must promote opportunities for youngsters with vision impairment to work at home, at school and in the community. They need to encourage children and adolescents to do chores at home and school that are commensurate with those being performed by their same-aged sighted peers and their siblings. In order to make these experiences meaningful, the adults may need to learn alternatives to performing the activities with sight such as following a grid pattern when sweeping, mopping or vacuuming a room or using raised markings on appliances to help young people with vision impairments find and secure their first voluntary and then paid positions in their communities. Children and youth learn about work rules and responsibilities through engagement in work activities, including chores. Research has shown that work, preferably multiple work experiences, is a strong predictor for employment as an adult with vision impairment (Capella-McDonnall, 2011; Conners et al., 2014; Shaw, Gold and Wolffe, 2007; Wolffe 2014).

Career education activities

Career education activities help prepare youngsters who are blind or partially sighted for success in life. These activities begin in children's homes through caregivers and other family members engaging with infants and toddlers and teaching them basic skills to prepare them to enter pre-school programmes. The following sections detail early competencies that need to be taught and reinforced from birth.

Learning to listen

This competency includes encouraging young children with vision impairment to find and attend to sound sources (music, voices, clapping, toys that make noises, etc.), then to make sense of what they hear. Adults and older children can facilitate in teaching blind or partially sighted infants and toddlers to listen by using the vision impaired children's names when addressing them, reinforcing them when they pay attention to people speaking to them, encouraging children who cannot see to orient toward others when they are speaking and to show that they are attending through nonverbal cues such as smiling, frowning, nodding or shaking one's head (as appropriate). It's also important to ask children questions such as, "Where's the music coming from?" or "Can you find the toy that's making noise?" Then as children get older to ask open-ended questions such as, "What do you hear in this room?" or "What did you hear me say?" and expect responses from them.

Learning to follow directions

This competency involves teaching children first to follow simple, one-word directives (no, sit, stand, come, etc.) and then to follow more complex directions ("get your coat", "pick up your toys", "wash your face"). Caregivers and service providers are encouraged to start their efforts to teach children to follow directions with nursery rhymes and simple songs (One, two, buckle my shoe . . . ; This little piggy went to market . . .) and then proceed to those simple directives (one/two-word commands). To help children follow oral instructions, parents and caregivers may need to add demonstration via hand-under-hand or hand-over-hand tactual cues. Adults need to tell children what they want them to do and then give children the time to perform.

Learning to be responsible

This competency focuses on children learning to take turns at games, put their clothes and toys where they belong and follow rules. Teachers and parents will want to encourage children with vision impairment do the same tasks as their same-aged peers do, such as picking up after themselves (toys and personal items), taking turns at play or in group activities (not being allowed to cut-in or interrupt), sharing their toys, snacks and adults' attention and following home, community and classroom rules such as not hitting others or raising one's hand for permission and so forth. Some of these skills such as raising one's hand for permission may require adults to pre-teach the skill, if necessary to help with compliance, because the child with a vision impairment will not have a visual referent for such behaviours.

Learning basic organisational skills

Children without good sight must be exposed to organisational systems and allowed to explore those systems to understand them. Concerned adults will want to teach children to distinguish between items by touch, smell, taste or use of any remaining functional vision. Adults will need to allow children with vision impairments to examine dividers in drawers that separate knives, folks and spoons; compartmentalised boxes and shelves for storing clothes, toys, books and equipment; and specialised containers for storing tools, jewellery, shoes or other items. They also need to show and demonstrate the systems they use for labelling, finding and retrieving items.

Learning to play and fantasise

Without the ability to casually observe other children and adults playing, children with vision impairment may need to be pre-taught board and playground games, how to build with items like LEGO or Lincoln Logs or blocks, and what movements are required to actively participate in group songs or activities such as singing and playing "If You're Happy and You Know It", "Ring Around the Rosy", "London Bridge Is Falling down" and similar childhood songs and nursery rhymes. Likewise, while most children with full sight naturally gravitate to fantasy play, children without good vision may not. They may need to be guided in these activities and shown how to manipulate representative items such as fake or imaginary food and drink, trollies or appliances to engage in fantasy play with others.

To encourage active participation in play groups, parents and instructional staff will need to pre-teach games, movement songs and how to use toys. When possible, participation in creative dramatics classes can help facilitate the understanding of imaginary play for blind and partially sighted children. Parents and service providers may want to overtly support pretend play by making available costumes in home or school settings, modelling the behaviours anticipated and demonstrating the use of props and costumes.

During primary school, there are many career education competencies that children with impaired vision must master. The expectation is that in primary school children learn the basics that will prepare them to enter secondary school settings needing a minimum of adult supervision so that they can focus their energies on the refinement of academic skills and knowledge to be successful as adults in the larger community. The competencies that primary school students need to acquire are detailed in the following sections.

Following more complex instructions

By the time that children enter primary school, there is an expectation that they will be able to follow verbal instructions. During primary school they learn to follow multi-step instructions in a variety of formats, including spoken, signed, pictorial and written instructions. Teachers and parents will want to provide oral (or signed) instructions first, then introduce written instructions for students to follow. These instructions may include standard directions for completing homework or class work, ordering school materials or supplies and corresponding with others via letters, cards, email or texting.

Working individually and in a group

Primary students are expected to work with others (peers and adults) as well as work on their own when requested to do so. Concerned adults need to ask students to initiate and work unassisted on chores at home and classroom assignments, while the adults monitor their efforts. At school and in the community, it is particularly important to encourage active participation in group projects (academic and extracurricular efforts).

Responding appropriately to adults and peers

It is anticipated that primary students can speak and engage with peers and adults in a socially acceptable fashion. This competency is evidenced by students greeting others, responding to queries and conforming to classroom and community social rules and mores. Adults need to model for visually impaired primary students how to engage in chit-chat (not gossip), then expect students to interact with classmates and instructors in casual conversations that centre on the weather, upcoming school or community events and so forth. Concerned adults may want to use examples from television, movies, videos or books to demonstrate the skill of chit-chatting with others and to help children understand the differences in responding to adults versus peers.

Being responsible for one's actions

Youngsters with and without disabilities are supposed to act according to society's rules and assume responsibility for their actions and behaviours. Teachers and related service providers must require students with vision impairment to bring their adapted tools and devices to class and use them to accomplish tasks. It is wise to reward students with verbal praise or tangible rewards, when appropriate, who keep their materials and work stations orderly, who submit their assignments in a timely fashion and who generally meet an instructor's expectations. Concerned adults need to expect socially responsible behaviours such as covering sneezes or coughs, asking forgiveness when bumping into another person or tripping someone, thanking another for a kindness, etc. from children whether they are able-bodied or not.

Assuming responsibilities at home and at school

This competency involves performing age-appropriate chores assigned by parents and caregivers at home; while at school, responsibility is demonstrated by keeping up with one's possessions, following school rules and regulations, respecting others' property, turning in assignments and a student's attendance and punctuality. Encourage parents to have children do chores at home, share information with parents about the kinds of chores other students their age are performing, assign students chores at school and encourage students to help one another and younger students. It can be helpful at home and at school to chart students' efforts over time by preparing charts using wikki sticks or puff paint to create raised line drawings or using tactile markers (stars, smiley faces or the like) to note their efforts on a wall calendar (also marked with raised lines, if the student has no vision).

Identifying different work roles and assuming them in fantasy and play

Children in primary school are expected to engage in fantasy play involving adult-like roles and responsibilities: Role-playing teacher, doctor, storekeeper, police officer, etc. Encourage children to talk about their dream jobs (astronaut, ball player, musician, ballerina, whatever) and encourage them to play out those roles during free time or on holidays such as Halloween (provide costumes and props). Concerned adults may also want to have students read books about various careers of interest and submit book reports to document their career exploration efforts.

Recognising community workers

The study of various community workers (police officers, firefighters, librarians, medical personnel, etc.) helps primary students distinguish different work being performed in their communities. Techniques for teaching this competency include going out to visit sundry sites (field trips) or bringing in community workers to discuss and demonstrate their jobs and responsibilities for students. Have children interview workers, read about their jobs in books and online, then report on such workers (what they do, where they work, when and how to contact them).

Understanding the rewards of work

Through chores at home and assignments at school, children learn that good work is rewarded with praise, compensation (an allowance or payment, grades, etc.), tangible rewards such as grades or certificates and acknowledgement from others (parents, teachers and peers). Teachers and caregivers will want to discuss the fiscal and emotional rewards of working, talk with youngsters about the consequences of missing work or not producing a quality product and ask them about their understanding of the value of their efforts. Specialist teachers need to advocate with general educators to ensure that those teachers are assigning appropriate grades for the work students with vision impairment are producing in comparison to the work their classmates without vision impairment are producing for the same grades.

Learning to solve problems

When adults step back and allow children to grapple with the challenges of life, children learn to sort through the alternatives known to them and determine how to resolve concerns or problems. Ask youngsters to look for lost items before helping to find them, encourage students to consider the array of choices available to them when they ask for assistance (how others solve such problems, what the student has tried, what they think might work to resolve the problem), try not to do for students with vision impairment anything they might be able to do independently: wait to see if they can perform a task, before assuming that they can't.

Developing good communication skills

Students in primary school settings need to learn what constitutes good communication skills (listening when spoken to and responding with understanding and care towards others, being polite and politic in dialogues with other children and adults, greeting others and responding to their salutations in kind and so forth) and be able to demonstrate these skills. Techniques to facilitate with this competency include: reinforce students for attending to others (looking at them or orienting toward them); responding appropriately (using facial expressions and body language such as nodding or shaking one's head to respond nonverbally, staying on-topic in conversations, indicating interest in others by not interrupting them or changing the focus of the dialogue and responding politely); using gestures properly in greetings and closing salutations; and learning to converse with peers and adults.

Developing basic academic skills

Primary school is the time and place for the acquisition of basic literacy and numeracy skills (language arts such as reading and writing, mathematics), as well as the time to gain the fundamentals of other content area subjects taught in the core curriculum (science, history, geography, health and physical education, fine arts and technology). For students with vision impairment, this is also the time to learn and refine disability-specific skills to access the mainstream or core curriculum (use of braille, optical devices, assistive technology for reading and writing; use of abacus, talking calculators, tactile graphics for mathematics, mapping and graphing; and use of adapted tools and devices).

By the time that young people are in secondary school settings, the expectation is that they will have mastered their basic academic and disability-specific skills and have knowledge of the fundamental life skills taught in primary schools and at home. They are expected to be able to

167

demonstrate the advanced competencies described in the following sections when they exit from secondary school settings and be ready to exit out of secondary into either postsecondary training or employment and adult life.

Meet increased demands for organising time

Youth in secondary settings are expected to follow schedules that require them to move between classes and extracurricular activities without supervision. They need to note when assignments are due and testing will occur so that they can prepare accordingly. If they are encouraged by their parents and caregivers, they will be setting their own social and medical appointments, planning holiday or vacation activities and structuring their schedules to include voluntary or paid work responsibilities.

Meet increased responsibility at home and in the community

Young adults are often given responsibilities at home such as monitoring or babysitting younger siblings, caring for family pets or communal animals on farms or ranches, taking on additional chores or work assignments and so forth. In addition, many young adults are asked to assist members of the community who may be in need, such as extended family members or neighbours.

Show a full understanding of the work performed by adults

Secondary students ought to be able to articulate the major occupational categories represented in their communities and describe the work being performed by any of the adults they know in detail. They should be able to express general information about the workforce such as minimum wage, typical working schedules, the difference between gross and actual earnings; understand what benefits such as vacation time and medical insurance are associated with the jobs they are interested in performing; and describe how jobs are secured.

Show a beginning notion of work he or she wants to do as an adult

By the time young people enter secondary settings, they ought to have some idea of the type of work or career they'd be interested in and able to pursue. They should have clearly articulated their interests, abilities, values, work personality and limitations with relation to their future vocational aspirations. Ideally, they will have read about careers of interest, interviewed adults performing in those jobs and visited either actual worksites or training facilities preparing workers in their career fields of choice.

Investigate identified areas of interest

During the secondary experience, it is anticipated that students will research their interests for both avocational and vocational pursuits and then engage in activities that help them develop or refine natural talents in those areas of interest.

Well-developed academic skills

The secondary setting enables students to refine and strengthen their academic skills in preparation for work and/or further educational or vocational training. Unless there are extenuating circumstances, secondary school graduates are expected to have the full literacy and numeracy skills to function as adults in society independently.

Well-developed thinking skills

Lower-order thinking skills: remembering, understanding and applying are reinforced in secondary, while the higher-order thinking skills: analysing, evaluating and creating are developed and refined during students' secondary school experiences.

Well-developed work behaviours

These are the soft skills that employers are concerned about for all new employees: dependability, honesty, initiative, cooperation, amiability and the like. These soft skills or work behaviours are expected to be fully developed when students exit secondary settings.

Participation in work activities

Secondary students with and without disabilities need to participate in work and work-related activities while they are in school to ensure they have the work skills and behaviours to succeed post-graduation.

Young adults exiting out of secondary school need to have action plans that incorporate their personal and vocational goals to succeed in life.

Assessment

There are few normative assessment tools that specifically focus on the career education needs of individuals with vision impairment; however, there are a few tools that are criterion-referenced and have been found to be effective in school and vocational settings (Wolffe 2014, 2017). To assess the career education knowledge and skills of youngsters with vision impairment there is the *Career Education Competencies Checklist* (Wolffe 2011, 2014, 2017), which reflects the competencies described in the preceding sections. For young adults preparing to exit out of secondary settings and enter postsecondary activities or work, there is the *Transition Competencies Checklist* (Wolffe 2011, 2014, 2017), which is also available in an online format upon request from the author. Finally, there are two tools that may prove beneficial to use as assessment tools for adults with vision impairment to determine their competence in this content area: The *Strengths/Problems Checklist* (Wolffe, 2012a) and the *Employment Assessment Toolkit* (Royal National Institute of Blind People, 2016b), which is used with the *Employment Action Plan* (Royal National Institute of Blind People, 2016a).

Assessment tools that are used in the general population to assess career interests, abilities and values such as the *Self-Directed Search* (Holland, 1994), *World of Work Inventory* (WOWI, 2017), and *My Next Move* (ONET, 2017) are also handy assessment tools for students with vision impairment who have assistive technology that enables them to access these tools online. Although the former are for-fee services, the latter, *My Next Move*, is a free tool available through the US Department of Labor's ONET site. Young adults and children with vision impairment can benefit from using these assessment tools to determine both their interests, abilities and values and how those personal attributes link to their career goals.

The career education area is one that stretches from birth through adulthood with particular relevance during childhood and into adolescence. Children and youth with vision impairment can benefit from structured learning in this content area and readers are encouraged to assist them both at home and at school. A listing of career education resources follows to help concerned parties in this endeavour:

- American Foundation for the Blind's CareerConnect website: www.afb.org/info/living-with-vision-loss/for-job-seekers/12.
- *ECC Essentials: Teaching the Expanded Core Curriculum to Students with Visual Impairments* (Allman and Lewis, 2014).
- *Foundations of Education, Volume II: Instructional Strategies for Teaching Children and Youths with Visual Impairments* (3rd ed.) (Holbrook et al., 2017).
- *Skills for Success: A Career Education Handbook for Children and Adolescents with Visual Impairments* (Wolffe, 1999).
- *Transition Tote System: Navigating the Rapids of Life* (Wolffe, 2012b).
- World Blind Union's Project Aspiro employment resources website: www.projectaspiro.com.

Conclusion

This chapter detailed the career development process for individuals working with children and adolescents who are blind or have partial sight. Practical training suggestions were included for caregivers and service providers to convey high expectations; develop blindness-specific skills for literacy, numeracy, independent living and mobility; promote socialisation, including recreation and leisure involvement with others; provide youngsters with realistic feedback concerning their performance in comparison to others; and promote opportunities for paid and voluntary work at home, school and in the community. Readers were introduced to internal and external barriers impeding career development and were offered solutions. Finally, career assessment tools were introduced.

References

Allman, C. and Lewis, S. (eds). 2014. *ECC essentials*. New York: AFB Press.

Brolin, D.E. 1995. *Career education: A functional life skills approach* (3rd ed.). Englewood Cliffs, NJ: Merrill.

Brolin, D.E. and Kokaska, C.J. 1995. *Career education for handicapped individuals* (3rd ed.). Englewood Cliffs, NJ: Merrill.

Capella-McDonnall, M. 2011. Predictors of employment for youths with visual impairments: Findings from the second National Longitudinal Transition Study. *Journal of Visual Impairment & Blindness*, 105(8), 453–466.

CEC. 2012. *Life-centered career education*. Accessed 20 September 2017. https://lce.cec.sped.org/public/main.

Conners, E., Curtis, A., Emerson, R.S.W. and Dormitorio, B. 2014. Longitudinal analysis of factors associated with successful outcomes for transition-age youths with visual impairment. *Journal of Visual Impairment & Blindness*, 108(2), 95–106.

Hatlen, P. 1996. The core curriculum for blind and visually impaired student, including those with additional disabilities. *RE: view*, 28(1), 2–32.

Holbrook, M.C., Kamei-Hannan, C. and McCarthy, T. (eds). 2017. *Foundations of education: Volume II instructional strategies for teaching children and youths with visual impairments* (3rd ed.). New York: AFB Press.

Holland, J. 1994. *Self-directed search*. Odessa, FL: Psychological Assessment Resources.

Kelly, S. and Wolffe, K. 2012. Internet use of transition-aged youth with visual impairments in the United States: Assessing the impact. *Journal of Visual Impairment & Blindness*, 106, 597–608.

Kokaska, C.J. and Brolin, D.E. 1985. *Career education for handicapped individuals* (2nd ed.). Englewood Cliffs, NJ: Merrill.

ONET. 2017. My next move: ONET Interest Profiler. Accessed 12 October 2017. www.mynextmove. org/explore/ip

Royal National Institute of Blind People. 2016a. *Employment action plan*. Accessed 5 July 2017. www.rnib. org.uk/sites/default/files/Employment_Action_Plan.pdf.

Royal National Institute of Blind People. 2016b. *Employment assessment toolkit*. Accessed 5 July 2017. www.rnib.org.uk/sites/default/files/v7Employment%20Assessment%20Tool.pdf.

Shaw, A., Gold, D. and Wolffe, K. 2007. Employment-related experiences of youths who are visually impaired: How are these youths faring? *Journal of Visual Impairment & Blindness*, 101, 7–21.

Wolffe, K.E. 1996. Career education for students with visual impairments. *RE: view*, 28(2), 89–93.

Wolffe, K.E. (ed.). 1999. *Skills for success: A career education handbook for children and adolescents with visual impairments*. New York: AFB Press.

Wolffe, K.E. 2011. *Pre-employment programme trainer's manual*. London: Royal National Institute of Blind People.

Wolffe, K.E. 2012a. *Career counseling for people with disabilities: A practical guide to finding employment* (2nd ed.). Austin, TX: PRO-ED.

Wolffe, K.E. 2012b. *The transition tote system: Navigating the rapids of life* (2nd ed.). Lousiville, KY: American Printing House for the Blind.

Wolffe, K.E. 2014. Career education. In C. Allman and S. Lewis (eds), *ECC essentials: Teaching the expanded core curriculum to students with visual impairments* (pp. 411–469). New York: AFB Press.

Wolffe, K.E. 2017. Career education. In M.C. Holbrook, C. Kamei-Hannan and T. McCarthy (eds), *Foundations of education: Volume II instructional strategies for teaching children and youths with visual impairments* (3rd ed., pp. 831–874). New York: AFB Press.

Wolffe, K. and Kelly, S. 2011. Instruction in areas of the expanded core curriculum linked to transition outcomes for students with visual impairments. *Journal of Visual Impairment & Blindness*, 105, 340–349.

World of Work Incorporated. 2017. *World of work inventory*. Accessed 12 October 2017. www.wowi.com.

Part IV

Sport and physical exercise for people with visual impairment

12

Teaching children who are deafblind in physical education, physical activity and recreation

Lauren J. Lieberman and Justin A. Haegele

Fernando is a 14-year-old young man who is deafblind from Usher syndrome type I. He grew up deaf and is slowly losing his vision due to Retinitis Pigmentosa. Fernando signs and is fully immersed in his school with his hearing peers and also with the deaf community in his city. He did not know he had Usher syndrome until he was 12 due to night blindness and the loss of some of his peripheral vision.

He has always gone to his typical elementary and middle school and used an interpreter. There are four other children in his school with different degrees of hearing loss and three of them utilise interpreter services. The other two have multiple disabilities and do not have the language development to use interpreters.

Fernando has always loved sports and played on his community basketball team and was in a summer swimming team. He has always participated fully in physical education with some modifications when necessary. His new high school physical education teacher Mr Ball knows that as Fernando loses more vision over the course of his time in high school, he will need to include more and more accommodations. But for now Fernando is a major part of the school and has many friends. His multidisciplinary team has agreed that with their cooperation and support none of that will change for Fernando.

As can be seen in the above scenario, it is not difficult to ensure a child who is deafblind is fully included in all aspects of his school. It is important, however, to be connected to the multidisciplinary team and work together on all aspects of the educational programme to ensure the student can access all areas of education. Therefore, the purpose of this chapter is to do the following:

1   Define and describe deafblindness.
2   Describe some causes of deafblindness and characteristics that may be seen with children who are deafblind.
3   Describe communication methods that may be used with children who are deafblind.
4   Describe important modification considerations for physical activity for children who are deafblind.

5 Ensure team multidisciplinary team collaboration throughout the school year.
6 Review strategies to help increase socialisation for children who are deafblind.
7 Lastly, share some role models who are deafblind who are involved in physical activity, sports and recreation.

Introduction

Definition of deafblindness

Deafblindness can be defined as "concomitant hearing and visual impairments, the combination that creates such severe communication and other developmental and educational needs that they cannot be accommodated in special education in programmes solely for children with deafness or children with blindness" (US Department of Education, n.d.).

Characteristics and causes of deafblindness

People who are deafblind do not have effective use of either of the distance senses (vision and hearing), causing difficulties in communication, access to information and mobility (Simms, 2004). Although the term *deafblind* suggests that these people can neither hear nor see, this is rarely the literal truth. Most people who are deafblind receive both visual and auditory input, but information received through these sensory channels is usually distorted. So, the term deafblind is often misleading – it is frequently more accurate to say that these people are both hard of hearing and partially sighted. Only in rare instances, such as with Helen Keller, is a person totally blind and profoundly deaf. Each person with the label deafblind has a unique history, and it is important to gather information about each student to understand what she/he might be able to see and hear (see Box 12.1 for considerations when teaching students with deafblindness).

Deafblindness has many causes. Understanding the cause might give an indication of the age of onset and whether remaining vision and hearing are likely. Following are explanations of several of the more common causes of deafblindness.

Usher syndrome

Usher syndrome is one major cause of adult-onset deafblindness, and when students have Usher syndrome, it is important to know the amount of hearing and vision they have. Usher syndrome is a congenital disability characterised by hearing loss present at birth or shortly thereafter and the progressive loss of peripheral vision. There are three types of Usher syndrome. Usher syndrome type I is congenital deafness and progressive retinitis pigmentosa, whereas type II is adventitious deafness and progressive retinitis pigmentosa. Lastly, individuals with Usher syndrome type III experience progressive hearing and vision loss, beginning in the first few decades of life.

CHARGE syndrome

The leading cause of child-onset deafblindness is CHARGE syndrome. The diagnosis of CHARGE syndrome is clinically based on the medical features of the child. An evaluation for possible CHARGE syndrome should be made by a medical geneticist who is familiar with the syndrome. The clinical diagnosis is made using a combination of major and minor features. Major features are characteristics that are common in CHARGE syndrome but relatively rare in other conditions and are, for the most part, diagnosable in the newborn period. Minor features are characteristics that are also common in CHARGE but not quite as helpful in distinguishing CHARGE from other syndromes. Major features in children with CHARGE include vision problems, swallowing and nasal issues, hearing difficulties and growth delays. CHARGE syndrome is a leading cause of deafblindness at birth. Because children with CHARGE experience so many medical complications, it is imperative that they be taught to their functional ability. As they get stronger and experience fewer visits to the hospital, the instructor can increase the length, duration and intensity of activities offered.

Other causes

Deafblindness can also be associated with meningitis, prematurity, parental use of drugs, sexually transmitted diseases (STDs), other syndromes and unknown causes. People who have both vision and hearing loss often have additional disabilities. These disabilities may include cerebral palsy, intellectual disability, autism or a combination of several disabilities. No matter what disabilities are present, it is most important to focus on the student's functional ability and communication. For example, if Megan has low vision and is hard of hearing, the instructor would need to provide demonstrations at close distances with plenty of explanation, physical assistance and feedback. For many children, this level of instruction would necessitate a one-on-one teaching situation (Lieberman, 2017).

General considerations

Though there is often a tendency for caregivers to focus on the medical aspects of deafblindness, physical educators can help parents begin to focus on the quality of life of their child with deafblindness. Physical educators can work to introduce students who are deafblind to activities that they may come to enjoy. They can help these students experience joy in life rather than focus only on survival. Teaching students who are deafblind is a unique experience that requires hands-on work; it is a topic that is difficult to cover comprehensively in the limited time allotted in professional preparation courses. Camp Abilities, a developmental sport camp for young people with visual impairments and deafblindness, is held for one week each summer at State University of New York (SUNY) at Brockport and in other locations throughout the United States. This camp is an excellent opportunity for pre-service teachers to learn how to teach young people who are deafblind. For more information on Camp Abilities, see www. campabilities.org. See the resource list in Box 12.1 for more great resources for educating students who are deafblind.

A major consideration with students with deafblindness is isolation. Many people who are deafblind experience a great amount of social isolation (McInnes, 1999). Some people who are deafblind move to communities where there are several others who are deafblind. Many attend camps for people who are deafblind. However, research suggests that they participate in little specific and regular leisure time physical activities (Sterbova and Kudlacek, 2014). Physical education and sport can provide opportunities to reduce this isolation and introduce the person who is deafblind to activities such as in-line skating, swimming, biking and gymnastics to increase socialisation. Deafblindness presents limited opportunities for *incidental learning*. This means that the student needs to be specifically taught everything. It is becoming more common to use an intervener, a person who works one on one with the student, signing exactly what is happening in the environment (Morgan, 2001). For example, the intervener signs when a child is on the swings over there, when a certain classmate recently entered the room, or who is saying what in a discussion. The range of communication methods is similar to the range for children who only have hearing loss. The exception with a child who is deafblind is that signing may need to be done in the child's limited field of vision. This may be close up to the child's face, far away from the child or in a limited space. If there is no vision, signing may be done tactually in the child's hand. See Figure 12.1 for an example of tactile sign language (Lieberman, 2017).

Communication and deafblindness

People who are deafblind have many different ways of communication. The methods they use vary, depending on the causes of their combined vision and hearing loss, their backgrounds and their education. Below are some of the most common ways that people who are deafblind communicate.

Sign language and modifications

Some deaf or hard of hearing people with low vision use sign language (e.g. American Sign Language, English-based sign language). In some cases, people may need to sign or fingerspell more slowly than usual so the person with limited vision can see signs more clearly. Sometimes the person with low vision can see the signs better if the signer wears a shirt that contrasts with his or her skin colour (e.g. a person with light skin needs to wear a dark-coloured shirt). Some people who are deafblind with restricted peripheral vision may prefer the signer to sign in a very small space, usually at chest level. Some signs located at waist level may need to be adapted (e.g. signing "belt" at chest level rather than at waist level).

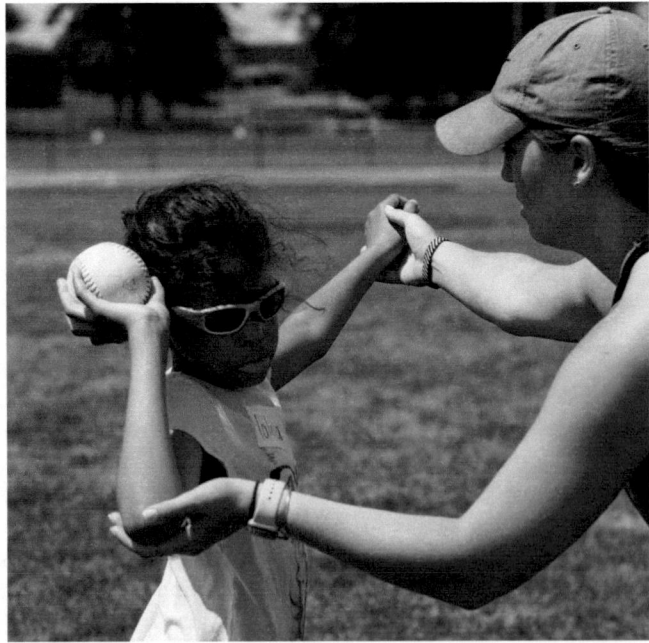

Figure 12.1   Student who is deafblind learning how to throw with her intervener using tactile sign language.

Tactile sign

The person who is deafblind puts his or her hands over the signer's hands to feel the shape, movement and location of the signs. Some signs and facial expressions may need to be modified (for example, signing "not understand" instead of signing "understand" and shaking one's head; spelling "dog" rather than signing "dog"). People can use one-handed or two-handed tactile sign language. People who grew up using sign language in a deaf community may prefer tactile versions of that specific sign language (e.g. American Sign Language). It is important for people working with those who are deafblind to discuss which language the student prefers, and attempt to adopt this preference.

Tracking

Some deafblind people with restricted but still usable vision (e.g. tunnel vision) may follow signs by holding the signer's forearm or wrist and using their eyes to follow the signs visually. This helps them follow signs more easily.

Tactile fingerspelling

Usually blind or visually impaired people who lose their hearing later, or deaf or hard of hearing people who have depended on their speech reading and do not know how to sign, prefer tactile fingerspelling because sometimes sign language can be difficult to learn. The deafblind person may prefer to put his or her hand over the fingerspelling hand, or on the signer's palm or cup his or her hand around the signer's hand.

Face-to-face communication systems

Some deafblind people use a Screen Braille Communicator (SBC). This is a small, portable device that enables them to communicate with sighted people. The device has a QWERTY keyboard with an LCD display on one side, and an eight-cell braille display on the other side. The sighted person types short text on the QWERTY keyboard. The deafblind person reads the printed text by placing his or her fingers on the braille display. He or she then uses the braille display to type back text. The sighted person can read the text on the LCD display.

Communication during physical activity

Communication during physical activity with a child who is deafblind can be difficult unless it is planned and discussed. Arndt, Lieberman and Pucci (2004) suggest the following steps for setting up clear, planned communication during physical activities:

1   *Allow the child to explore the equipment and environment to gain a better understanding of the activity.* This may include a bicycle, canoe, volleyball court and ball or pool. Exploration time will help the child understand the environment and equipment before beginning to learn skills or an activity. The tactile exploration needs to be accompanied by clear terminology of what is being felt. For instance, a bike would open up the concepts of wheels, chain, handlebars, seat and frame.

2   *It is important to listen to the expert, including the child, paraeducator and intervenor or interpreter.* When children have a question or concern, or if they are apprehensive about a new

activity, their feelings and communication must be addressed. For example, if a child is swimming in the shallow end of the pool with a life vest and he points to the deep end, it is likely that he has experienced swimming and is skilled enough to swim in the deep end. Ask questions and explore what the child's communication is conveying.

3   *Make sure that new continuous activities are made discrete until the child feels comfortable.* Continuous skills are those that do not have a clear beginning or ending, such as biking, running, rock climbing, swimming and in-line skating. On the other hand, discrete activities include those that have a definite beginning and ending, such as the shot put, bowling roll or free throw in basketball. When children who are deafblind engage in a continuous activity for the first time, it may be scary and they may not know when they can stop, when they will have a chance to communicate what they need or when they will get feedback. Making a continuous activity discrete will allow the child to choose to continue, ask a question or receive important feedback. For example, if a child is swimming in the deep end and she is afraid, she can swim for five strokes and then stop and get feedback, rest or ask a question. Planning ahead of time when communication will happen will minimise fears and allow the child to get more feedback as well as increase opportunities for communication.

4   *Make sure the child has the opportunity to receive and express communication with others.* This will take careful planning, discussion and often positioning before the activity, but it is vital to success. For example, if the physical education teacher plans for the child to pull himself prone on a scooter and he uses tactile signing, the teacher, intervenor (interpreter) and child will need to plan time for instruction, activity and feedback before the child starts moving (Lieberman, Ponchillia and Ponchillia, 2013).

Teaching physical education to students with deafblindness

Children with deafblindness have unique and specific needs that must be met in order for them to be successful in physical education. Because of this, a number of items must be taken into consideration by their physical educations. This section describes guidelines and tips for physical education teachers who have students with deafblindness in their classes. Because the deafblind population is extremely heterogeneous (Kamenopoulou, 2012), it is essential to keep in mind that some of these tips may be better for some students than others. Teachers should discuss each concept with the student prior to beginning.

Pre-teaching

Pre-teaching involves teaching elements of an upcoming activity prior to engaging in the activity in a class. This can be very beneficial for children who are deafblind. Pre-teaching includes knowing the perimeter of the court or fields using a tactile board, knowing the equipment, rules, scoring, terminology and strategy (see Figure 12.2). This must be completed well before each unit being taught. In addition, the students must learn not only the signs for each part of the unit but also how it is spelled and what it means. For example: a three-point line in basketball means what in the game? A triple threat in basketball is signed how and what does it mean and when is it used?

Modifications

Many students who are deafblind will need modifications to successfully participate in regular activities. Teaching tips for children with visual impairments and for deaf children can also

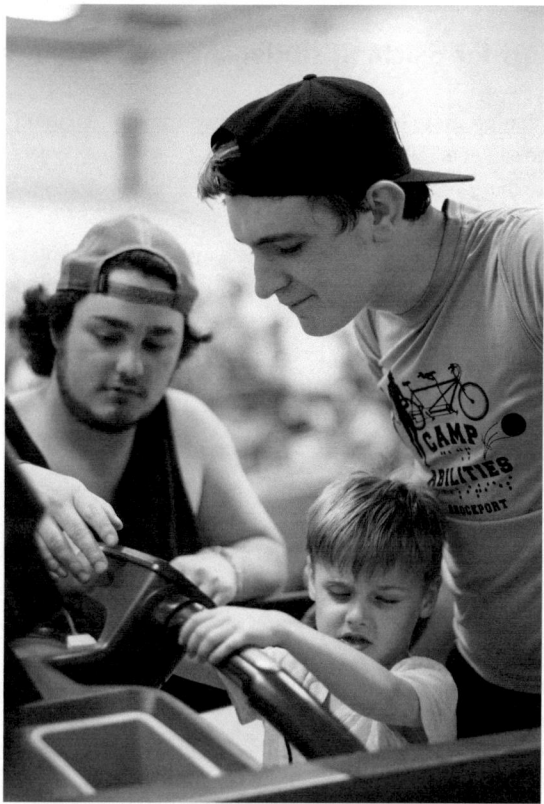

Figure 12.2   Student feeling the whole treadmill with all of the signs and terminology before the bike unit starts.

apply for students who are deafblind. Refer to the list below for additional considerations when teaching students with deafblindness. Keep in mind that a multisensory approach is preferred when teaching these students (Grenier and Lieberman, 2018). Modifications might include changing the rules, equipment, instruction or environment, as described in Chapter 13.

Students with deafblindness, who do not have additional disabilities, can participate in most sports at both a competitive and recreational level. Weightlifting, dance, in-line skating, swimming, skiing, bowling, hiking, goalball, track and field, cycling and canoeing are some of the possibilities. Like students who are visually impaired, it is important to teach a combination of open and closed skills. Deafblind athletes wishing to compete might choose to compete in sports for people who are blind (e.g. via the International Blind Sports Association or the Deaflympics).

An experience with a student named Eddie illustrates the importance of not placing ceilings on expectations for students who are deafblind. Eddie was a 15-year-old student with deafblindness who asked to learn to ride a unicycle. Using the same task analysis his physical education teacher had used to learn to ride, Eddie learned to ride the unicycle independently. Teaching students who are deafblind challenges physical educators to adapt appropriately to enable these students to learn. To meet Eddie and learn about this process, view the video at the following link: www.youtube.com/watch?v=lLYp4b_p_wg.

Box 12.1 10 tips for teaching students with deafblindness

1   Offer activities that promote movement, such as swimming, swinging, biking, walking and climbing (Lieberman et al., 2013).
2   Use multiple teaching modes, such as explanation, demonstration, tactile modeling and physical assistance.
3   Encourage choice making, such as choice of activity and equipment.
4   Set up the environment to accommodate the student's strengths. For example, if the student will be batting, offer bats and balls in a variety of sizes, colours and textures as well as several ways to deliver the ball, such as on a string, on a tee or from a pitch. This way the student can choose the size, weight and colour of the bat and ball and the preferred trajectory of the ball.
5   Be flexible, patient and creative.
6   Facilitate socialisation because students who are deafblind often experience isolation and loneliness (Lieberman and MacVicar, 2003). This can be done by implementing a peer tutor programme, teaching the student's mode of communication to classmates or encouraging the student who is deafblind to become involved in after-school programmes and community activities.
7   Provide all incidental information.
8   Link movement to language. Teach the word for each skill learned and explain the purpose of each sport and activity.
9   Learn the student's form of communication, including gestures and body language.
10 Help students find activities in their homes to engage in with and without siblings and peers (Lieberman and Pecorella, 2006).

(Modified from Lieberman, 2017)

Teaching environment

Research has noted that a number of environmental barriers can affect the social and physical participation of children who are deafblind (Lieberman, Haegele and Marquez, 2016; Lieberman, Kirk and Haegele, 2018). More specifically, Moller and Danermark (2007) noted that bad lighting conditions, poor labelling of school areas and difficulties with transportation to and from class are among the most challenging barriers. Furthermore, students in their study reported that physical education was the most challenging subject to navigate (Moller and Danermark, 2007), likely because of the open and free-flowing nature of the subject. Taking these barriers into consideration when structuring the physical education environment can help students who are deafblind be more successful when participating in activities and engaging in social inclusion (Kamenopoulou, 2012). Follow this link to see more information about other environmental and communication practices to successfully include those who are deafblind: www.youtube.com/watch?v=gKvEA4fM o68&feature=youtu.be.

Collaboration with the team

A multidisciplinary team consisting of the student's parents, educational specialists and medical specialists in the areas in which the child requires services should work together to ensure the best possible services and collaboration (Grenier and Lieberman, 2018; Lieberman et al., 2018). Descriptions of the unique team members are below although they will always have a physical educator on the team.

Deafblind (DB) specialist

A DB specialist may provide direct services to the child or consultation/training to teachers and support staff. DB specialists understand the unique effects of combined vision and hearing loss in communication, learning, orientation and mobility, social skills, etc.

Teacher of students with visual impairments (TVIs)

TVIs can help a child with deafblindness use optical (low vision) and non-optical devices (e.g. reading stands); identify appropriate visual materials; make modifications to visual materials (e.g. large print); and acquire materials from the American Printing House for the Blind (APH).

Teacher of the deaf/hard of hearing

A child with deafblindness may need direct or consultant services from a teacher who can help in the use of appropriate communication and assisted listening devices and address literacy issues related to hearing loss.

Orientation and mobility (O&M) specialist

Instruction will help the child with deafblindness develop skills to understand and navigate his/her environment, including developing independent travel skills. The O&M specialist must be able to communicate with the child in his/her primary mode of communication (sign language, touch or object cues or alternate communication forms).

Intervener

An intervener, a one-to-one service provider with training and specialised skills in deafblindness, facilitates access to environmental information usually gained through vision and hearing; the development and use of receptive and expressive communication skills; and positive relationships to promote social and emotional well-being.

Paraprofessionals

One-on-one paraprofessionals, also known as instructional aides or assistants, will likely support services, and there must be effective allocation of responsibility, identification of the appropriate qualifications for personnel responsible to carry out each function and coordination among all professionals. In order to be effective in physical education for children who are deafblind they must be trained (Lieberman, Haibach and Schedlin, 2012).

Other members

Other members of the multidisciplinary team may also be the speech therapist, physical therapist, occupational therapist and the nurse if the child has any medical issues. Collaboration of all of these individuals is tantamount to ensure appropriate programming for children who are deafblind.

Socialisation

One of the major goals for physical education is often socialisation. This goal for children who are deafblind is important to coordinate for, as it is not easily incorporated without careful planning (Bruce et al., 2016). The first step to take is to determine the child's communication mode.

Communication mode

As mentioned earlier in this chapter it is important to determine the communication mode of the child who is deafblind in order to know how to approach socialisation whether it is with the teacher, paraeducator, peers or staff. The communication mode will also help determine the student's set-up and positioning during each activity. For example, if a child uses tactile communication a specific communication method will need to be set up for them when they are riding a tandem bike. Tactile signs, touch and signals will need to be incorporated during biking so they know when there will be a turn, stop or any dangerous areas. In addition, expressive signs must be set up as well in order to ensure the student can express their questions or comments such as how far to go or can they stop to use the bathroom. Infusing communication into the class can help ensure the student is self-determined.

Self-determination

Self-determination among people who are visually impaired (Robinson and Lieberman, 2004) or deafblind (Lieberman and Stuart, 2002) has been shown to be low (Lieberman et al., 2018). In other words, in many cases other people decide *for* people who are deafblind related to choices in their lives. Incorporating a quality physical education programme with choices provides the child with many opportunities to talk about typical things. For example, if a child has the opportunity to swim, play baseball, basketball and do yoga they have much to talk about with their peers and family. This can increase their socialisation and life satisfaction. In order to do this effectively we must educate their peers about their communication and modifications needed.

Educate peers

The idea of disability awareness is not new (Lieberman and Houston-Wilson, 2018). Educating the peers about the specific way that a child can communicate and showing them how to facilitate expressive and receptive communication can increase socialisation tremendously. In addition, showing the peers how to modify activities for the child can increase participation and the opportunity to socialise as well. Lastly, socialisation will only be effective if incidental learning is ensured throughout the child's day.

Incidental learning

Incidental learning is anything that happens in the environment that must be intentionally taught to the child who is deafblind. This can be anything from an announcement on the loudspeaker to the principal showing up to observe the class. Anything that the peers can gain from sight or sound must be intentionally taught to the child who is deafblind. Without the intentional communication of the incidental information the child will often be left out of the most basic information. Incidental information also includes role models who are like them. Individuals who are deafblind have accomplished great feats in the past ten years.

Role models/case study

Just as able-bodied children look to Abbey Wambach or Michael Jordan as role models for soccer and basketball respectively, children who are deafblind also need to have role models like themselves. Some case studies from *Possibilities: Recreation Experiences of Individuals Who Are Deafblind* (Lieberman et al., 2016) show how children themselves are to be the role models that other deafblind and non-deafblind children admire and look up to.

Cody Colchado

My name is Cody and I currently work as a motivational speaker, strength and conditioning coach, high school trainer and assistant manager for my family's ranch, Santa Rita Farms, in San Manuel, Texas. I have always had hearing loss but in 1981, I had a freak football accident that brought on vision loss as well. After the accident I had only five degrees of vision left and was diagnosed with Usher syndrome type II.

For many years I was in denial about my deafblindness and felt a great deal of anger and frustration over my loss of vision; this is when I began power lifting and found that I loved it. Power lifting is an individual sport that you can do anywhere (you don't even need a ride to the gym if you have your own equipment); it doesn't take much equipment to get started and you can always build on what you have. This made it the perfect sport for me and the perfect outlet for my emotions. I soon began attending a gym where I met my coach, Clint, who taught me the basics of power lifting and gave me a job there.

I practised regularly at the gym and taught myself how to get around, quickly becoming accustomed to the placement of the different exercise machines and memorising where each item was. Luckily, the equipment was kept in the same place and was well organised and; if something was out of place, I learned how to look for it. I worked with a spotter for heavy lifting and used my anger as motivation; the angrier I got, the more I lifted.

As I continued lifting, I began to power lift competitively and later joined the United States Association of Blind Athletes (USABA). I am currently a 30-time world champion in power lifting for the blind as well as sighted in the ATA, IBPF, IBSA and WADAL Power Lifting Federations. I have won approximately 15 Texas state championships and numerous national championships. In 2012, I was inducted into the World Association of Bench Press and Dead Lifters Association (WABDL) Hall of Fame, becoming the first person with a disability to receive that honour. I also participated in strong man competitions and became the first American to become the World's Strongest Disabled Man, Standing Division.

In addition to lifting, I have participated in other sports including fishing, hunting, shooting, running and even Taekwondo. In 2014, I entered a fishing competition in Galveston, Texas, the Turning Point National Disability Fishing Tournament, and got first place in the adult division and *was named angler of the year! That same year, I entered a target shooting competition, the South Texas Pistol Shooting Championship, and won first place. I also participated in the Challenged Sportsmen of America Shotgun Shooting Challenge. These experiences allowed me to meet other Sportsmen with disabilities and helped boost my confidence in trying new things. I have competed in track and field as well and have gone on to many competitions, winning three National Championships for the Blind in track and field in the pentathlon event and also participating in the 100- and 200-metre run, the 1500 metre run, shot put, long jump and javelin discus throw. I even won the Taekwondo CTF Competition in Board Breaking, Able Body Division.*

I still lift in my home gym, but will only do light weights unless I have someone to spot me. I lift and also run to build my cardio; at home, there is an open area where I can run; I use ropes to keep me within the right area. I have had wonderful training partners who have been patient in working with me; I could never have accomplished all I have without their help and the help of many others. I practice a skill until I get it right and then build on it. I have had many, many failures, but I never give up.

Lifting weights has opened up the world to me and made it a far less threatening place. I have not only travelled to different states such as Colorado, South Carolina, Nevada, Washington, Florida, Oklahoma and California, but have also been abroad to Canada, Mexico, Czechoslovakia, Austria and Holland representing Team USA. Physical fitness will always be part of my life because it helps me release stress, maintain my weight (because I love to eat) and makes me feel young.

Rachel Weeks

When I was growing up, the question would often arise: "If given a choice, would you rather be blind or deaf?" As a hearing impaired child, not aware of the cause of my impairment, the question was not an easy one to answer. Little did I know that at age 19, I would have to face losing both my hearing and sight with a diagnosis of a rare genetic condition called Usher syndrome. Because Usher syndrome is a degenerative disease, it requires the person to constantly adapt, adjust and persevere. It is also genetic and I continually worried about my daughters, my sister and my nieces. None of them show signs of the disorder; for that, I am grateful.

As a child, I was only aware of having a hearing impairment and was very active as a dancer, gymnast, horseback rider and cheerleader. I wore hearing aids, took speech therapy intensively and did quite well in mainstream classrooms. When I attended elementary school in Nashville, Tennessee, where I was born, I had an aide in class and the attitude of my classmates was that of acceptance. There were other schools that I attended where the students were less accepting and I experienced bullying and indifference. It was not until I went to high school that I found a group of peers who accepted me and, in some cases, forgot that I had a hearing impairment all together. My teachers in high school were thoughtful and inclusive, helping me become an honour and advanced placement student. I eventually received a full ride to the University of South Florida and received my master's in counseling. I now work with youth and adults, helping them in their jobs, classrooms and daily living activities so that they can be at their highest functioning.

After graduating from high school, I remained physically active until I became more sedentary during my master's programme. After I received my degree, my sister mentioned that she was participating in a half marathon with her college roommate, which is when I became interested in running and discovered guide running. A guide runner is a partner who runs alongside runners who are visually impaired or blind, providing guidance for them during a race. Guidance can involve running in front of the athlete, running beside the athlete and giving verbal cues or running with a wrist or waist tether between the runner and guide. My sister was my first guide and we found the waist tether to be the best support for me. I went on to finish races in the 5K, 10K and half marathon distances. While I loved running, my first desire was to participate in the Ironman Triathlon.

I first heard about the Ironman Triathlon from a professor at the University of South Florida. She was in her sixties, had lost a lot of weight, quit a drinking habit, got her PhD and went on to complete a triathlon which involved a 2.4-mile swim, a 112-mile bike ride and a 26.2-mile run. I remember sitting in her classroom, six months pregnant, visually and hearing impaired, saying to myself, "I want to do that!" I eventually learned that I could participate in Ironman competitions with a guide in the same way that I could participate in running with a guide. This is when my journey truly began.

Since I was already running, all I needed to learn was swimming and biking. I began swimming laps, which was not easy at all; I was used to swimming with full vision and to swim as an adult with no peripheral vision was extremely difficult. However, with each lap I grew stronger and after months of practice I gained my rhythm. Biking was an even greater test of patience. I had no clue what a derailleur, cassette or cycling name brand was and I had to navigate the world of tandem cycling.

After receiving a grant from the Challenged Athletes Foundation towards a tandem bike, I began to test tandems out. I found my first tandem in Greenville, South Carolina at TTR Bikes. My sister and I named it the Beast and soon began launching, stopping, learning the gears and hill climbing. We combined tandem biking with swimming and running and this prepared me for my first triathlon in June of 2012. I have since gone on to compete in multiple races of varying distances including Ironman Texas 2013, my biggest race to date.

The world of sports has not been a place of barriers for me but one of huge opportunities. The primary challenges have been financial costs, which include shipping large equipment as well as two people to races and the fact that race directors often have no experience with athletes who are blind or visually impaired. Many times it is up to the athlete to educate directors and those involved with the races about visually impaired and blind racing techniques. Luckily, there are many organisations in place for visually impaired and blind athletes, as well as athletes who are deafblind. These organisations include Challenged Athletes Foundation, Achilles International, Team RWB, Team with a Vision, USAT Paratriathlon and Dare2Tri Paratriathlon to name a few.

My goals for the future are to compete in the 70.3 and 140.6 World Championship Ironman races as well as to work towards a designated championship race for physically challenged athletes in the 70.3 and 140.6 distances. I would also like to coach youth who are visually impaired, blind and deafblind in the sport of triathlon. I have partnered with Camp Abilities and started my own team, Light Up the Darkness, in the Tampa Bay Area. I'm excited about coaching, raising awareness in youth and adults and promoting health and wellness through sports.

Conclusion

Children with deafblindness have unique needs that must be met in order for them to successfully participate in physical activity and physical education. The purpose of this chapter was to shed light on teaching children who are deafblind in physical education, and provide useful information to help these students be successful. With some careful planning, collaboration, modification and creativity, they can reach their potential in their chosen sport or activity.

References

Arndt, K.L., Lieberman, L.J. and Pucci, G. 2004. Communication during physical activity for youth who are deafblind. *Teaching Exceptional Children Plus*, 1(2), Article 1.

Bruce, S.M., Zatta, M.C., Gavin, M. and Stelzer, S. 2016. Socialization and self-determination in different-age dyads of students who are deafblind. *Journal of Visual Impairment and Blindness*, 110(3), 149–161.

Grenier, M. and Lieberman, L.J. (eds). 2018. *Physical education for children with moderate to severe disabilities*. Champaign, IL: Human Kinetics.

Kamenopoulou, L. 2012. A study on the inclusion of deafblind young people in mainstream schools: Key findings and implications for research and practice. *British Journal of Special Education*, 39(3), 137–145.

Lieberman, L.J. 2017. Visual impairments. In J.P. Winnick and D. Porretta (eds), *Adapted physical education and sport* (6th ed., pp. 235–252). Champaign, IL: Human Kinetics.

Lieberman, L.J., Haegele, J.A. and Marquez, M. 2016. *Possibilities: Recreation experiences of people who are deafblind*. Louisville, KY: American Printing House for the Blind.

Lieberman, L.J., Haibach, P. and Schedlin, H. 2012. Physical education and children with CHARGE Syndrome: Research to practice. *Journal of Visual Impairment and Blindness*, 106(2), 106–119.

Lieberman, L.J. and Houston-Wilson, C. 2018. *Strategies for inclusion: Physical education for everyone* (3rd ed.). Champaign, IL: Human Kinetics.

Lieberman, L.J. and Stuart, M.E. 2002. Self-determined recreation and leisure choices of individuals with deaf-blindness. *Journal of Visual Impairment and Blindness*, 96(10), 724–735.

Lieberman, L.J., Kirk, T.N. and Haegele, J.A. 2018. Physical education and transition planning experiences relating to recreation among adults who are deafblind: A recall analysis. *Journal of Visual Impairment and Blindness*, 112(1), 73–86.

Lieberman, L.J. and MacVicar, J. 2003. Play and recreation habits of youth who are deaf-blind. *Journal of Visual Impairment and Blindness*, 97(12), 755–768.

Lieberman, L.J. and Pecorella, M. 2006. Activity at home for children and youth who are deafblind. *Deaf-Blind Perspectives*, 14(1), 3–7.

Lieberman, L.J., Ponchillia, P. and Ponchillia, S. (2013). *Physical education and sport for individuals who are visually impaired or deafblind: Foundations of instruction*. New York: AFB Press.

McInnes, J. (1999). *A guide to planning and support for individuals who are deaf-blind*. Toronto, ON: University of Toronto Press.

Moller, K. and Danermark, B. 2007. Social recognition, participation, and the dynamic between the environment and personal factors of students with deafblindness. *American Annals of the Deaf*, 152(1), 42–55.

Morgan, S. 2001. "What's my role?" A comparison of the responsibilities of interpreters, interveners, and support service providers. *Deaf-Blind Perspectives*, 9, 1–3.

Robinson, B. and Lieberman, L.J. 2004. Effects of visual impairment, gender, and age on self-determination. *Journal of Visual Impairment and Blindness*, 98(6), 351–366.

Simms, B. (2004). *European guidelines on combating the social exclusion of deafblind people*. London: Sense International.

Sterbova, D. and Kudlacek, M. 2014. Deaf-blindness: Voices of mothers concerning leisure-time physical activity and coping with disability. *Acta Gymnica*, 44(4), 193–201.

US Department of Education (n.d.). IDEA Regulations: Part 300/A/300.8. Accessed 4 January 2019. http://idea.ed.gov/explore/view/p/%2Croot%2Cregs%2C300%2CA%2C300%252E8%2C.

13

Movement and visual impairment

Research and practice

Justin A. Haegele and Lauren J. Lieberman

Introduction

Children with visual impairments are born with the same potential as their sighted peers, and having a visual impairment itself does not affect the ability of children to be physically active (Lieberman, 2011; Lieberman and Runyan, 2016). However, research suggests that youth with visual impairments tend not to meet recommended physical activity levels and are less likely to be physically active than their sighted peers (Augestad and Jiang, 2015; Haegele and Porretta, 2015a). Because of low physical activity participation, youth with visual impairments also demonstrate higher rates of poor health-related fitness and can be at a high risk for developing mental health conditions (Brunes, Flanders and Augestad, 2015; Lieberman et al., 2010). Although youth with visual impairments describe physical activity as being fun and enjoyable, and report being confident in their abilities to be active (Ward et al., 2011), they experience a number of barriers to participation that inhibit their activity within and outside of school settings (Perkins et al., 2013). Namely, a lack of physical activity opportunities, encouragement from parents and trained physical educators (Stuart, Lieberman and Hand, 2006) are commonly described barriers, which impede physical activity participation.

Additional factors that must be considered include the role that fundamental motor skill competence and perceived motor skill competence play in physical activity (Stodden et al., 2008). Conceptually, both motor skill competence and perceived motor skill competence contribute to one's ability to perform tasks related to physical activities. Motor skill competence is considered proficiency in fundamental motor skills; building blocks of more complex movements that are typically classified as either object control (e.g. throwing, kicking) or locomotor skills (e.g. running, jumping). Research suggests that motor skill competence has a dynamic relationship with physical activity (Stodden et al., 2008) and is important in promoting activity throughout the lifespan. For those with visual impairments, motor skills are as important for daily living and sport activities as they are for any other children (Houwen, Hartman, Jonker and Visscher, 2010). Current research, though, demonstrates that youth with visual impairments tend to demonstrate significantly worse motor skill competence than sighted peers (Haegele, Brian and Goodway, 2015; Wagner, Haibach and Lieberman, 2013), and those with more severe visual impairments tend to have worse motor skill competence than those with less severe impairments (Haibach, Wagner and Lieberman, 2014).

Perceived motor skill competence is defined as an individual's personal perception of his/her physical strength, movement capability, capacity for sport and fitness levels (Fox and Corbin, 1989). Young children often demonstrate a limited ability to accurately perceive their motor skill competence, and tend to overestimate their abilities. Because of this, they are persistent and willing to engage in activities because they believe they are being successful (Brian, Haegele and Bostick, 2016). As children grow older, however, their perceived motor skill competence is more directly related to the likelihood of them being physically active. As such, when children have low perceived motor competence, they believe they are not as advanced as their peers and may withdraw from activity (Stodden et al., 2008). Recent research suggests that youth with visual impairments tend to demonstrate poor to very poor levels of perceived motor competence (Brian, Haegele and Bostick, 2016; Brian, Haegele et al., 2018), which may also impact their desire to be physically active.

In summary, research suggests that youth with visual impairments tend to demonstrate lower physical activity participation, motor skill competence and perceived motor skill competence than their sighted peers. Because of this, they tend to experience higher rates of low health-related physical fitness and mental health concerns. Having a visual impairment may impact some of these delays (for example, having a visual impairment may slow down motor acquisition because of a lack of visual input of appropriate models), fortunately, adequate amounts of movement experiences can reverse these delays (Houwen, Hartman, Jonker and Visscher, 2010). Rather, low levels of physical activity, motor competence and perceived motor competence are most likely due to barriers in participation that youth with visual impairments experience. Therefore, additional support and careful planning in physical education, recreation or other movement-related fields can make the difference for these students.

Teaching physical education to students with visual impairments

The most likely environment for students with visual impairments to participate in and learn about physical activity is school-based physical education. In most cases, students with visual impairments are included in general physical education classes with their typically developing peers (Lieberman, Ponchillia and Ponchillia, 2013). In order for these experiences to be successful, general physical education teachers must have the appropriate knowledge and skills in order to make activities accessible (Conroy, 2012; Perkins et al., 2013). This section describes a number of guidelines and tips for physical education teachers who have students with visual impairments in their classes. Because each child is different, it is important to keep in mind that some of these ideas may be better for some students than others and it is essential for teachers to discuss each of these strategies with the student prior to implementing them.

Pre-teaching/tactile maps and boards

For students with visual impairments, the ability to understand the spatial layout of the playing area of a sport or activity is an important instructional consideration (Renshaw and Zimmerman, 2008). One technique used to teach students with visual impairments about the layout of playing areas is tactile mapping/boards. Tactile mapping is commonly accepted as being an effective medium for teaching students how to move through space (Renshaw and Zimmerman, 2008). Tactile maps consist of a piece of paper or other surface that utilises raised lines and symbols to indicate where landmarks are located, such as boundaries, obstacles, equipment, participants or targets. Tactile boards are tactile mapping material that is

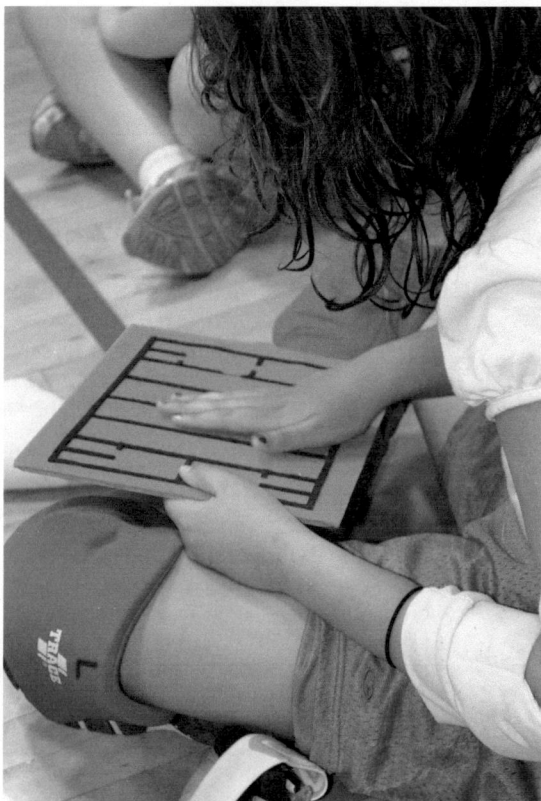

Figure 13.1   Student using a tactile board to learn goalball.

mounted on a sturdy surface (e.g. clipboard, see Figure 13.1). When utilising tactile maps or boards, teachers should describe and explain the playing area using the board while the student explores the playing area physically.

Tactile maps and board can be particularly helpful during pre-teaching activities. Pre-teaching is the concept of teaching elements of an upcoming unit or activity prior to actually engaging in that activity. Important information for students with visual impairments to learn prior to a unit may be the physical layout of a playing area, equipment used in that game, all terminology related to that game or sport, the scoring systems, the player positions involved in an activity, strategy and other background information on a game. Utilising tactile maps and boards, physical educators can pre-teach content related to the physical layout of the playing area and player positions prior to the unit starting so students with visual impairments are up to speed during class instruction and activities. In addition to the physical educator, other professionals such as the student's orientation and mobility instructor or teacher aids can assist with pre-teaching and tactile mapping activities.

Activity modifications

With proper modifications, students with visual impairments have the ability to participate in most of the same activities as their sighted peers. Physical education teachers can modify the rules and regulations (including equipment) of any game or sport necessary in order to assure that

Table 13.1 Activity modifications.

Modification type	Example
Equipment modifications	• Use a larger ball
	• Use a bright or high-contrast ball
	• Use a softer ball
	• Deflate a ball to slow it down
	• Use balloons or scarves that are light and will stay in the air longer
	• Add sound sources
	• Add a beeper or bells to the ball
	• Lower goals or make them larger
	• Tie a plastic bag around a ball to make noise
Rule modifications	• Give player on the offensive more space between himself and defender
	• Bounce passes or roll the ball only during basketball
	• Forgive technicalities
	• Allow more bounces
	• Assign player roles
	• Everyone must touch the ball before scoring
	• Give everyone a turn before changing possession
Boundary modifications	• Increase or decrease playing area
	• Put rope under tape to give rise to boundaries
	• Use caution tape or flag-rope to make off-playing area
	• Put sound sources behind goals or other target areas
	• Use bright tape or high-contrast colours on floor to make boundaries
	• Use larger cones to mark area

Note: Adapted from Haegele and Mescall (2013).

learning takes place in the physical education environment (Brian and Haegele, 2014). Within each activity, equipment, rules and boundaries can be modified in many simple and creative ways to ensure active participation. Table 13.1 displays examples of each of these types of modifications.

The modifications needed for each student will be different based on his/her unique needs. Prior to modifying activities, the physical education teacher should speak with the student's teacher for the visually impaired, paraprofessional, orientation and mobility instructor or directly to the student to ensure that modifications are appropriate and desired. A modification may be as little as a baseball hat and sunglasses for a child with albinism, or rule modifications for someone who is completely blind that allow them to walk to a net and feel it before striking in volleyball. It is important for physical educators to take into consideration the needs of each child individually when considering modifications to ensure success. Lastly, it has been shown that the modifications to activities do not affect the performance of sighted children so everyone in the class can used the modified equipment if so desired (de Schipper, Lieberman and Moody, 2017).

Instructional approaches

The most significant instructional barrier between a physical educator and a student with a visual impairment tends to occur when students need to learn complex skills (Lieberman et al., 2013). This may be because physical educators typically teach complex skills utilising visual modelling techniques that are inherently challenging for students with severe visual impairments. For instruction to be meaningful, physical educators must choose carefully which method to use depending on the skill being taught and the student's learning preferences (Lieberman and

Runyan, 2016). A number of instructional approaches have been devised that make observation and demonstration accessible for those with little or no vision. These instructional approaches can be used in isolation, or in combination with one another. These include (a) verbal instruction, (b) tactile modelling, (c) physical guidance and (d) tactile mapping/boards.

Verbal instruction

Verbal instruction includes verbally describing what a learner must do in order to successfully complete a task. Verbal instruction is a useful tool for many lessons, especially those that include simple skills or with students who have previous experience with similar skills (Lieberman et al., 2013). When using verbal instruction, it is especially important for teachers to use precise and consistent language. Precise language is particularly important when performing more complex skills, and typically general language will not suffice. Furthermore, teachers should ensure that they are consistent with their cues within and across units to ensure consistent movements based on those words. However, words may not provide enough information for students with visual impairments to successfully perform complex skills, and modelling techniques (described below) are essential for teaching the entire skill.

Tactile modelling

Modelling is essential when teaching students new physical activities. Modelling provides a mental picture of how a particular skill or activity is performed, which guides a student's actions when

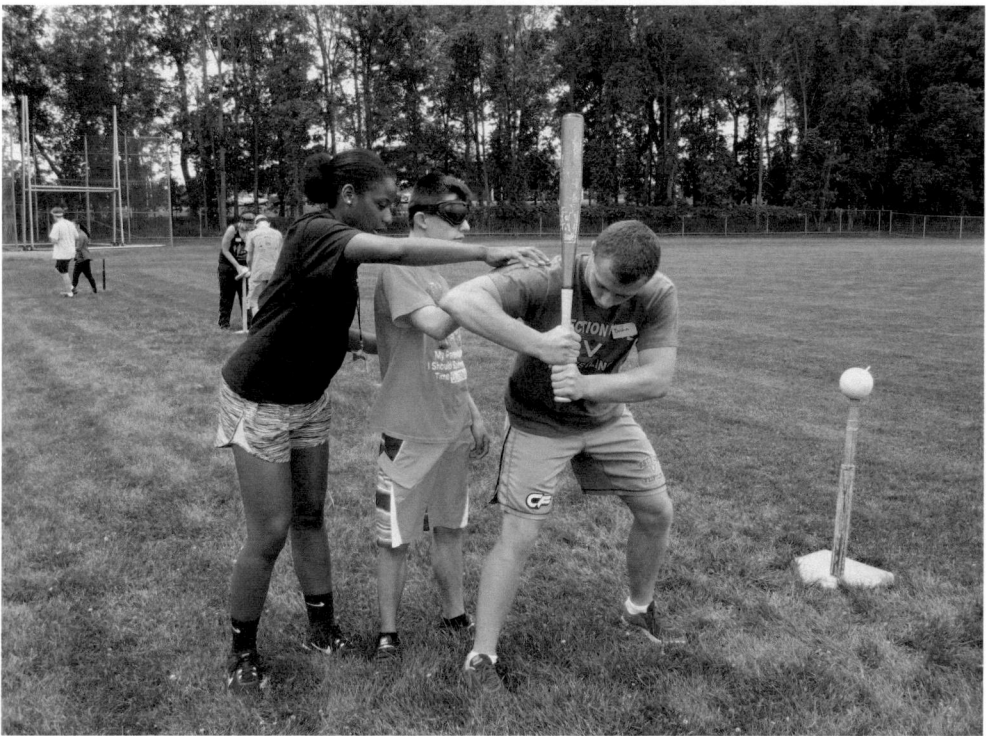

Figure 13.2 Student learning to hit a ball through tactile modelling.

they are asked to reproduce the skill (Haegele et al., 2014). Tactile modelling, or hand–under–hand instruction, is defined as an exhibition of a motor activity that is presented by touch to make it comprehensible to individuals with visual impairments (O'Connell, Lieberman and Petersen, 2006). This modelling technique allows students with severe visual impairments to appropriately feel and explore a movement by touching a model's (or teacher's) body while the model demonstrates the skill (O'Connell et al., 2006) (see Figure 13.2). This technique is helpful because it can help clarify misunderstandings of a movement more comprehensively than verbal descriptions alone. Also, students can control his or her learning by deciding which parts of the movement to focus on.

Physical guidance

A second modelling technique is called physical guidance. Physical guidance, or hand–over–hand instruction, is defined as performing a particular movement with a student in order for him or her to understand the rhythm and motion of the action (O'Connell et al., 2006). Physical guidance is distinct from tactile modelling in that tactile modelling involves the athlete touching the model, whereas physical guidance involves the teacher actively moving the athlete to perform the skill. Importantly, teachers must actively communicate with students during physical guidance so that students are comfortable with being touched and understand what is about to happen. Typically, teachers can begin teaching complex activities using physical guidance or tactile modelling, then refine these movements using verbal instruction.

Please note that any time tactile instruction is used it must be well documented. The purpose is to ensure shared knowledge of the preferred and successful techniques as well as to let the multidisciplinary team know why the child is being touched or touching others.

Support personnel

Paraprofessionals

Paraprofessionals, or teacher assistants, work alongside teachers who educate children with disabilities who are in need of support (Haegele and Kozub, 2010). They typically have ambiguous roles in physical education and are not trained specifically for physical education classes (Bryan, McCubbin and van der Mars, 2013; Lieberman and Conroy, 2013). However, they have a wealth of knowledge pertaining to each student because they spend more time with their students than anyone else in the school system (Lee and Haegele, 2016). Trained paraprofessionals who are engaged in activities can be instrumental in ensuring that students are actively participating in class, and can perform a number of tasks related to pre-teaching, modelling or providing supplementary verbal instruction. In order to effectively work with paraprofessionals, physical educations are encouraged to (a) actively and reciprocally communicate with paraprofessionals about the needs of students, (b) share lesson plans to ensure everyone is on the same page and (c) showe the paraprofessional that you value their contributions to the physical education environment (Lee and Haegele, 2016). A paraeducator training video to teach techniques for physical education for children with visual impairments can be found at www.youtube.com/watch?v=77fyMsRWrYs.

Trained peer tutors

Like paraprofessionals, trained peer tutors can also provide important support within a classroom. Peer tutors are age-appropriate partners who can navigate the gymnasium and physical activities with students with visual impairments. Research suggests that the utilisation of trained peer tutors with children with visual impairments can provide positive role models and honest feedback (Wiskochil et al., 2007). Like paraprofessionals, it is essential that peer tutors are properly trained in order to be effective, and these individuals can also perform a number of tasks regarding modelling and providing supplemental instruction. A number of specific training programmes are available that can help train paraprofessionals and peer tutors to be effective and meaningful members of the physical education team (see Lieberman and Runyan, 2016).

Teaching for generalisation

As mentioned, youth with visual impairments tend to be less active than their sighted peers. One reason youth may be inactive outside of school is because of difficulties transferring skills learned during physical education to other settings (Haegele, 2015). In order to expect students with visual impairments to use skills learned in physical education to be active outside of school, teachers must plan to train students to generalise those skills. Generalisation is defined as the use of newly acquired skills or behaviours in non-training environments (Cooper, Heron and Heward, 2007). Haegele (2015) has identified a number of strategies that can be used by physical educators to help train students with visual impairments to generalise skills to promote physical activity outside of school. A summary of those strategies are presented in Table 13.2.

Fitness activity modifications

As mentioned, youth with visual impairments tend to demonstrate low levels of health-related fitness (Lieberman et al., 2010). For many children and adolescents, this may be due to not

Table 13.2 Generalisation tactics.

Tactic	Meaning	Physical educators can . . .
Recruiting reinforcements for physical activity participation	Asking individuals (e.g. parents) outside of school to reinforce physical activity participation in order to increase the likelihood of participation	• Inform parents of the physical activities taught in school and how to reinforce them at home • Use class-wide emails or announcements to promote reinforcement at home
Teaching students to recruit reinforcement	A student calling attention to his or her accomplishments to obtain praise or assistance for those efforts from significant others	• Teach students to perform skills correctly before attempting to recruit attention • Teach students to limit the number of times their recruit attention • Model simple recruiting sequences for students
Teaching sufficient stimulus examples	Teaching students to perform a behaviour correctly in response to more than one prompt or condition	• Change dimensions of the skill, activity or environment of instruction from one instructional setting to the next • Allow those other than the physical educator to deliver physical activity instruction
Teaching self-management skills	Teaching skills that students personally apply to produce desired behaviours	• Instruct students to use physical activity journals • Embed homework or pedometers into physical activity programmes

Note: Adapted from Haegele (2015).

Table 13.3 Fitness activity modifications.

Activity	Modification	Description	Activity	Modification	Description
Running	Sighted guide	Runner grasps the guide's elbow, shoulder or hand, depending on what is most comfortable	Bicycling	Stationary bike	Biker rides a stationary bike with no modifications
	Tether	The runner and guide grasp a short string, allowing the runners to have a full range of motion		Tandem bike	Biker can ride a tandem bike with no modifications. The sighted person acts as the pilot (front seat), and the individual with a visual impairment acts as the stoker (back sear)
	Guide wire	The runner holds a fixed wire and runs independently for time or distance		Side-by-side bike	Biker can ride with no modifications. Two bikers can ride sitting next to each other. Little balance or communication issues
	Sound source from a distance	The runner runs toward a sound source (clap, bell)	Swimming	Tapper	A sighted person taps the swimmer on the shoulder with a large pole when he/she is about eight feet from the wall as a signal to turn
	Sound source	The guide rings bells or shakes a noisemaker while running side by side		Sprinkler system	A sprinkler can be set up to land water about eight feet from the wall in order to signal for swimmers of the approaching wall
	Circular running	The runner runs in a large circular motion hold a rope that is staked into the ground		Counting strokes	Swimmers keep track of how many strokes it takes to get from one side of the pool to the other and count strokes while swimming
	Sighted guide shirts	The runner runs behind a guide wearing a bright shirt (low vision)		Side of the pool	Swimmers can use the side of the pool or lane lines to guide them to swim in a straight line

Note: Adapted from Hodge, Lieberman and Murata (2012).

having proper modifications available for common fitness activities, such as running, cycling or swimming. Table 13.3 provides examples of a number of commonly used modifications for each of these fitness activities. It is important to teach each technique to each youth with a visual impairment so that he or she can choose the best one for each situation. For example, some youth may choose one technique for shorter distances, and others for further distances. Also, they may use one for recreational activities, and others for competition.

For older students (high school-aged), an additional fitness activity that is important to teach are skills related to frequenting an exercise facility. Teaching students to use weight training and fitness equipment, such as treadmills, elliptical machines, exercise bikes, can help promote lifelong fitness outside of schools. Also, these are the types of fitness activities that other students this age are learning, and it is important to teach the same curriculum. Exercise equipment can be made accessible to youth with visual impairments through braille markers and tactile cues (Lieberman et al., 2014). By teaching these activities in schools, it increases the likelihood of students having the skills needed to continue to be physically active and exercise at home or in their community (Lieberman et al., 2013).

Assessments

Assessments are essential in determining the strengths and weaknesses of students regarding their physical activity participation, health-related fitness, motor competence and perceived motor competence. All students with disabilities, including those with visual impairments, must be properly assessed for referral, eligibility and placement in physical education. A variety of types of assessments are used in physical education environments to assess students' physical activity, health-related fitness, motor skill competence and perceived motor skill competence. For example, a recent trend in physical education classes is to assess the amount of physical activity students participate in during class using pedometers. Currently, several assessment tools are validated for children with visual impairments, including:

- *Brockport Physical Fitness Test (health-related fitness)*: A health-related, criterion-referenced physical fitness test designed specifically for use among students with disabilities aged 10 to 17 (Winnick and Short, 2014). One unique feature of this assessment instrument is that it provides options for test administrators to personalise testing. Because of this, the test includes a battery of 27 test items, but typically students complete 4 to 6 items in order to attain a health-related physical fitness estimate. This is the only health-related physical fitness assessment that is validated for youth with visual impairments.
- *Centrios Talking Pedometer (physical activity)*: Pedometers are small devices that can be worn unobtrusively on the belt or waistband that provides users with feedback via a digital screen that displays accumulated step counts. Talking pedometers, designed specifically for individuals with visual impairments, provide auditory feedback in addition to visual feedback. The Centrios Talking Pedometer is a spring-levered device that includes an automatic voice-announcement feature with announcement options such as number of steps taken, distance travelled, calories burned and time elapsed. This talking pedometer is the only currently commercially available device that has been validated for individuals with visual impairments (Beets et al., 2007; Haegele and Porretta, 2015b; Holbrook et al., 2011). In addition to being a physical activity measure, research suggests that talking pedometers can be motivating for youth with visual impairments to set goals for increasing daily physical activity (Lieberman et al., 2006).

- *Modified-Pictorial Scale for Perceived Competence and Social Acceptance (PSPCSA) (perceived motor competence)*: The PSPCSA is a six-item scale that measures children's perceived motor competence and typically includes pictorial representations of motor skills (Harter and Pike, 1984). The six motor skills featured within this scale include running, skipping, hopping, swinging, typing shoelaces and climbing. The modified-PSPCSA has replaced pictorial representations into standard verbal scripts that describe and explain each picture. The modified-PSPCSA has been tested for content and face validity (Brian, Haegele, Lieberman and Bostick, 2016) and construct validity and reliability (Brian et al., 2017) for assessing perceived motor competence for youth with visual impairments.
- *Test for Gross Motor Development-2 (TGMD-2) and -3 (TGMD-3) (motor skill competence)*: The TGMD-2 (Ulrich, 2000) is a qualitative measure to assess the motor skill competence of children aged 3–10. Twelve skills are subdivided into two areas: locomotor (run, gallop, hop, leap, horizontal jump and slide) and object control (two-hand strike, dribble, catch, kick, overhand throw and underhand roll). More recently, the TGMD-3 (Webster and Ulrich, 2017), an updated version of the TGMD-2, was released. The updated version of the assessment utilises the same structure, with some skills being changed. More specifically, the underhand roll was removed, and two new object control skills, the underhand throw and one-hand strike, were added. In addition, the leap was replaced with skipping. The TGMD-2 (Houwen, Hartman, Jonker and Visscher, 2010) and TGMD-3 (Brian, Taunton et al., 2018) are the only motor skills assessments that have been validated for students with visual impairments.

Inclusion example: Brittany

Brittany is a 13-year-old student in Oliver Middle School who is blind from Retinopathy of Prematurity (ROP). She is in her typical eighth-grade class and has been with the same peers since second grade. She has been going to physical education with her peers since second grade as well and they are all used to the modifications necessary to include her. For example, when they played tag in elementary school she had a peer guide her around and help her to locate her peers. When they played parachute she was pre-taught the dimensions of the parachute and given ideas on how the game would be played before class started. One of her peers helped her to know what colour she was holding and helped guide her through the parachute games.

In middle school, she has a paraprofessional named Ms Hopple. Ms Hopple has been her paraprofessional since sixth grade and has worked with the physical education teacher, Mrs Houston, on inclusion strategies for each unit. The current unit they are doing is volleyball and as usual Brittany will be fully included. Two weeks before the unit Brittany was pre-taught the dimensions of the court, positions of the players, the different ways to hit the ball, the rules of the game and the variations that she could choose to utilise. She was also given choices of various balls to use as well as distances from the net to serve and play. When the unit started she worked with her trained peer tutors, although Ms Hopple was still available if she needed her during the class. They started out with a cooperative game to see how many times they could get the ball over the net in a row without stopping. Mrs Houston taped rope on the floor throughout the perimeter of the court so Brittany would know the boundaries of the court during the game. For the game, Brittany chose to use several modifications, including (a) a beach ball with bells inside (equipment modification), (b) to let the ball bounce once if necessary (rule modification) and (c) to let her peer tutor catch the ball and hand it to her (rule modification). She also chose to stand at the mid-court line to serve the ball (rule modification). Her teammates could choose to use the same rules as Brittany or play with typical volleyball rules. Lastly, one player from the other team was blindfolded so the playing field was equal. This player rotated among her class and there was a waiting list to be blindfolded!

Conclusion

Internationally, approximately 1.4 million youth have irreversible conditions that cause visual impairments. Unfortunately, youth with visual impairments tend to participate in less physical activity than their sighted peers (Haegele and Porretta, 2015a) and demonstrate low levels of motor skill competence (Haegele et al., 2015), perceived motor skill competence (Brian, Haegele and Bostick, 2016) and health-related fitness (Lieberman et al., 2010). But, having a visual impairment in and of itself does not mean children need to be inactive. By carefully planning instruction and utilising successful modifications, supporting personal and instructional approaches, physical education teachers can ensure that children with visual impairments, like Brittany, have positive and meaningful physical education experiences with their sighted peers.

References

Augestad, L.B. and Jiang, L. 2015. Physical activity, physical fitness, and body composition among children and young adults with visual impairments: A systematic review. *British Journal of Visual Impairment*, 33(3), 167–182. http://dx.doi:10.1177/0264619615599813

Beets, M., Foley, J.T., Tindall, D.W.S. and Lieberman, L.J. 2007. Accuracy of voice-announcement pedometers for youth with visual impairment. *Adapted Physical Activity Quarterly*, 24(3), 218–227.

Brian, A., Bostick, L., Taunton, S. and Pennell, A. 2017. Construct validity and reliability of the test of perceived motor competence for children with visual impairments. *British Journal of Visual Impairment*, 35(2), 113–119.

Brian, A. and Haegele, J.A. 2014. Including students with visual impairments: Softball. *Journal of Physical Education, Recreation, and Dance*, 85(3), 39–45. http://dx.doi:10.1080/07303084.2014.875808

Brian, A., Haegele, J.A. and Bostick, L. 2016. Perceived motor competence of children with visual impairments: A preliminary investigation. *British Journal of Visual Impairment*, 34(2), 151–155.

Brian, A., Haegele, J.A., Lieberman, L.J. and Bostick, L. 2016. Examining the content and face validity for assessing perceived motor competence of individuals with visual impairments: A Delphi study. *British Journal of Visual Impairment*, 34(3), 238–247.

Brian, A., Haegele, J.A., Nesbitt, D., Lieberman, L., Bostick, L., Taunton, S. and Stodden, D. 2018. A pilot investigation of the perceived motor competence of children with visual impairments and those who are sighted. *Journal of Visual Impairments and Blindness*, 112(1), 118–124.

Brian, A., Taunton, S., Lieberman, L.J., Haibach-Beach, P., Foley, J. and Santarossa, S. 2018. Psychometric properties of the test for gross motor development-3 for children with visual impairments. *Adapted Physical Activity Quarterly*, 35(2), 145–158.

Brunes, A., Flanders, W.D. and Augestad, L.B. 2015. The effect of physical activity on mental health among adolescents with and without self-reported visual impairments: The young-HUNT study, Norway. *British Journal of Visual Impairment*, 33(3), 183–199. http://dx.doi:10.1177-02346196156022998

Bryan, R., McCubbin, J. and van der Mars, H. 2013. The ambiguous role of the paraeducator in the general physical education environment. *Adapted Physical Activity Quarterly*, 30(2), 164–183.

Cooper, J.O., Heron, T.E. and Heward, W.L. 2007. *Applied behavior analysis* (2nd ed.). London: Pearson Education.

Conroy, P. (2012). Supporting students with visual impairments in physical education. *Insight: Research and Practice in Visual Impairment and Blindness*, 5(1), 3–7.

De Schipper, T., Lieberman, L. and Moody, B. 2017. "Kids like me, we go lightly on the head": Experiences of children with a visual impairment on the physical self-concept. *British Journal of Visual Impairment*, 35(1), 55–68.

Fox, K.R. and Corbin, C.B. 1989. The physical self-perception profile: Development and preliminary validation. *Journal of Sport and Exercise Psychology*, 11(4), 408–430.

Haegele, J.A. 2015. Promoting leisure-time physical activity for students with visual impairments using generalization tactics. *Journal of Visual Impairment and Blindness*, 109(4), 322–326.

Haegele, J.A., Brian, A. and Goodway, J. 2015. Fundamental motor skills and school-aged individuals with visual impairments: A review. *Review Journal of Autism and Developmental Disorders*, 2(3), 320–327. http://dx.doi:10.1007/s40489-015-0055-8

Haegele, J.A. and Kozub, F.M. 2010. A continuum of paraeducator support for utilization in adapted physical education. *Teaching Exceptional Children Plus*, 6(5), 2–11.

Haegele, J.A., Lieberman, L.J., Lepore, M. and Lepore-Stevens, M. 2014. A service delivery model for physical activity in students with visual impairments: Camp Abilities. *Journal of Visual Impairment and Blindness*, 108(6), 474–484.

Haegele, J.A. and Mescall, M. 2013. Inclusive physical education. *Division of Visual Impairment Quarterly*, 58(3), 7–16.

Haegele, J.A. and Porretta, D.L. 2015a. Physical activity and school-age individuals with visual impairments: A literature review. *Adapted Physical Activity Quarterly*, 32(1), 68–82. http://dx.doi:10.1123/apaq.2013-0110

Haegele, J.A. and Porretta, D.L. 2015b. Validation of a talking pedometer for adolescents with visual impairments in free-living settings. *Journal of Visual Impairment and Blindness*, 109(3), 219–223.

Haibach, P., Wagner, M. and Lieberman, L. 2014. Determinants of gross motor skill performance in children with visual impairments. *Research in Developmental Disabilities*, 35(10), 2577–2584. http://dx.doi:10.1016/j.ridd.2014.05.030

Harter, S. and Pike, R. 1984. The pictorial scale of perceived competences and social acceptance for young children. *Child Development*, 55(6), 1969–1982.

Hodge, S., Lieberman, L. and Murata, N. 2012. *Essentials of teaching adapted physical education: Diversity, culture, and inclusion*. Scottsdale, AZ: Holcomb Hathaway.

Holbrook, E., Stevens, S., Kang, M. and Morgan, D. 2011. Validation of a talking pedometer for adults with visual impairments. *Medicine and Science in Sports and Exercise*, 43(6), 1094–1099.

Houwen, S., Hartman, E., Jonker, L. and Visscher, C. 2010. Reliability and validity of the TGMD-2 in primary school-aged children with visual impairments. *Adapted Physical Activity Quarterly*, 27(2), 149–159.

Houwen, S., Hartman, E. and Visscher, C. 2010. The relationship amoung motor performance, physical fitness, and body composition in children with and without visual impairment. *Research Quarterly for Exercise and Sport*, 81(3), 290–299.

Lee, S.H. and Haegele, J.A. 2016. Tips for effectively utilizing paraprofessionals in physical education. *Journal of Physical Education, Recreation, and Dance*, 87(1), 46–48.

Lieberman, L.J. 2011. Visual impairments. In J.P. Winnick (ed.), *Adapted physical education and sport* (5th ed., pp. 233–249). Champaign, IL: Human Kinetics.

Lieberman, L.J., Byrne, H., Mattern, C.O., Watt, C.A. and Fernandez-Vivo, M. 2010. Health-related fitness of youths with visual impairments. *Journal of Visual Impairment and Blindness*, 104(6), 349–359.

Lieberman, L.J. and Conroy, P. 2013. Training of paraeducators for physical education for children with visual impairments. *Journal of Visual Impairment and Blindness*, 107(1), 17–28.

Lieberman, L.J., Ponchillia, P. and Ponchillia, S. 2013. *Physical education and sports for people with visual impairments and deaf blindness: Foundations of instruction*. New York: AFB Press.

Lieberman, L.J. and Runyan, M. 2016. Visual impairment and deaf blindness. In M.E. Block (ed.), *A teacher's guide to adapted physical education* (4th ed., pp. 231–243). Brookes.

Lieberman, L.J., Stuart, M.E., Hand, K. and Robinson, B. 2006. Motivational effects of talking pedometers among children with visual impairments and deaf-blindness. *Journal of Visual Impairment and Blindness*, 100(12), 726–736.

O'Connell, M., Lieberman, L.J. and Petersen, S. 2006. The use of tactile modeling and physical guidance as instructional strategies in physical activity for children who are blind. *Journal of Visual Impairment and Blindness*, 100(8), 471–477.

Perkins, K., Columna, L., Lieberman, L. and Bailey, J. 2013. Parents' perceptions of physical activity for their children with visual impairments. *Journal of Visual Impairment and Blindness*, 107(2), 131–142.

Renshaw, R.L. and Zimmerman, G.L. 2008. Using a tactile map with a 5-year-old child in a large-scale outdoor environment. *RE: view*, 39(3), 113–120.

Stodden, D., Goodway, J.D., Langendorfer, S., Roberton, M., Rudisill, M., Garcia, C. and Garcia, L. 2008. A developmental perspective on the role of motor skill competence in physical activity: An emergent relationship. *Quest*, 13(1), 16–26.

Stuart, M., Lieberman, L. and Hand, K. 2006. Beliefs about physical activity among children who are visually impaired and their parents. *Journal of Visual Impairment and Blindness*, 100(4), 223–234.

Ulrich, D. 2000. *Test for gross motor development* (2nd ed.). Austin, TX: Pro-Ed.

Wagner, M., Haibach, P. and Lieberman, L. 2013. Gross motor skill performance in children with and without visual impairments: Research to practice. *Research in Developmental Disabilities*, 34(10), 3246–3252. http://dx.doi:10.1016/j.ridd.2013.06.030

Ward, S., Fansworth, C., Babkes-Stellino, M. and Perrett, J. 2011. Parental influences and the attraction to physical activity for youths who are visually impaired at a residential day school. *Journal of Visual Impairment and Blindness*, 105(8), 493–498.

Webster, E.K. and Ulrich, D.A. 2017. Evaluation of the psychometric properties of the Test of Gross Motor Development (TGMD-3). *Journal of Motor Learning and Development*, 5(1), 45–58.

Winnick J. and Short, F. 2014. *Brockport physical fitness test manual: A health-related assessment for youngesters with disabilities*. Champaign, IL: Human Kinetics.

Wiskolchil, B., Lieberman, L., Houston-Wilson, C. and Petersen, S. 2007. The effects of trained peer tutors on the physical education of children who are visually impaired. *Journal of Visual Impairment and Blindness*, 101(6), 339–350.

Part V
Assistive technology

14

Foundations and recommendations for research in access technology

Yue-Ting Siu

Introduction

The author is a sighted educator whose work involves direct instruction with visually impaired students across the lifespan, preparing teachers to work with this demographic and consulting in the design and dissemination of accessible educational materials including multimedia and use of technology. Despite maintaining a professional and research agenda focused on technology for individuals with visual impairments, the author's expertise remains limited due to being a sighted individual. The author's experience and insights could never replace those of a visually impaired end-user who depends upon technology to access everyday information; while the author could certainly advise on pedagogical aspects of visual impairment, it would be presumptuous to feign a blind user's experience. All research activities that ultimately impact blind or visually impaired users must begin and end with individuals who are blind or visually impaired. This premise includes understanding what visually impaired individuals actually need, variations in sensory needs and preferences, and how information might be conceptualised differently for low vision or nonvisual interpretation. The greatest pitfall in researching technology for low vision or nonvisual use is the exclusion of visually impaired individuals in every step of the process from conception to conclusion.

Given this sentiment, why not have a blind technology user write this chapter? This question could fortify a series of conversations among mixed company, so this author offers just this: understanding visual impairments and related needs and considerations requires a holistic approach. Any one person's singular perspective of technology will yield a limited scope of study. Although this chapter inherently presents one author's views, recommendations will focus on connecting with a range of stakeholders including multiple individuals with visual impairments. For more information about the importance of including stakeholders from related disability groups, readers are encouraged to study literature from the *Nothing About Us Without Us* movement.

The purpose of this chapter is to offer a conceptual framework for approaching research in the area of access (or more traditionally referred to as "assistive") technology. It is not prescriptive and will not assign any particular methodology. However, it will present concepts and recommendations that can be applicable to any methodology. Common pitfalls will also be discussed alongside suggestions for best practices in carrying out research in the area of technology for individuals with visual impairments. Ultimately, research in this area must be action-oriented. Technology innovates faster than the research, so there is no value for theoretical conjectures without actionable outcomes. Research focused on the user side of technology (for example, studying individuals' perceptual abilities or preferences) might inform the development of future technology features. Research focused on the usability side of technology (for example, how well a particular tool meets learning or assessment objectives) might focus more on the fit of the technology to the task at hand and the impact of a particular technology on one's quality of life. It is impossible to advise what research is or is not worth carrying out; rather, the implications of a research project will distil the purpose of any proposed agenda and advise investigators on designing a meaningful study.

Foundational concepts

Role of technology for individuals with visual impairments

If you are a sighted reader, take a moment to look up from this text and consider all the information you see as you look around the room: information posted on the walls, restaurant menus, what people are wearing, perhaps a notification on your smartphone about a bank deposit or upcoming appointment? Outside, there might be street signage that identifies buildings or special promotions, a bus stop with arrival times that update every minute or even a display that lists movie times. As sighted people, we take all of this information for granted because we assume it is our *right* to access freely available information. When we review personal information such as medical or bank records, we expect confidentiality because it involves our *right* to privacy. During leisure activities, sighted individuals also assume the privilege of choosing where and how to travel and what community events to engage with. In all, most of us take for granted our independent, primary and timely access to information.

For individuals who are blind or visually impaired, technology can play a critical role in facilitating equitable access to information, privacy and individual rights. Consider all the instances of looking around a room and assuming ease in accessing seemingly inane information; visually impaired individuals might otherwise depend on sighted assistance to access the same information yet do so at the cost of sacrificing privacy and independence. In practicality, the visually impaired individual instantly loses their right to independent, primary and timely access to information.

When technology is well designed to meet a visually impaired person's needs, it reduces previous barriers, improves one's quality of life and facilitates achievement of the same academic, employment or leisure goals as sighted peers. Technology can be a critical component of a larger toolkit that delivers a positive solution to a stated need. Researching and designing technology for individuals with visual impairments is no different from designing for sighted users; the best solutions begin with a user need and end with satisfying this need from the perspective of the end-user. At times, research and development of technology for low vision or nonvisual accessibility deviate from this basic premise and results in limited or no impact despite a researcher's good intentions. To avoid this pitfall, the chapter will dedicate significant discussion to help researchers develop a mindset for conducting research in this particular area of need: access to information as mediated by technology. Technology-based interventions for "curing" blindness will not be discussed; rather, research and interventions will focus on how technology can enhance low vision or nonvisual access and reduce barriers including those found in physical and digital environments. Taking this approach can help the researcher reduce any pre-existing negative perceptions of blindness. With adequate education, training and tools, people who are blind or visually impaired can mediate information independently and efficiently and be seen as equals rather than a demographic that is dependent on sighted assistance.

User experiences in access and assistive technology

When discussing technology for users who are blind or visually impaired, the following question inevitably arises: *Is technology replacing braille?* In short, the answer is: *No!*

To fully answer this question, the role of technology must be re-visited in the context of the user needs it is meant to serve. This requires understanding how low vision or nonvisual access to information is inherently different from "retino-centric" experiences (Abrahamson et al., 2018). Teachers of the visually impaired (TVIs) are particularly conversant in this area and exercise pedagogical knowledge of how a visual impairment can impact a student's learning and global development. In particular, TVIs are responsible for teaching the expanded core curriculum (ECC) (Hatlen, 1996; Huebner et al., 2004; Sapp and Hatlen, 2010), which encompasses skills in nine areas of development that are impacted by vision impairment. These areas of development are typically learned incidentally through visual observation, but students who are visually impaired require direct instruction. The areas include compensatory skills, orientation and mobility, social skills, independent living skills, recreation and leisure, career education, use of assistive technology, sensory efficiency skills and self-determination. For school-age students, prioritisation of instruction in various areas of the ECC will dictate an intervention plan and dictate what types of access and assistive technology will be most beneficial (Huebner et al., 2004).

In understanding how the ECC guides instruction for school-age students, it becomes evident how low or nonvisual access requires differentiated conceptualisations of information. Visually impaired individuals must develop alternative strategies for interacting with information in a visual world, which in turn dictates how technology must function for these end-users (Barclay, 2011; Morash et al., 2014; Presley and Siu, in press).

Most individuals with visual impairments use more than one sensory channel to access information. The effectiveness of each sensory channel (visual, auditory, tactile) differs across individuals and changes depending on the task at hand and the modality that is most efficient in a particular moment (Holbrook et al., 2017; Koenig and Holbrook, 1995). For example, a person with low vision might use vision primarily to access short reading tasks such as lists or word problems, but switch to auditory access for reading a novel and tactile access for carrying out activities of daily living. A functionally blind person might use their auditory channel primarily to access mobile reading tasks such as text messages or leisure reading such as novels, but switch to tactile access for reviewing memos and editing papers in braille or exploring tactile graphics (raised line drawings). Regardless of the sensory channel and number of modalities an individual might utilise to carry out a task, access to information depends on two general constructs: how the media is formatted for multimodal access and what features of technology can be utilised to support multimodal access (Miyashita et al., 2007; Siu, 2016).

In some instances, information translates seamlessly across sensory modalities. For example, when printed text is translated to accessible digital text, textual information can be represented with similar integrity in visual, auditory or tactile formats. However, non-textual information does not necessarily translate with similar ease. Images, graphics and environmental information in both physical and digital formats require pedagogical understanding to adequately represent data spatially for nonvisual interpretation. Consider the following examples.

Images

Information about some images can be adequately conveyed with a concise description (Morash et al., 2015; Packer, Vizenor and Miele, 2015). More complex images might require a tactile graphic or 3D model. Deciding how to represent an image depends on understanding what information the image is meant to convey and how this information is meaningful in a nonvisual format (Braille Authority of North America, 2010; Diagram Center 2014). A common practice when creating tactile graphics is to render raised line drawings as exact replicas of the visual drawing. However, simply feeling the lines of a drawing might not convey the information that the drawing is meant to convey. For example, while a simple square might be adequately represented with four raised lines, it is impossible to raise the lines of a drawn 3D cube and tactually convey the 3D-ness of a cube. In this instance, the cube would be better represented for tactile learning as a handheld model. The provision of 3D models might also require additional consideration to ensure the model is adequately representative; keeping in mind that most 3D printed models have a generic plastic feel with limited capacity to distinguish details, it is important to consider what is appropriate for 3D printing (for low vision or nonvisual accessibility) and when to provide an actual object or use alternative mixed media (Buehler, Kane and Hurst, 2014).

Scientific notations and data visualisations (charts and graphs)

Some of the biggest differences between visual and nonvisual access is the ease of previewing an overview of data including spatial relationships. Although scientific notations can be described or converted into a digital format for reading with a screen reader or refreshable braille display, the auditory format conveys information in a purely linear fashion that cannot adequately convey how equations might be laid out spatially (Alajarmeh, Pontelli and Son, 2011; Bouck and Meyer, 2012; Noble et al., 2018). Instead, information is only accessible as it is read aloud or shown on a traditional refreshable braille display that displays a single line at a time. Emerging technologies are showing great promise, however; sonification resolves the problem of linearity by providing an auditory landscape of how data are laid out (Belardinelli et al., 2009; Brown et al., 2003; Walker and Mauney, 2010), which is supplemented by a drill-down approach that describes specific data points. Multi-line refreshable braille and tactile graphics displays are highly desirable in order to present dynamic spatial layouts that refresh as data refreshes, with early prototypes on the horizon.

Tactile graphics can be an effective strategy for visualising data and providing a tactile overview. However, labelling data on a tactile graphic can require a delicate balance between conveying information and cluttering the tactile integrity of the graphic (Amick and Corcoran, 1997). Multimodal technologies such as audio-tactile graphics and models are a simple yet sophisticated method for joining sensory modalities via audio labels that speak when tactually activated. The combined approach leverages the benefits of each modality without the limitations (Miele, Landau and Gilden, 2006).

Environmental information

Accessibility in physical and digital environments often transcends conventional approaches of presenting information visually, auditorially or tactually. Haptic interfaces, kinesthetic and proprioceptive feedback and even olfactory senses can convey an incredible amount of information about one's environment. When researching technology in this area of access, it is important to recognise how an individual most organically gains information about the environment and identify where specific limitations exist. Consider the example of a white cane, which is a time-honoured no-tech tool for nonvisual mobility. Despite minimal technology adaptations to the cane since its inception in the 1920s (Strong, 2009), the white cane continues to be a successful tool for savvy travellers who are visually impaired (Bourquin et al., 2017; Sauerburger and Bourquin, 2010). White canes can transmit an abundance of environmental information if an end-user has developed skills to access this information. The cane is meant to provide feedback on elevation changes and low-lying obstacles, and can give the traveller a sense of the surrounding space depending on how the cane sounds as it moves across a walking surface. It does not, however, detect high-lying obstacles and is less successful on surfaces that restrict cane movement. Understanding the affordances and limitations of the white cane will help specify needs for technology aimed at improving nonvisual mobility. Any technology that interrupts an existing successful flow of information from the cane therefore creates a disruptive experience that further divorces the traveller from naturally accessing the environment. Technology that respects an end-user's natural inclinations are most effective when the tools augment rather than intercept intuitive information gathering. As with any area of access technology, usability is critical; technology that delivers information remains ineffective when the user experience is unpleasant or ostracising.

Another example relates to the usability of orientation and navigation technologies. As global positioning system (GPS) apps have become more accessible with assistive technologies, visually impaired travellers might select tools for navigation based on the ease and extent of sensory feedback needed. Although most GPS apps have features for auditory navigation, how a traveller accesses that information may help or hinder the travel experience. Headphones or earbuds might occlude environmental sounds needed for street crossing and orientation, braille displays that present turn-by-turn directions might be cumbersome if hands are needed to use a cane or dog guide and visual interfaces might become unusable if map elements fail to display with colour-contrast adjustments. These factors will affect which tools a blind traveller chooses to use in different situations. The latest technology innovations in haptic feedback for dictating where to turn (Rodriguez, Conwell and Digimarc Corp., 2014; Ye et al., 2014) or visual interpreter applications (Fleet, 2017) that provide remote sighted assistance highlight some examples of how technology can solve a particular aspect of a user need that results in a more independent and less disruptive workflow.

Usability is particularly relevant when accessing digital environments such as a website, electronic documents or online curricula that include multimedia. Despite the development of web and digital accessibility standards (Caldwell et al., 2018) and automated accessibility checkers (Vigo, Brown and Conway, 2013), usability ultimately dictates the user experience and accessibility of the digital landscape (Olalere and Lazar, 2011; Petrie and Kheir, 2007; Power et al., 2012). For example, a document that is readable by a screen reader but is not formatted correctly with a logical structure of headings is not truly accessible. Online curricula and assessments that include images and videos are only accessible if visually impaired students can meet the same learning objectives as sighted peers using their preferred method of access.

To return to the question of *does technology replace braille?* Technology merely supports the end-user in accessing information using the modality of choice for visual, auditory and/or tactile access. Braille is the tactile equivalent to reading print. As long as print is a viable medium for sighted readers, braille remains a tactile medium for those who read tactually.

Technology potentially delivers more immediate options via visual, auditory *and* tactile access if the media is formatted in an accessible digital format. Great flexibility also becomes available if the end-user can quickly switch between various sensory access channels at will. Without technology, a visually impaired individual is limited to only visual access (if provided with enlarged paper copies), only auditory access (if provided with an audio file) *or* only tactile access (if provided with embossed braille or graphics on paper). Using no tech, each of these modes of access might require additional time and dependence on sighted assistance.

The flexible modes of access as described are dependent on a digital workflow that delivers information in multimedia formats for multimodal accessibility. User experiences therefore focus on efficiency, customisation and equity in accessing information. Ideally, people should have the option to choose how they want to engage with information at any given time and be empowered to be in charge of their own accessibility. By designing along the tenets of ensuring independent, primary and timely access to information, technology can improve the quality of living for individuals with visual impairments.

As digital information and computing have become more ubiquitous (Billah et al., 2017), the term "assistive technology" generally refers to technology that is specially made for disabled people's use and has become less popular among end-users. Rather, the term "access technology" is emerging as the more preferred term due to the evolution of mainstream technology to incorporate features that support a greater variety of user preferences (Presley and Siu, in press). Considering how technology can ensure equitable access to information regardless of an end-user's abilities, the following section will focus on how technology can be seamlessly integrated into learning environments and adopted into lifelong practice. Understanding of these processes will guide the development of an action-oriented research agenda.

Best practices for technology integration

When embarking on new research or implementation of technology, how the prototype will be adopted by end-users might seem like a concept that is far enough off to address later in the research process. However, consideration of such logistical pieces can impact the efficacy of one's research and development beginning with the initial stages of inception. How technology might be integrated into practice will dictate design elements, usability testing and fit of the technology into user workflows.

Technology adoption processes in the United States can be very different between primary and secondary school students, students in higher education, employed versus retired personnel and adventitiously versus congenitally blind individuals. Adoption processes include technology acquisition and training, identification of goals the technology will help a user meet and sustainability of the technology in the greater scope of solving a user-specific problem. The following subsections summarise how adoption processes might differ between user groups.

Primary and secondary school students

In the United States, students from kindergarten to age 22 are entitled to federally funded education resources, included technology needed to access instruction. However, students with visual impairments rely on a teacher of the visually impaired (TVI) for identifying and acquiring needed tools and intervention plans. The TVI takes on the role of gatekeeper for technology for visually impaired students, so it is critical that easily accessible resources for training and troubleshooting are made available to teachers when new technologies are introduced (Morash and Siu, 2016; Siu and Morash, 2014). Parental involvement also plays a key role in these students' adoption of technology, so recognition of parents as a major stakeholder for educational technologies can be a major boon (Kelly, 2011).

Postsecondary students in higher education

Upon graduation from secondary school, students in higher education are supported by a federally funded department of rehabilitation for funding technology and additional services (job coaching, orientation and mobility) as needed. Other accessibility needs for instructional media are typically met by a campus-wide office for disability services, but no additional intervention is provided. These students must assume responsibility for learning and troubleshooting their own technology, identify what technology they need and seek out services as needed.

Employed versus retired personnel

Employed individuals are also supported by a federally funded department of rehabilitation, including technology needed to carry out employment tasks and job coaching or orientation and mobility services as needed. Once an individual retires or is unemployed, however, scarce funding is available for technology purchases and additional services. Retirees must personally fund any technology purchases and seek out services if/when needed.

Adventitiously versus congenitally blind individuals

Although service delivery and funding options vary depending on the aforementioned demographics, technology research and design can be influenced by how a blind individual has developed their senses for accessing information. Those who are visually impaired from birth will have developed strategies for accessing and conceptualising information auditorally and tactually; those who are adventitiously visually impaired might have more visual mental maps to reference with developing auditory and tactile skills. Depending on the age of onset of a visual impairment, tactile skills might need specific training and practice to develop the haptic perceptual skills that were previously not as well utilised with vision.

Engagement in communities of practice

Regardless of the demographic a new technology might target, the role of a community of practice (CoP) in learning, acquiring and troubleshooting technology is invaluable. This is particularly true for anyone who experiences isolation in accessing and developing technology expertise. In particular, TVIs are often gatekeepers to primary and secondary students' technology adoption and the most susceptible to challenges in accessing a community of practice (Morash and Siu, 2016; Siu and Morash, 2014). Most TVIs work in an itinerant setting and travel across multiple school sites with minimal opportunities to update their technology knowledge with fellow colleagues (Correa-Torres and Johnson, 2004; Kapperman, Sticken and Heinze, 2002). End-users in postsecondary education and employment or homemaker programmes are also tasked with finding their own resources for accessing technology options, evaluation and adoption. TVIs as well as end-users benefit from a CoP to develop technology proficiency and evaluate which tools will work best for a given task (Mishra and Koehler, 2006; Morash and Siu, 2016).

Given the value of a CoP when implementing technology, the shift from assistive to universally designed technologies has great potential in engaging a larger community movement around accessibility (Siu, 2016). Universally designed materials are meant for mainstream adoption and dissemination, and do not require further remediation to ensure accessibility by all members of a community. In other words, universal design can promote how media can be "born accessible" (Summers et al., 2012). Understanding how the environment, task demands and technology affordances interact with user needs (Mishra and Koehler, 2006; Zabala, 1995) can help prioritise what is most relevant for research and development at any given time.

On a practical note, grant opportunities will often favour project proposals that align with principles of universal design due to the promise of scalability, impact factor and cross-field collaboration. The most exciting research in assistive technology solves a problem not just for people with disabilities but also improves usability for all members of a community. Exercising an inclusive mindset in research will facilitate successful technology adoption and inform shared practices that support all individuals' access to information.

The next section will guide the reader on developing a research plan for carrying out research in technology for individuals with visual impairments.

Designing a research plan

Embarking on a new research project in the area of assistive technology can be very exciting! There is the promise of solving an accessibility issue, hopefully engaging with other communities and lines of inquiry and ideally bringing awareness to accessibility as an advocacy effort. Research in this area generally focuses on the development of new technology or evaluating the efficacy of technologies for specific tasks, and results in implications for practice. Conducting research in technology is inherently action-oriented; there is limited value in researching theories of technology unless they link to clear recommendations for future practice.

The next section of this chapter will identify some key components of designing an effective research plan as well as some common pitfalls to be aware of. For researchers who are new to assistive/access technology for individuals with visual impairments, this process might seem as much daunting as it is exciting. However, with an appropriate framework to guide the researcher, problems to be solved in this area of inquiry can become relatable to common research questions. The following recommendations will focus on developing a research plan that will be impactful and benefit technology users who are blind or visually impaired.

Recommendation 1: begin at the beginning (start with the problem, not the technology)

One of the thrills of working in technology also makes research in this area the most challenging: It changes *so fast!* As a result, it is tempting to begin with a technology innovation and then hunt for a problem to solve. While it might seem counterintuitive to resist this temptation (especially when working in assistive technology), it is important to keep an open mind regarding what potential solutions might look like and widen the scope of questioning and problem-solving potential prior to selecting a specific technology. Consider how a designer or builder in other fields might approach a new construction project; there is usually an extensive process of identifying what has already been done, how things were built previously and what has and hasn't worked well in existing models. The tools (aka technology) used for a construction project are then decided according to what the project requires. Less often will a builder start with a particular tool and then decide what to make with it. When this occurs, the end product tends to function more as a showcase for how a tool can work rather than solving an actual problem.

At times, researchers can become so enamoured with a particular technology that the focus becomes more on the technology and less on solving a problem of practice. When wanting to make an impact with assistive technology, research must always start with a problem of practice *before* identifying how technology will fit the problem. Recall that the most meaningful research in access technology relates directly to implications for practice! Critical errors are made when skipping the initial step of identifying what has been done, what current practices are and what problems remain unsolved. Recommendation #2 addresses how to carry out this preliminary research.

Recommendation 2: conduct a thorough needs assessment (who are my end-users and what do they need?)

If the researcher is unfamiliar with the pedagogical aspects of visual impairment (i.e. how visually impaired individuals access and interact with information), it becomes impossible to identify what problems beg a solution. The first step must therefore involve connecting with stakeholders who can distil the most pressing needs, provide guidance on what's been done and what the current problems of practice are and provide any related pedagogical expertise. Stakeholders in the field of visual impairments must always include the end-users, the practitioners who might provide the technology training and determine adoption practices and related personnel who shape intervention priorities for the field. A comprehensive needs assessment will capture information specific to end-users, potential workflows the technology will influence, factors that will impact usability of the proposed technology and stakeholders' priorities that identify which needs would most benefit from technology intervention.

Understand the end-user

Visual impairment is not a homogenous category. Individuals who are visually impaired range from total blindness, to functional blindness with some vision but more utilisation of tactile and/or auditory skills, to having low vision and utilising a combination of visual, auditory and tactile skills for most tasks. Problems of practice might vary across different individuals with visual impairments because information must be presented and understood differently depending on low vision versus nonvisual representations. One cannot fully understand the nuances of a problem without comprehensive observations and interviews with a range of possible end-users. Even individuals who share similar levels of visual impairment will have different preferences in how they interact with various kinds of information within various tasks. Recall that when working with younger individuals, a visual impairment will significantly impact typical learning and developmental processes as described in the ECC (Hatlen, 1996; Huebner et al., 2004). As a result, age of onset of a visual impairment and preferences for learning media will greatly influence an end-user's needs. Because of the variability across end-users, their sensory preferences and how information must be represented, it will be strategic to identify the type of user a technology is designed for and relate research questions to particular user needs.

Understand the workflow the technology is designed to support

To keep the research action-oriented, the researcher must understand the typical workflow for a particular end-user and how the proposed technology will improve the user experience in this workflow. Recall that the best interventions facilitate a visually impaired individual's ability to access information independently and equitably. To do so, it is important to understand how a task can be carried out more efficiently while maintaining the highest quality of life. Too often, technologies are introduced that might offer better accessibility but further stigmatise an individual in his or her community. For example, wearable technologies can be particularly precarious when they are cumbersome to wear or render the individual hopelessly unfashionable. Educational technologies can also be difficult to adopt if it sets a student apart from his or her peers and disrupts an inclusive learning environment. Finally, logistical issues about one's workflow can be a deciding factor in the efficacy of proposed technologies; individuals who are visually impaired often do not have enough hands to manage everything! Between a mobility device (such as a white cane or dog), mobile devices (such as a smartphone), access technologies (refreshable braille displays) and low-tech tools (such as a handheld magnifier or slate and stylus), it is strategic to consider the value of adding a single- versus multi-function device to an end-user's existing arsenal of tools.

Understand advantages and limitations of technology application

Similar to any other field of research that involves a product, tool or device, it is of utmost importance to understand the different factors that influence an individual's usage of any technology regardless of visual ability. In addition to the most typical usability factors a researcher might consider, individuals with visual impairments might have additional usability factors that include one's sensory access to information (visual, auditory, haptic, kinaesthetic, olfactory), or differentiated representational and spatial concept development to interpret information through low or nonvisual means. Work efficiency is often the greatest consideration due to the increased time it often takes for nonvisual access to information; auditory access can be more tedious if media are not formatted for easy navigation to explore content, and tactile access can require more time if media are not formatted properly to render on a refreshable braille display. As mentioned earlier, fit of the technology into an individual's workflow is a critical usability factor if it impacts the time and effort required to employ the tool.

Understand available resources and intervention priorities

One of the greatest pitfalls is encountered when a researcher assumes an area of need that is not actually a priority for blind or visually impaired people. This can sometimes happen when a researcher does not realise the amount of information a visually impaired person can gain through nonvisual means. For example, a blind person could likely identify a preferred sweater in his or her closet based on how it feels – as a result, a high-tech labelling device using a camera system would be unnecessary and incorrectly assume that vision is needed for such a task. If well developed, a visually impaired individual can often use alternative sensory skills to access information that others might access visually. Technology solutions don't necessarily require a synthetic visual solution or need to solve a problem that is already solved with nonvisual strategies. Carrying out a gap analysis can help a researcher avoid this critical error by identifying how much information an end-user can already access and what information remains inaccessible. Based on this initial analysis, the accessibility gaps can be discussed with stakeholders to determine which information are most valuable, what solutions have already been tried and what needs continue to persist. Identification of specific advantages and limitations of previous solutions is advantageous to develop a focused and productive research plan.

Recommendation 3: consider the technology learning curve (how technology proficiency can confound evaluation measures)

All technologies require some learning curve to achieve proficient use. While an end-user develops proficiency, previous tools and strategies might continue to be the most efficient way an end-user completes a particular task. This is especially prevalent in education interventions where technology research defaults to an evaluation of a student's or teacher's technology proficiency rather than how well a technology supports learning objectives. This pitfall can be avoided with a research design that reconsiders the definition of efficacy based on what stakeholders would deem successful. Take for instance Freeland et al.'s (2010) study on the use of a braille notetaker for increasing test scores. The initial research question focused on students' academic performance as the dependent variable when using a notetaker for test-taking based on the assumption that the device would provide improved access to the content. However, academic performance was actually not the dependent variable because students' proficiency in using the device was a limiting factor. Outcomes found that students performed just as well on the test without the device using the low-tech methods they were accustomed to.

The research and development of the iBraille Challenge app met a similar fate (Kamei-Hannan, McCarthy and Pomeroy, 2015); the investigators conceptualised an app that would allow more students in rural areas to participate remotely in the Braille Challenge rather than travel to a contest centre. However, upon launching the ambitious project, it became apparent that students' app usage was impacted by their teachers' ability to set up a refreshable braille display. The researchers' efforts required more focus on teachers' needs for technology training in addition to an evaluation of how well the app functioned for students' engagement in the Braille Challenge.

Recall that the role of technology is to facilitate independent, timely and equitable access to information. Might these factors be a more impactful measure of a tool's efficacy? As demonstrated in the aforementioned studies, achievement measures such as test scores are not necessarily variables that rely on technology. If a student or teacher has not yet achieved the technology proficiency to carry out a task intuitively using the tool at hand, the technology itself could confound evaluation of learning outcomes.

Recommendation 4: differentiate research methods for low-incidence disabilities and visual impairment

Clear research agendas begin with a hypothesis that informs what research method is employed. In the case of designing a research study focused on technology usage by blind or visually impaired individuals, the initial methodological planning is no different. However, as with any research that involves technology for task completion, the following questions beg additional consideration:

- Does the research design evaluate how well the technology functions versus the individual's ability to operate the tool?
- How is efficacy defined? Is a successful trial dependent on:
  - Tool operation (how well the tool works as intended)?
  - Ease of operation and individuals' skills (usability factors)?
  - Inclusion (social factors or fit with mainstream applications)?
  - Achievement of learning or employment objectives (workflow factors)?
  - Implementation into practice (likelihood of adoption)?

Additional considerations when carrying out research with blind or visually impaired individuals relate to general challenges when conducting research in low-incidence disability areas (Odom et al., 2005). These considerations impact participant demographics, sample sizes, statistical power and generalisability of findings.

Comparison of blind versus sighted

Due to the pervasive impact of visual impairment on many aspects of learning, development, access to and interpretation of information, *it is impossible to compare blind and sighted participants as if vision is an independent variable* (Warren, 1994, 1978). Technology is best evaluated within groups across participants with matched levels of visual impairment or sensory use depending on the research question. Any research design that compares blind versus sighted use will have limited validity in addressing the efficacy of the technology for blind individuals. The comparison of sighted and blindfolded sighted participants also invalidates generalisations to blind or visually impaired individuals because participants who are typically sighted and blindfolded will not have developed the compensatory and sensory skills that a naturally visually impaired person would utilise for the same tasks. Despite challenges in recruiting participants with visual impairments, such efforts can be well rewarded with meaningful research outcomes that actually add value to technology practices.

Recruitment and sampling

When recruiting participants, recall that visual impairments is a heterogenous population. Specifying the research goals will help guide decisions to recruit participants based on visual functioning, literacy medium or even age of onset of visual impairment. These decisions will depend on understanding how a visual impairment impacts an individual's access to information and what objectives the research intends to evaluate. Remember that any sampling biases will require discussion in terms of limitations in generalisability and recommendations for practice.

Managing small sample sizes

Also recall that visual impairment is a low-incidence disability. There are usually limited numbers of participants who meet the established participant criteria, which calls for understanding which research methodologies are more appropriate when working with small sample sizes. In the United States, the two methodologies that are considered "gold standard" are randomised controlled trials and single-case subject design (Horner et al., 2005). Of these methodologies, single-case subject design is more appropriate for small, heterogenous samples. Researchers who choose to undertake this methodology are advised to study the nuances of this approach including considerations for replicating and generalising findings. When carrying out any statistical analyses of a small sample, the significance of findings can be enhanced by triangulating quantitative data with qualitative measures from multiple data sources for a robust mixed-methods presentation (Collins, Onwuegbuzie and Sutton, 2006; Creswell and Creswell, 2017).

Conclusion

Conducting technology research for the benefit of individuals with visual impairments is an ongoing adventure that requires humility, patience and strategic foresight. Unless a researcher is reporting on one's own technology usage, this area of inquiry involves sensitive mediation between investigators' assumptions and practical usability factors. Hopefully, the chapter has given the researcher some foundational concepts to address his or her assumptions and create a plan that recognises the most pertinent user considerations.

First and foremost, research in technology requires a different mindset; hypotheses must take into consideration how information is processed differently in nonvisual or low vision formats. Sighted researchers are encouraged to move away from retino-centric perspectives and consider how different senses can convey equitable experiences in learning, interactions and information exchange. These experiences must then be designed to support alternative spatial representations that facilitate visually impaired individuals' synthesis of information. Sighted and visually impaired researchers alike are encouraged to expand their own perspectives of information.

Recall that end-users of access technology can have a range of needs, technology proficiency and flexibility in using various senses to access information. Workflows might also differ between various end-users. To accommodate this great variability, researchers must budget for an iterative research and design process. Initial identification of end-users, related stakeholders and gatekeepers is critical so that these extended team members can be called upon for regular feedback and input from the beginning to the end of the research endeavour. The ensuing designs and/or evaluation of technology applications requires periodic (formative) evaluation of the efficacy of the research process. When configuring the validity of technology to meet users' needs, automated evaluation tools such as accessibility checkers are insufficient. Extensive usability testing with a varied sample of visually impaired individuals will always yield more actionable data and support recommendations for practice.

Ultimately, the most impactful research incorporates a plan for sustainable technology use in an individual's workflow. Outcomes of effective research also help identify potential adoption trends. Merely focusing on theoretical use cases will inevitably lead to a limited scope of understanding and short-lived recommendations. With these tips in mind, conducting research in technologies for people who are blind or visually impaired can be most rewarding when thought experiments manifest in tangible products that improve an individual's independence and quality of life.

References

Abrahamson, D., Flood, V.J., Miele, J.A. and Siu, Y. 2018. Enactivism and ethnomethodological conversation analysis as tools for expanding universal design for learning: The case of visually impaired mathematics students. *ZDM*, 1–13. https://doi.org/10.1007/s11858-018-0998-1

Alajarmeh, N., Pontelli, E. and Son, T. 2011. From "reading" math to "doing" math: A new direction in non-visual math accessibility. In *International Conference on Universal Access in Human–Computer Interaction* (pp. 501–210). Orlando, FL: Springer.

Amick, N. and Corcoran, J. 1997. *Guidelines for the design of tactile graphics*. Louisville, KY: American Printing House for the Blind. Accessed 9 August 2018. www.aph.org/research/guides.

Barclay, L.A. 2011. *Learning to listen/listening to learn: Teaching listening skills to students with visual impairments.* New York: American Foundation for the Blind.

Belardinelli, M.O., Federici, S., Delogu, F. and Palmiero, M. 2009. Sonification of spatial information: Audio-tactile exploration strategies by normal and blind subjects. In *International Conference on Universal Access in Human–Computer Interaction* (pp. 557–563). San Diego, CA: Springer,.

Billah, S.M., Ashok, V., Porter, D.E. and Ramakrishnan, I.V. 2017. Ubiquitous accessibility for people with visual impairments: Are we there yet? In *CHI Conference on Human Factors in Computing Systems* (pp. 5862–5868). New York: ACM.

Bouck, E.C. and Meyer, N.K. 2012. eText, mathematics, and students with visual impairments: What teachers need to know. *Teaching Exceptional Children*, 45(2), 42–49.

Bourquin, E.A., Emerson, R.W., Sauerburger, D. and Barlow, J. 2017. The effect of the color of a long cane used by individuals who are visually impaired on the yielding behavior of drivers. *Journal of Visual Impairment & Blindness*, 111(5), 401–410.

Braille Authority of North America. 2010. Guidelines and standards for tactile graphics. Accessed 9 August 2018. www.brailleauthority.org/tg.

Brown, L.M., Brewster, S.A., Ramloll, S.A., Burton, R. and Riedel, B. 2003. Design guidelines for audio presentation of graphs and tables. In *International Conference on Auditory Display* (pp. 284–287). Boston, MA: ICAD.

Buehler, E., Kane, S.K. and Hurst, A. 2014. ABC and 3D: Opportunities and obstacles to 3D printing in special education environments. In *Proceedings of the 16th International ACM SIGACCESS Conference on Computers & Accessibility* (pp. 107–114). Rochester, NY: ACM.

Caldwell, B. et al. 2018. *Web content accessibility guidelines overview.* Accessed 9 August 2018. www.w3.org/WAI/standards-guidelines/wcag.

Collins, K.M., Onwuegbuzie, A.J. and Sutton, I.L. 2006. A model incorporating the rationale and purpose for conducting mixed methods research in special education and beyond. *Learning Disabilities: A Contemporary Journal,* 4(1), 67–100.

Correa-Torres, S.M. and Johnson, J. 2004. Facing the challenges of itinerant teaching: Perspectives and suggestions from the field. *Journal of Visual Impairment and Blindness,* 98(7), 420–433.

Creswell, J.W. and Creswell, J.D. 2017. *Research design: Qualitative, quantitative, and mixed methods approaches.* Thousand Oaks, CA: Sage.

DIAGRAM Center. 2014. *Image description guidelines.* Accessed 9 August 2018. http://diagramcenter.org/table-of-contents-2.html.

Fleet, C. 2017. Need vision on demand? There's an app for that. *Braille Monitor,* 60(7). Accessed 9 August 2018. https://nfb.org/images/nfb/publications/bm/bm17/bm1707/bm170702.htm.

Freeland, A.L., Emerson, R.W., Curtis, A.B. and Fogarty, K. 2010. Exploring the relationship between access technology and standardized test scores for youths with visual impairments: Secondary analysis of the National Longitudinal Transition Study 2. *Journal of Visual Impairment & Blindness,* 104(3), 170–182.

Hatlen, P. 1996. The core curriculum for blind and visually impaired students, including those with additional disabilities. *RE: view,* 28(1), 25–32.

Holbrook, M.C., McCarthy, T.S., Kamei-Hannan, C. and Zebehazy, K.T. (eds). 2017. *Foundations of education. Volume II: Instructional strategies for teaching children and youths with visual impairments* (3rd ed.). New York: AFB Press.

Horner, R.H., Carr, E.G., Halle, J., McGee, G., Odom, S. and Wolery, M. 2005. The use of single-subject research to identify evidence-based practice in special education. *Exceptional Children,* 71(2), 165–179.

Huebner, K.M., Brunhilde, M.-A., Stryker, D. and Wolffe, K. 2004. *National agenda.* New York: AFB. Accessed 9 August 2018. www.afb.org/info/national-agenda-for-education/introduction-2464/25.

Kamei-Hannan, C., McCarthy, T. and Pomeroy, B. 2015. *Methods in creating the iBraille Challenge mobile app for braille users.* San Diego, CA: CSUN Assistive Technology Conference.

Kapperman, G., Sticken, J. and Heinze, T. 2002. Survey of the use of assistive technology by Illinois students who are visually impaired. *Journal of Visual Impairment & Blindness,* 96(2), 106–108.

Kelly, S.M. 2011. The use of assistive technology by high school students with visual impairments: A second look at the current problem. *Journal of Visual Impairment & Blindness,* 105(4), 235.

Koenig, A.J. and Holbrook, M.C. 1995. *Learning media assessment of students with visual impairments: A resource guide for teachers.* Austin, TX: Texas School for the Blind and Visually Impaired, Business.

Miele, J.A., Landau, S. and Gilden, D. 2006. Talking TMAP: Automated generation of audio-tactile maps using Smith-Kettlewell's TMAP software. *British Journal of Visual Impairment,* 24(2), 93–100.

Mishra, P. and Koehler, M.J. 2006. Technological pedagogical content knowledge: A framework for teacher knowledge. *Teachers College Record,* 108(6), 1017.

Miyashita, H., Sato, D., Takagi, H. and Asakawa, C. 2007. Making multimedia content accessible for screen reader users. In *Proceedings of the 2007 International Cross-Disciplinary Conference on Web Accessibility (W4A)* (pp. 126–127). Banff, Canada: ACM.

Morash, V.S., Pensky, A.E.C., Tseng, S.T. and Miele, J.A. 2014. Effects of using multiple hands and fingers on haptic performance in individuals who are blind. *Perception,* 43(6), 569–588.

Morash, V.S. and Siu, Y.-T., 2016. Social predictors of assistive technology proficiency among teachers of students with visual impairments. *ACM Transactions on Accessible Computing (TACCESS),* 9(2), 4.

Morash, V.S., Siu, Y.-T., Miele, J.A., Hasty, L. and Landau, S. 2015. Guiding novice web workers in making image descriptions using templates. *ACM Transactions on Accessible Computing (TACCESS),* 7(4), 12.

Noble, S., Soiffer, N., Dooley, S., Lozano, E. and Brown, D. 2018. Accessible math: Best practices after 25 years of research and development. *Journal on Technology and Persons with Disabilities,* 6(30), 284–296.

Odom, S.L., Brantlinger, E., Gersten, R., Horner, R.H., Thompson, B. and Harris, K.R. 2005. Research in special education: Scientific methods and evidence-based practices. *Exceptional Children,* 71(2), 137–148.

Olalere, A. and Lazar, J. 2011. Accessibility of US federal government home pages: Section 508 compliance and site accessibility statements. *Government Information Quarterly,* 28(3), 303–309.

Packer, J., Vizenor, K. and Miele, J.A. 2015. An overview of video description: History, benefits, and guidelines. *Journal of Visual Impairment & Blindness,* 109(2), 83–93.

Petrie, H. and Kheir, O. 2007. The relationship between accessibility and usability of websites. In *Proceedings of the SIGCHI Conference on Human Factors in Computing Systems* (pp. 397–406). San Jose, CA: ACM.

Power, C., Freire, A., Petrie, H. and Swallow, D. 2012. Guidelines are only half of the story: Accessibility problems encountered by blind users on the web. In *Proceedings of the SIGCHI Conference on Human Factors in Computing Systems* (pp. 433–442). Austin, TX: ACM.

Presley, I. and Siu, Y. In press. *Assistive technology for individuals with visual impairments.* New York: AFB Press.

Rodriguez, T.F., Conwell, W.Y. and Digimarc Corp. 2014. *Mobile devices and methods employing haptics.* US Patent 8,798,534.

Sapp, W. and Hatlen, P. 2010. The expanded core curriculum: Where we have been, where we are going, and how we can get there. *Journal of Visual Impairment & Blindness*, 104(6), 339–340.

Sauerburger, D. and Bourquin, E. 2010. Teaching the use of a long cane step by step: Suggestions for progressive, methodical instruction. *Journal of Visual Impairment & Blindness*, 104(4), 203–205.

Siu, Y. 2016. Designing for all learners with technology. *Educational Designer*, 9(3), n.p.

Siu, Y.T. and Morash, V.S. 2014. Teachers of students with visual impairments and their use of assistive technology: Measuring the proficiency of teachers and their identification with a community of practice. *Journal of Visual Impairment & Blindness*, 108(5), 384–398.

Strong, P. 2009. The history of the white cane. *Paths to Literacy*. Accessed 9 August 2018. www.path stoliteracy.org/sites/pathstoliteracy.perkinsdev1.org/files/The%20History%20of%20the%20White%20 Cane.docx.

Summers, E., Langston, J., Allison, R. and Cowley, J. 2012. *Using SAS/GRAPH to create visualizations that also support tactile and auditory interaction.* Raleigh, NC: SAS Global Forum.

Vigo, M., Brown, J. and Conway, V. 2013. Benchmarking web accessibility evaluation tools: measuring the harm of sole reliance on automated tests. In *Proceedings of the 10th International Cross-Disciplinary Conference on Web Accessibility* (p. 1). Rio de Janeiro: ACM.

Walker, B.N. and Mauney, L.M. 2010. Universal design of auditory graphs: A comparison of sonification mappings for visually impaired and sighted listeners. *ACM Transactions on Accessible Computing (TACCESS)*, 2(3), 12.

Warren, D.H. 1978. Childhood visual impairment: Perspectives on research design and methodology. *Journal of Visual Impairment and Blindness*, 72(10), 404–411.

Warren, D.H. 1994. *Blindness and children: An individual differences approach.* Cambridge: Cambridge University Press.

Ye, H., Malu, M., Oh, U. and Findlater, L. 2014. Current and future mobile and wearable device use by people with visual impairments. In *Proceedings of the SIGCHI Conference on Human Factors in Computing Systems* (pp. 3123–3132). Toronto, ON: ACM.

Zabala, J. 1995. The SETT framework: Critical areas to consider when making informed assistive technology decisions. In *Florida Assistive Technology Impact Conference and Technology and Media Division of Council for Exceptional Children* (pp. 2–5). Orlando, FL: CEC.

Part VI

Understanding the cultural aesthetics

15

Classical philosophies on blindness and cross-modal transfer, 1688–2003

Simon Hayhoe

Introduction

This chapter surveys classical philosophies on blindness and cross-modal transfer, and how these philosophies' methods have negatively affected our understanding of visual impairment. The study is designed to help the reader understand why we think sense data from low or no vision can only be enhanced or substituted through touch. The survey's discussion is necessary for those working with people who are visually impaired, to understand the epistemology of learning theory and visual impairment in practice.

This chapter is written with professionals, researchers and students of education and related fields in mind – either those developing informal education in social settings such as museums or workplaces, or formal education through institutions such as schools, colleges or universities. Although this survey is far from the complete story of understanding cognition and blindness, it is a foundation on which future research on blindness and learning can be designed.

Importantly, in this chapter I develop an argument from a previous study, which examined the philosophical influences on English schools for the blind (Hayhoe, 2015), to ask the question: *Has the methodology of cross-modal transfer affected our theory of cognition and blindness to the detriment of the majority of people with visual impairments?*

In this chapter, I discuss this question in relation to two approximate academic periods of philosophy: the first spanning the century following 1688, the second spanning the half-century following 1950. In discussing this question, I argue philosophies on blindness have unnaturally divided people into two artificial categories: the sighted and the sightless. Furthermore, I argue these categories have become connected in ways that are unrelated to eyesight and the social needs of people with visual impairments.

I call this epistemological process of categorisation passive exclusion, and this historical development of philosophies an epistemological model of examining blindness. In my discussion, I shorten this latter long title to the epistemological model of blindness for brevity. In this chapter, I focus on epistemology as a tool to study knowledge development, with a specific emphasis on its social, historical and cultural influences.

The epistemological model of blindness is largely inspired by two sources of literature. The first source is centred on an understanding that the natural sciences are premised on the existence of evolution in the traditional sense. It also examines the philosophical belief in a pre-determined natural order, in which impairments such as blindness exist. The modern source inspiring this refinement is Nagel's (2012) theory that: "The mind–body problem is not just a local problem, having to do with the relation between mind, brain and behaviour in living animal organisms, but that it invades our understanding of the entire cosmos and its history" (p. 3). Consequently, I argue we have tried too hard to classify blindness through a reductionist, unified theory of material philosophy. In doing so, we have over-simplified multifaceted impairments and social categories of impairment, and illogically conflated visual and aesthetic beliefs to construct a *visual disability*.

My second source of inspiration in forming this argument is Popper's (1998, 1979, 2010) argument that our understanding of material is not a phenomenon that can be located in the physical world. Instead, this understanding can only be interpreted through our perceptual and cognitive need to simplify and categorise human physiology, belief and behaviour. This need motivates philosophers to develop artificial categories through crude scientific classes and methodologies. As Popper (1979, pp. 23–24) states:

> It was first in animals and children, but later also in adults, that I observed the immensely powerful need for regularity – the need which makes them seek for regularities; which makes them sometimes experience regularities even where there are none.

I argue these two influences help us understand how cross-modal transfer has been used by theorists to emphasise sightlessness in people with visual impairment. This philosophy has been used to develop a theory of material philosophy, link blindness to physical disability and damage rather than the promotion of ability and adaptation.

Consequently, philosophies have helped to reduce and classify blindness into an ethic of ability, inability, disability, handicap and impairment according to its most extreme, prototypical features. During the Enlightenment, these philosophies were not just attempting to understand how humans consciously process the material world, they were also moral philosophies – these philosophies were trying to understand if morality is developed internally or communicated as images of the outer world are.

This study starts with a discussion on the nature and importance of cross-modal transfer.

The study of cross-modal transfer

In the modern era, two theories of multi-sensory learning have had particular significance on the methodology of learning theory and visual impairment: (1) what can be referred to as cross-modal linkage, in which different forms of sensory data – such as vision, sound and touch – are processed together in the mind to form a single mental "image" (see for example, Driver and Spence, 2004); and (2) cross-modal transfer, in which sensory experiences associated with one sense can be understood through the stimulation of another sense (Gregory, 1974).

Since the late twentieth century, the psychological theory of cross-modal transfer is recognised as having a significant effect on a general theory of human learning. For example, research on child development by Gottfried, Rose and Bridger (1977) discovered babies' earliest experiences of touch and taste affect their later understanding of other forms of perception.

There is also evidence that, despite an early reliance on touch and taste, adult humans' visual data changes other sensory data when immediate sensory attention is needed. Spence (2010) refers to this as cross-modal attention. For instance, studies of the so-called Colavita effect (Colavita, 1974; Spence, 2009), finds that the mind gives priority to visual information over auditory sensory data during events where auditory and visual data conflict – e.g. if a person's mouth appears to visually mouth one word yet the voice says another, the mind will tend to hear the mouthed word.

Similarly, studies of so-called cross-modal plasticity, where vision is removed and the mind has to rely on other sensory data, shows that sensory images can adapt to rely on other sensory data. For example, research with people who have significant visual impairments has shown that what is called the visual cortex in the brain can be stimulated by touch (Sathian and Stilla, 2010) – this research subsequently questions whether the visual cortex is designed to process vision alone, as was traditionally thought.

So how did this theory of cross-modal transfer come about? Moreover, how has its theory helped us to understand the learning of people with visual impairments?

To answer these questions, it is vital to understand the historical context of this early period of the Enlightenment. For instance, writers who have observed the contemporary study of blindness and cross-modal transfer often refer to the Protestant English and Irish enlightenment (Gregory, 1974, 1987; Hayhoe, 2003, 2015; Jay, 1994; Paulson, 1987) – although Hayhoe (2015), Paulson (1987) and Jay (1994) also argue that similar political philosophies existed in the earlier period of French enlightenment, dating back to what is now referred to as the mind–body problem, or Cartesian-duality (Descartes, 1984).

These writers observe that this philosophical revolution of thinking began with a question posed to the English legal and moral philosopher John Locke by the Irish natural philosopher William Molyneux. This question is reproduced below:

Pour Les Auteurs de la Biblioteque

Monsieur Waesberg

March and Librair

a

Amsterdam

Per Lond. 62

6th July 88

Dublin July 88

A problem proposed to the author of the Essai Philosophique Consernant L'Enteneem

A man being born blind and having a globe and a cube, nigh of the same bigness, committed into his hand, and being taught or told, which is called the globe and which the cube, so as easily to distinguish them by touch or feeling; then both things taken from him, and laid on a table. Let us suppose his sight restored to him; whether he could, by his sight, and before he touch them, know which is the globe and which the cube? So whether he could not reach them though they were removed 20 or 1000 feet from him?

If the learned and ingenious author of this fore mentioned treatise think this problem worth his consideration and answer, he may at any time direct it to one, that much esteem him, and is, his humble servant,

Will: Molyneux

High Ormond's Gate in Dublin, Ireland

(Letter from William Molyneux to John Locke, 7 July 1688.
From the correspondence of John Locke, John Locke Collection,
Bodlean Library, Oxford University)

Molyneux's question was later reproduced in edited form under the heading "On Perception", in the second edition of Locke's (2001) *Essay Concerning Human Understanding*. This second edition of the essay was published on Locke's return to England after a period of political exile in France – the first edition was published in French in 1688, and the reference to the essay at the start of Molyneux's letter refers to this original essay.

At the time, this form of studying human perception remained untested by natural philosophers. In its range, however, this question did not simply address the narrow study of a relationship between touch and sight. This question was fundamental to understanding the perception and comprehension of a material consciousness separate to the external physical and moral world.

However, the focus of this study was also not simply inspired by a material and cognitive understanding of perception, as Gregory (1974) later argued. Its origin was part of a more complex philosophy of mind, morality and metaphysics that questioned what was known in the human mind (Hayhoe, 2015). This philosophy was designed to challenge the conservative elements of the Anglican Church in England, and to undermine the theological dogmatism of the Roman Catholic Church.

To understand the motivation for this challenge, it is important to recognise the hypothetical discussion of blindness as philosophy of mind on sightlessness. In addition, it is essential to understand the illustration of blindness in Molyneux's original letter to Locke was only part of a discussion on the experience of blindness in Locke's essay.

Consequently, to fully understand the development of cross-modal transfer, I have divided the evolution of this theory into two classical periods of study in the field of cognition and blindness: the first period begins with John Locke's first essay in 1688; the second begins with a renaissance of this philosophy by Richard Gregory in the 1950s. Both periods are essential for teaching us how the epistemology of cross-modal transfer and learning has philosophically evolved, and the mistakes that were made in our assumptions about blindness and learning. I argue that only through critically analysing the epistemology of these studies can we begin to understand the true learning potential of people with visual impairments.

Lockean blindness in the study of philosophy

John Locke courted political and religious controversy in the early 1680s and began to encourage debate among more radical philosophies of this era. Although staying loyal to the broader cause of the Anglican Church, he formed a circle of philosophers with a similar aim, philosophers who had influence on the drafting of his essay (Hayhoe, 2015).

As Locke associated with politically dangerous political philosophies – religion and politics were entwined in this era – an order was made for his arrest and he was forced to leave England for Holland. A year later, Charles II also publicly expelled Locke from Christchurch College, Oxford, where Locke was a fellow. Thus, Locke's philosophy of mind became politicised and his methodology of study became associated with the questioning of theological orthodoxy, power and government.

Rather than dampening his influence, Locke's arrest warrant encouraged his political and academic philosophies, and became a focal point for a political counter-culture in England. Importantly, Locke also engaged in a secret theological dialogue with Isaac Newton (1959), who also challenged the truth of vision, and more particularly the place of visions in the Bible (Hayhoe, 2015).

In his essay, Locke used examples of non-sighted blindness in a number of passages beyond Molyneux's question. In particular, rather than questioning this notion of blindness as inherent punishment of immorality, Locke argued morality was learnt after birth, i.e. inherited blindness was not a punishment for sin, as many orthodox and dogmatic theologies argued.

For example, under the heading "Further Considerations Concerning Innate Principles Both Speculative and Practical", Locke argued that the experience of all sensory modalities was learning. More importantly, in this chapter he identified memory as the foremost mode of understanding, rather than a more inward notion of inherent deliberation released through meditation. This inherent deliberation was previously held to be the key to human understanding. As he stated in his text:

> [A] blind man I once talked with, who lost his sight by the smallpox when he was a small child [had] no more notion of colours than one born blind. I ask whether anyone can say this man had any ideas of colours in his mind, any more than one born blind? And I think nobody will say that either of them had in his mind any idea of colours at all . . .
>
> [The] truth is, ideas and notions are no more born in us than arts and sciences, though some of them indeed offer themselves to our faculties more readily than others and are therefore more generally received, though that too be according as the organs of our bodies and powers of our minds happen to be employed: God having fitted men with faculties and means to discover, receive, and retain truths, accordingly as they are employed.
>
> *(Locke, 2001, pp. 41–42)*

Eighteenth-century philosophies on blindness and touch

Early in the eighteenth century, the philosopher and Anglican bishop, George Berkeley (1899) also offered an answer to Molyneux's question. Like Locke, Berkeley concluded that seeing was not an inherent, God-given function, and that what we call sight was learnt rather than inherent. What's more, Berkeley argued that sensory experiences must be discrete, with vision being processed separately from sound and touch, and subsequently certain mental concepts could only be understood by sight. As he wrote on this answer:

> [A] man born blind, being made to see, would at first have no idea of distance by sight; the sun and stars, the remotest objects as well as the nearer, would all seem to be in his eye, or rather in his mind.
>
> *(Berkeley, 1899, p. 187)*

More importantly, however, in this era a possible empirical test to this solution was offered. Some 15 years after Berkeley, the philosopher and surgeon William Cheselden (1839) developed a procedure for removing cataracts, allowing him to observe a boy born with no usable sight after surgery. Although prior to surgery the boy would have some understanding of light – he was said to be able to distinguish day from night – his vision was sufficiently impaired that he was unable to see objects through what light perception remained. What's more, as sensory data from light was so abstracted in the boy's mind, it could not provide a visual image, rendering colour patterns from objects vague and flat at best.

Consequently, the boy's relationship with physical objects before surgery was largely through holding and feeling them, and not usefully through understanding their shape visually. Similarly, the boy's understanding of his environment was also through his non-visual senses, through physically moving through his environment or sensing his reflection of noise. Subsequently, the boy had no understanding of space through sight, as the light in his world was two-dimensional.

After the boy's eyes had sufficiently recovered from surgery, it soon became clear to Cheselden the boy could not understand the concept of distance or objects by sight alone. What's more, when Cheselden showed the boy objects that were out of reach and that he'd previously held before surgery, the boy did not recognise them at first. It was only when the boy re-held the objects that he began to recognise them by what he assumed was by sight.

However, following this early period of confusion Cheselden observed the boy could associate his experiences of handling objects to identifying the objects while seeing them alone. After a period of learning by sight what he had held by hand, the boy learnt to recognise many of these objects by sight alone, as if the boy was learning objects for the first time. Subsequently, Cheselden made the following observation:

> When he first saw, he was so far from making any judgement about distances that he thought all objects whatever touched his eyes (as he expressed it) as what he felt did his skin . . . He knew not the shape of anything, nor any one thing from another, no matter how different in shape or magnitude: but on being told what things were, whose form he before knew from feeling, he would carefully observe them that he might know them again; but having too many objects to learn at once he forgot many of them.
>
> *(Cheselden, 1839, p. 11)*

Following Berkeley and Cheselden, and using a method of intuitive observation, Denis Diderot's (2001) "Letter on the Blind for Those Who Can See" promoted the intellectual equality of people with visual impairments. Significantly, Diderot's philosophy was particularly important for its consequences on the development of schools for the blind later in the century, and the French politicisation of blindness (Paulson, 1987). Through Diderot, material philosophies also began to normalise touch as an ethically, emotionally and intellectually driven sensory modality. Furthermore, defying Roman Catholic orthodoxy, Diderot argued morality was developed internally, and morals were learnt without recourse to specific or finite senses. As Diderot observed on this issue:

> How different is the morality of the blind man from ours? And how different would that of a deaf man from his? And how to one with an extra sense, how deficient would our morality appear – to say nothing more? Our metaphysics and theirs agree no better.
>
> *(Diderot, 2001, p. 156).*

Like Locke's earlier essay, Diderot's letter also challenged the cultural power of the Roman Catholic Church, by arguing visually impaired people become physically attached to the arts through touch and hearing. In making this argument, Diderot looked beyond simple intellectual classifications, and asserted touch was not simply perceptual, but could be a mode of social justice.

However, in arguing for an equality of the senses, Diderot also did not believe the senses were equivalent, or that sensory data had cognitive parallels through other senses. Instead, Diderot believed that senses were naturally created to comprehend discrete forms of packaged sensory data, or the temporal difference between objects and the space that surrounded them.

For example, Diderot argued that touch could be important for understanding a person's very existence, as without tactile contact the world had a different sensory quality. What's more, and unlike sight, without touch the nature of the world is not experienced as a sense of being connected to the earth, but as an abstract notion. Consequently, Diderot felt touch could be a more honest modality for understanding the true nature of our environment.

Nurses help [babies] to acquire the notion of a continuance of absent persons by playing a game which consists in hiding the face, and showing it again. Thus, they learn a hundred times in a quarter of an hour that what ceases to appear does not necessarily cease to exist. From this it follows that we owe the notion of the continuous existence of objects to experience, of their distance to the sense of touch; that it would be surprising should the aid of one of the senses be necessary to another; and that touch, which ascertains the existence of objects exterior to ourselves when present to our eyes, is similarly the sense to which the confirmation not only of these figures, and other details of these objects, but even their presence is reserved.

(Diderot, 2001, p. 181)

However, despite promoting social justice for people with visual impairments, Paulson (1987) later argued Diderot seemed to create a new form of romanticised mythology about blindness; Paulson observed that Diderot went as far as to suggest sightlessness could be advantageous to the human mind's understanding of the outer world. This claim later inspired French writers in the nineteenth century to elevate fictitious blind characters to an almost fabled status.

Undeniably, this philosophy was not unique and similar mythologies existed from antiquity, with a belief in sightless inner-vision in ancient Greece in particular (Barasch, 2001). However, Diderot's material philosophy differed as it further separated the development of consciousness through perception from a belief in the direct interference of God. As a consequence, and as Jay (1994) argued, it is without doubt that Diderot's essay was epistemologically important, as it became the seedbed for general philosophies of both material and language.

Diderot's first argument concerned the value of touch, which he claimed was as potent a source of knowledge as vision. One recent French commentator, Elizabeth de Fontenay, has gone so far as to say that in the Letter "The great victor in this carnival of the senses established on the ruins of the castle of the eye and consciousness is touch" . . .

For a materialist like Diderot, the dethroning of vision was especially appealing, for although he sarcastically calls idealism "an extravagant system which should to my thinking have been the offspring of blindness itself', he recognised the tendential linkage between privileging ideas in the mind and the putative superiority of vision.

(Jay, 1994, pp. 100–101)

Early philosophies of cross-modal transfer also inspired the first published proposal for the education of people with visual impairment in the style of Diderot's letter. This proposal was published in an open letter in 1774 by Thomas Blacklock, a Presbyterian Minister and philosopher who was later to create Edinburgh's Asylum for the Blind – for the purposes of his letter, Blacklock wrote under the pseudonym Demodocus, a blind bard in Homer's *Odyssey*, who was deprived of sight by the Muses, the ancient Greek goddesses (Hayhoe, 2015).

Blacklock was born in the rural county of Dumfries and Galloway, and died in Edinburgh in 1791, obtained a doctorate from Marischal College, Aberdeen, and preached in Edinburgh. Blacklock's letter was published in a well-known political journal from the Enlightenment, the *Edinburgh Magazine and Review* (Demodocus, 1774). Blacklock himself was blinded at the age of 6 months from smallpox, and he referred to his blindness at several points in this letter.

In his letter, Demodocus cited the cross-modal use of touch as a substitute for vision, and to promote an academic, musical and vocational education and a liberal pedagogy. As with Diderot, the aim of Demodocus' letter was to develop an ethical treatment of a blind social underclass that was often found begging in the major cities of Europe. Drawing from moral philosophy, Demodocus also saw the cause of the population of people with visual impairments as overtly political, and one that affected religious belief.

> The data which they explore may be presented in such a manner, as to render discoveries easier; but still let invention be allowed to co-operate. The internal triumph and exultation which the mind feels free from the attainment and conviction of new truths, heightens their charms, impresses them deep on the memory, and gives them an influence in practice, which they could not otherwise have boasted.
>
> *(Demodocus, 1774, p. 680)*

In his letter Demodocus also gave examples of successful people with visual impairments in the aristocracy, commerce, government and academia. Most notable among these examples was Nicholas Sanderson – Sanderson, a protégé of Isaac Newton, was a recent Lucasian professor of mathematics at Cambridge University, and invented a system of mathematical pin-prick language.

However, despite his belief in the academic ability of people with visual impairments, Demodocus still saw total blindness – his own form of blindness – as a form of moral disability. Consequently, and like his colleague Hume (1748), Demodocus stressed the person who lived "in darkness" still felt threatened in daily life and struggled to overcome a moral dread.

> Those philosophers who have attempted to break the alliance between darkness and spectres, were certainly inspired by laudable motives. But they must give us leave to assert there is a natural and essential connection between night and oreus. Were we endowed with senses to advertise us of every noxious object before its congruity could render it formidable, our panics would probably be less frequent and sensible than we really feel them. Darkness and silence therefore have something dreadful in them, because they supersede the vigilance of those senses which give us the earliest notices of things.
>
> *(Demodocus, 1774, p. 679)*

Contemporary replications of Cheselden's study

Although empirically moving on from the political and religious enlightenment of the seventeenth and eighteenth centuries, contemporary philosophies of blindness replicated earlier methods and categorisation. The most widely cited of these studies began in the late 1950s, when Richard Gregory and his research assistant Jean Wallace re-problematised Molyneux's question (Gregory, 1974) – although previous studies, such as one by the phenomenologist von Senden, had tested Molyneux's questions, Gregory and Wallace were the first to use a method much like that of Cheselden. As with Cheselden's case study, Gregory and Wallace studied a 52-year-old man, SB, who had recently been successfully treated for congenital cataracts and had no previously usable vision.

Drawing on Cheselden's method, Gregory and Wallace observed SB's experiences in the period immediately after his eyes physically recovered, seeing SB's response to his environment. Furthermore, Gregory and Wallace contrived situations in which SB could be presented with structured, empirical tasks including visits to museums and city centres to gauge SB's recognition of objects, drawing familiar objects when he had never tried this art before and the recognition of objects he'd previously felt when he was visually impaired. Subsequently, Gregory and Wallace were the first to describe the observations that transpired as *cross-modal transfer*.

Gregory and Wallace's observations and tests were recorded qualitatively, with the remainder of their data coming from health and school records provided by SB. For example, in Gregory and Wallace's later publication of the case study, it was said: "[SB] found that when looking down from a high window (about 30–40 feet above the ground) he thought that he could safely lower himself down by his hands" (Gregory, 1974, p. 101).

Many of Cheselden's original observations were replicated in SB's case study, with Gregory and Wallace finding that SB could appreciate objects aesthetically by sight – casting doubt on previous phenomenological studies by the likes of Revesz (1950) and von Senden (1932), which favoured Hume's philosophy that sensory information had discrete values (Hayhoe, 2015). Subsequently, in their concluding remarks Gregory and Wallace argued of Berkeley's boy and of SB:

> One may even say that their attempt to see was made long before their eyes were opened to the light, and in this respect they differ not only from most other cases in the literature but also of course from infants.
>
> *(Gregory, 1974, p. 117)*

However, despite SB's ability to become used to his environment through sight, Gregory and Wallace also observed the emotional problems that this transition caused. This difficulty appeared to illustrate not only a psychological difference of cognition, but also a cultural difference between a largely sighted and a largely tactile world that SB never reconciled.

For example, Gregory and Wallace observed SB became depressed because of this transition. Although this depression was at its strongest just after his operation, it lingered far longer than was healthy – this depression was a new phenomenon, something that had not been reported before SB's surgery. After keeping in touch with him after he left hospital, Gregory and Wallace also found SB tried to recreate a non-visual world in private, often sitting at home in darkened rooms. In the long term, he never seemed comfortable or happy with his new visual world and died not long after Gregory and Wallace's contact finished. Understandably, Gregory and Wallace found SB's death disturbing, particularly after becoming close to him during their study, and Gregory subsequently recorded the following in his diary:

> On 2 August 1960, S.B. died.
>
> His story is in some ways tragic. He suffered one of the greatest handicaps [sic], and yet he lived with energy and enthusiasm. When his handicap was apparently swept away, as by a miracle, he lost his peace and his self-respect.
>
> We may feel disappointment at a private dream come true: S.B. found disappointment with what he took to be reality.
>
> *(Gregory, 1974, p. 114)*

Later in the twentieth century, Gregory's observations were replicated by Oliver Sacks (1995) in his study of a middle-aged person recovering from surgery to gain sight for the first time. Sacks began this study after he was approached by the family of a 50-year-old man, who he gave the pseudonym Virgil. Sacks described Virgil as someone "who had been virtually blind since early childhood. He had thick cataracts, and was said also to have retinitis pigmentosa, a hereditary condition that slowly but implacably eats away at the retinas" (Sacks, 1995, p. 63). In his study, Sacks borrowed from Gregory's methodology, going as far as to consult Gregory about his and Wallace's work with SB. Subsequently, Sacks collected educational and medical records from Virgil, observed Virgil not long after his surgery and conducted tests on his ability to recognise objects by sight. In addition, Sacks had a significant extra advantage, as he was also given permission to refer to the diaries of Virgil's sister, collected from childhood to the time of the study.

As a physician himself, Sacks observed Virgil's medical records provided little usable or objective results, and so largely these documents remained unused in his analysis. Instead, Sacks found Gregory's methodology of observation and structured tasks more useful, and discussed qualitative data, constructing a narrative case study.

On publishing his results, Sacks found many similarities with Cheselden's and Gregory and Wallace's observations, and cast further doubt on the phenomenological studies criticised by Gregory and Wallace. The most notable similarity with SB was that even after his eyes recovered from surgery, Virgil would still rely on touch to familiarise himself with objects. For example, after their first meeting at the airport, Sacks observed "[Virgil pointed] to all of the cars we passed . . . 'Look at that one' he exclaimed once. 'I have to look down!' and bending felt it" (Sacks, 1995, p. 66).

Furthermore, Sacks also agreed with Gregory and Wallace's earlier finding that a transition from blindness to sightedness could disrupt Virgil's mental health. For example, Sacks found that during his study Virgil became depressed and would often recreate his earlier blindness at home, switching off lights and sitting in a darkened room. However, in a paradoxical change of fortune, and following further illness, Virgil lost his sight for a second time shortly afterwards, an event that improved his mental health. As Sacks noted in his case study:

> [Now] a final blindness – a blindness he received as a gift. Now, at last, Virgil is allowed to see, allowed to escape from the glaring and confusing world of sight and space, and to return to his own being, the touch world that has been his home for almost fifty years.
>
> *(Sacks, 1995, p. 73)*

Material philosophies after Gregory and Wallace

In the latter years of the twentieth century, the philosophy of blindness had a renaissance and material philosophers found themselves inspired by the epistemology of enlightenment. Importantly, like Gregory and Wallace, material philosophers in the twentieth and twenty-first centuries also attempted to replicate the methodology and classification of moral philosophies.

For instance, as Rene Descartes (1984) used the analogue of a cat to represent superior vision, Thomas Nagel (1991) used the analogue of a bat to represent experiences of sightlessness. And like Descartes, Nagel's aim in doing so was to show the subjectivity of the experience of sightlessness, arguing it provided a unique experience of objects and the environment.

Drawing on Hume's (1748) theory of the colour red, Nagel's philosophy was in common with Diderot's (2001) belief that the senses were equal but discrete. Consequently, Nagel theorised visual concepts such as colour could only be understood through direct experiences of seeing colour; the only exception being when light and dark shades of the same colour are seen, and the mind can imagine the individual shade in between.

However, and unlike Hume and Diderot, Nagel argued there were two types of understanding: objective and subjective sensory concepts. Subjective understanding, Nagel argued, could only be understood through direct experience, whereas objective understanding could only be communicated through language.

More particularly, Nagel observed that language cannot be used as an analogue for subjective experiences, which cannot be imagined as others see them, finding sensory analogies with synthesisia – where a colour is heard or smelt, rather than seen – were misappropriated. What's more, Nagel argued that using language with direct links to a visual vocabulary – such as describing bread as "looking warm" or sky that "looks cold" – with people who are born blind cannot lead to subjective understanding.

For Nagel, if a person never saw they would never be able to understand a sense they had never experienced, even when vision was presented as an analogy. Thus, Nagel argued, blindness is a subjective deficiency in a sighted world, but not an objective one. Therefore, cross-modal thinking can only be based on direct experiences of phenomena, and language or symbolic knowledge merely elucidates objective visual concepts – i.e. experiences render these concepts understandable only by their subjective and direct experience.

> One might try . . . to develop concepts that could be used to explain to a person blind from birth what it was like to see. One would reach a blank wall eventually, but it should be possible to devise a method of expressing in objective terms much more than we can at present, and with much greater precision. The loose inter-modal analogies – for example, "Red is like the sound of a trumpet" – which crop up in discussions of this subject are of little use. That should be clear to anyone who has both heard a trumpet and seen red. But structural features of perception might be more accessible to objective description, even though something would be left out. And concepts alternative to those we learn in the first person may enable us to arrive at a kind of understanding even of our own experience which is denied us by the very ease of our description and lack of distance that subjective concepts afford.
>
> *(Nagel, 1991, p. 179)*

Taking inspiration from the correspondence of philosophers such as Locke and Molyneux, Bryan Magee and Martin Milligan (1998) formed contrasting opinions on cross-modal transfer. Milligan, who was himself visually impaired and campaigned for the rights of visually impaired people, argued that his own experiences through touch provided a unique view on the world. Like Diderot, Milligan felt these experiences, although different, were no less morally or intellectually deficient than those of people with sight.

Conversely, and similar to Nagel and Hume, Magee argued that lacking sight also led to a deficit of subjective experience, of semantics of language and of an understanding of visual imagination. What's more, Magee argued blindness could not allow Milligan to comprehend the experiences of sighted people. Instead, Magee argued Milligan's experience of the world was segmented and uncontinuous, as Milligan could only touch a single object at a time. For instance, Magee observed, Milligan could not conceptualise visual concepts requiring distance beyond his reach.

Although similar to Diderot in agreeing touch was segmented, Milligan felt sight could be dishonest, describing it as a *hungry* sense, which must experience everything all the time. Consequently, Milligan suggested, people with vision needed to see aesthetically and greedily while they were awoken, and rarely distinguished between experiences and aesthetics. Contrariwise, touch was selective, and therefore took time to carefully discriminate between different sensory experiences. Touch is subsequently less greedy, and more of a *gourmand* of the aesthetics and the world it encounters. As Milligan argued:

> By the sighted, seeing is felt as a need. And it is the feeding of this almost ungovernable craving that constitutes the ongoing pleasure of sight. It is as if we were desperately hungry all the time, in such a way that only if we were eating all the time could we be content – so we eat all the time.

Because the realization seems to be lacking, your conception of the pleasures of sight appears altogether too aesthetic, as if someone were to suppose that the only pleasures involved in eating and drinking were those of the gourmet. There are, of course, aesthetic visual pleasures, but for most of us these are associated with rare or special occasions – looking at a painting or a landscape, seeing a beautiful woman, going to the ballet. Not many of us are lucky to see beautiful objects every day, whereas the normal pleasures of seeing, which is some sort of hungered-for and deeply needed satisfyingness, accompanies us all the time we are awake.

(Magee and Milligan, 1998, p. 135)

In common with Nagel and Magee, Robert Hopkins (2000, 2003) argued that people who are sighted differ from people who are blind quantitatively, as they have superior sensory experiences. Through a review of studies on the comprehension of tactile pictures by people with visual impairments, Hopkins hypothesised that distance and perspective have different qualities to those without sight.

Therefore, people with sight have an advantage when touching the features of objects that are associated with vision, such as foreshortening in tactile pictures – the concept of faraway objects feeling smaller than those in the foreground. Their experience of vision, Hopkins argued, allows people without visual impairments to experience touch through their visual experience as well as their tactile sensation.

Consequently, Hopkins argued, sculpture is the only exceptional art form for people who have no sight and no visual experience. This is because sculpture simulates space more completely than a tactile picture could, as it does not involve metaphors or visual symbolism. Sculpture is a unique form of art, which lends itself to further interpretation beyond that of mere sightedness. Where pictures are created primarily for vision, sculpture is a more democratic reproduction of the real world, lending itself to little interpretation.

[Sculpture] is able to straddle the divide between the represented and representing, as painting does not, precisely because it does not incorporate a perspective on what it represents . . . [Sculpture's] fundamental source is our awareness of our own possibilities for movement and action. That awareness is not something we derive from any particular sense, so much as something which informs experience in every sense modality. Thus, in offering us the form of engagement [Suzanne] Langer describes, sculpture is neither visual, nor tactile, but a complex mixture of the sensory, as standardly conceived, with our awareness of our own bodies, and their possible interactions with the world.

(Hopkins, 2003, pp. 25–26)

Discussion

In the introduction to this chapter, I asked the following question: *Has the methodology of cross-modal transfer affected our theory of cognition and blindness to the detriment of the majority of people with visual impairments?*

I would argue that it has.

The methodologies of early philosophical studies of cross-modal transfer mostly lacked imagination in developing an epistemology of blindness, or in promoting the social inclusion of people with visual impairments. Instead, the categorisation and ontology of cross-modal transfer was conflated with moral philosophy and used enlightened thinking as a tool to challenge orthodox religion and political power.

Importantly, Molyneux's question was not asked in isolation. Neither was this question the only instance of a consideration of blindness by Locke or his circle of philosophers; nor was it the only use of a methodology that can be referred to as *political blindness* by the philosophers that followed Locke in the eighteenth century. Importantly, the methodological assumption that experiences of blindness were wholly sightless was repeated elsewhere in Locke's essay, and discussed and examined more than other perceptual impairments as an example of ignorance. Consequently, the motivation for a so-called enlightened study of blindness was in part to show a lack of an inherited visual ability alone as evidence of internal morality.

The biased and ill-conceived methodologies of enlightened philosophies were to have consequences for later material philosophies of blindness. Following the Enlightenment, material philosophies repeated the miscategorisation of people as either sighted or sightless. Subsequently, the use of blindness and touch as a symbol of philosophy and equality also elevated people without sight to case studies of visual impairment, rather than as exceptions to the norm. This use of cross-modal transfer also made the plight of the wholly sightless infamous, and an object of moral fascination, singling such people out as examples of inequality.

Consequently, enlightened philosophies of cross-modal transfer and non-visual perception were not based on the practical logic of supporting or teaching people with visual impairments. What's more, their understanding of non-visual perception was often concentrated on developing a belief that non-visual perception could only partially make up for vision loss – even Diderot and Blacklock believed touch had a different cognitive as well as perceptual quality.

This categorisation of blindness thus brought prejudice as much as it developed useful knowledge. Subsequently, in the twentieth century although through observations Gregory and Sacks empirically illustrated learned perceptions, they also repeated the stereotype of blindness as sightlessness. This belief was yet again repeated by the material philosophies of Nagel, Magee and Milligan and Hopkins.

Consequently, educators who are influenced by these studies develop their own theories in the belief that touch is a primary mode of learning (Hayhoe, 2015). This largely explains why *institutions for the blind* have focused on handwork, touch, vibration and audible communication in the past – these were often the only medium of communication, imagination and vocation for over 200 years. These philosophies of cross-modal transfer also had the inadvertent effect of producing reductionist and biased ideas about blindness in the development of touch languages and technologies.

For instance, the use of such symbols as braille labelling and literature have come to be seen as inclusion for people who are blind. However, this stereotyping of people who are visually impaired serves them badly, as it is estimated that the majority of people with visual impairments have little need or want for braille – for instance, in 2012 it was found that the great majority of British people registered blind do not read braille and rely on audio books or digital readers either to speak or enlarge text (Creaser and Spacey, 2012; RNIB, 2012).

Subsequently, this sole reliance on braille in traditional education, buildings and reading materials produced for people with visual impairments has promoted passive exclusion (Hayhoe, 2015, 2016). What's more, this reliance on touch in colleges and the workplace has also restricted life chances and often led people with visual impairments to believe they are incapable of vocational, intellectual or artistic activities (see for example, Hayhoe, 2008, 2011).

Conclusion

It is undeniable that the philosophies discussed in this chapter provided a body of theory on perception that was testable through empiricism, and these philosophies have motivated inclusion in education. Without cross-modal transfer, children with visual impairments would not have received an education, strategies of teaching would not be considered important and building accessibility and accessible technologies would not have developed. As importantly, these theories also provide us with a discourse for informed debate on inclusion and disability. Philosophies from the Enlightenment in particular have given us our contemporary moral values of social justice and equality and raised such moral issues in the public consciousness.

However, the original philosophies of the Enlightenment were not just trying to raise the status of people with visual impairments they were also trying to create a general moral and political philosophy. Consequently, it suited these philosophers to categorise people with visual impairments as a sightless population rather than a population with restricted sight.

This problem has improved little in the modern era: whereas the understanding of these philosophies evolved significantly, and our understanding of human capacity has improved through a critical evaluation of previous generations of philosophy, methods have evolved little. Subsequently, modern material philosophies – and psychologies – of blindness still focus on blindness as sightlessness and see the support of people with visual impairment as largely being premised on touch. This has hampered the progress of inclusion and the pedagogical strategies we need to teach people with visual impairments alongside people with full sight.

Consequently, a potential solution to this problem is twofold. First philosophies, particularly philosophies that inform cognitive studies of blindness, need an updated methodology. This methodology needs to see the ontology of people with visual impairments as a spectrum of needs based on different forms of perception, as well as different social and broader cultural needs. Second, philosophers should only consider creating philosophies of blindness if their aim is to promote the inclusion and understanding of blindness itself, and not make broader points about the mind. Only when people with visual impairments are not regarded as this separate perceptual species will blindness be seen largely as a human issue rather than a cognitive novelty and deficit.

Acknowledgement

This project has received funding from the European Union's Horizon 2020 research and innovation programme under grant agreement No 693229 – Appendix A.

References

Barasch, M. 2001. *Blindness: The history of a mental image in Western thought.* London: Routledge.

Berkeley, G. 1899. *Selections from Berkeley* (5th ed.). Oxford: Clarendon Press.

Cheselden, W. 1839. *An appendix to the fourth edition of the anatomy of the human body.* London: W. Bowyer.

Colavita, F.B. 1974. Human sensory dominance. *Perception & Psychophysics*, 16(2), 409–412.

Creaser, C. and Spacey, R. 2012. *Assessing the impact of reading for blind and partially sighted adults.* London: RNIB.

Demodocus. 1774. On the education of the blind (open letter, dated 10 September 1774). *Edinburgh Magazine and Review*, 2, 673–686.

Descartes, R. 1984. *The philosophical writings of Descartes.* Cambridge: Cambridge University Press.

Diderot, D. 2001. *Thoughts on the interpretation of nature and other philosophical works.* Manchester, UK: Clinamen Press.

Driver, J. and Spence, C. 2004. *Cross modal space and cross modal attention.* Oxford: Oxford University Press.

Gottfried, A.W., Rose, S.A. and Bridger, W.H. 1977. Cross modal transfer in human infants. *Child Development*, 48(1), 118–123.

Gregory, R.L. 1974. *Concepts and mechanisms of perception.* London: Duckworth.

Gregory, R.L. 1987. *The Oxford companion to the mind.* Oxford: Oxford University Press.

Hayhoe, S. 2003. The development of the research of the psychology of visual impairment in the visual arts. In E. Axel and N. Levent (eds), *Art beyond sight* (pp. 84–95). New York: American Foundation for the Blind.

Hayhoe, S. 2008. *Arts, culture and blindness: Studies of blind students in the visual arts.* Youngstown, NY: Teneo Press.

Hayhoe, S. 2011. Non-visual programming, perceptual culture and mulsemedia: Case studies of five blind computer programmers. In G. Ghinea, F. Andres, and S.R. Gulliver (eds), *Multiple sensorial media advances and applications: New developments in MulSeMedia* (pp. 80–98). Hershey, PA: IGI Global.

Hayhoe, S. 2015. *Philosophy as disability & exclusion: The development of theories on blindness, touch and the arts in England, 1688–2010.* Charlotte, NC: IAP.

Hayhoe, S. 2016. The epistemological model of disability, and its role in understanding passive exclusion in eighteenth and nineteenth century Protestant educational asylums. *International Journal of Christianity and Education*, 20(1), 49–66.

Hopkins, R. 2000. Touching pictures. *British Journal of Aesthetics*, 40(1), 149–167.

Hopkins, R. 2003. *Painting, sculpture, sight and touch* [Professorial lecture]. Sheffield University, UK, 1 March.

Hume, D. 1748. *Essay concerning human understanding.* Oxford: Oxford University Press.

Jay, M. 1994. *Downcast eyes: The denigration of vision in twentieth-century French thought.* Berkeley, CA: University of California Press.

Locke, J. 2001. *An essay concerning human understanding.* London: Everyman Library/J.M. Dent.

Magee, B. and Milligan, M. 1998. *Sight unseen.* London: Phoenix.

Nagel, T. 1991. *Mortal questions.* Cambridge: Canto.

Nagel, T. 2012. *Mind and cosmos: Why the materialist neo-Darwinian conception of nature is almost certainly false.* Oxford: Oxford University Press.

Newton, I. 1959. *The correspondence of Isaac Newton.* Cambridge: Cambridge University Press.

Paulson, W.R. 1987. *Enlightenment, romanticism and the blind in France.* Princeton, NJ: Princeton University Press.

Popper, K. 1979. *Objective knowledge: An evolutionary approach* (revised edition). Oxford: Clarendon Press.

Popper, K. 1998. *Conjectures and refutations: The growth of scientific knowledge.* London: Routledge.

Popper, K. 2010. *The logic of scientific discovery.* London: Routledge.

Revesz, G. 1950. *Psychology and art of the blind.* London: Longmans Green.

RNIB. 2012. Braille [e-publication]. Accessed November 2012. www.rnib.org.uk/professionals/accessible information/accessibleformats/braille/Pages/braille.aspx.

Sacks, O. 1995. *An anthropologist on Mars.* London: Picador.

Sathian, K. and Stilla, R. 2010. Cross modal plasticity of tactile perception in blindness. *Restoratory Neurology and Neuroscience*, 28(2), 271–281.

Spence, C. 2009. Explaining the Colavita visual dominance effect. *Progress in Brain Research*, 176(0), 245–258.

Spence, C. 2010. Cross modal attention. *Scholarpedia*, 5(5), 6309.

von Senden, M. 1932. *Space and sight: The perception of space and shape in the congenitally blind before and after operation.* Glencoe, Illinois: Free Press.

16

In vision and touch, pictures trigger equations for surfaces and edges

John M. Kennedy

Introduction

Tactile pictures make sense to the blind (Kennedy, 2014b; Picard and Lebaz, 2012). Some have thought this ontologically impossible (Hopkins, 2003, 2008). Indeed, Yvette Hatwell (2003) noted that "touch is a modality whose function . . . has given rise to diverse and even contradictory appreciations" (p. 1). Here, I will argue that blind people can indeed use outline pictures. In vision and touch, the explanation goes, a line acts as if it triggers one equation for an edge and two for surfaces. One equation supplies information for an edge, and a surface needs two – one for azimuth, one for elevation.

A pitfall in the theory of perception, dominant today, which holds that a bundle of features in the world triggers single cells in the perceptual cortex is that a single cell only offers firing rates, not meaning. Other theories suggest we only observe an image of the world, but these are homunculus theories. Accounts of perception sorely need a new analogy. Here, I note that equations could be useful.

Tactile pictures

Is tactile perception of lines so cumbersome, slow and inaccurate that outline pictures are unusable? The truth is quite the opposite. Tactile picture recognition is actually quite easy if the pictures are simple and large with salient details (Heller et al., 2006). Accuracy scores reach 100% if test items are changed from hard to easy, or accompanied by hints or merely increased in size to fit with tactile resolution (Kennedy, 1993; Kennedy and Bai, 2002; Wijntjes et al., 2008a). Tactile perception only takes seconds to identify a picture of the Eiffel Tower, the Taj Mahal or Edinburgh Castle. By selecting objects wisely, tactile pictures can have enormous scope and deal with goals, thoughts, good, evil, politics and esthetics (Eriksson, 1998; Hanslick, 1854/1986; Hayhoe, 2008; Lopes, 2005). Given evidence of their use and value, major advocacy groups like Art Education for the Blind (Axel and Levent, 2003), educators such as Bogusław Marek, and museums and schools from London and Paris to Manila and Melbourne have begun offering pictures to the blind. In the United States, the National Federation of the Blind helps provide drawing kits to all blind children.

Tactile pictures clearly show shapes. They naturally show A is to the left or right of B. Left and right is the azimuth dimension. They also reveal which is higher, the elevation dimension. They offer foreground and background impressions (Kennedy, 1993). They can readily provide simple, straightforward geometrical information about depth and slant, so with practice there is reason to expect tactile pictures could yield depth and slant impressions. "Touch may be slower than vision at extracting spatial information, but is not inferior in the representations it produces" (Morash et al., 2012, p. 87). In essence, every doom and gloom opinion about tactile pictures has failed to ask how outline works, in vision as well as haptics, and underestimated the range of touch (Chao and Kennedy, 2015; Heller, Brackett and Scroggs, 2002; Heller et al., 1996).

Some argue that tactile pictures only work indirectly by means of images in the observer's head (Wijntjes et al., 2008b). This is a homunculus argument, akin to Plato's allegory of shadows on a cave wall seen by prisoners who can only guess at what they mean. Such arguments are off the wall indeed! A positive theory of outline pictures holds that both vision and touch readily perceive surfaces and spontaneously take lines in pictures as depicting relief – edges of surfaces facing a vantage point (Koenderinck and van Doorn, 2003). On this point, I am most grateful to Hatwell and Martinez-Sarrochi (2003) for their generous remark that to my partners and I, "we owe the most astonishing demonstration of the congenitally blind capacities to draw in relief" (p. 261). In this light, I present here reliefs portrayed by EW, a blind adult, self-taught, who started drawing in her thirties.

For decades, experiments on tactile pictures recruited groups of blind novices (Heller, Kennedy and Joyner, 1995; Kennedy, 1974, 1983). Later some very helpful informants from Turkey (Joan Eroncel), Italy (Paola Di Giulio) and Germany (Elke Zollitsch), to whom scholarship is deeply indebted, kindly let me know about blind people who were experienced in making pictures (Kennedy, 2003, 2014a, 2014b; Kennedy and Juricevic, 2003, 2006; Kennedy and Merkas, 2000). Blind people hear comments about pictures, and ask questions about pictures, so hearsay could explain some of their abilities, but not many, and my case histories include novel problems designed to test understanding of space beyond what rote memory can accomplish (Burke, 2016). The tests often reveal spontaneous facility with outline, apt reference, use of distinctive shapes, reliance on vantage points, comprehension of 3D space, appreciation of azimuth (width) and elevation (height) in the picture plane and invention of sensible metaphoric devices.

Complete novices identify tactile pictures (Heller and Gentaz, 2014; Heller and Kennedy, 1990; Kennedy, 1993; Picard and Lebaz, 2012). Heller (1989) argued that though the late blind have skill in touch plus prior visual experience to fall back on, the congenitally blind, without any visual experience at all, can identify tactile pictures. D'Angiulli, Kennedy and Heller (1998) found that blind children about 9 years old outscored sighted blindfolded children on tactile picture identification, despite having virtually no previous experience. Most telling of all, D'Angiulli et al. (1998) found that blind children retained correct identifications and changed incorrect ones when given a second run-through with a set of tactile pictures.

We still sorely need to test some blind people who have had years of practice identifying pictures. That day will surely come, as more and more institutions offer experience with tactile pictures. In Berlin, for example, docent Heike Hamann at the Bode Museum and Alte Nationalgalerie has classes on pictures for blind adults (Kennedy, 2012). What will result? Like visual reading, practice makes braille reading increase in speed and sensitivity by orders of magnitude. There is every reason to expect similar improvement with tactile pictures.

The observer needs to detect lines and examine shapes in pictures. The lines need to be taken as representations. Lines can have several meanings and visual inspection of a picture allows quick checks back and forth to compare parts. One line's significance should accord with the others, usually. It follows that recognition of a tactile picture is improved by sketching it as it is examined, all the while (or subsequently) looking at the sketch (Cechetto and Lawson, 2015; Wijntjes et al., 2008b), because tactile recognition will never catch up with visual recognition's quick checks to and fro. Furthermore, for most purposes, visual acuity is much greater than tactual acuity, so tactile pictures need to be relatively large and simple, taking seconds to examine, a longer time than the quick glance that is all that many visual pictures need. The orientation of lines is more acutely assessed by vision. But, speed and acuity aside, as the shape is gathered by perception, the principles being applied by vision and touch to lines are the same, I suggest. Not speed and not acuity, it is the principles that define pictures. Accordingly, many pictures in touch deserve and repay careful examination (the same can be said for subtle pictures for vision).

What is a picture?

The headline "Robbie Burns image in burnt toast" (pun intended) only means an accident has produced a blot with a very slight resemblance to the bard. Pictures with much fidelity to their referent did not exist until they were made by Ice Age *Homo sapiens sapiens* – Cro-Magnons in France and aborigines in Australia. A picture is a surface on which lines, contours and graded features (such as gradients of texture or colour) have been deliberately arranged to deliver projections of aspects of the environment (Koenderink and van Doorn, 2003). In the simplest case, the projection is orthogonal to the picture surface and the picture shape is congruent with the target's form, like an imprint (Hammad and Kennedy, 2017; Kennedy and Hammad, 2011). The process creating the artifact, be it drawing or photography, is one meant to create a projection of an aspect of the environment.

Chiefly, what lines and contours in pictures do is copy surface edges, features that are visible and tangible. If so, outline drawing does not have to be taught as a convention to the sighted or the blind, contra Deregowski (1984). A picture with forms that copy shapes in the environment, such as shapes of leaves, uses similarity geometry. In it, forms can be repeated at different scales. Blind people readily understand the change of scale. Though a 1 to 1 scale may be helpful, a drawing of the shape of a tower in miniature is not difficult in principle.

Projections in perspective geometry also offer scale changes (Hopkins, 2003; Reid, 1764). Projections from an object inward towards an observer are the exact inverse of the observer reaching outwards and pointing toward the object. Reaching to near objects and pointing to distant objects is in the domain of touch, so projection and perspective have a comfortable place in touch. For example, if we point to the top and bottom parts of a very distant object, the angle between our pointing arms is modest compared to pointing to the same spots when the object is quite near (Morash et al., 2012). Understanding how directions to fixed targets change as we walk about is a matter of perspective and change of scale (Loomis and Philbeck, 2008).

Bird and windmill: drawings from EW

In support of the theory of lines and surface, the lines in Figures 16.1 and 16.2 show edges of surfaces. They imply a vantage point and projection to it. In addition, by representing sound and wind they require an extension to the theory of surface edges.

Figure 16.1 is part of a raised-line picture, "Birds Paradise", made by a ballpoint pen on a plastic sheet resting on a rubberised board. The ballpoint puckers the sheet, producing a line one can feel. "Birds Paradise" was drawn by EW. She was blind as an infant, and is a self-taught artist. Due to retinal blastomas, her eyes were surgically excised, the right at 11 months, the left six months later. Encouraged by Elke Zollitsch (2003), a grade-school teacher she met at a

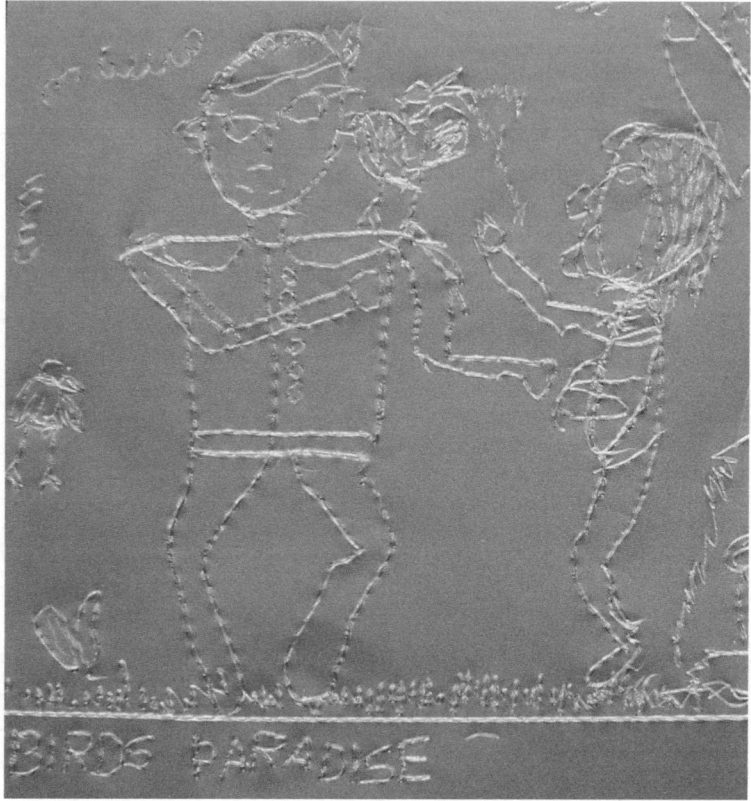

Figure 16.1   Part of a raised-line drawing, "Birds Paradise" (August, 2008), by EW, a blind adult.

conference in 2003, she began drawing frequently in her thirties. She drew Figure 16.1 on a trip to Australia, August 2008. It shows two people and birds. A woman is beside a man wearing spectacles and a cap. A bird is perched on the man's shoulder. Showing the artist's vantage point on the scene, the man faces front, and the woman is shown from the side, her head in profile, with long hair. The woman appears to reach toward the bird, and two small thin zigzags, one descending toward her arm, suggest, "the warning sound and pecking from the bird, and the pain and the associated sense of surprise I felt at the bird's sudden reaction – the overall unexpected experience. And it was quite a sharp pecking for something that small" (EW, email to the author, 26 April 2017).

Figure 16.2, dated 13 August 2008, is from the same trip to Australia. EW shows a windmill (centre) in Oatlands, Tasmania, a person (right, mill owner), horses (left), a stable, a house (right, the mill owner's) and wind, turning the sails, shown by long thin lines running left to right, in the top half of the picture and in an arc in the top centre of the picture. Lines attached to the sails suggest "the air pressure created by turning vanes" and zigzag lines near the sails "indicate the wailing noise the wind was actually making on the day we visited there" (EW, email to author, 29 September 2016). Ground is suggested by the base line, and height above the ground by converging lines in the lower right coming to the house. Of note, the drawing of the upper horse is about 10% smaller than the horse sketched below it, and the drawing of the bird walking on

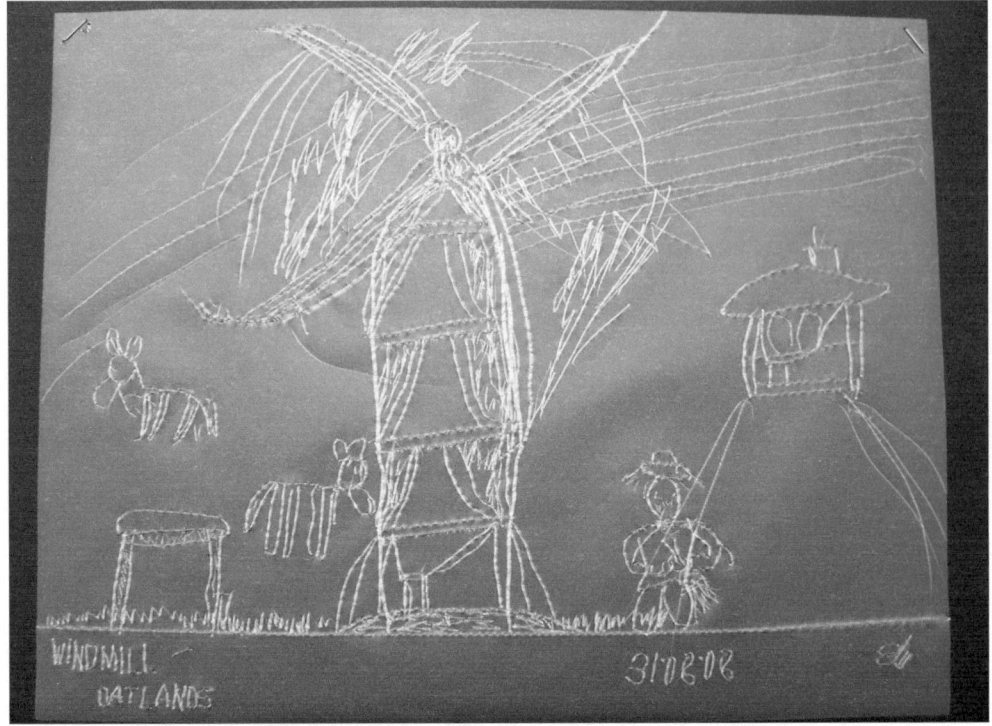

Figure 16.2 "Windmill, Oatlands" (31 August 2008). Drawing by EW, a blind adult.

the ground (left) is 15% smaller than the drawing of the bird perched on the man's shoulder. In a drawing of a desert, made on the same trip, the more distant the rock, the smaller the sketch, higher up the picture.

Lines, edges and six kinds of foregrounds

EW's lines stand for edges of surfaces. They stand for the rounded occluding bounds of people, including the shoulders of the male figure in Figure 16.1 and the nose and chin of the female figure. Edges of fairly flat surfaces include the sails, the roof of the house, its chimney, the openings of the man's shirt and the buttons. In all of these cases, one side of the line shows foreground surface, and on the other is background, sometimes close behind. Besides surface edges, lines also show skinny elements such as the legs of birds and the left arm of the spectacles in Figure 16.1. These have background on both sides of the line, and the skinny elements are foreground.

Foreground can be shown on one side of a line, or both sides, or by the line itself, and the line itself can show background. Options are shown in Figure 16.3. These are combinations of a foreground surface and a background, with the background sometimes being another surface. The yield is a "wee" set of six. The "wee six", from the top, are as follows:

1 A post (a slim foreground surface, with background on both sides).
2 An edge of the cap of the block (a foreground surface ends at an edge, with no defined background surface).

3   An edge of the front surface of the block (a foreground surface ends at an edge that has a background surface, the top of a platform).

4   An edge of a foreground surface (the front of the block) with another foreground surface – the platform's top – slipping under the front.

5   Two foreground surfaces meeting at a crack – their edges have a background between them. The line could show the background as dark.

6   Two foreground surfaces meeting (a convex corner of the platform) – their edges have no space between them. The darkness or lightness of the line is irrelevant.

A combination of foreground and background that is impossible is: two background surfaces nestle against each other. A background requires a foreground. (For the vantage point used in Figure 16.3, the rightmost face of the block, if it were transparent, would overlap the rear and bottom faces of the block. Also, the front face would overlap the back face, the bottom face and a side face.)

    The lines in Figure 16.3 have two contours. Each line is a thin ribbon with two sides or contours, its thickness indicating the thickness of posts and cracks. The contours show the borders of the posts or cracks. In lines standing for the edges of the top and side of the block, the outer contour of the line is readily taken as the outer limit of the block, the inner contour is irrelevant. In contrast, neither contour of a line showing the convex corner of the platform is taken as an edge. Instead, a middle of the line is readily taken as indicating the corner, the thickness of the line is irrelevant.

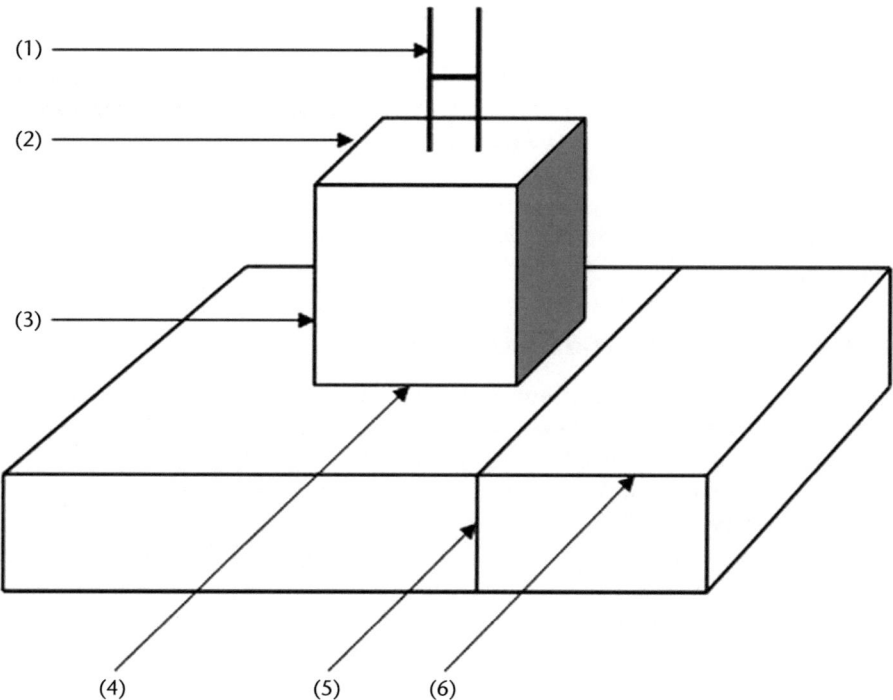

Figure 16.3 A set of six options for lines, showing a block on a platform.

Evidently, outline uses individual contours as representations of edges on occasion, and sometimes the width of the line represents the width of the referent. But also, width can be irrelevant and a contour can be irrelevant.

As they do in pictures for vision, lines and their contours can show edges in tactile pictures. In order from top left in Figure 16.3, the lines stand for (1) a post, background both sides; (2) an edge with background empty; (3) an edge with a background surface; (4) a corner between a foreground vertical surface that terminates at another foreground surface, the top of the platform, which continues under the block; (5) a crack with foreground on both sides; and (6) a convex corner between two foreground surfaces terminating at the corner. Like (6), edges have no width, though posts and cracks do.

Wind and wail

Lines, surfaces and edges can show the world realistically. But a ship on fire with a crew of leaders frantically manning pumps can be realistic in its parts but metaphoric overall. Is this the ship of state? A complete theory of outline needs to consider lines that may be metaphoric (Kennedy and Gabias, 1985).

Lines for wind can show surface borders, even if wind is invisible. Likewise, borders of a current flowing under a water surface would be tangible. EW described such lines as metaphoric for the sighted (Kennedy, 2008, 2009, 2013), but literal for the blind. We can feel invisible edges of streams of water in water. Around a windmill's sails (Figure 16.2), EW drew lines showing wind. Borders of wind currents would also be tangible. Additionally, she drew noises, wailing from wind moving the sails and, in Figure 16.1, warnings from birds. Noises and surprises are not surfaces or edges, not tangible or visible. In these instances, I suggest, the use of lines is metaphoric. It is akin to taking trails made in dust behind a sliding object and putting them in the sky behind a superhero in flight.

EW's extended jagged lines stand for extended wails. Metaphors like "jailors have hearts of stone" tell us the topic (jailor) and a vehicle (stone) share significant features. If the features are highly relevant, the metaphor is apt. Several features of jagged lines (a vehicle) could be apt for wails (a topic). The jagged lines go up and down, like wailing or chirping increasing and decreasing in volume. Sometimes they change direction abruptly, and are dense, which could suggest a short burst of intense noise, volume changing suddenly and surprisingly. Continuous lines of zigzags, all the same size, can suggest continuous noise.

Studies on blind people and space

In Figure 16.1, EW drew the man from the front and the woman from the side. In the windmill picture the man shows his front and the horses their sides. Surfaces and vantage points are fundamental to 3D space. Hence, blind people should have an effective grasp of 3D. Studies with Hsin-Yi Chao and Marta Wnuczko support this claim (Chao and Kennedy, 2014; Chao, Kennedy and Wnuczko, 2013).

We studied blind and sighted observers tackling Jean Piaget's "Three Mountains" tabletop scene (Figure 16.4). A square mat on a table has on it a cone, a sphere and a cube. The observer is on one of the four sides of the mat. From the vantage point of the observer, the objects might be arranged with the cone on the near left corner, the sphere at the back of the mat in the middle of the side and the cube on the right side halfway along the side. Ergo, in an elevation, the cone is to the left, the sphere is in the middle and the cube is on the right (Figure 16.4, bottom). The observer is asked to imagine moving to the left side of the mat, or across to the far side,

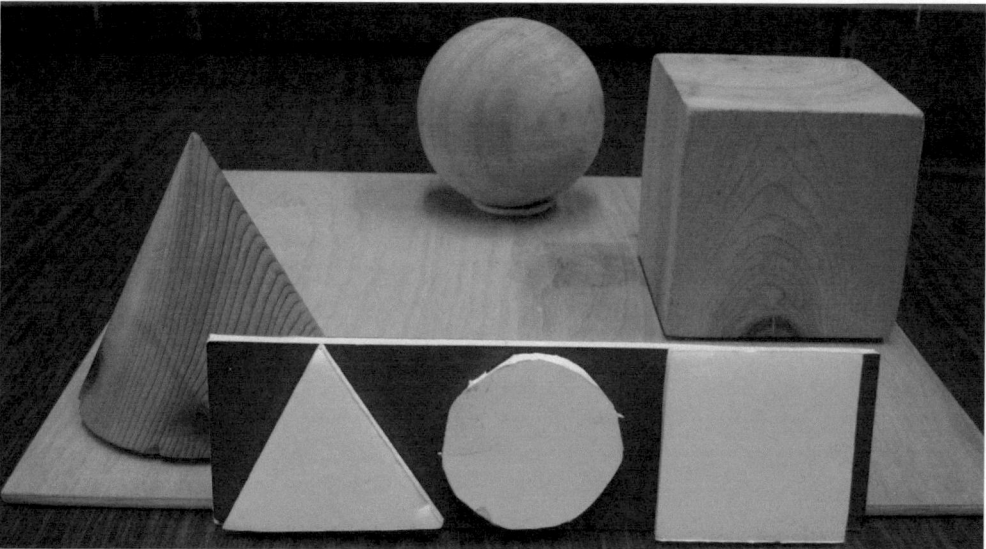

Figure 16.4   Piaget's "Three Mountains" task, with a cone, a sphere and a cube, and an elevation, with a triangle, a circle and a square fitting the observer's vantage point.

or to the right side. The task is to decide how the three objects would be arranged in an elevation (as in Figure 16.4, bottom) or a plan (Figure 16.5) for each of the four sides. The elevation shows the shape of the object in height, and the plan shows the shape from above. For example, in an elevation from directly across the mat, a square shows the cube is to the left, a circle for the sphere sits in the middle and a triangle shows the cone is to the right.

Of interest, there are two impossible side elevations. There are six ways to arrange three objects left to right but only four sides to the mat. Two arrangements are impossible – the elevations that put the triangle in the middle. The cone is at a corner, and from no side can it be in the middle of the left to right arrangement. Figure 16.4 (bottom) includes a correct elevation, and Figure 16.5 shows an incorrect "plan". Figure 16.6 shows one impossible and two possible elevations.

Blind adult observers were slightly more accurate than sighted blindfolded observers on elevations (Chao et al., 2013). (An always-sighted group of undergraduates tested had 24 participants; a similar group shown the displays sighted and then tested blindfolded also had 24; an always-blindfolded group had 19. The early blind group had 6 participants. All were totally blind prior to 3 years old.). Of interest, tested on "plans" of the display, the blind group again performed better than the blindfolded.

On a task with "impossible" elevations the blind and blindfolded were about equal and both were more accurate than observers trying the task sighted (Chao and Kennedy, 2014; an experiment with 48 Toronto undergraduates, 24 tested with sight, 24 blindfolded and 19 blind adults, of which 7 early blind were 1 totally blind and 6 with only light perception before the age of 2 years old; of 12 later blind volunteers, 4 were totally blind and 8 had only light perception).

Marta Wnuczko and I reported a study on blind and sighted observers pointing to objects set along the ground (Figure 16.7). Blind and blindfolded observers pointed to target circles in a path on the ground, in two parallel rows, after viewing the circles or touching them with a

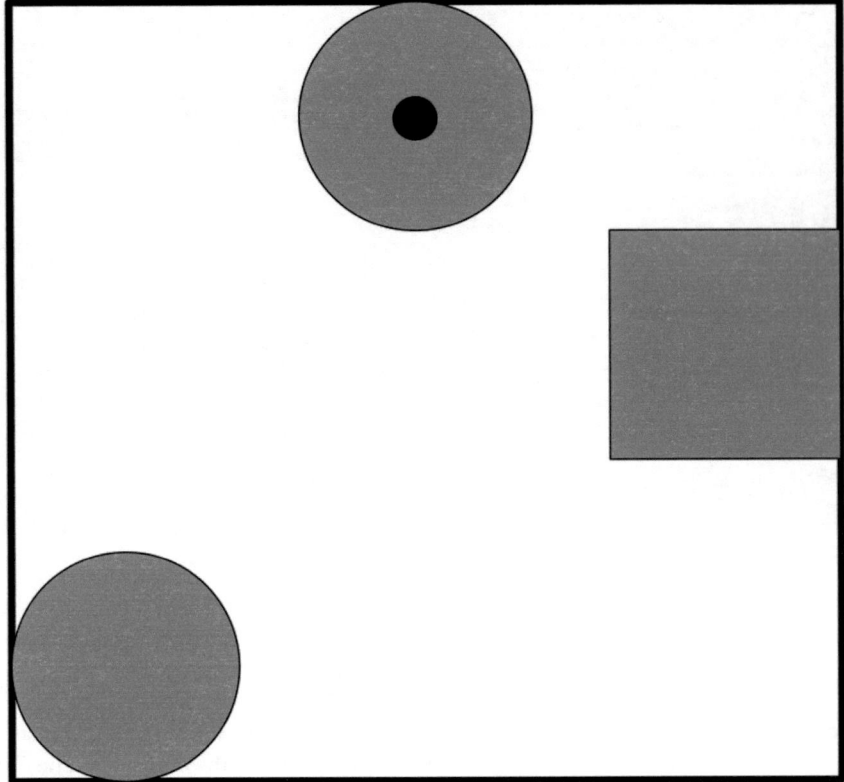

Figure 16.5 A plan of Piaget's "Three Mountains". This is an "impossible" option for Figure 16.4's array because it shows a sphere on the left (near corner), a cone in the middle (and near the top) and a cube on the right (at mid-distance). No plan or elevation for Figure 16.4 can show the cone in the middle of a side.

stick while walking past them (Wnuczko and Kennedy, 2014). The stimuli were 12 cardboard circles, glued on a 6 m long and 2 m wide plastic sheet. Two paths of six equidistant circles stretched in front of an observer. The paths were separated horizontally, in azimuth, by 1 m. Adjacent circles were separated from each other by 1 m in depth (generating differences in elevation). The nearest pair of circles was set 50 cm distant from the observers at their pointing location. The circle's centres served as targets. The participants were 14 sighted undergraduates who viewed the targets and were then blindfolded before pointing to the circles. A total of 13 sighted-but-blindfolded undergraduates and 6 blind adults participated in the task without vision. After they explored the targets with a stick, the participants walked back to base and then were asked to point to the circles. With distance, pointing by all groups diminished in azimuth and increased in elevation. Performance by the blind and blindfolded participants was close to indistinguishable. The ground is a plane that can support distance and size perception (Al Hazen, 1039/1939; Gibson, 1979), and evidently it can take this role for touch and the blind as well as vision and the sighted.

Surface-perception theories hold that the principles of space govern touch, and hence the perceptual skills of the blind. With Alison Eardley, Geoffrey Edwards and Francine Malouin, I

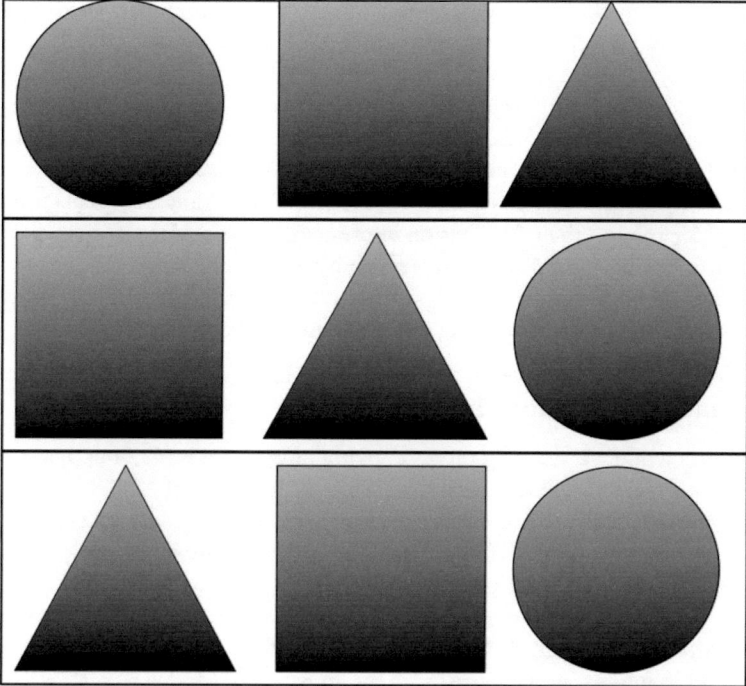

Figure 16.6   Two "possible" elevations of Figure 16.4, and an "impossible" option (the middle row).

wondered if blind people are equal to the sighted on tasks to do with plans as maps of a region (Eardley et al., 2016). Previous research on this issue often included individuals with retinopathy of prematurity (RoP, and, as a result, over-oxygenation at birth) in the study sample. However, RoP is confounded with prematurity. Prematurity, per se, has been associated with spatial difficulties. In this experiment, blindfolded sighted participants and two groups of functionally

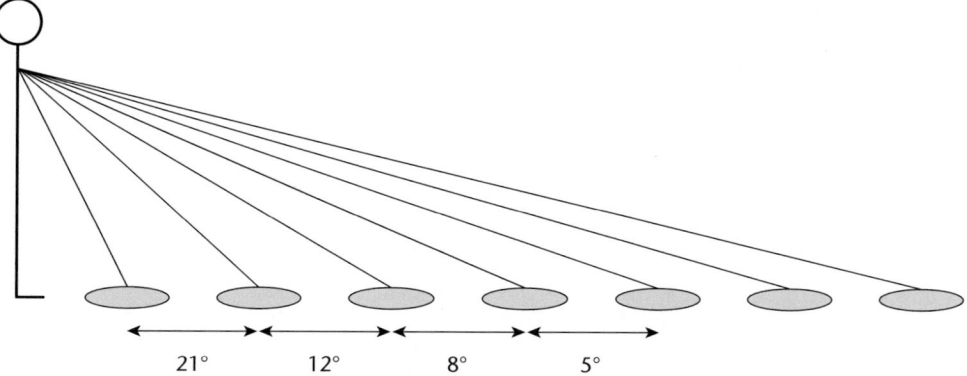

Figure 16.7   Pointing to a row of targets spaced equal distances apart. With distance, elevation increases. The angle subtended by the spaces between two adjacent targets decreases with distance.

totally blind participants heard text descriptions from a plan (allocentric) or route (egocentric) perspective. One blind group lost their sight due to RoP and a second group before 24 months of age. The accuracy of participants' understanding of the text descriptions was assessed via questions and maps. The RoP participants had lower scores than the sighted and early blind, who performed similarly. In other words, it may not have been prolonged visual impairment alone that diminished performance on plans in this task but visual impairment together with prematurity and possibly neural damage from too much oxygen. This finding may explain contradictions in the existing literature on the role of vision in processing spatial plans. (Alison Eardley was the lead researcher in this study, and advice was given by Morton Heller.)

Some research supports the theory that touch accesses vantage points in 3D, offers directions to points on an extended surface and supports plans and egocentric routes.

Surface equations or images in the head

People sometimes wonder if drawing means copying how things look, or copying visual images in the head (Scocchia, Stucchi and Loomis, 2009; Wijntjes, et al., 2008b). The idea is that observers are copying intermediaries, way-stations such as looks and images, not the actual objects. Such way-stations are little more than conundrums wrapped in riddles because the first and primary task in drawing is for people to get information about the world. Occam's razor requires that we do not multiply intermediary entities – offer as few way-stations as possible. To this end, it is surely best to assert that tactile information for surfaces is understood directly, and needs no translation into imagery before it can be appreciated. Models of surface perception can hold that comprehension is best represented by equations that contain information for target features. The models are well exemplified by a picture made of dotted lines, because a dotted line fits a linear equation, and this suggests several stages in perception: dot grouping, then shape finding and finally surface representation (Feldman, 1997; Kubovy and Wagemans, 1995).

Imagine Figure 16.3 is full of rows of dots such as, ... , a line of eight dots. Physically, the dots fit a linear equation. To move towards the equation, the first order of business in perception is to detect the individual dots and somehow to take them as a group. To achieve this, first, dots that are physically close together could form simple, small perceptual packages, such as pairs. Dot 1 is close to and could be recognised as along with 2, 2 with 3, 3 with 4, etc. Second, the links for each dot need to be noted. Dot 1 is a terminal but it is allied with one other dot, namely dot 2. Dot 2 joins with both 1 and 3, 3 with 2 and 4, etc., and the result is that the full set of dots, 1 to 8, are found to be chained together. Third, perception needs to respond to the chain's physical fit to an equation. In the present instance, the set of 8 fits an equation such as $y = ax + b$, suitable for a straight line.

A word of caution, and an optimistic note: At first thought, displays made of a few dots may seem far removed from perception of the ordinary environment, for our world is a place of solid textured surfaces, things we can see and touch, matter in the round, not flat on a picture surface. But the texture of a surface is a set of elements, repeated (forming a gradient from the vantage point of an observer). So too is a dotted line, meaning it is a texture reduced to its essence, and, furthermore, the information for slant and depth has to do with equations fitting texture gradients, and if these are fair assumptions, dotted displays are perhaps to be taken as miniature and highly simplified versions of the textured world. They may be able to show us perception's use of the informative equations generally supplied by ordinary real-world surfaces.

The giant advantage of an equation over a list of the pairs of dots and a commonsense description of a chain of dots is that the equation can say something about the shape between the dots. It can fill the empty space between each pair of dots and say that a line formed by the dots is a straight and continuous shape. To be continuous, a function must be able to indicate values between the dots, such as 1.1, 1.11, 1.111 etc., all the way to 2, if needed. Dots 1 and 8 anchor the function, and once the chain from 1 to 8 triggers the equation, the function operates independently of dots 2 to 7. An infinite number of equations fit a finite set of dots, but in practice perception notes only one or two, and vision and touch commonly concur.

In this model, gaps between dots are filled. The filler is a shape. Just a shape, it does not appear as if sketched by a pen on the sheet or board or screen on which the dots are evident. The shape is virtual, mathematical, invisible and intangible – merely a shape, like the smile on a Cheshire cat. A Gestalt, it joins dots, like the invisible but highly effective lines of force between two magnets.

An equation, which can be put generally as $y = F(x)$, is a property of solid lines like _____ just as it is of lines of dots. In perceptual processing, both the dotted line and the solid line resonate with the shape defined by $y = F(x)$ – the dots fit the function, and the function describes the dots as a single ensemble.

In perception, if the part of a line in Figure 16.3 that is of interest is one of its contours, then it is the contour that triggers the equation. A clear example is option 2 in Figure 16.3, the outer contour of the line standing for the edge of the top of the block. Of special significance for picture perception, the perceptual function can also be triggered by edges of surfaces. They too fit an equation, physically. This is a key to outline representation: $F(x)$ is triggered by elements in pictures and by elements along surface edges. A full description of the elements is needed to develop this promising theory, but this much is obvious: We can tell that a line, dotted or solid, and an edge have the same shape.

The equation $y = ax + b$ is an effect of dots 1 to 8, but the equation is not entirely beholden to dots 1 to 8, as it could have been caused by dots at 1, 1.5, 2, 2.5, etc. As a result, once it is caused in perception, an equation carries no information about the actual dots that triggered it, and it becomes independent of dots 2, 3, 4, 5, 6 and 7 that it fits. However, equations generally need to run no further than from one end of a shape to another, which can be summarised for the dot 1 to dot 8 shape as $y = Dot1[F(x)]Dot8$. This function states that $F(x)$ applies from dot 1 to dot 8, and fits intermediate dots, but it does not specify that it was triggered by the specific dots 2 to 7. In cortical terms, a part of the brain that holds $y = ax + b$ deals with shape and continuity, but has lost information about dots 2 to 7. Dots 2 to 7 have been left behind in earlier cortical processes. Likewise, the equation for the shape of a convex corner (such as option 6 in Figure 16.3) is triggered in perception by a line with two contours, but contains no information about the line's contours. And also, just so, similar shape equations triggered by elements along surface edges hold no information about the edge elements.

Graduate student Peter Coppin asked me, why dots tell us about a line, but a line does not tell us about dots. The answer is that the causal arrow points one way: elements trigger the equation, in this case. The equation does not make us perceive dots 2 to 7, and neither does it suggest extra dots between dots 1 to 8. The equation allows us to perceive continuity between 1 and 8, nothing more. Dots 2 to 7 are on one side of an event horizon, the equation is on the other. A useful analogy is that any entanglement is between terminal dots 1 and 8 and the equation.

Continuous functions such as $y = F(x)$ fit dots in the world, and neural versions allow surface edges to be perceived, and bring outline pictures to life. In this account, dots that fit a linear equation, physically, trigger a function in perceptual processing, and in turn the function supports surface perception. The surfaces are virtual, perceived (Rubin, 1915), but known by the observer to be represented and not real.

To support perception of a surface and its edge, in addition to describing a linear shape of the edge, the equation $y = F(x)$ must support the shape of an area alongside the linear shape. A surface alongside is defined by two further equations, one for azimuth and one for elevation. Many factors supply physical information about surfaces and can trigger these equations in perception (Kennedy, 1993; Peterson, 2015; Rubin, 1915). The equations needed are an azimuth and an elevation equation, applying simultaneously to an area to one side of the $y = F(x)$ shape. Two equations are needed since they describe an area, not a line. But further, areas on both sides of the linear function need to be described (as in option 6 in Figure 16.3). In other words, the linear function for an edge in perceptual processing allows two functions per side, four side functions in all.

In this model of the workings of tactile pictures, elements such as dots, contours and lines fit continuous linear shapes and trigger linear functions in both touch and vision. Next, functions for areas act alongside the linear shape, an idea that might be especially controversial for tactile pictures, even more than it is novel for pictures for vision. But the evidence it describes is that rank beginners take tactile lines as showing profiles, and profiles tell us about surfaces of foreheads and noses and chins off to the side of the line.

Let us be clear that the functions suggested by $y = F(x)$ are more than a mere summary of pairs of dots. A set of eight equally spaced dots is perceived as a circle, not an octagon, though on their own each pair of dots is linked by a straight line. A curve takes precedence. It overrides the straight links, and defines a circle. As a demonstration, it is worth observing a pair of dots from the 8, on their own, noting that they appear to be joined by a straight link. Then, one should expose an adjacent dot, a third dot and then the next dot in the series, forming a quartet, then a fifth and so on. The initial two dots appear as if joined by a straight imaginary line. The trio may suggest a triangle, the fourth a trapeze, but by the fifth dot, the circle takes precedence generally. The curve supplants the straight links.

In the $y = F(x)$ model of outline pictures made of dots, the equation requires no mental image of a link joining dots, like a wire joining pearls in a necklace. The link is virtual. There is no image to be seen by an imaginary interior eye or touched by an interior finger – no homunculus. Instead, the observer is aware of links, aware of the virtual shape, aware of edges and aware of surfaces.

Mental images

In mental images of common objects or scenes, lines of any kind are usually conspicuous by their absence. Consequently, we do not draw outline drawings of objects by copying images that are composed of lines. Also, all the angles in an image of a cube are right angles, by definition, but the drawing of a cube has lots of acute and obtuse angles, and therefore is not a copy of the image. In most people's mental life, mental images are found in abundance, but that does not mean that images are what we draw. The heart of the matter is that we draw the object because we get information about it, then pose the question how to draw its parts and fit them together. This is not straightforward. Drawing entails thinking about several factors: how to select and draw the shapes of particular features, the orientation of the features, their links to other features and the space containing the object, bearing in mind the observer's vantage point. Should the picture be a stick figure, we ask, or should we first sketch it with rough balloon shapes, ovals and circles or should we try to draw a line following the object's external contour, like a profile? Images, should we entertain them, are more about the object than the way to draw them. Drawing is a separate skill from imagery, in several respects. This helps explain why, in two impressive studies, several measures of imagery ability did not predict rates of tactile picture identification (Picard et al., 2010; Thompson, Chronicle and Collins, 2003). Imagery is too vague an explanation of picture use, and has very little handle on the different factors entailed in drawing.

Equation theory of perception objects to imagery theory as a "way-station" argument, and in a similar vein it goes toe to toe with "enactive" theories (Noe, 2005, 2008). These are children of Plato's analogy for perception that we stare at shadows of objects on the wall of the cave cast by a fire behind us, and know the world only indirectly via the shadows. Indirect-perception theory holds that we have internal "sense data," or maps or models, much like Plato's shadows, and then guess that they tell us about the external world. Helmholtz (1911/1925) argued we act "as if" guessing on the "evidence" of our senses. "As if" means he offers an analogy, much as a theory of equations in the head is an analogy. He argued that internal sensations are "symbols" for our imagination, and perception of an external object is due to a judgement. However, are data in our head evidence to be "observed" and "judged" by a third party, an internal observer? That would be an infinite regress, alas. Certainly we do not want to say neurons take on the character of our percepts, such as continuity, and observation of these shows us the world. Neurons do not copy the world this way. If that was true our neurons would have to turn green to have us see green. That would be straight from the Ministry of Silly Theories. Neurons do not take on the character of what they signify.

A popular indirect theory today is "enaction": we see via predispositions to act — potential sensorimotor events (Noe, 2008). A large size is something to reach up to. A small object we reach down to. Distance is perceived as the number of steps or energy we think we require to reach an object. (Alas for pictures, they call for different actions and energy than real objects.) For William James, to attain perfect clarity in our thoughts of an object, we should consider what conceivable effects of a practical kind the object may involve — especially what reactions we must prepare (James, 1907).

Like enactions, "reactions we must prepare" is a non-starter. James fails to prepare for the infinite. The rub is, any object can call for an infinite number of reactions. We can walk up to it. We can run from it. We can dance to it. We can rock it, we can roll it. Often, the actions to get information are not the same as the acts an object affords. We get information about a hammer's shape from a tactile picture, if, say, we explore it with one finger (Morash, Pensky and Miele, 2013; Morash et al., 2014; Symmons and Richardson, 2000), even though we might explore the real object by holding it in one hand and running our other hand over it (Lederman and Klatzky, 2009) or wielding it (Cabe, 2013; Carello and Turvey, 2017).

To draw an object, what we need to do in essence is to get information about it. Many incidental acts or mental images or maps accompanying the gathering of useful information are just that, incidentals. We need to distinguish the happenstances from the accurate information for the object. If our only basis for drawing was any and all mental activity that accompanied looking at or touching an object, complete irrelevancies would sidetrack us and be added to the drawing. The object might be a box. It might remind us of striking matches or using an eraser and such acts might pop up in our consciousness, fodder for images. But we need to use the information from the object to ward off distractions. The object gives off information — we need to gather that. If the information we gather is that the object is round — if it triggers $X^2 + Y^2 = C$, a constant — we should draw a picture that reveals something is round. If the information is that the object is tilted, we might try to show that it is tilted. The shapes, locations and orientations of objects are the target for a picture. In the midst of a stream of mental activities, drawing cognition selects targets from the information supplied by the world, setting aside what is irrelevant.

Conclusion

Touch feels surfaces and their edges. Visual and tactile pictures use lines, including dotted lines, to stand for the edges. Continuity is given by equations such as $y = ax + b$, triggered by the dots and lines. Broadly, ^{m}[ax^p +b]^n is a shape that runs from point m to point n, with a curvature defined by an exponent p. The shape equation offers a shape for the surface edge, and similar pairs of equations show the shapes of surfaces alongside edges.

A visible picture can be scanned superficially in a second, and a tactile picture takes longer to scan. Its shapes have to be found, which takes longer than a second, and the shapes have to be taken as representations. Recognition follows, even for novices with the medium. Both the visible and the tangible picture rely on the same depiction principles.

References

Al Hazen, I. 1039/1989. *The optics of Ibn-Hatham* (vol. I). A.I. Sabra (trans.). London: University of London and Warburg Institute.

Axel, E. and Levent, N. 2003. *Art beyond sight*. New York: AEB and AFB Press.

Burke, R. 2016. *Painting in the dark*. Weston, MA: Tumblehome Learning.

Cabe, P.A. 2013. Haptic distal spatial perception mediated by strings: Size at a distance and egocentric localization based on ellipse geometry. *Attention, Perception & Psychophysics*, 75(2), 358–374. http://dx.doi./org.10.3758/s13414-012-0389-6

Carello, C. and Turvey, M. 2017. Useful dimensions of haptic perception: 50 years after *The Senses Considered as Perceptual Systems*. *Ecological Psychology*, 29(2), 95–121. http://dx.doi./org.10.1080/10407413.2017.1297188

Cechetto, S. and Lawson, R. 2015. Simultaneous sketching aids the haptic identification of raised line drawings. *Perception*, 44(7), 743–754. http://dx.doi./org.10.1177/0301006615594695

Chao, H.-Y. and Kennedy, J.M. 2014. 3-mountains, impossible responses: Blind and blindfolded more accurate than sighted. *55th Annual Conference of the Psychonomics Society*. Long Beach, CA. Nov. 20–23.

Chao, H.-Y. and Kennedy, J.M. 2015. Metaphoric car drawings by a 12-year-old congenitally blind girl. *Perception*, 44(12), 1349–1355. http://dx.doi./org.10.1177/0301006615596916

Chao, H.-Y., Kennedy, J.M. and Wnuczko, M. 2013. Elevation easier than plan for sighted and early-blind adults in a perspective-taking task. *Attention, Perception & Psychophysics*, 75(6), 1186–1192. http://dx.doi./org.10.3758/s13414-013-0469-2

D'Angiulli, A., Kennedy, J.M. and Heller, M.A. 1998. Blind children recognizing tactile pictures respond like sighted children given guidance in exploration. *Scandinavian Journal of Psychology*, 39(3), 189–190. http://dx.doi./org.10.3758/BF03205550

Deregowski, J.B. 1984. *Distortion in art: The eye and the mind*. London: Routledge & Kegan Paul.

Eardley, A.F., Edwards, G., Malouin, F. and Kennedy, J.M. 2016. Allocentric spatial performance higher in early-blind and sighted adults than in retinopathy-of-prematurity adults. *Perception*, 5(3), 281–299. http://dx.doi./org.10.1177/0301006615607157

Eriksson, Y. 1998. *Tactile pictures: Pictorial representations for the blind 1784–1940*. Gothenburg, Sweden: Gothenburg University Press.

Feldman, J. 1997. Regularity-based perceptual grouping. *Computational Intelligence*, 13(4), 582–623. http://dx.doi./org.10.1111/0824-7935.00052

Gibson, J.J. 1979. *The ecological approach to visual perception*. Boston, MA: Houghton-Mifflin.

Hammad, S. and Kennedy, J.M. 2017. The picture surface illusion: 3D biases 2D. In Arthur Shapiro and Dejan Todorovic (eds.), *The Oxford compendium of visual illusions* (pp. 209–213). Oxford: Oxford University Press.

Hanslick, E. 1854/1986. *Vom Musikalisch-Schönen* [*On the musically beautiful*]. Leipzig, Germany: Rudolph Weigel. (English edition translated by G. Payzant. London: Hackett.)

Hatwell, Y. 2003. Introduction: Touch and cognition. In Y. Hatwell, A. Streri and E. Gentaz (eds), *Touching for knowing* (pp. 1–16). Paris: Presses Universitaires de France.

Hatwell, Y. and Martinez-Sarrochi, F. 2003. The tactile reading of maps and drawings and the access of blind people to works of art. In Y. Hatwell, A. Streri and E. Gentaz (eds), *Touching for knowing* (pp. 255–274). Paris: Presses Universitaires de France.

Hayhoe, S. 2008. *Arts, culture and blindness*. Youngstown, NY: Teneo Press.

Heller, M.A. 1989. Picture and pattern perception in the sighted and the blind: The advantage of the late blind. *Perception*, 18(3), 379–389. http://dx.doi.org/10.1068/p180379

Heller, M.A., Brackett, D.B. and Scroggs, E. 2002. Tangible picture matching by people who are visually impaired. *Journal of Visual Impairment & Blindness*, 96(5), 349–353. http://dx.doi.org/10.1177/0264619613512838?

Heller, M.A., Calceterra, J.A., Burson, L.L. and Tyler, L.A. 1996. Tactual picture identification by blind and sighted people: Effects of providing categorical information. *Perception & Psychophysics*, 58(2), 310 323 http://dx.doi.org/10.3758/BF03211884

Heller, M.A. and Gentaz, E. 2014. *Psychology of touch and blindness*. London: Psychology Press.

Heller, M.A. and Kennedy, J.M. 1990. Perspective taking, pictures, and the blind. *Perception & Psychophysics*, 48(5), 459–466. http://dx.doi.org/10.3758%2FBF03211590

Heller, M.A., Kennedy, J.M., Clark, A., McCarthy, M., Borgert, A., Fulkerson, E., Wemple, L.A., Kaffel, N., Duncan, A. and Riddle, T. 2006. Viewpoint and orientation influence picture recognition in the blind. *Perception*, 35(10), 1397–1420. http://dx.doi.org/10.1068/p5460

Heller, M.A., Kennedy, J.M. and Joyner, A.D. 1995. Production and interpretation of pictures of houses by blind people. *Perception*, 24, 1049–1058. doi: 10.1068/p241049

Helmholtz, H. von. 1911/1925. *Treatise on physiological optics* (3rd ed.). J.P.C. Southall (trans. and ed.). Washington, DC: Optical Society of America.

Hopkins, R. 2003. Perspective, convention and compromise. In H. Hecht, R. Schwartz and M. Atherton (eds), *Reconceiving pictorial space* (pp. 145–166). Cambridge, MA: MIT Press.

Hopkins, R. 2008. Personal communication. 19 June, Gargnano, Italy.

James, W. 1907. *Pragmatism: A new name for some old ways of thinking*. Project Gutenberg [e-book]. Accessed October 2016. www.gutenberg.org/files/5116/5116-h/5116-h.htm.

Kennedy, J.M. 1974. *A psychology of picture perception*. San Francisco, CA: Jossey Bass.

Kennedy, J.M. 1983. What can we learn about pictures from the blind? *American Scientist*, 71(Jan.–Feb.), 19–26. http://dx.doi.org/10.3758/BF03211590

Kennedy, J.M. 1993. *Drawing and the blind*. New Haven, CT: Yale University Press.

Kennedy, J.M. 2003. Drawings from Gaia, a blind girl. *Perception*, 32(3), 321–340. http://dx.doi.org/10.1068/p3436?id=p3436

Kennedy, J.M. 2008. Metaphoric drawings devised by an early-blind adult on her own initiative. *Perception*, 37(11), 1720–1728. http://dx.doi.org/10.3758/APP.71.2.217

Kennedy, J.M. 2009. Outline, mental states and drawings by a blind woman. *Perception*, 38(10), 1481–1496. http://dx.doi.org/10.3758/APP.71.2.217

Kennedy, J.M. 2012. What is an outline picture in vision and touch? Blind and palaeolithic artists. In H. Bredekamp, M. Lauschke and A. Artega (eds), *Bodies in action and symbolic forms: Essays in honour of John Krois* (pp. 239–252). Berlin, Germany: Akademie Press.

Kennedy, J.M. 2013. Tactile drawings, ethics and a sanctuary: Metaphoric devices invented by a blind woman. *Perception*, 42(6), 658–668. http://dx.doi.org/10.1068/p7480

Kennedy, J.M. 2014a. Esthetics, "Aida" and "re-entry shock": Fountains in a blind woman's drawings. *Psychology & Neuroscience*, 7(3), 341–347. http://dx.doi.org/10.3922/j.psns.2014.049

Kennedy, J.M. 2014b. Tactile drawing aesthetics and a blind woman's drawings of sounds. *British Journal of Visual Impairment*, 32(1), 33–43. http://dx.doi.org/10.1177/0264619613512838

Kennedy, J.M. and Bai, J. 2002. Haptic pictures: Fit judgments predict identification, recognition memory, and confidence. *Perception*, 31(8), 1013–1026. http://dx.doi.org/10.1068/p3259

Kennedy, J.M. and Gabias, P. 1985. Metaphoric devices in drawings of motion mean the same to the blind and the sighted. *Perception*, 14(4), 189–195. http://dx.doi.org/10.1068/p150189

Kennedy, J.M. and Hammad, S. 2011. Foldout includes foreshortening in drawings by a blind man. *Rivista di Estetica*, 47(2), 31–45. https://dialnet.unirioja.es/ejemplar/308326

Kennedy, J.M. and Juricevic, I. 2003. Haptics and projection: Drawings by Tracy, a blind adult. *Perception*, 32(9), 1059–1071. http://dx.doi.org/10.1068/p3425

Kennedy, J.M. and Juricevic, I. 2006. Blind man draws using diminution in three dimensions. *Psychonomic Bulletin and Review*, 13(3), 506–509. http://dx.doi.org/10.3758/BF03193877

Kennedy, J.M. and Merkas, C. 2000. Depictions of motion devised by a blind person. *Psychonomic Bulletin and Review*, 7(4), 700–706. http://dx.doi.org/10.3758%2FBF03213009

Koenderink, J.J. and van Doorn, A.J. 2003. Pictorial space. In H. Hecht, R. Schwartz and M. Atherton (eds), *Looking into pictures: An interdisciplinary approach to pictorial space* (pp. 239–299). Cambridge, MA: MIT Press.

Kubovy, M. and Wagemans, J. 1995. Grouping by proximity and multistability in dot lattices: A quantitative Gestalt theory. *Psychological Science*, 6(4), 225–234. http://dx.doi.org/10.1111/j.1467-9280.1995.tb00597.

Lederman, S. and Klatzky, B. 2009. Haptic perception: A tutorial. *Attention, Perception & Psychophysics*, 71(7), 1439–1459. http://dx.doi.org/10.3758/APP.71.7.1439

Loomis, J.M. and Philbeck, J.W. 2008. Measuring perception with spatial updating and action. In R.L. Klatzky, M. Behrmann and B. MacWhinney (eds), *Embodiment, ego-space and action* (pp. 1–43). Mahwah, NJ: Erlbaum.

Lopes, D. 2005. *Sight and sensibility: Evaluating pictures*. Oxford: Oxford University Press.

Morash, V.S., Pensky, A.E.C., Alfaro, A.U. and McKerracher, A. 2012. A review of haptic spatial abilities in the blind. *Spatial Cognition & Computation*, 12(2–3), 83–95. http://dx.doi.org/org/10.1080/13875868.2011.599901

Morash, V.S., Pensky, A.E.C. and Miele, J.A. 2013. Effects of using multiple hands and fingers on haptic performance. *Perception*, 42(7), 759–777. http://dx.doi.org/10.1068/p7443

Morash, V.S., Pensky, A.E.C., Tseng, S.T.W. and Miele, J.A. 2014. Effects of using multiple hands and fingers on haptic performance in individuals who are blind. *Perception*, 43(6), 569–588. http://dx.doi.org/10.1068/p7712

Noe, A. 2005. *Action in perception*. Cambridge, MA: MIT Press.

Noe, A. 2008. Précis of action. *Perception, Philosophy and Phenomenological Research*, 76(3), 660–665. http://dx.doi.org/10.1111/j.1933-1592.2008.00161.x

Peterson, M.A. 2015. Low-level and high-level contributions to figure-ground organization: Evidence and theoretical implications. In J. Wagemans (ed.), *The Oxford handbook of perceptual organization* (pp. 259–280). Oxford: Oxford University Press.

Picard, D. and Lebaz, S. 2012. Identifying raised-line drawings by touch: A hard but not impossible task. *Journal of Visual Impairment & Blindness*, 106(7), 427–431. http://dx.doi.org/org/p/89181/

Picard, D., Lebaz, S, Jouffrais, C. and Monnier, C. 2010. Haptic recognition of two-dimensional raised-line patterns by early-blind, late-blind, and blindfolded sighted adults. *Perception*, 39(2), 224–235. http://dx.doi.org/10.1068/p6527

Reid, T. 1764. *An inquiry into the human mind, on the principles of common sense*. London: A. Kincaid & J. Bell.

Rubin, E. 1915. *Synsoplevede figurer* [*Visually experienced figures*]. Copenhagen, Denmark: Gyldendals.

Scocchia, L., Stucchi, N. and Loomis, J. 2009. The influence of facing direction on the haptic identification of two-dimensional raised pictures. *Perception*, 38(4), 606–612. http://dx.doi.org/10.1068/p5881

Symmons, M. and Richardson, B. 2000. Raised line drawings are spontaneously explored with a single finger. *Perception*, 29(5), 621–626. http://dx.doi.org/10.1068/p2964

Thompson, L., Chronicle, F. and Collins, A. 2003. The role of pictorial convention in haptic picture perception. *Perception*, 32(7), 887–893. http://dx.doi.org/10.1068/p5020

Wertheimer, M. 1922/1938. Untersuchungen zur Lehre von der Gestalt II. *Psychologische Forschung*, 1(1), 301–350. (Republished as: Principles of perceptual organization, in D.C. Beardslee and Michael Wertheimer (eds), *Readings in perception* (pp. 115–137). New York: D. Van Nostrand.

Wijntjes, M.W.A., van Lienen, T., Verstijned, I. and Kappers, A. 2008a. The influence of picture size on recognition and exploratory behaviour in raised-line drawings. *Perception*, 37(4), 602–614. http://dx.doi.org/10.1068/p5714

Wijntjes, M.W.A., van Lienen, T., Verstijnen, I.M. and Kappers, A.M.L. 2008b. Look what I have felt: Unidentified haptic line drawings are identified after sketching. *Acta Psychologica*, 128(2), 255–263. http://dx.doi.org/10.2991/978-94-6239-133-8_15

Wnuczko, M. and Kennedy, J.M. 2014. Pointing to azimuths and elevations of targets: Blind and blindfolded-sighted. *Perception*, 43(2–3), 117–128. http://dx.doi.org/10.1068/p7605

Zollitsch, E. 2003. *I know where I am*. Waldkirchen, Germany: SüdOst-Verlag.

17

Art, visual impairment and the gatekeepers of aesthetic value

David Feeney

Introduction

This chapter positions the creative output of individuals with visual impairment within a review of the social processes commonly identified as underpinning the determination of value within the domain of the arts. The basis of my analytical framework is established by means of a preliminary outlining of interpretative approaches to the arts, which have been characterised by institutional contextualisation since the 1960s. In keeping with this approach, art is treated here as an entity that assumes its value within a certain type of institutional framework. The roles of "gatekeepers" at the periphery of this formal domain receive particular attention here, as the processes underpinning the bestowal of credibility on an artwork's candidacy for appreciation are scrutinised through the critical lens of an ableist framework borrowed from cultural disability studies.

The reorientation of art theory prompted by the reconceptualisation of art in terms of its sociological and relational underpinnings is presented here as being indicative of a certain alignment between that field and the socially oriented discipline of cultural disability studies. However, the opportunities for cross-disciplinary conversations scaffolded by the common principles of social constructivism have yet to be comprehensively exploited. Celebratory accounts of the therapeutic and rehabilitative benefits of art practice and, even more abundantly, accounts of what the clinically monitored practices of disabled artists can tell us about the nature of human brain activity, wield what is presented here as a disproportionate and ultimately regrettable influence among studies of art and visual impairment. Concentrating on the second of these two approaches, this chapter takes critical issue with the performative contingencies underpinning the affirmation of the creative output of artists with visual impairment from within the field of perceptual psychology. Bringing Howard Becker's (1974, 1982) identification of the "point of contact" between the humanities and the social sciences into service as a means of politicising the forms of critical reception regularly afforded to painting produced by artists with visual impairment, I outline the debilitating impact of the ostensibly affirmative championing of these artworks according to normative and visually charged evaluative criteria.

David Feeney

Institutional theories of art and the art world

Much of the critical interpretation to which the domain of visual art has been subjected since the 1960s has been informed by institutional forms of contextualisation. By the mid-point of the last century, the influence wielded by the writings of Morris Weitz (1950, 1956) and others was such that the long-established philosophical project of compiling characteristics deemed essential to artfulness had begun to be undermined. At this time a number of core aesthetic theorists lost what had remained of their collective patience with the time-honoured philosophical endeavour of formulating an exhaustive definition of art. The objective of formulating categorical delimitations of the defining characteristics of artworks and the experiences afforded by properly informed engagement with them started to be dismissed, at this time, as a thankless and ultimately wrong-headed venture. Concern for procedural and relational characteristics of art started to displace earlier attempts to account for its function and to categorically delimit its proper experiential yield. In the perturbed theoretical aftermath of this challenge to the age-old orientation of aesthetic theory, Maurice Mandelbaum (1965) suggested that if there is an essential characteristic of art, then that characteristic might be akin to the relational character of a family dynamic, rather than rooted in distinct features intrinsic within artworks. This line of thought culminated in the institutional theory of art, and in the positing of an "art world" at the core of this institutional framework. The primary value of this shift in theoretical approach, for the purposes of this chapter, is to serve as a framework within which to expose the ableist and debilitatingly normative habits of appraisal to which the creative output of artists with visual impairment is regularly subjected.

The institutional theory of art is commonly traced back to Arthur Danto. Writing at a time when the artefacts that were being accepted as artworks demonstrated an increasingly diverse range of characteristics, Danto's approach to art theory was underpinned by the contention that the theoretical framework within which art is generated, exhibited and interpreted is critical to the project of arriving at a meaningful understanding of the value of art. Danto's concern for the relational and sociological aspects of artworks informed his most celebrated and often quoted observation, to the effect that "[t]o see something as art requires something the eye cannot decry – an atmosphere of artistic theory, a knowledge of the history of art: an art world" (1964, p. 580). The influence wielded by this institutional dynamic is such that a Brillo Box positioned within a gallery might have characteristics attributed to it that are not considered to have anything to do with an identical box when encountered in the aisle of a supermarket. The question of whether claims to artfulness convince or collapse, Danto held, can be reduced to matters of institutionalised presentation.

What Danto calls "the art world", Terry Diffey conceives of as a "republic". He reflects that a republican metaphor generates connotations of submissiveness to authority, while also conceding that an ambiguity surrounds the precise location and identity of the authority within whose gift resides art-conferring powers (Diffey, 1991, p. 46). Drawing on the work of John Searle, Diffey argues that the proposition "x is a work of art" is not a brute fact but an institutional fact, as the status of "work of art" must be granted by the public's judgement (1991, p. 41). Diffey also openly divulges that articulation of the rationale underpinning consensus that artworks merit that status is beyond the scope of his theory. The identification of an essential set of circumstance within which designations of artfulness are deemed merited is equally beyond the scope of this chapter. What is of primary concern for our current purposes is the epistemological alignment of these conceptions of the art world as a relational and socially constructed domain, and conceptions of disablement as a socially constructed phenomenon.

For George Dickie, the characteristics that constitute the aesthetic object are neither inherent within the object itself, nor in our experience of it. They are socially (or institutionally) determined (Dickie, 1974, pp. 86–87). Considered within this relationally oriented framework, art registers itself as an incessantly negotiated social phenomenon. Within the art world conceived as institution, established practice is the accepted currency – it is granted art-status conferral privileges. Dickie (1974) argues that "some social system or other must exist as the framework within which the conferring takes place" (p. 35). The conferral of "arthood" on diversely styled representations has much less to do with any particular aesthetic elements that they may have in common, than with the existence of an overarching institutional framework. The domain of cultural disability studies could, it seems to me, add a valuable dimension to its existing approaches to the arts and inclusion, if it were to map this institutional framework of art evaluation on to the sociological framework that emerged roughly contemporaneously as a means of distinguishing disablement from impairment.

The disabling leverage of normative appraisal

As an extension of this sociological approach to art theory, the conventional critical approach of regarding artworks as the products of individual artists has been repeatedly and persuasively challenged. It is not uncommon for the generation of artworks to be attributed to a considered division of labour among an array of individuals who populate the art world. Working within the sociological tradition of art theory considered above, Howard Becker (1974, 1982) conceives of artworks as the product of the cooperative activity of an assortment of stakeholders, not all of whom exemplify the figure of artist as conventionally imagined. Artists often work with an entourage comprising such figures as curators, gallery managers, marketing staff, printmakers, framing and installation professionals and so on. Similarly, Pierre Bourdieu (1992) argues that the art world evolves in line with transformations in the artistic field of production. Different inhabitants of the art world are engaged in different ways in the formulation and attribution of value within the domain. For the purposes of this chapter, these figures are referred to as "gatekeepers" by virtue of the command they collectively wield over the "proper" constitution of art, and over the distinctions between art and non-art and good and bad art. Gatekeepers include art critics, curators, museum and gallery directors, teachers and researchers. Members of this assemblage have key roles in setting the art world agenda. Outlining the increasingly large ensembles who are allocated roles in the production of artworks, Bourdieu singles out the relationship between artists, artworks and those who interpret or critique the work: "The discourse on the work is not a simple side-effect, designed to encourage its apprehension and appreciation", Bourdieu (1992) stresses, but a moment that is part of the production of the work, of its meaning and its value (p. 170). The role of the theorist within the art world is singled out for attention here – in particular, what I describe as the "value-gatekeeping" responsibilities attendant on that role. It will, no doubt, be noted that the criticism here is not free of wardenal characteristics of its own. The argument presented here, however, is not that theorists should be expelled from the "republic" of the art world, but that we need wider diversity of theoretical views and objectives. The creative output of blind theorists tends to be of theoretical interest in terms of the opportunities it presents for the generation of contemporary responses to questions asked by such figures as John Locke and Denis Diderot about the nature of human knowledge and perception. While these responses have yielded impressive advances of such knowledge, they tend to gauge the achievements of artists with visual impairment according to visually charged criteria. I will attempt to illustrate here the detrimental impact of this theoretical trend for the disability arts movement, and to outline the need for approaches that are premised on a concept of capacity that goes beyond the replication by blind and visually impaired painters of the achievements of their celebrated fully sighted counterparts. In keeping with a compelling line of argument developed by Rosemarie Garland-Thomson (2012), it is suggested here that at the basis of approaches to visual impairment and art we need a conception of visual impairment as a generative rather than a replicative resource.

Addressing the authority commanded by art theorists, Ashley Holmes (2008, n.p.) contends that "the discourse that precedes, envelopes, and exists in art creates both its meaning and value". When considered within an institutionalised framework, artists are "more than ever tributaries to the whole accompaniment of commentaries and commentators who contribute directly to the production of the work of art by their reflection on an art" (Holmes, 2008, n.p.). The relationship between the artworks produced by painters with visual impairments and the theoretical/critical response these works have generated is an extremely interesting case in point. The sizeable body of academic affirmations of the mastery of visual convention demonstrated by the creative output of blind painters seems to me to be particularly noteworthy in this regard. While linear perspective and related pictorial conventions featured heavily in traditional renderings of landscape, these representational conventions are encountered much less frequently within the contemporary art world and critical evaluation of the illusions afforded by these traditional skillsets no longer assumes anything like a salient role in contemporary discourse. As will become evident below, however, it is not uncommon for blind artists whose candidacy for art world affiliation has been sanctioned to be granted entrance on the strength of their demonstrated mastery of these conventions. The creative output of painters with visual impairment, therefore, is being held to task by an outmoded convention that has a dubious experiential bearing on either their art practice or their everyday lives. The critical endorsement of their entrance into the needlessly "selectivised" art world, in other words, seems predicated on the conformity of their art with a convention that has long been abandoned with impunity by non-disabled artists.

Convention and creative expression

The formal introduction of pictorial convention of linear perspective is widely attributed to the Italian Renaissance architect Filippo Brunelleschi in the early part of the fifteenth century. Over time, the acknowledged limitations of perspective gave rise to a range of supplementary conventions such as foreshortening and anamorphosis. Becker (1974) introduces the notion of pictorial convention by observing that rather than deciding things "afresh", people who produce works of art tend to "rely on earlier agreements now become customary, agreements that have become part of the conventional way of doing things in art" (p. 770). He goes as far as to say that "the possibility of artistic experience arises from the existence of a body of conventions that artists and audiences can refer to in making sense of the work" (p. 771). In the course of volunteering a representative inventory of conventions across several art forms, he asserts that conventions "dictate the abstractions to be used convey particular ideas or experiences, as when painters use the laws of perspective to convey the illusion of three dimensions" (p. 770). Convention, for example, makes it possible for viewers of an artwork to read "essentially arbitrary marks as shadowing" (p. 771), or, with more relevance to our current subject, to read a three-dimensional scene from a two-dimensional plane. Remarking on the part played by convention within the institutional theory of art, Holmes (2008) notes how Becker "placed emphasis on the shared knowledge of conventions current in a medium and the 'networked' nature of the intersecting groups who use this knowledge to create socially shared meaning" (n.p.).

A considerable proportion of the existing literature on the creation and reception of artworks by individuals with visual impairment focuses primarily on the capacity of these individuals to appreciate or master a variety of visual conventions. Of these conventions, linear perspective tends to receive the most attention, but the ability of artists with visual impairments to engage in practices of foreshortening, to appreciate the concept of point of view and to incorporate perspective convergence into their pictorial output is also regularly contemplated. The ability of blind painters to factor the vantage of the beholder into the draughting of their representation also finds considerable favour. John Kennedy, for example, acclaims the abilities of blind individuals to recognise and generate paintings that resemble those produced by their fully sighted counterparts. This capacity, Kennedy holds, although generally untaught, can be developed (1980, p. 301). Elsewhere within the sizeable body of work that Kennedy has produced on this topic, we encounter instances where the idea of drawing an object from a particular point of view does not occur to blind painters, but where they prove themselves capable of demonstrating an understanding of perspective once they have been conceptually initiated into the convention (Heller and Kennedy, 1990). When considered within a cultural disability studies framework, the effort invested in identifying examples where blind people prove themselves capable of appreciating how fully sighted people conceive of the phenomenon of depiction, and of understanding and applying visual convention, seems dubious.

The contention, as I believe Kennedy's ultimate argument to be, that the principles of pictorial representation are broadly perceptual rather than being confined to vision is positive in a lot of ways that are not at all difficult to discern. However, the impact of these affirmations of the ability of blind painters to produce paintings that might have been produced by fully sighted painters, and to render landscape in a way that is purposefully tailored to the vantage point of the fully sighted beholder appears to me to be hugely problematic. A brief consideration of these forms of affirmation within the framework that has become known as the affirmative model of disability will help to elucidate the nature of my misgivings.

Visual impairment, art and the discourse of "real super humanism"

People who are better and more intimately versed in this body of literature addressing the psychology of pictorial convention are better positioned than I am to present a faithful outline of the rationale that underpins it and the advances of knowledge that it has doubtlessly secured. For illustrative purposes, I will dwell briefly here on an experience I had in 2017 as a delegate at a conference on the theme of art and visual impairment. Delegates were treated to a screening of a short documentary about the artist Eşref Armağan, entitled *Extraordinary People: The Artist with No Eyes, Eşref Armağan* (2008). The film was produced by the Discovery Channel as part of a series entitled *The Real Super Humans and the Quest for the Future Fantastic*. When it aired on television viewers were urged to "witness the amazing stories of real people with extraordinary super powers". I am electing to focus on this rendering for two reasons: (1) its emphasis on perspective remains a feature of many contemporary investigations of visual impairment and art; and (2) having been downloaded over 400,000 times (www.provost.utoronto.ca/awards/uprofessors/complete/johnmkennedy.htm) it seems a more definitive indicator than academic journal articles of the influence wielded by theorists within the art world.

"In Turkey", the narrator of the film begins, "lives the most extraordinary painter", before pitching the phenomenon in the ocular-centric rhetoric that recurs throughout the narration – an artist with no eyes, we are informed, proves that you do not need eyes to see. Within the referencing of Eşref, the term "painter" is unfailingly mentioned alongside the adjectives "blind" and "astounding". He is so good, we are told, he arguably draws better than most sighted people. The interest in Eşref's creative expression is firmly rooted in the contention that his practice "changes everything science has assumed about vision". His work is described as "astounding" on the strength of its use of colour, shade, composition "and, most importantly, perspective". His ability to depict objects receding into the distance "mystifies scientists", whose response takes the form of a desperate compulsion to scan his brain. Eşref's art demonstrates what scientists had always assumed was "locked in the visual brain", and his command of three-dimensional space has them particularly excited. The documentary is structured around an experiment undertaken to determine whether Eşref "truly understands perspective". We are informed that the experiment will involve transporting Eşref to Florence and sitting him in front of the octoganonal Roman baptistry that spawned the pictorial convention of perspective. The challenge is laid down at this point: if Eşref can appreciate the complex geometry of the ancient building, incorporate the three dimensions of space within his rendering of it, and "get them right", then this man is – you guessed it – "astounding". First, however, a team of scientists need to see the artist's brain lit up.

On route to Florence – from Turkey – Eşref is hastily ferried to Boston where a neurology team can monitor the functioning of his brain as he contemplates scale and perspective. The artist is put into an MRI scanner so that the neurologists can observe the remarkable goings-on in his brain as he draws. The scientists are riveted. Regions of Eşref's brain that shouldn't host any activity due to his congenital blindness react in an "extraordinary" way. "The visual parts of the brain", we are informed – "the parts that for normal sighted people light up like Christmas trees when we're looking at things – those became alive and excited and incredibly dynamic when Eşref was thinking of drawing in perspective". The frequently expressed astonishment not prompted by any of the aesthetic qualities of the rendering produced in the MRI scanner that is brought into innovative service as a makeshift studio, but rather by the groundbreaking realisation that "we have misunderstood vision". And in this way the value and purpose of Eşref's artistry is heralded as its role in disabusing us of the assumption that pictures are "creatures of vision".

Onwards, full speed, to Florence. A blind man from Turkey is going to try to outdo Filippo Brunelleschi. A curious agenda, one might think, for "a blind artist from Turkey", but one that has been attributed to him nonetheless. What Eşref "must do", we are told, is to draw the sides of the baptistry upwards and downwards so that the lines converge on the horizon. As tests go, it seems a particularly harsh and arduous one – surely few among us, whether blind or sighted, would fancy being subjected to it in such a public manner. The justification for the setting of such a demanding agenda takes the form of the assertion that "this is what Brunelleschi did, and this is what even now most sighted people get wrong". One notes that the transferral of the rhetoric of getting things either right or wrong from the scientific to the aesthetic domain feels a little awkward, but one crosses one's fingers and volunteers a prayer to Saint Anthony for the artist nonetheless. Detailed instructions are administered to Eşref so that he can be under no illusion about what is expected of him, and he is dramatically urged to "go for it". A sizeable crowd gathers in the piazza and holds their collective breath while Eşref, in a demonstration that his mastery of pictorial perspective is accompanied by nerves of steel, continues diligently with the undertaking of his assessment. "For Eşref", the narrator informs us, "this is the moment of truth. He must draw the bottom two lines converging upward towards the top". Just when the anticipation threatens to become too much the narrator reassures us that "Eşref Armağan has just set his place in history. He has outdone Filippo Brunelleschi, a Renaissance master". Cue tears, applause and a celebratory chorus of "bravo Eşref". The concluding assertion reminds us that "this is a moment that happened first 600 years ago. The next time it happened was today".

Having replicated what a fully sighted draughtsman accomplished well over half a century previously, and produced an architectural rendering that looks for all the world as though it might have been generated by a fully sighted artist, Eşref, metaphorically flanked by a team of neurologists serving as the guard of honour through which he is paraded, has secured his passage into the art world. But what, one cannot help but wonder, would have happened had Eşref failed the perspective test? Would the up-lipped trumpets have sounded anyway? Or would derogatory catcalls have replaced the round of applause afforded to him upon "getting it right"?

Ableist gatekeeping of aesthetic value

One of the benefits of conceiving of art within a sociologically oriented institutionalised analytic framework is that it cautions theorists like myself to be mindful of certain responsibilities attendant on our role within the art world. The theories of Danto, Diffey, Dickie, Becker and others, remind us that, as theorists, we become, however inadvertently, arbiters of value. In this capacity, we need, more specifically, to be mindful of the dynamic reflected in James Winchester's contention that cultural understanding across cultural divides requires sustained sensitive attention to the worlds out of which the sensibilities in question emerge (Winchester, 2002).

Environmental engagement assumes multiple forms, and contemporary art reflects a diversity of such forms in its increasingly assorted representational configurations. The fixation on perspective, conveyed in the documentary as a seemingly mandatory characteristic of pictorial representation, betrays, it seems to me, distinct features of an ableist evaluative framework. Within such a framework a certain essentialness is attributed to favoured abilities. Perceived deviation from or lack of these essentialised abilities becomes labelled as regrettably problematic. One gets the sense that Eşref's completion of a sketch in a way that demonstrated a working knowledge of the laws of perspective was essential to the prospect of his attempt to find favour with his team of well-wishing neurologists and with the initiated throng that assembled around him in the piazza.

From a cultural disability studies perspective, a certain spuriousness appears to characterise the celebratory treatment Eşref's creative output is afforded. He is not, I think it is fair to say, subject in any obvious or direct way to disablism, a process whereby those without the abilities and skill sets deemed to be essential are "othered" and therefore invariably subjected to prejudicial treatment. He is not excluded from the art world – he is, on the contrary, ushered into it with a triumphant and the type of hyperbolic bravado that we have come to expect from interpretive accounts pitched within a supercrip narrative. However, as will be argued in more corroborating detail below, his admittance into the art world seems contingent on his meeting of a functional precondition to which his fully sighted counterparts are rarely subjected. The performative contingency that underpins Eşref's jubilant initiation into the art world seems anomalous within the context of a contemporary art world that prides itself on a lack of prescriptiveness (Silvers, 2002). What is in question here seems much more literal and exacting than the vague "atmosphere" that Dickie (1974, 1997) posits at the core of the art world. The "success" or "failure" of Eşref's rendering – of his candidacy for the title of (good) artist – seems to hinge on his capacity to demonstrate a working knowledge of painstakingly unequivocal laws and conventions of pictorial representation.

The documentary's treatment of Eşref's artistic accomplishment definitely seems affirmative in relation to some of the unremittingly bleak judgements delivered by some of Kennedy's precursors in the field of perceptual psychology. Géza Révész, for example, expressed resolute misgivings about the capability of the sensory network that remains to blind people of facilitating a truly aesthetic experience. Because of the rigid nature of haptically based appraisals, and what Révész sees as the crudeness of haptic reception of the subtleties of aesthetic form, he claims that blind people "cannot force their way" into the aesthetic domain (Révész, 1950, p. 205). In his *Psychology and Art of the Blind* (1950), Révész argues that the appreciation of form is a predominantly visual function, and that the aesthetic significance of the world of forms is "brought home in full consciousness only to the sighted" (pp. v, 77). Among the most notable observations Révész makes are that "the aestheticians who trace [the] aesthetic pleasure [in plastic works] back to a haptic or kinaesthetic element make a great mistake", that "aesthetic attitude and aesthetic experience are . . . a field to which a person working haptically has no access or only a restricted one" and that "all the principles of form creation, all the forms of aesthetic contemplation, all the criteria of aesthetic appreciation are based on visual perception" (pp. 206–205).

The ableist framework within which Kennedy's affirmative and Révész's less than enthusiastic arguments are arrived at becomes clear when we compare their conflicting accounts of geometric form. One of Révész's chief reservations about the ability of people who cannot see for the nurturing of an aesthetic awareness through the sense of touch is the inevitable emphasis within haptic appreciation on the accuracy of the artist's execution. The quality of a work of art is assessed by blind persons in terms of the extent of the divergence of the object under consideration from the "norms" of beauty, the criteria for which are established by their aesthetic tuition. Sighted persons also approach the aesthetic object with an ideal of beauty in mind, but when the reality does not coincide with the ideal, sighted beholders can exercise a degree of improvisation unavailable to their unsighted peers and hastily revise the terms of the treaty by which the satisfaction of their aesthetic expectations is secured. The rigid form of evaluation thus enforced on blind people is not conducive to an appreciation of the subtle, intricate ways in which artistic expression can deviated from pre-established convention. The "norms" of "the blind", to adopt Révész's parlance, exemplify a stubborn conventional imperative that impedes their capacity to appreciate novel manifestations of beauty. Principles of Greek sculpture, for example, were regularly applied in the aesthetic education of blind pupils at the time Révész was devising his theory. The emphasis of these principles on geometry and symmetry constitute, according to Révész, the limits of what can be evaluated through haptic perception. This education, as Révész sees it, results in the rejection of a lot of fine art, which, having been conceived according to alternative aesthetic principles, do not meet the aesthetic demands of the educated blind person. Much of the vitality of modern art stems from the impulse of the artist toward the disruption of continuity of line and pattern, the avoidance of hackneyed expression and the departure from preconceived shapes and plans (Ehrenzweig, 1961, pp. 121–133). The characteristic feature of much contemporary art, in other words, is its undermining or spoiling of the surface coherence that, according to Révész, exhausts the spectrum of haptic perception.

As an ideology, ableism represents a value system employed by social groups that manifests in the promotion of certain abilities and the disregarding of others. Its influence is such that individual self-conception tends to be rooted in proven or disproven capacity to demonstrate normatively favoured abilities. Social groupings who enjoy certain privileges, rights and status, have been known to sustain their elevated social standing on the strength of demonstration of proficiency in the approved skill sets. Eşref Armağan is a wonderful painter. Yet, I suspect that were his paintings included among an anonymised selection of pictorial renderings of landscape it would be unlikely that his use of perspective would be identified by an expert as the most exemplary. While several aspects of the artistry of Eşref's creative output merit critical acclaim, it is knowledge of his blindness that renders his use of perspective so "remarkable" or "astounding". I am not personally acquainted with Eşref and so I have no way of knowing how he feels about this. I have, however, worked with a number of artists with visual impairments who have gone to considerable lengths to ensure that their visual impairment is not afforded a disproportionate degree of attention in the critical appraisal of their creative output. I am reminded here of Matthew Arnold's cautionary rejoinder to interpreters of the Wordsworthian canon: "We must be on our guard against the Wordsworthians", Arnold (1879) counsels, "if we want to secure for Wordsworth his due rank as a poet. The Wordsworthians are apt to praise him for the wrong things, and to lay far too much stress upon what they call his philosophy" (pp. 138–146). Eşref's talent, I repeat, seems to me to be beyond reasonable dispute. However, reduction of his talent to his capacity to replicate the achievements of his sighted predecessors seems to me to do both him and his creative output a disservice. The privileging of the abilities of blind painters to produce work that looks as though it has been produced by sighted painters also has problematic implications for the disability arts movement more generally. Within the related domain of literary representation, David Bolt (2006) volunteers an analogous suggestion when he argues that the deceptively affirmative attribution of skills to blind characters situates accomplishment in a causal relationship with blindness, thereby demonstrating a seeming disregard for the individual who happens to be blind.

I have hinted at a similarity between the approaches of Révész and Kennedy that belies the obvious forms of superficial contrast that characterise the inter-relationship of the verdicts they deliver. However, I would argue that the enthusiasm that greets Eşref's demonstrated mastery of perspective can be traced back to an older precedent. William Paulson, in his *Enlightenment, Romanticism, and the Blind in France* (1987), accounts for some of the reasons behind the captivating influence exercised by blindness on the minds of well-renowned thinkers from a variety of disciplines. The preoccupation reached new heights, according to Paulson, with the surgical advances in the eighteenth century that led to the possibility of cures for some congenital cataracts. The study of blindness, Paulson (1987) suggests, "brings us face to face with some of the major and by now well-known problems that have undermined confidence in traditional histories of ideas" (p. 16). The study of the behaviour of the blind person made to see meant that theoretical speculation about the nature of philosophical sensationalism could finally be supplemented or replaced by experimental verification. Locke and his followers were granted a practical means of illustrating the contention that the mind's ideas derived from its "contact with earthly reality" and of dismissing the suggestion that these ideas were innate or traceable back to ideal origins (Paulson, 1987, p. 10). The absence of sight was regarded by such thinkers primarily as "a means of producing a moment of first sight" (Paulson, 1987, p. 26). To prove that understanding is acquired through experience, the philosophers of the eighteenth century were in need of minds deprived of bodies of experience, and in "the blind" they discovered exactly what they needed:

> Summoned to bear witness before the bar of philosophy, the blind man is of interest to his hearers for his prior sensory lack, for his negativity, for the unused portion of his understanding where certain acquisitions have not yet been made. He also interests them insofar as he can be cured, made suddenly like (and yet unlike) one of the seeing.
>
> *(Paulson, 1987, p. 26)*

Although interest in Eşref's art clearly has nothing to do with cure, or with the granting of sight, the theoretical treatment afforded to it seems to me to be rooted in an expediency or scholarly opportunism akin to that represented by the first cataract operations. Whereas blind people were of value to Locke and his counterparts because of the opportunity they presented for the advancement of knowledge about the nature of knowledge, the Discovery Channel documentary gives the impression that Eşref's creative output is of value for the opportunity it presents to advance our existing understanding of the psychology of pictorial representation. The documentary is very positive, in the sense that it exudes enthusiasm and excitement for Eşref's achievements. It is notable, however, that the enthusiasm seems to be a response to the parts of Eşref's brain that "light up like a Christmas tree" when he is contemplating or demonstrating linear perspective, rather than any particular aesthetic qualities of his creative output. In seems telling, in this regard, that beyond their status as replications of Brunelleschi's accomplishments, the aesthetic qualities of Eşref's work remain unremarked upon.

Convention revisited: how one artist's liberty becomes another artist's failing

Howard Becker (1974, 1982) recounts how the existence of convention brings with it the potential for playing with it in order to manipulate the emotional engagement of an audience. Referring to musical composition, for example, Becker describes how calculated delays and deviations from conventional organisations of tones within a scale, elements of tension, frustration and relief can be wilfully factored by a musician into the experiences of listeners familiar with the appropriate musical conventions. Within the domain of the visual arts, Ernst Gombrich (1960) famously accounts for the role of the taking of well-considered liberties with pictorial convention in the generation of emotionally charged encounters with art. "Though standardized", Becker (1974) notes, "conventions are seldom rigid and unchanging". The conventions inherent within an art world or within a particular form of art practice "do not specify an inviolate set of rules everyone must refer to in settling the question of what to do" (p. 772). Convention is rarely so prescriptive as to preclude negotiation within the processes of production or interpretation. As a means of illustrating this point, Becker refers to the practice of Italian Renaissance painters. Although the adherence to convention at the core of their use of content, symbolism and colouring "allowed viewers to read much emotion and meaning into the picture", the fact that customary interpretation of convention had in itself become part of the convention of viewer engagement, liberated artists "to do things differently, negotiation making change possible" (p. 772).

Becker's (1974) general observation that "conventions place strong constraints on the artist" (p. 772) would appear to contain a heightened degree of relevance when considered in the context of the art practices of artists with visual impairments. As does his later remark that

> breaking with existing conventions and their manifestations in social structure and material artifacts increases the artist's trouble and decreases the circulation of his work, on the one hand, but at the same time increases his freedom to choose unconventional alternatives and to depart substantially from conventional practice.
>
> *(Becker, 1974, p. 773)*

However, it would appear that in the case of artists with visual impairment whose paintings do not comply with visual convention, entries within this cost–benefit analysis are weighted to an untenably extreme extent on the side of expense. Such instances of departure from convention, the documentary appears to suggest, will be received as a failure of execution, rather than an innovative form of creative departure. "Every convention carries with it an aesthetic", Becker (1974) observes, "according to which what is conventional becomes the standard by which artistic beauty and effectiveness is judged" (p. 773). Despite the fixation of the professionals who interrogate the value of Eşref's art on compliance with certain conventions of pictorial representation, it has been a very long time since the aesthetics of landscape representation have been deemed within the art world to begin and end with compliance with these prerequisites of competent draughtsmanship. Despite the celebratory tone of the documentary, I would argue, the disabling composite of ableist and anomalous evaluative criteria to which the creative output of artists with visual impairment are subject is problematic in a variety of ways.

It may not be directly evident how keen attentiveness to the creative output of a blind painter might be anything less than affirmative. However, the generation of this interest by the painter's capacity to master linear perspective appears to betray an alignment of sorts with Penketh's (2016) suggestion that "creativity appears to be put beyond the reach of those of us who may not 'master' particular skills in drawing, painting and sculpture" (p. 439). I have suggested elsewhere (Feeney, 2007) that the environmental engagement of people with visual impairments might be constructively conceived as the basis of a differential aesthetic, outlining, in the process, a certain generative kinship between it and a feminist aesthetic. My issue with the emphasis on the ability of blind painters to render landscape as though they could see it is the implicit incentivisation of what Penketh refers to as "typical productivity". Penketh (2016) conceives of such rewarding of aesthetic complicity as a form of "epistemic invalidation" that entails "the devaluing of what one might know through one's experience when it is set against official dominant knowledge forms" (p. 433). The tendency for the most celebrated blind artists to be the ones whose output coincides representationally to the greatest degree with that of their fully sighted counterparts seems to me to be a source of concern. The anxiety is that aspiring blind artists might be prompted by the acclaim earned by normative renderings and by the critical rejoicing in pictorial convention, to devalue certain epistemological, aesthetic and phenomenological aspects of their experience that could very conceivably prove vital to their creativity and artistic orientation.

Pluralistic conceptions of capability and non-normative forms of appreciation

The debilitating forms of "othering" and marginality that have traditionally accompanied difference are rigorously challenged within such fields as disability, feminist and post-colonial studies. As the grand narratives of universal convention have given way to appreciation of the legitimacy of individual difference, non-normative forms of appraisal have emerged, which, were they to be applied to Eşref's paintings, would yield responses that are likely to be as ostensibly celebratory as those expressed by the professionals who monitor his brain activity in the documentary. The difference, however, is that these alternative evaluative frameworks are not configured in a way that rewards disabled artists for purging all indications of their impairment from their creative output. The capability approach devised by Amartya Sen (1992) and Martha Nussbaum (2000), for example, and David Bolt's (2015) application of the tripartite model of disability, could be brought into very effective service in this regard, although limitations of space here do not afford a thorough operationalism of either.

- Lorella Terzi (2005) describes capabilities as "the real freedoms people have to achieve the valued functioning's that are constitutive of their well-being (p. 449). Social environments should, according to Terzi, be evaluated in relation to the degree to which they accommodate a diversity of capabilities. At the core of Terzi's suggestion for how diversity might be valued on its own terms is the pluralistic concept of "functioning's", which she describes as "the beings and doings that individuals have reason to value" (p. 449). The capabilities framework derived by Terzi from Amartya Sen represents possibly the most succinct means of conveying the nature of the reservations expressed in this chapter about the impact of the considerable emphasis that has been placed on affirming the art produced by blind painters in relation to its demonstrated mastery of visual convention. Reduced to its rudimentary tenets, an application of a capabilities framework to the appraisal of the creative output of painters with visual impairment might go as follows.

Everybody is talented, in one way or another. We have every reason to be proud of our talents. However, we often find ourselves operating within environments that prioritise some talents over others, and actually disregard many very legitimate talents. Blind and visually impaired painters (needless, perhaps to say) have talents. As contemporary artists, they are working within a domain that cherishes diversity as an enlivening influence and eschews prescriptiveness. However, the most celebrated blind artists are celebrated on account of a demonstrable mastery of various visually charged pictorial conventions that enable them to replicate the output of celebrated fully sighted masters. While these talents are undoubtedly genuine, they are not the only talents that artists with visual impairment might possess. To value these talents more than any other talents an artist with a visual impairment might possess is ableist in the sense that other artists with visual impairments are likely to appraise their own artistic capabilities in relation to the distinction between possession and lack of this extremely limited skill set. The distal qualities inherent in perspective do not tend to characterise the everyday modes of environmental engagement consciously enjoyed by blind people. Yet the creative output of blind artists is less likely to be critically acclaimed if certain traditionally acclaimed visually charged conventions are not manifest within it. This may lead, in some cases, to a lot of innovative work by artists with visual impairment being under-appreciated, or, in other cases, generate a demotivating influence that discourages artists with visual impairments from attempting to capture moments of environmental engagement on canvas either for the simple purpose of sharing these moments or becoming excellent artists.

Bolt brings the model into service as a means of interrogating the affirmation of socially accepted standards (ablism), and of critically probing the all-too-often problematic consequences of deviation from them (disablism). To these two intricately interconnected forms of response to convention, which Bolt (2015) terms, respectively, "normative positivism" and "non-normative negativism," he adds a third – "non-normative positivism". This third component of the model relates to "affirmed deviations from socially accepted standards" (p. 1106). Applied to the evaluation of the creative output of artists with visual impairment, for example, the relevance of Bolt's subsequent claim – that "it is not enough to recognise disability along a continuum of difference that defines human variation" (p. 1107) becomes clear. If mastery of visual convention is the criterion according to which we attribute value to paintings produced by painters with visual impairment, it seems likely that, exceptional cases notwithstanding, the renderings of these painters, however impressive, will be considered to be less exquisitely or accurately rendered than the more recognisable landscapes portrayed by their fully sighted counterparts. For my own part, I can say that I have attended several presentations on art and visual impairment where the paintings deemed to be best were those renderings of buildings, people or whatever, that corresponded most closely to how the original referents of these images are perceived by fully sighted people. I have also come across instances where a negligible degree of such correspondence generates agreement that the paintings under review are non-representational. I would argue, however, that the mis-placed prescriptiveness informing such verdicts is akin to the hubris demonstrated by a traveller who voyages to a country where he/she does not speak the language and considers the natives to be non-communicative. Just as a painting is not non-representational because it represents something other than what the beholder expects to see or is accustomed to seeing, paintings by artists with visual impairment are not inevitably good because they demonstrate a mastery of visual convention or bad because they are uninformed by such customary modes of representation. Visual language – to use a one loaded term – allows a variety of communicative notation – to use another. If a representation of a landscape does not portray the landscape as it presents itself to the beholder, it seems unreasonable to dismiss it as a representational failure.

In the Discovery Channel documentary, Eşref is unqualifiedly hailed as a success. On the strength of his ability to replicate the standards of draughtsmanship demonstrated by a Renaissance master, he is allowed entry in the art world. The contingency underpinning his sanctioned admittance, however, seems to me to exemplify the distinction interrogated by Bolt between inclusion and inclusionism. Describing what he means by the latter term, Bolt (2015) says that "opportunities may well have opened to formerly excluded groups, which must be commended, but for inclusion to become truly worthwhile it must involve recognition of disability in terms of alternative lives and values that neither enforce nor reify normalcy" (p. 1107). This element of Bolt's argument is aligned with James Winchester's (2002) description, considered above, of meaningful forms of aesthetic appreciation across cultural divides. It is heartening, to a degree, to witness a blind painter being the recipient of such unqualified acclaim. However, the admittance of a blind artist into the art world on the strength of his demonstrated mastery of linear perspective will do little – or at least little of truly affirmative substance – for the experiences of blind artists more generally.

The non-normative approaches pioneered within disability studies were not devised with any particular orientation towards the art world. Yet the principles informing them are not at any great argumentational remove from those underpinning the emergence of a feminist aesthetics towards the end of the last century. Rita Felski (1989), for example, claims that one of the most important achievements of the woman's movement has been to "repoliticize art on the level of both production and reception" (p. 175). Writing at the turn of the century, Penny Florence and Nicola Foster (2000, p. 2), describe how a plethora of emerging discourses on the experience of marginality disrupts the allegedly "universal" applicability of aesthetic principles (see also Battersby, 1991, pp. 31–44; Benjamin and Osborne, 1991). Maurice Berger points out that throughout the 1990s the postmodern interrogation of the discipline of history and the subsequent scrutinising of relationships between knowledge, representation, ideology and power, began to permeate the fields of art history, criticism and curational practice and to challenge the "narrow ideological basis" upon which they are traditionally constructed (cited in Kelly, 1998, p. 21). "The postmodern task of witnessing those who are different and forging dialogue between such persons", Berger contends, "cannot rest assured by previous acts of legitimation, since the point is to find and invent modes of listening, speaking, and connection that are . . . not captured by existing rules" (cited in Kelly, 1998, p. 61). The sizeable body of existing literature on the creative output of artists with visual impairments that prioritises the capacity of these artists to apply the laws of perspective, foreshortening, horizon convergence and other visually charged conventions seems to me to demonstrate an inapposite prescriptiveness and an anomalous regard for what within the wider art world has long been an outmoded representational precept. The admission of blind painters into the art world is being negotiated on visual terms. Inclusion is vital. But, as Bolt puts it, it "can become transformative and more comprehensively productive when disability is recognised as a site for alternative values" (cited in Kelly, 1998, p. 1107).

The final point to be made here about Eşref's admittance into the art world is that the "convention test" he is required to ace before entering is completely unnecessary. Becker makes it clear that deviation from convention, rather than adept compliance with it, is the hallmark of artistic noteworthiness. Becker (1982, p. 353) asserts that

> [many people] may, by following the rules which govern the making of artworks, produce creditable musical performances, readable novels, and not entirely uninteresting paintings. By following the conventions, such workers will produce work others will recognize as competent. One might thus write a tragedy, using Aristotle's *Poetics* as a guide. Of course, that would not necessarily (or even likely) result in an important work. The theory holds, however, that people with special gifts can manipulate the available conventions, perhaps change them or invent new ones, and so produce works which are not just so-so or ho-hum but, rather, are extraordinary. Those works will stand out from the mass the way Dickens' novels stand out from the thousands of roughly similar works produced in nineteenth-century England, the way the recordings of Louis Armstrong stand out from thousands of similar performances by early jazz trumpet players. They have more, a lot more, of whatever characterizes beautiful or profound works than does most work.

My abiding impression of the Discovery Channel documentary is of teams of perceptual psychologists and sundry medical professionals stationing themselves as sentinels at the periphery of the art world, like so many Saint Peters at the pearly gates admitting only those blind artists deemed to have made a commendable effort at simulating the creative output of fully sighted artists, while bouncing the remainder back into some form of perspectiveless purgatory. Although the trope of blind artists being allowed to pass through the art world gates is being volunteered here as an admittedly facetious metaphor, it is aligned with a very real phenomenon, namely the practice of "passing", which has received considerable attention within the field of critical disability studies. It is central to my misgivings about the ableist premise underpinning many affirmative valuations of the creative output of artists with visual impairments.

Art as an exemplification of the needlessness of passing

As alluded to above, the screening of the Discovery Channel documentary at the conference I attended was preceded by a talk about Eşref's work. At the outset of this talk two of his paintings were presented to the audience. Not knowing at this point who had painted the scenes we were dutifully contemplating, we were encouraged to consider whether it might be possible for a congenitally blind person to comprehend a verbal description of the presented images. While we delegates were still debating this question among ourselves we were treated to the grand reveal – the paintings in question had been produced by Eşref Armağan, a congenitally blind painter from Turkey. The disclosure generated the presumably desired reaction from the audience as gasps of disbelief circulated around the lecture theatre at such an achievement – considered exceptional only after the identity and the circumstances of the painter were disclosed. The atmosphere in the conference theatre indicated that the value of the paintings was considered anew in light of this belatedly divulged information. My own reaction – and I sensed that I represented a distinct minority among conference delegates, was that the demonstrated mastery of perspective was worryingly indistinguishable from a mastery of "passing". This phenomenon, explored in a collection of essays edited by Jeffrey Brune and Daniel Wilson in 2013 refers to the concealment of markers of impairment as a means of avoiding stigma and generating a convincing simulation of "normal". Brune and Wilson's edited volume, alongside texts by Tobin Siebers (2004), Brenda Bruegemann, (1997), and others, illustrate various scenarios in which disabled individuals are faced with choices between concealing their impairment and drawing attention to it.

Let us forget, momentarily, about the particular case of Eşref, and broaden the debate to a more general consideration of the artwork produced by individuals with visual impairment and the evaluative frameworks to which it tends to be subjected. When watching the documentary, I could not help but think about the many blind and visually impaired artists I have had the pleasure to work with in an artistic context, and the others I have gone for walks with. Knowing how these artists work, and how they engage with the assorted environments through which we have passed together, for some of these individuals, aspiring to demonstrate a mastery of perspective and horizon convergence would entail a certain denial of the very selfhood that art generally helps them to express. In a different, but not entirely unrelated context, Rod Michalko (2002) observes that when a blind child attends a (re)habilitation service, the focus is invariably on cultivating a capacity to "pass" as sighted: "teaching techniques to stop blind children from enacting unsociable behaviour (such as head rocking, rolling eyes, hand flapping)", Michalko suggests, "all attempt to create a sighted imaginary for blind children" (p. 133). I am troubled by the affirmative nature of the emphasis placed within the perceptual psychology literature consulted in an admittedly perfunctory manner above on the similarity between drawings produced by blind and fully sighted individuals, and on the capacity of blind individuals to be taught how to understand and demonstrate perspective. I suspect that my misgivings are akin to those expressed by Michalko in relation to the purpose of rehabilitation initiatives. There seems something wrong about an evaluative framework structured around a positive correlation between the quality of a painting produced by a blind artist, and the degree to which the painting serves as a means of concealing the fact that the painter cannot see. The consequences for the disability arts movement, and for artists with visual impairment more generally, of the fact that the most celebrated art is that which serves as the most convincing means of passing, do not, in my opinion, bear thinking about. To emphasise, my argument here is not that Eşref deliberately uses his art as a form of passing. Even if this were the case (and it clearly is not), it would surely be more appropriate to take issue with the forces of ableism that make disabled individuals feel compelled to attempt to pass, than to judge or denounce disabled individuals who elect to do so.

We have very good reason for not treating art as a passing facilitator. Among considerations factored into decisions about whether or not to attempt to pass is the question of whether the form of diversity one represents is likely to be received as an enlivening form of variance or as a regrettable deviation from a fixed/idealised norm. The irony is that artists with visual impairment are operating within a domain whose history is arguably (but it is an argument for another day) the very embodiment of embracing difference and innovation as an enlivening entity. Within the field of cultural disability studies, Anita Silvers is among the clearest and most compelling advocates of this feature of artistic endeavour. Silvers volunteers a convincing account of the marked discrepancy between the orders of significance attributed to normality in art and in everyday society:

> For the idea of the normal holds so much less sway in art than in ordinary life. While everyday practical discourse is disturbed by anomaly, aesthetic discourse revels in the shock of the new. Understanding this capacity of aesthetic discourse can lead us to an aesthetic that makes disability powerful.
>
> (Silvers, 2002, p. 230)

The suggestion that the same deviations from convention that prove problematic in everyday life are perceived as cause for celebration when encountered in art would appear to have obvious implications for celebrations of blind artists by virtue of the fact that they comply with traditional pictorial convention. Normalcy, Silvers (2002) continues "appears to be a regulatory ideal" in our everyday lives but has little purchase within the art world (p. 238). Silvers points to a significant discrepancy between the rigidity of the "prescriptiveness" with which individuals are expected to conform with precedents in their quotidien social affairs, and the excitement with which radically new forms of identity and expression are embraced within the art world. Innovative art, Silvers suggests, "calls into question the prescriptive authority of the historical contingencies that shape our expectations", and in the process prompts a revisioning of our conception of "normalcy" (p. 239). Being "interpretive" rather than "coercive", art's history does not repudiate diverse forms of perception, of representation, or of being in the world in the way that human history does. Ashley Holmes (2008) expresses a similar point – although without any explicit reference to the issues of disability or impairment, when asserting that "there is a need for art to be, by defini- tion, non-prescriptive of what constitutes art in itself to enable its reflective and socially interpre- tative component to remain invigorated and renewable (n.p.). When considered in this context, pitching mastery of linear perspective as a prerequisite for entry of blind artists into the art world is arguably as detrimental for the art world as it is for the sense of self harboured by blind people.

Forward-facing reflections

In keeping with the spirit of the lines of argument developed above, I deviate here from the established practice of summarising and synthesising preceding lines of argument in conclud- ing reflections. I feel that I have only begun to describe the scope of the debilitating impact of applications of normative forms of appraisal to artworks produced by individuals with visual impairment. Had I successfully resolved the entire inventory of issues raised above, I would happily recap these accomplishments here. I am stealing the space that would conventionally be afforded to a conclusion and bringing it into service as a repository for (a) a brief clarification of some of the issues presented above as being an inevitable outcome of ableist approaches to evaluating the creative output of individuals with visual impairment; and (b) the signalling of problems arising from such evaluative approaches not considered in any depth here as a means of targeting areas where further research is required.

Classificatory and evaluative approaches

I am aware that the commentary presented here on the critical reception of the artworks pro- duced by individuals with visual impairment quite vaguely straddles classificatory and evaluative frameworks. The aestheticians associated with the institutional theory of art and the concept of the "art world" around which it is structured, were torn on this issue. However, especially within a context in which the art practices of disabled people tend to have therapeutic rather than aesthetic connotations, I feel that clarification of this distinction will prove valuable. No doubt this will deepen the conundrum that perceptual psychologists have elected to appropriate as they resolve whether they should distinguish between art and non-art, or between good and bad art.

Practitioner as researcher

I am very much addressing this chapter when I say that research is too often something that is done to individuals with visual impairment, rather than something that is done with them, or, better still, something that they do themselves. In the field of critical disability studies, the social relations underpinning the production of knowledge about impairment and disablement has been heavily discussed within an emancipatory framework for some time now (see, for example, Barnes, 2008; Oliver, 1997). There are analogies here with current trends in art education institutions where the conception of artist as researcher is becoming increasingly familiar (Holmes, 2008). The time-honoured distinction between practitioner and theorist/critic is becoming fragmented as a composite conception of art practice and research has begun to permeate the curricula of institutions of higher education. This subsumption of theory within practice is not as commonly encountered in the case with disabled artists, however, as exemplified perfectly by this chapter. The motivations underpinning the maintenance of this distinction needs to be critically interrogated, as do the apparent assumptions that, unlike their non-disabled counterparts, disabled artists are not capable of critically interrogating their own experience through their own practice. Pursuit of this line of thought would result in interrogations of the social relations underpinning the production of art and aesthetic value. The emancipatory framework that characterises an increasing amount of contemporary disability studies research undertakings would, I feel, freely accommodate such an approach.

Art as an expression of identity

Although concern for identity was an implicit theme throughout this chapter, the consequences for the sense of self harboured by artists with visual impairments, of being made to feel answerable to the diktats of visual convention, are in need of further research. General studies of the impact of art practice on the self-identity of marginalised groups are relatively plentiful (see, for example, Barnes and Mercer, 2001; Choi Caruso, 2005; Eisenhauer, 2007). However, the process of arriving at self-understanding through art practice, and, conversely, of compromising one's identity through art practice that is targeted at meeting predefined normative criteria, are under-researched phenomena. Equally, exploration of the potential for image-making practices to be associated with particular ways of being human and being in one's environment might be fruitfully undertaken within the context of further study of the practice of "passing" considered above of a resolved sense of identity that this process connotes. These discussions might be effectively facilitated within wider debates in relation to attitudes of artists with visual impairment towards the disability arts movement.

Reputation

Becker (1982) extends his sociological exploration of art into a consideration of reputation as a social process. "Art worlds", he observes, "in a variety of interwoven activities, routinely make and unmake reputations – of works, artists, schools, genres, and media" (p. 352). It is important to consider the idea of an art world making or unmaking a reputation in relation to approaches to art evaluation that result in the reputation of artists like Eşref Armağan being based on their demonstrated mastery of visual convention. The consequences for artists with visual impairments more generally of the knowledge that the most reputed blind painters are the ones whose output most closely resembles that of their fully sighted counterparts also merit further investigation.

The funding implications of normative forms of art appraisal

Many of the philosophers associated with the institutional theory of art conceived art as a collective undertaking that needs contributions from an array of professionals such as curators, theorists, gallery managers, installation engineers and so on. In this chapter, the role of theorist was granted particular emphasis. All members of this collective are agenda setters and, directly or indirectly wield an influence over the criteria that need to be satisfied before public funding can be allocated to artists and arts organisations. It is not inconceivable that, should the type of normative criteria explored in this chapter become more widely applied to disabled artists, those among this group whose work does not resemble the creative output of their non-disabled peers could find themselves threatened with withdrawal of whatever meagre degree of public funding they are currently deemed to be entitled to. I suspect that the professionals I depicted above as gatekeepers of aesthetic value do not see themselves as such. They are, however, in a definite way, arbiters and determiners of value. Agendas are set in accordance with prevailing values, and agenda setting within the domain of arts funding is a serious business indeed. It makes little sense to discuss value in isolation from the experience of value. We need to remember that within the domain of the arts, the most meaningful forms of value rarely manifest themselves through convention.

The need for creative responses to ableist affirmations

It has been widely claimed that media representations of disability regularly serve as a first point of contact in terms of the generation of public awareness, and that engagement with these representations inform attitudes towards and treatments of people with impairments in a very direct manner. Sharon Snyder and David Mitchell (2006), for example, argue that interrogation of these representations "is necessary and even paramount to influencing the ideological agenda of disability" (p. 201), while Ato Quayson (2007) argues that representations of disability have "a direct effect on the social views of people with disability" (p. 19). The terms "crip" and "supercrip" have been appropriated by disabled people and applied in a variety of thoughtful and innovative ways as a means of generating empowerment and reflection. In light of these developments, Sami Schalk argues (2016) that "nuanced engagement" with supercrip representations is "critical to the rigor and vitality" of the field of disability studies. Whatever their representational inaccuracies, however incalculable the vastness of their potential for miseducation and however dubious their provocation and rationale, supercrip narratives need to be taken seriously. "By not having a flexible theoretical framework to address supercrip representations and take seriously their ideological influences", Schalk (2016) warns, "disability studies risks missing out on important cultural conversations about disability occurring outside of the academy" (p. 72). The ultimate word on the issues addressed in this chapter needs to be that of artists with visual impairment. What we need much more than theoretical musings like this one, is a creative response from artists with visual impairments to the tendency for their admittance into the art world being contingent on their ability to replicate the achievements of their fully sighted counterparts.

References

Arnold, M. 1879. Wordsworth. *Appleton's Journal: A Magazine of General Literature*, 7(2), 138–146 [e-resource]. Accessed May 2018. https://quod.lib.umich.edu/m/moajrnl/acw8433.2-07.002?node=acw8433.2-07.002:6&view=text&seq=147.

Barnes, C. 2008. An ethical agenda in disability research: Rhetoric or reality? In D.M. Mertens and P.E. Ginsberg (eds), *The handbook of social research ethics* (pp. 458–473). London: Sage.

Barnes, C. and Mercer, G. 2001. Disability culture: assimilation or inclusion? In G. Albrecht, K. Seelman and M. Bury (eds), *Handbook of disability studies* (pp. 515–534). London: Sage.

Battersby, C. 1991. Situating the aesthetic: A feminist defense. In A. Benjamin and P. Osborne (eds), *Thinking art: Beyond traditional aesthetics* (pp. 31–44). London: Institute of Contemporary Arts.

Becker, H.S. 1974. Art as collective action. *American Sociological Review*, 39(6), 767–776.

Becker, H.S. 1982. *Art worlds*. Berkeley, CA: University of California Press.

Benjamin, A. and Osborne, P. (eds) 1991. *Thinking art: Beyond traditional aesthetics*. London: Institute of Contemporary Arts.

Bolt, D. 2006. Beneficial blindness: Literary representation and the so-called positive stereotyping of people with impaired vision. *New Zealand Journal of Disability Studies*, 12, 80–100.

Bolt, D. 2015. Not forgetting happiness: The tripartite model of disability and its application in literary criticism. *Disability & Society*, 30(7), 1103–1117.

Bourdieu, P. 1992. *The rules of art: Genesis and structure of the literary field*. S. Emanuel (trans.). Cambridge, MA: Polity Press.

Brune, J. and Wilson, D. 2013. *Disability and passing*. Philadelpha, PA: Temple University Press.

Bruegemann, B.J. 1997. "On [almost] passing". *College English*, 59(6), 647–660.

Choi Caruso, H.Y. 2005. Art as a political act: Expression of cultural identity, self-identity, and gender, by Suk Yun and Yong Soon Min. *Journal of Aesthetic Education*, 19(3), 71–87.

Danto, A.C. 1964. The art world. *Journal of Philosophy*, 61(19), 571–584.

Dickie, G. 1974. *Art and the aesthetic: An institutional analysis*. Ithaca, NY: Cornell University Press.

Dickie, G. 1997. *The art circle: A theory of art*. London: Spectrum Press.

Diffey, T.J. 1991. The republic of art. In R. Ginsberg (ed.), *The republic of art and other essays* (pp. 39–52). New York: Peter Lang.

Discovery Channel. 2008. *Extraordinary people: The artist with no eyes, Eşref Armağan* [e-resource]. Accessed May 2018. www.youtube.com/watch?v=8nXAsHnaoxk.

Ehrenzweig, A. 1961. The hidden order of art. *British Journal of Aesthetics*, 1(3), 121–133.

Eisenhauer, J. 2007. Just looking and staring back: Challenging ableism through disability performance art. *Studies in Art Education*, 49(1), 7–22.

Feeney, D. 2007. *Toward an aesthetics of blindness: An interdisciplinary response to Synge, Yeats and Friel*. New York: Peter Lang.

Felski, R. 1989. *Beyond feminist aesthetics: Feminist literature and social change*. London: Hutchinson Radius.

Florence, P. and Foster, N. (eds). 2000. *Differential aesthetics: Art practices, philosophy, and feminist understandings*. Farnham, UK: Ashgate.

Garland-Thomson, R. 2012. The case for conserving disability. *Journal of Bioethical Inquiry*, 9(3), 339–355.

Gombrich, E. 1960. *Art and illusion: A study in the psychology of pictorial representation*. Princeton, NJ: Princeton University Press.

Heller, M.A. and Kennedy, J.M. 1990. Perspective-taking pictures and the blind. *Perception and Psychophysics*, 48(5), 459–466.

Holmes, A.M. 2008. Art world: Changing gatekeepers? Working Papers in Art and Design 5 [e-resource]. Accessed March 2018. www.herts.ac.uk/__data/assets/pdf_file/0011/12422/WPIAAD_vol5_holmes.pdf.

Kelly, M. (ed.). 1998. *Encyclopaedia of aesthetics*. Vols 1–4. Oxford: Oxford University Press.

Kennedy, J.M. 1980. Blind people recognising and making haptic pictures. In M.A. Hagen (ed.), *The perception of pictures* (pp. 263–304). Cambridge, MA: Academic Press.

Mandelbaum, M. 1965. Family resemblances and generalization concerning the arts. *American Philosophical Quarterly*, 2(3), 219–228.

Michalko, R. 2002. *The difference that disability makes*. Philadelphia, PA: Temple University Press.

Nussbaum, M. 2000. *Women and human development: The capabilities approach*. Cambridge: Cambridge University Press.

Oliver, M. 1997. Emancipatory research: realistic goal or impossible dream? In C. Barnes and G. Mercer (eds.), *Doing disability research* (pp. 15–31). Leeds, UK: The Disability Press.

Paulson, W.R. 1987. *Enlightenment, romanticism ad the blind in France*. Princeton, NJ: Princeton University Press.

Penketh, C. 2016. Special educational needs and art and design education: plural perspectives on exclusion. *Journal of Education Policy*, 31(4), 432–442.

Quayson, A. 2007. *Aesthetic nervousness: Disability and the crisis of representation*. New York: Columbia University Press.

Révész, G. 1950. *Psychology and art of the blind*. London: Longmans, Green & Co.

Schalk, S. 2016. Re-evaluating the supercrip. *Journal of Literary and Cultural Disability Studies*, 10(1), 71–86.

Sen, A. 1992. *Inequality re-examined*. Oxford: Clarendon Press.

Siebers, T. 2004. Disability as masquerade. *Literature & Medicine*, 23(1), 1–22

Silvers, A. 2002. The crooked timber of humanity: Disability, ideology and the aesthetic. In M. Corker and T. Shakespeare (eds), *Disability/postmodernity: embodying disability theory* (pp. 228–244). London: Continuum.

Snyder, S.L. and Mitchell, D.T. 2006. *Cultural locations of disability*. Chicago, IL: University of Chicago Press.

Terzi, L. 2005. Beyond the dilemma of difference: The capability approach to disability and special educational needs. *Journal of Philosophy of Education*, 39(3), 443–459.

Weitz, M. 1950. *Philosophy of the arts*. Cambridge, MA: Harvard University Press.

Weitz, M. 1956. The role of theory in aesthetics. *Journal of Aesthetics and Art Criticism*, 15(1), 27–35.

Winchester, J. 2002. *Aesthetics across the color line: Why Nietzsche (sometimes) can't sing the blues*. Lanham, MD: Rowman & Littlefield.

18

Using expressive movement and haptics to explore kinaesthetic empathy, aesthetic and physical literacy

Wendy Timmons and John Ravenscroft

The purpose of the chapter is to:

(a) show how existing technology can be applied in novel ways to support the learning and experience of children and adults with visual impairments; and

(b) propose a potentially new scheme of communication using expressive movement and haptic feedback.

Introduction

Aesthetic and physical literacy, communication and expression

The term *aesthetic* originates in the Greek language and word αισθητικός, or "perceiving through ones senses". The simplest and clearest way to appreciate this term in the English language is to consider "anaesthetic", its antonym (something that renders us without feelings or senses). Chatterjee (2014) suggests that the term "aesthetic" refers to particular attention given to reality and he argues that the "core of aesthetic experiences is sensations, emotions, and meaning" (cited in Savoie, 2017, p. 56). This opposes the idea that perception is built from purely logical and criteria-based observations that describe reality from the standpoint of value and functionality (Feldman, 1970; Parsons and Blocker, 1993; Swanger, 1990). Indeed, Dewey also refers to this notion of criteria-based perception as "the anaesthetic in experience", or a perception of reality made of habits, routines and automatic reflexes (Greene, 1995). If we consider for a moment what our perception of the world around us would be like without our sensory capacity then the notion of an *aesthetic perception* takes on an importance that may well be otherwise overlooked. The concept of *aesthetic literacy* (as explained by Lussier, 2010) has grown also from Dewey's philosophical standpoint and his differentiation between *experience* and *aesthetic experience*, and thus his influence contributes to our current understanding of art as experience.

Within the physical environment the different, yet associated, concept of *physical literacy* is now widely acknowledged and largely attributed to the work of Whitehead (2010). Among other physical competencies, physical literacy includes overall body management and an "aesthetic" that can also be described as grace or poise. Physical literacy gives a person an embodied dimension of assurance and the capacity to respond to the demands of everyday life (Whitehead, 2010). Within the somatic literature, physical literacy is recognised and understood as learning through personal experience and active engagement through our body (Eddy, 2002) or the "doing and being" that is associated with the "accommodation and convergence" phases within in Klob's (1984) "processing continuum" and experiential learning. Aesthetic experience as argued by Fenner (2003) also gives meaning and value to not only *what* but *how* we perceive through our bodily senses in everyday encounters and this perception allows us to judge and differentiate between mere experience and quality experience.

The development of aesthetic literacy through the inclusion of expressive arts in the curriculum can enable the development of the child's motor, psychological and socio-cognitive skills, including those of reflection, comprehension, knowledge acquisition, concentration, the expression of emotions, and the sense of originality and of course creativity (Savoie, 2017, p. 54). Similarly, within an educational environment the development of physical literacy through the inclusion of aesthetic activities, such as expressive dance, can have a significant impact on assimilating the body, artistic, intellectual, creative and social abilities (Chappell et al., 2008). Best (1982) certainly distinguishes dance from other physical activities for its potential to be meaningful in a way that goes beyond aesthetic value. Emotions and feelings are paramount in the aesthetic experience and the dancing body is truly a vehicle through which feelings, meaning and emotions are expressed and communicated to the audience (Carr, 1997).

Visual impairment, aesthetic and physical literacy

Reiser and Mason (1990) discuss how social models of disability do not refute that some individual differences can result in limitations. However they go on to explain that these are not the cause for exclusion, rather it is, societies' lack of ability to accommodate disabled people's needs, which is the most significant limiting factor (cited in Whitehead, 2010, p. 131). Undeniably, individuals with visual impairment face more psychomotor difficulties and challenges than their sighted peers (Skaggs and Hopper, 1996) and many people with visual impairment attribute their inability to appreciate arts, such as dance and expressive movement, to a deficit in public acknowledgement and accommodation to their needs (Duckett and Pratt 2001; Kleege 2014). Often the lack of access excludes individuals with visual impairments from many cultural and recreational activities and this prevents people with vision loss from interfacing with others and becoming actively involved with the world (Lieberman, Houston-Wilson, and Kozub, 2002; Sherrill, Rainbolt and Ervin, 1984). The negative impact in turn affects aesthetic and physical literacy, fitness and ultimately also social interaction. This often results in a lower quality of life; indeed, research indicates that accessibility of dance programmes for people with visual impairment is very limited. Seham and Yeo (2015) report that 60% of children have been excluded from physical activity (that includes dance) because of visual impairment.

There are, however, some existing good practice models for expressive movement and dance that provide training and performance opportunities specific to the needs of people with visual impairment. These include Touchdown Dance across England; the Association of Ballet and Arts for the Blind (ABAB) in Sao Paolo; Canadian National Institute for the Blind and DZouk

Productions in Toronto (Vision Dance, 2014); Association for India (AID) and Articulate Ability; Greater London Fund for the Blind (Extant, 2014). The Royal Ballet (RB), Scottish Ballet (SB), Northern Ballet Theatre (NBT) and others have made significant progress in increasing access and including visually impaired populations within the dance audience. In spring 1998, SB was the first major ballet company in Europe to audio-describe performances of dance live via audio equipment during the performance event. The multidimensional pattern information associated with dance is, however, difficult to transmit through verbal description, and this form of information potentially also detracts from the important audience experience of the dance music accompaniment. Scottish Ballet also include sensory experiences prior to a performance where individuals are invited to touch the costumes and set designs. Furthermore, there have been a number of dance education pioneers (Alvin Ailey, Martha Graham and Jacques d'Amboise) who have also successfully communicated through their distinct artistry (integrating physical guidance, tactile modelling, descriptive verbal instruction and concept development), surmounting social barriers with their teaching of dance to the blind.

Kinaesthetic empathy

It has been argued that dance, though it has a visual component, is fundamentally a kinesthetic art (Warburton, 2011), however the apperception of this kinaesthetic art is grounded in both the eye and the entire body (Daly, 1992). This grounding suggests that when we observe dance there is a coupling and sophisticated synchronisation of movement and emotional display between the dance movement that resonates within our motor systems and the mapping of the observed dance actions (Warburton, 2011, p. 73).

Warburton (2011) also suggests that the source of empathetic experience in dance is fundamentally somatic, he also articulates somatic empathy being a "feeling for" the movement, which dancers themselves describe as connecting to the choreography and by extension the audience (Warburton, 2011, p. 74). When discussing art forms, Hal Foster (1995) identifies the dynamic interaction between artefacts and the language that reanimates their cultural significance. He establishes that the term "empathy" was introduced by German participatory aestheticians who wanted to emphasise the physical connection (also associated with aesthetic experience) between viewer and artwork in the late nineteenth century. Susan Leigh Foster (1995) suggests that "[o]nce the historian's body recognizes the value and meaning in kinaesthesia it cannot dis-animate the physical action of past bodies it has begun to sense" (p. 7) and defines kinaesthetic empathy as an affiliation apparent between the living and the imagined. Likewise, John Martin (1939/1965) previously interpreted kinaesthetic empathy as having an emotional impact on the viewer because it encouraged dance audiences to respond kinaesthetically by internally experiencing the movements they watch and their associated emotions. Neurophysiologists (Brown, Martinez and Parsons, 2005; Calvo-Merino et al., 2006) propose the theory of mirror neurons as a scientific explanation for this phenomenon and suggest that this region of the brain becomes activated in the same way it would if the viewer was performing the movements they watch. A collaborative project called "Watching Dance" explored the experiences of dance audiences in relation to different dance styles across a variety of viewers and also provoked an interest in the cultural specificity of kinaesthetic empathy (Reynolds and Reason, 2010; Grosbras and Pollick cited in McConachie et al., 2013, pp. 2008–2011). In John Martin's (1939/1965) interpretation, *kinaesthetic empathy* has an emotional impact on the viewer because it encourages dance audiences to respond kinaesthetically by experiencing internally the movements they watch, as well as their associated emotions.

When attending to dancer performance, external perceptions provided are largely through viewing and audio and to a lesser extent through the olfactory system. Within this immersion perceived information includes the following:

(a) The dynamic energy in the body, gesture, movement and lights that is received through the visual system.
(b) The auditory information within the sounds and rhythms made by the moving body and the musical accompaniment (although music is not always necessary or appropriate) that are audibly sensed in the performance.
(c) The odours of the theatre or performance space and the dancers.

Kinaesthetic empathy and visual impairment

Research suggests that locomotive milestones for the visually impaired at an early age are significantly delayed, their understanding and personal experience in movement is potentially limited and this also transfers from child to adulthood (Aki et al., 2007, p. 1329). This suggests that a person with visual impairment will potentially also have limited responsiveness to kinaesthesia. Foster (2010, 2011) and Martin's (1939/1965) notion of kinaesthetic empathy infer that a person with visual impairment attending a dance performance will only perceive external sensations of the performance that are delivered through audio description, potentially also through the olfactory system and ultimately visual feedback will be absent. This concludes that kinaesthetic empathy and the experience of the performed movement (onstage) will be at best limited, defined by the extent of the visual impairment and in the case of blindness would be non-existent.

Choreo-haptic experiments

Haptic technology and visual impairment

The body's haptic system is used, in the context of blindness, to actively explore a shape or spatial dimension with the hands (Davidson, 1976). In human–computer interaction, active engineered haptic devices provide dynamic computer-controlled sensory information to perceivers typically in the form of dynamic forces (Hayward et al., 2004). Gibson (1966, p. 111ff) also refers to kinaesthesia as a part of the body's haptic system and the perception of the body's movement that cuts across several perceptual systems. This sensory perception is embodied and is experienced through re-afferent feedback that is received as a synergetic conjunction of visceral sensation and external perception (Paterson, 2009, p. 769). Tactile information is indeed an important means for people with visual impairment to understand and participate in their immediate environment and haptic technology is now readily used (for example braille technology) within the environment for people with visual impairments.

Haptic technology that supports tactile devices is increasingly employed for persons with visual impairment to assist, negotiate, understand and investigate their immediate surroundings. Tactile devices engage users through their sense of touch, by combining tactile perception with kinaesthetic sensing (i.e. the position, placement and orientation) through appropriate haptic interfaces. This technology has not been used to assist access of visually impaired persons to movement-related events and spectacles, such as dance performances or sports events. The concept behind the device was that it would provide people with visual impairments unique access to the dynamic feelings associated with expressive movement (dance). The prototype technology comprised of three separate deliverable components: (i) tracking technology (Kinect sensors); (ii) mapping software (bespoke); and (iii) a haptic interface (vibro-tactile motors), which made it inexpensive, novel and accessible. The device would provide audiences with visual impairments access to the affective phenomenon of kinaesthetic empathy (Reason and Reynolds, 2010) when attending expressive movement.

These existing concepts were the basis for the authors of this chapter to engage in thought experiments resulting in a hypothesis to be challenged – that haptic feedback is a means to access kinaesthic empathy and the dynamics of dance – and thought-provoking questions:

1   Can a person with visual impairment attending dance experience kinaesthesia and kinaes-thetic empathy through haptic technology?
2   Can the dynamic forces of haptic information enrich the "watching dance" experience and replicate the dynamic visual information received?
3   Can this experience in turn inform the sighted audience by providing information about what it is we actually see when we attend to dance?

A series of case study experiments were devised to challenge these questions and a sum-mary of each of these experiments follows. The experiments were carried out over a period of one year. A constructivist ontological approach was taken and data was collected through semi-structured interview discussions and participant observations, the data collections were recorded and analysed by the research team after each session. This allowed the research-ers to reflect on the intimate experiences, actions and opinions of the participants in each discreet experiment and use the findings to inform the next stage in the development of the research. This cyclical organic process was driven by the conceptual nature of the choreo-haptic experiments and allowed the researchers to fully explore the potential of the research and scope new ideas about how and what we attend to when viewing dance performance. This interactive research design meant that the researchers came into direct contact with the participants during the data collections and ethical dilemmas were a continual consideration. Ethical permission was granted for the choreo-haptic experiments by the ethical committee at the researchers' academic organisation.

Choreo-haptic experiment I: designing and building the choreo-haptic interface

The aims of experiment 1 were to scope the design and the size of a choreo-haptic interface.

The hypothesis for the design was that the choreo-haptic would be representative of the way that a sighted viewer explores the stage or performance space with their vision, scanning and extracting selected information while viewing. The size and design of the interface will allow the users with visual impairments to interactively explore the choreo-haptic surface with their hands. A highly inductive and relatively loosely planned approach to the design of the haptic interface was adopted as the concept under investigation was itself unexplored and unknown.

A large sheet (60 cm x 40 cm x 5 cm) of dense polystyrene, 30 mechanical vibro-tactile motors (MVTM), self-adhesive Velcro ribbon, insulating tape and textiles to cover the choreo-haptic surface (silk, velvet, silicone, lace and satin) were used to construct the device and an Apple mac laptop was used to drive the micro vibro-tactile motors (MVTMs). Two participants were chosen to inform the prototype design process. Participant A, a VI veteran theatregoer (male, 60 years old) who had been non-sighted from a very early stage in life and had no practical dance experience. Participant A had an advanced understanding of assistive technology for the visually impaired (e.g. Optacon and electronic braille devices). Participant B was a student with visual impairment and theatregoer (female, 18 years old) who had very limited peripheral vision and little experience of using tactile technology (braille) used for visual impairment. Participant B had practical experience in dance through taking part in dance classes, performances and also as an audience member. Researchers were present at each of the sessions to collate information and feedback through observation and questioning of the participants and one haptic technician operated the system.

The participants were briefed about the proposed use of the choreo–haptic interface and their experience in both viewing and participating in dance was discussed. The testing was carried out as informal trials during two sessions over two consecutive weeks. The participants were initially consulted about the "size and shape" of the interface. Next the MVTM placing and interface surface were discussed and various prototypes were considered and tested. At each stage in the design prototyping the MVTM matrix was temporarily attached to the interface with Velcro ribbon for testing. To avoid confusion at this "design stage", the complexities of the dance medium were not introduced and the data flow of the MVTM matrix was operated manually by the haptic technician. A range of amplitudes were manually transmitted to the participants in order to determine the lower and optimum threshold range for the vibro-tactile feedback. Once the size of the device and configuration of the MVTMs had been decided, surface textiles were tested for sensitivity and preference. Feedback and observations from the two sessions were collated and analysed.

The testing session was planned to last 90 minutes, however this was extended to 150 minutes (with mutual agreement from all) as it became apparent to the researchers that the participants were, in their words, "eager, curious and intrigued" to see if the device could provide them with information about movement. The previous and very different movement experience that the two participants had also appeared to influence their perception of the device. For example, participant A, the more experienced theatregoer, was interested to see if the device could give an impression of movement and suggested that this together with the regular audio description may provide an even richer viewing experience to persons with visual impairment. Participant A also followed the research briefing by attempting to explore the interface with his fingers. During one of the manual data flow trials he commented, "Oh yes I can see how this might represent the fluttering of movement". Participant B was clearly influenced by her personal experiences participating in dance classes, which she commented were "frustrating because the dance teacher moved too fast for her to keep up with the dance material being delivered". She wanted to know "how will this help me learn more about specific techniques and dance steps?" Participant B also had a different way of interacting with the device and a tendency to "flop" both palms around the interface in an attempt to "randomly capture" the tactile feedback. Both participants had very different thresholds to the vibratory feedback; participant A (lower threshold = 0.4, comfortable at maximum 1) required more intense feedback than participant B (lower threshold = 0.2, comfortable at 0.7).

Choreo–haptic experiment I allowed the researchers to consider how accessible the interface might be to persons with visual impairments. The limitation was that at this stage only two participants were used. This stage, however, was merely to construct a prototype interface to test the broader concept of the overall research. Further modifications following additional participant testing with real-time data flows were considered as the choreo–haptic experiments project progressed. The participants' level of experience with assistive tactile devices appeared to influence how they interacted with the interface. Participant A explored the choreo-haptic surface with his fingertips more than participant B. Participant A's experience using braille and a tactile scanning/reading device (Optacon) may have given him this understanding whereas participant B (with no experience in braille or other) was less able to follow the instructions and remit, and preferred to pat the device with the whole palm of the hand. Participant B also described how she would prefer to use the device to "find out more about movement techniques" (referring to body positions in relation to herself and others around her as opposed to the holistic dynamics of the dance phrases). Her conception of the device possibly stemmed from the practical experience she had in a dance class and a desire to know more about the codified technique, steps, postures and gestures of the movement form that she had been introduced to during this experience as opposed to sensing the overall dynamic visceral content of movement. The important issues such as the dimensions of the prototype and the arrangement of the sensing area were achieved. These dimensions, however, remained at this stage as scoped according to the researchers briefing (i.e. that the user would explore the surface as a sighted viewer explores the stage with their eyes). Participant A's decreased sensitivity to the vibrations were considered and it was hypothesised that this was due to loss of tactile sensitivity through use of tactile devices, aging or both. The significant difference in the participants' optimum and lower MVTM tactile threshold was considered important for the future testing and this was addressed by modifying the device and adding a vibration intensity control button so that the vibration could be optimised for each user.

Choreo-haptic experiment II: testing the prototype

The choreo-haptic prototype scoped in experiment 1 was subsequently modified and a more compact version including a vibration intensity control was taken forward for the testing in experiment 2. For this development in the research dynamic data was also collected from dancers, mapped and transmitted over an internal network on to the choreo-haptic device. Previously (in experiment 1) the data streams had been provided manually by the haptic technician. Prior to the data collections, each dancer spent time exploring and preparing solos that were individual to them. The concept of the improvised pieces was that they were not "composed" (i.e. the use of set codified steps or movements in the sequences) but each dancer merely created, interpreted and expressed movement's dynamic qualities in accordance with the categories and framework of movement discussed by dance theoretician Rudolf Laban (1879–1958). Laban discussed the concept of kinaesthetic sense as a sense "by which we perceive muscular effort, movement and position in space" (Laban and Vial, 1988, p. 111). Laban's ideas originate from efficiency studies and observation of movement carried out for post-war industry in the UK and Germany. The term effort (or Antrieb in German) was the term Laban assigned to the noticeable changes workers made in the quality of exertion in movement. In a similar vein, the idea of shape as a correlate of effort later lead to Laban's study of space harmony in his book *Choreutics* (Laban, 1966). Effort/shape became a method of describing changes in movement quality in terms of the kinds of exertions and body adaptions in space. Laban used effort to explore the dynamics of movement and how the body expresses through movement in the dynamosphere; he described how it is possible to relate feelings for dynamics to the space harmonics in trace forms and the areas through which these lead (Laban, 1966, p. 27). This theory was taken forward by Bartenieff (1965) and applied as an effort theory in her analysis of fundamental patterns of movement. Functional capacity and efficient movement patterns are critical to fundamental development in the brain and allow increased expressivity in the body (Hackney, 2003, p. 19). Movement quality can be considered a natural resultant of bio-psycho-sociological factors that can be refined and controlled in practices like dance to produce efficient, expressive and aesthetic movement patterns. Mind–body connection and using the power of mental and psychological processes to bear on physical movements was also pioneered by Todd (1937), this work was later furthered to include the use of imagery to produce dynamic qualities and alignments in movement (Sweigard, 1974) and dance (Franklin, 2012). We now understand these processes as embodied practices that illustrate how the aesthetic dimensions of quality, imagery, patterns, emotions and sensori–motor processes are central to our embodied activities (Johnson, 2007, p. 1). Describing movement in terms of quality or dynamics is different from describing the movement itself, in a stream of movement; quality has richness and variation that is difficult to define in terms of movement. Laban's (1966) methods for describing movement are a relatively simple framework using words such as slashing or whipping, gliding and beating. The dynamic qualities of dance that are addressed in the choreo-haptic experiments refer to this movement effort framework and the embodied sense of meaning and expressivity that these are associated with (Franklin, 2012; Johnson, 2007; Sweigard, 1974; Todd, 1937).

The improvised interpretation approach allowed the dancers maximum expressivity and a lesser focus on the actual individual steps, skills and techniques. The dynamics of the movement phrases were defined and named according to Laban's categorisation of effort and the choice of dynamic qualities for each dancer to use in this experiment was restricted to "slashing, whipping, gliding and beating" and the duration of the improvisation was restricted to 1 minute (approx.).

Five members of a theatre group for persons with visual impairments were selected as participants for the testing in experiment 2. Their only impairment was visual and the criterion for the level of their visual impairment was that they were non-sighted either from birth or from an early age. The movement participants were dance artists with a strong performance background. Experiment 2 comprised of four separate data collections; the procedure protocol was exactly replicated each session. Data were video and audio recorded throughout entire sessions and stages. Each participant was introduced to the dance studio, seated, verbally briefed about the project and asked to verbally consent to participate in the project. For each data collection the dance space was calibrated and demarked to ensure that the Kinect sensor would capture all of the movement data for each session. Each participant was familiarised with the choreo-haptic device and given time to ask questions about the device. The haptic technician tested a sample data flow to determine the participants' tactile threshold, their optimum vibratory sensory input level was set for the testing in accordance. All participants were asked about their viewing experience of dance in general. The participants were briefed to explore the choreo-haptic's surface with their hands once the dancer started to walk. The first dance artist then walked around the dance space following a random improvised pathway each time, this was carried out without musical accompaniment and the participant had no prior knowledge of the dancer's pathway. Once this dance artist had exited the space, the second dance artist repeated the process. This procedure was repeated four times by each dance artist. The participants' experience and interpretation of the dance artist's pathway was then discussed with the researchers and the feedback recorded. Next each dance artist announced a dynamic quality to the researchers that would represent the next improvisation before entering the dance space to perform. The dynamic qualities of the improvised solos were performed in an improvised "dialogue" type format in response to the previous dance artist's performance. The participant discussed the experience of the haptic feedback they received on the choreo-haptic device and their understanding of the dance movement after every two performances. This process was repeated four times until each dance artist had performed each of the four qualities once (slashing, whipping, gliding and beating). Each of the participants' background and experience of dance together with their experience and commentary during the data collection were collated and analysed.

The interpretations of the movement, commonalities, as well as unique experiences of the participants were noted. Each of the participants brought a slightly different experience of dance to the research; participant's 1 and 3 were male and had both only experienced dance through attending the theatre and accessing the audio commentary, which they both agreed was "better than nothing, however did have a tendency to be subjective". Participant 2 (female) had attended many dance performances at a younger age when she had limited vision, however she had since completely lost this vision. She commented how "the memories and experience that I have retained from the time when I had partial sight mean that I easily become 'disillusioned' by the audio commentary" and said that "I have since stopped going to dance performance because I become frustrated". Participant 5 had some experience of participating in ballroom dancing with his wife. All participants requested a slightly different volume for the vibratory tactile feedback, this ranged from (0.2 = lower threshold to 0.7 = comfortable level). All the participants were able to follow the dancer around the interface, recognising when the dancer was stage right, left, front and back. The movement sensations were described by all, however, not all specific qualities and dynamics were recognised by all. Smooth, flowing dynamics such as floating and gliding were the qualities that all five participants described as experiencing. Participant 2 described the experience as "a much more pleasurable interpretation of movement than the audio commentary as it let the imagination work". Participant 5 was not as convinced about what he was sensing as the other participants; he commented "I don't get it . . . I can't feel the dancers waltzing around the space". All participants commented that they thought it may be easier to determine what the dancers were expressing if they did not have to search with their fingers to find the source and location of the vibratory feedback. They also all suggested that after a while this searching was to an extent guided by the noise of the activated MVTMs. None of the participants mentioned being aware of experiencing audio feedback from the dancers as they moved around the dance space.

The number of participants tested in this experiment was limited, however during this experiment there appeared to be an implicit association between the participants' background experiences in dance and the way they interpreted the tactile feedback provided by the choreo-haptic device. For example, participant 2 appeared to associate the feedback with the limited yet pleasurable memories she had of viewing dance as a child. Participant 5, however, was not able to associate the feedback with the motor experience he had from participating in ballroom dance sessions. Ballroom dance is a codified technical type of dance that has specific rules, techniques and step sequences that are mastered before dynamic qualities can be explored. As with participant 2 in experiment 1, the observations may be because he (participant 5) was looking for codified and technical elements in the dance that he recognised from past motor experiences while participating in dance sessions. Further research is needed to verify and develop this theory. Limitations and future research plans were noted for the next experiment. At this stage in the research, financial and time constraints on the project meant that the scope of the technology was indeed relatively basic. This in turn meant that the haptic feedback the choreo-haptic device was able to provide was also potentially basic and unsophisticated. The limitations of the size and vibro-tactile noise noted in this experiment were considered and it was decided to rebuild and modify the choreo-haptic device to allow for a smaller and more condensed sensing area. This would allow the haptic feedback to be received using the whole surface of the palms of the hands, not just the fingers, and without moving them across the choreo-haptic surface. In an attempt to reduce the noise that the MVTMs emitted, it was also decided to us a softer "insulating" material to house the MVTMs and the wiring. The covering surface was modified from insulating tape to a silky silicone.

Choreo-haptic experiment III: pilot testing the modified choreo-haptic device

For the pilot testing of the modified device one participant was engaged in the testing. For this stage the most experienced participant who was totally non-sighted was recalled to take part in the pilot testing. The participant was given the new choreo-haptic device and asked to familiarise himself with its new adapted size and surface texture. Initial testing was carried out (as in experiment 2) to determine if the participant could trace the directional movement of the dancer walking in the space on the scale of the new, smaller device. Following this the researchers instructed the dance artist to move in to the space and express one of the improvised movement phrases he had worked on previously. The whipping phrase was chosen for this trial. The participant was not aware of the choice of the dynamics and quality of the phrase, he was then asked to seek and find the dynamic qualities he sensed with his hands placed on the choreo-haptic. The participant commented that he was more comfortable with the use and size of the modified device. As in the previous trials (experiment 2, stage 2), the participant was also able to experience and trace the spatial orientation of the dancer in the dance space. This time, however, this was done with little effort as the information was received without the participant having to move his hands around the choreo-haptic. When the participant was asked to comment on and interpret the feedback from the movement phrase during the procedures the participant hesitated for a moment and then announced, "Well, I think that I felt a turning, yes it was a twirling movement with arms swirling in the air". Indeed this was an exact description of the dance performance.

Choreo-haptic experiment IV: exploratory pilot workshop

Within the proof of concept project, a final exploratory pilot workshop was carried out at a school for visually impaired young people again using the modified choreo-haptic vibro-tactile technology. During this experiment, children with visual impairments worked with each other in pairs, one as a "dancer" and the other as an "audience member" who communicated via the device with impressive results. The drama teacher at the school was present at the session and remarked, "I have never seen the children discuss movement in this way before . . . it is usually so hard for them to externalise expressive movement". An example of this interaction was when one child moved in to the allocated dance space where the movement could be captured and another child had her hands on the choreo-haptic device, "I do not know what you are doing . . . but that is a very happy movement it makes me feel happy inside". The child was indeed witnessing and referring to the other child's star jumps, which she had no means of seeing. This work clearly evidences that the device also had potential to be used in a teaching and learning context to expand students' expressive movement and motivate learners with visual impairments to experience the kinaesthetic. This pilot corresponded to the work of Boud, Cohen and Walker (1993), who proposed that counterposing experience with something that is external to the learner enabled meaning to be created and the belief that learning required interaction either directly or symbolically with elements outside the learner. In doing so, the process represented bodily kinaesthetic intelligence in which the person's engagement within the learning environment was required (Aziz et al., 2010) and fostered the concept of active learning (Bonwell and Eison, 1991).

Conclusion

Visual impairment (meaning low vision or blindness) has an impact on a child's development (Warren, 1994), motor perception, learning and development and consequently quality of life and well-being (Poulsen et al., 2008; Skinner and Piek, 2001; Sleeuwenhock, Boter and Vermeer, 1995). Having no or impaired vision means that children cannot access and imitate movements made by others (Brambring, 2006). Reflective practice is the ability to look back at one's actions, discuss, describe, analyse and evaluate them in order to take responsibility for one's own learning and development as a state of mind and as an orientation for deeper learning (Moon, 2013, p. 63). Digital recording technology is increasingly used effectively for this purpose in dance and expressive movement contexts, digital recordings are not, however, accessible to people with visual impairments. The prototype choreo-haptic technology potentially has applications within a reflective learning environment that would allow persons with visual impairments to viscerally access their own (and others') performance and use this experience to develop and experience the expressive and emotive content.

Acknowledgement

The authors would like to acknowledge the work and input to the project this chapter details by Dr Sophia Lycouris, University of Edinburgh.

References

Aki, E., Atasavun, S., Turan, A. and Kayihan, H. 2007. Training motor skills of children with low vision. *Perceptual and Motor Skills*, 104(3 suppl.), 1328–1336. https://doi.org/10.2466/pms.104.4.1328-1336

Aziz, N., Roseli, N.H.M., Eshak, E.S. and Mutalib, A.A.. 2010. Assistive courseware for the visually impaired based on theory of multiple intelligence. In K. Liu and J. Filipe, *KMIS 2010: Proceedings of Knowledge Management International Conference*. Setúbal, Portugal: SciTePress.

Bartenieff, I. 1965. *Effort-shape analysis of movement: The unity of expression and function*. New York: Albert Einstein College of Medicine, Yeshiva University.

Best, D. 1982. The aesthetic and the artistic. *Philosophy*, 57(221), 357–372. https://doi.org/10.1017/S0031819100050968

Bonwell, C.C. and Eison, J.A. 1991. *Active learning: Creating excitement in the classroom*. ASHE-ERIC Higher Education Reports. Washington, DC: ERIC Clearinghouse on Higher Education, George Washington University.

Boud, D., Cohen, R. and Walker, D. 1993. *Using experience for learning*. Maidenhead, UK: McGraw-Hill Education.

Brambring, M. 2006. Divergent development of gross motor skills in children who are blind or sighted. *Journal of Visual Impairment & Blindness*, 100(10), 620–634.

Brown, S., Martinez, M.J. and Parsons, L.M. 2005. The neural basis of human dance. *Cerebral Cortex*, 16(8), 1157–1167.

Calvo-Merino, B., Grèzes, J., Glaser, D.E., Passingham, R.E. and Haggard, P. 2006. Seeing or doing? Influence of visual and motor familiarity in action observation. *Current Biology*, 16(19),1905–1910.

Carr, D. 1997. Meaning in dance. *British Journal of Aesthetics*, 37(4), 349–366. https://doi.org/10.1093/bjaesthetics/37.4.349

Chappell, K., Craft, A., Burnard, P. and Cremin, T. 2008. Question-posing and question-responding: The heart of "possibility thinking" in the early years. *Early Years*, 28(3), 267–286. https://doi.org/10.1080/09575140802224477

Chatterjee, A. 2014. *The aesthetic brain: How we evolved to desire beauty and enjoy art.* New York, NY: Oxford University Press.

Daly, A. 1992. Dance history and feminist theory: Reconsidering Isadora Duncan and the male gaze. In Laurence Senelick (ed.), *Gender in performance: The presentation of difference in the performing arts* (pp. 239–259). Hanover, NH: Tufts University Press.

Davidson, P.W. 1976. Haptic perception. *Journal of Pediatric Psychology*, 1(3), 21–25.

Duckett, P.S. and Pratt, R. 2001. The researched opinions on research: Visually impaired people and visual impairment research. *Disability & Society*, 16(6), 815–835.

Eddy, M. 2002. Somatic practices and dance: Global influences. *Dance Research Journal*, 34(2), 46. https://doi.org/10.2307/1478459

Extant. 2014. Accessed 18 December 2018. www.glfb.org.uk.

Feldman, E.B. 1970. *Becoming human through art: Aesthetic experience in the school.* Englewood Cliffs, NJ: Prentice-Hall.

Fenner, D.E. 2003. Aesthetic experience and aesthetic analysis. *Journal of Aesthetic Education*, 37(1), 40–53.

Foster, H. 1995. The artist as ethnographer? In G. Marcus and F. Myers (eds.), *The traffic in culture: Refiguring art and anthropology* (pp. 302–309). Berkeley, CA and London: University of California Press.

Foster, S.L. 1995. Ballerina's phallic pointe. In S.L. Foster (ed.), *Corporealities: Dancing, knowledge, culture, and power* (pp. 1–24). New York: Routledge.

Foster, S.L. 2010. *Choreographing empathy: Kinesthesia in performance.* London: Routledge.

Franklin, E.N. 2012. *Dynamic alignment through imagery.* Champaign, IL: Human Kinetics.

Gibson, J.J. 1966. *The senses considered as perceptual systems.* Boston, MA: Houghton-Mifflin.

Greene, M. 1995. *Releasing the imagination: Essay on education, the arts, and social change.* San Francisco, CA: Jossey-Bass.

Hackney, P. 2003. *Making connections: Total body integration through Bartenieff fundamentals.* London: Routledge.

Hayward, V., Astley, O.R., Cruz-Hernandez, M., Grant, D. and Robles-De-La-Torre, G. 2004. Haptic interfaces and devices. *Sensor Review*, 24(1), 16–29.

Johnson, M. 2007. *The meaning of the body: Aesthetics of human understanding.* Chicago, IL: University of Chicago Press.

Kleege, G. 2014. What does dance do, and who says so? Some thoughts on blind access to dance performance. *British Journal of Visual Impairment*, 32(1), 7–13.

Klob, D. 1984. *Experiential learning: Experience as the source of learning and development.* Princeton, NJ: Princeton University Press..

Laban, R. 1966. *Choreutics.* London: Macdonald & Evans.

Laban, R. and Vial, K. 1988. *Kunst der Bewegung.* Wilhelmshaven, Germany: Florian Noetzel Verlag.

Lieberman, L.J., Houston-Wilson, C. and Kozub, F.M. 2002. Perceived barriers to including students with visual impairments in general physical education. *Adapted Physical Activity Quarterly*, 19(3), 364–377.

Lussier, C. 2010. Aesthetic literacy: The gold medal standard of learning excellence in dance. *Physical & Health Education Journal*, 76(1), 40–44.

McConachie, B., Blair, R., Cook, A., Furse, A., Hood, E., Lutterbie, J., Machon, J., Pollick, F.E. and Trimingham, M. 2013. *Affective performance and cognitive science: Body, brain and being.* London: A&C Black.

Martin, J. [1939] 1965. *The dance in theory.* Princeton, NJ: Princeton University Press.

Moon, J.A. 2013. *A handbook of reflective and experiential learning: Theory and practice.* London: Routledge.

Parsons, M.J. and Blocker, H.G. 1993. *Aesthetics and education.* Champaign, IL: University of Illinois Press.

Paterson, M. 2009. Haptic geographies: Ethnography, haptic knowledges and sensuous dispositions. *Progress in Human Geography*, 33(6), 766–788.

Poulsen, A.A., Ziviani, J.M., Johnson, H. and Cuskelly, M. 2008. Loneliness and life satisfaction of boys with developmental coordination disorder: The impact of leisure participation and perceived freedom in leisure. *Human Movement Science*, 27(2), 325–343.

Reason, M. and Reynolds, D. 2010. Kinesthesia, empathy, and related pleasures: An inquiry into audience experiences of watching dance. *Dance Research Journal*, 42(2), 49–75.

Reiser, R. and Mason, M. (1990). *Disability equity in the classroom: A human rights issue.* London: Inner London Education Authority.

Savoie, A. 2017. Aesthetic experience and creativity in arts education: Ehrenzweig and the primal syncretistic perception of the child. *Cambridge Journal of Education*, 47(1), 53–66. https://doi.org/10.1080/0305764X.2015.1102864

Seham, J. and Yeo, A.J. 2015. Extending our vision: Access to inclusive dance education for people with visual impairment. *Journal of Dance Education*, 15(3), 91–99.

Sherrill, C., Rainbolt, W. and Ervin, S. 1984. Attitudes of blind persons toward physical education and recreation. *Adapted Physical Activity Quarterly*, 1(1), 3–11.

Skaggs, S. and Hopper, C. 1996. Individuals with visual impairments: A review of psychomotor behavior. *Adapted Physical Activity Quarterly*, 13(1), 16–26.

Skinner, R.A. and Piek, J.P. 2001. Psychosocial implications of poor motor coordination in children and adolescents. *Human Movement Science*, 20(1–2), 73–94.

Sleeuwenhock, H.C., Boter, R.D. and Vermeer, A. 1995. Perceptual-motor performance and the social development of visually impaired children [Review]. *Journal of Visual Impairment and Blindness*, 89(4), 359–367.

Swanger, D. 1990. Discipline-based art education: Heat and light. *Educational Theory*, 40(4), 437–442.

Sweigard, L. 1974. *Human movement potential*. New York: Dodd, Mead & Co.

Todd, M. 1937. *The thinking body*. Princeton, NJ: Princeton University Press.

Vision Dance. 2014. Vision dance encounter. Accessed 18 December 2018. www.visiondanceencounter.com/2014-event.

Warburton, E.C. 2011. Of meanings and movements: Re-languaging embodiment in dance phenomenology and cognition. *Dance Research Journal*, 43(2), 65–84. https://doi.org/10.1017/S0149767711000064

Warren, D.H. 1994. *Blindness and children: An individual differences approach*. Cambridge: Cambridge University Press.

Whitehead, M. 2010. *Physical literacy: Throughout the lifecourse* (1st ed.). London and New York: Routledge.

Part VII

Socio-emotional and sexual aspects of visual impairment

19

Social-emotional aspects of visual impairment

A practitioner's perspective

Joao Roe

Introduction

It is widely accepted that there is a dynamic interaction between social–emotional development and academic achievement (Aviles, Anderson and Davilla, 2006; Roe, 2008; Schneider, 2000). There is increasing recognition that emotions and feelings affect what we do and that our emotional abilities have a significant role in supporting the achievement of a fulfilling life (Dowling, 2014).

In this chapter, we will be focusing on the impact of vision impairment and how to promote social–emotional development from an early age. We will be looking at the role of peripatetic/ itinerary teachers working with children and young people (CYP) with visual impairment (VI), the role of families and peers and consider the views of some young people with VI (gathered through semi-structured interviews).

Early social relationships occur spontaneously in natural contexts, first during caregiving activities (Sroufe, 1995) and later on with other adults and peers as the child's social world expands and they go on to attend educational settings and participate in their wider community. We will be considering how children develop in the context of social relationships with others and the role adults play in promoting development (Rogoff, 1991; Vygostky, 1978).

As social interaction, play and the development of friendships often develop naturally between children there is often an expectation that CYP with VI are developing these naturally as well but this is often not the case. Establishing positive social interactions and making friends is a challenging skill for children with VI and those who are blind (Celeste and Grum, 2010; MacCuspie, 1992; Preisler, 1997; Sacks, 2006; Salleh and Zainal, 2010; Verdier, 2016). In educational settings, adults often only consider that there may be a difficulty in this area if there is evidence of conflict with others or visible signs of social–emotional difficulties. Although most adults would recognise the challenges CYP with VI face, social–emotional difficulties may be underestimated and only become evident later on. Adults are also less likely than children to consider that bullying has occurred (Harris et al., 2014).

Direct intervention in this area is not always successful and may actually interfere with the spontaneous natural relationships and interactions needed to promote development. Equally, skills learnt in controlled situations are not necessarily transferred to more natural contexts (Schneider, 2000).

Therefore, promoting social-emotional development, social skills, friendships and social relationships is not a straightforward process. The subtleties of social skills and relationships make this area of development quite challenging for professionals to understand fully (LaVenture, Lesner and Zabelski, 2006).

Children who do not develop these skills are more likely to go on to have difficulties throughout their lives and children with developmental disabilities are more likely to have social-emotional difficulties (Ladd, 2005; Squires et al., 2012).

It is crucial to develop understanding of social-emotional needs of CYP with VI and to support families and professionals to subtly monitor and intervene to promote social-emotional development.

Throughout this chapter references will be made to the impact of VI but in considering these, it is important to note that each child or young person is very individual and how they develop, respond and the social experiences they encounter will be very different (Webster and Roe, 1998). It also does not mean that all CYP with VI face significant difficulties in this area. Furthermore, those who may have difficulties in this area may perceive these difficulties differently; they may feel fine about it while others may feel isolated (Schneider, 2000).

Early social development

Human infants rely on social interactions to learn about themselves and the world around them. From a very early age babies are able and have a desire to interact with people (Fisher, 2016). It is through regular, consistent, responsive and highly reliable interaction with a caregiver that infants begin to understand themselves as distinct from others and develop secure attachments (Dowling, 2014; Lewis and Wolffe, 2006; Sroufe, 1995).

Adults who respond sensitively to the infant behave in ways that amplify, support and modulate the infant's response (Sroufe, 1995). Infants begin to make connections between what they do and what is done to them in return through contingent interactions. This in turn enables the development of intersubjectivity and joint attention (Gauvain, 2001; Webster and Roe, 1998) and helps the infant to start developing a predictable mental structure (Dowling, 2014).

Responsive adults are able to interpret the infant's behaviour and guide their attention in a rewarding way. Both adult and infant play an important role in these interactions. Infants do this by responding to adults' interactions and showing what interests them by maintaining attention (Gauvain, 2001).

Towards the end of the first year of life, children begin to show social referencing, i.e. looking at a more experienced social partner to seek confirmation on how to respond, what to think or feel about a particular situation, person or object (Fisher, 2016; Gauvain, 2001). Vision plays an important role here as subtle facial expressions and body language can provide useful clues in these situations (Fisher, 2016).

By developing children's awareness of emotion and supporting children to develop a range of effective emotion regulation strategies such as distraction, reappraisal, soothing and response modulation caregivers promote the development of emotion and the progression from co-regulation to self-regulation (Dowling, 2014; Silkenbeumer, Schiller and Holodynski, 2016).

For example, a toddler is much more able than the infant to regulate affect, e.g. fighting back tears. However, at times this ability to self-regulate may be overwhelmed and the child is not always able to self-manage themselves (Sroufe, 1995).

To establish effective social interactions it will be important to engage positively with peers and regulate emotions so that the child can manage their own and the needs of others during social interactions. For this to be possible, children need to have social competence skills such as self-regulation, social and emotional awareness, perspective problem-solving, empathy and pro-social behaviour (Aviles et al., 2006; Howes, 2009; Silkenbeumer et al., 2016; Sroufe, 1995).

Early social-emotional development of children with VI

The presence of vision impairment can disrupt the natural interactions between the young child and their caregiver as it may be harder for adults to tune into the child, to interpret the child's subtle attempts to interact and respond contingently (Dale and Salt, 2008; Roe, 1998; van den Broek et al., 2017; Webster and Roe, 1998). From birth, vision plays an important role in social interactive processes, for example in obtaining the infant's attention, interest in faces and mutual gazing, looking away to signal disengagement, etc. (Preisler, 1991; Roe, 1998). Although early interaction can be established through other means, families may not be aware of the infant's responses, infants may seem unresponsive that in turn may impact on caregivers who may feel unable to engage with their child (Salleh and Zainal, 2010). Adults' emotional responses can also impact on the nature of interaction with the child and the communication and parenting style they adopt (Andersen, Dunlea and Kekelis, 1993; Lewis and Wolffe, 2006).

Developing intersubjectivity and establishing joint attention are paramount in promoting development (Preisler, 1991; van den Broek et al., 2017). It is crucial that caregivers of infants with VI are able to interpret their subtle attempts to interact, are sensitive, able to respond contingently and scaffold the child. Infants with VI often stay still and listen attentively when interested in what is happening around them and they may not interact in ways caregivers would expect. This can make caregivers feel that they are not able to maintain the positive interest and involvement of their infant, which in turn is required to develop a sense of efficacy and satisfaction.

Specialist teachers (we will use this term to mean itinerant teachers and qualified teachers of the visually impaired (QTVIs)) can provide early intervention support to families during this very early stage of development. They have to be particularly sensitive to caregivers and promote their sense of efficacy by focusing on what they are already doing well (this may not be obvious to the caregiver themselves), provide information that can help caregivers interpret the infant's attempts to interact and promote their child's development.

The presence of vision impairment can disturb the natural interaction between child and caregivers who will vary in their ability or capacity at that moment to promote the child's development. The emotional state of caregivers acts as part of the relationship established with the child (Bailey, 2012; Preisler, 1997). Early intervention needs to focus on fostering positive interactions and bonding between child and adults while taking into account each individual family situation. To develop effective early intervention, Limbrick (2017) refers to the need to adopt approaches that support, value and respect families by developing effective partnerships and ways of working, which focus on active listening and consider the wider range of family needs.

Children who are seen as more passive tend to elicit more directive styles of communication (Webster and Roe, 1998) and interaction with children with VI has shown that they are often provided with more labels and requests for an action (declaratives and imperatives). On the other hand, they receive less descriptions and explanations compared to their sighted peers. Language directed to children with VI tends to focus on their activities or interests and to request specific actions; with adults showing a tendency for managing and controlling the interaction rather than facilitating in a contingent way (Andersen et al., 1993; Kekelis and Andersen, 1984; Perez-Pereira and Conti-Ramsden, 1999; Roe, 1998; van den Broek et al., 2017).

All young children enjoy familiar routines that are repeated over and over again and they require a high number of experiences to make sense of the world around them. For young children with VI these experiences may be more dependent on adults bringing them to the child. It is important that the infant and adult dyad experience positive interactions that maintain interest and promote development and well-being. If adults are also having difficulties tuning in with the child then these early experiences may not be as rewarding and may not occur as often, so young children with VI do not necessarily have the same amount and/or quality of experiences as their sighted peers.

In bringing the world to the young child with VI, adults should not only consider the physical world but also the social world. Through experiences and language interactions, adults can foster an interest in other people's minds, their feelings and emotions (Silkenbeumer et al., 2016). This will promote the development of theory of mind.

Styles of parenting that are high on the level of emotional conversations have been associated with developing emotion regulation. This emotional coaching style of parenting involves empathetic listening, validating the child's emotions, guiding emotion regulation and teaching the child problem-solving skills.

Families play a crucial role from the beginning and they need to understand how to develop supportive relationships and styles of parenting. Support needs to be provided in a sensitive way that meets the needs of the family, promotes their confidence and does not interfere with natural interactions and bonding with their child. Specialist teachers visiting families at home can raise awareness of the need to promote social understanding, helping their child understand social language and emotions and sharing their feelings, thoughts and intentions, which helps the child understand other people's perspectives. It can be beneficial to access opportunities to meet other families with CYP with VI.

Interacting with peers and the expanding social world

As they develop, young children's social worlds expand and they make significant progress in understanding other people's minds, their emotions and the links between what other people believe and how they act (Bruce, 2004; Dunn, 2004; Lavoie, 2005; Maguire and Dunn, 1997). "Social emotional competence is defined as cooperative pro-social behaviour, initiation and maintenance of peer friendships and adult relationships, management of aggression and conflict and emotional regulation and reactivity" (Squires, 2002 cited in Aviles et al., 2006, p. 33).

Being socially competent means that you are able to understand the social situation you are in and you are able to respond appropriately, adapt your behaviours and understand the impact of your actions on those around you. It is very fluid and not something you can practice unless you are living it.

Play has a significant role in children's well-being, social understanding, language development and conflict resolution as it provides a context for children to learn skills, which contribute to positive social interaction with peers (Coplan and Arbeau, 2009). It provides opportunities to practise flexibility and exploration of new ways of thinking (Bruce, 2004). Children present higher levels of cognitive functioning when playing with peers they like and are familiar with (Rubin, Fein and Vanderberg, 1983).

Pretend play provides opportunities for children to develop social understanding, use language to reason with peers and resolve conflict in real contexts, as well as an opportunity to enjoy the company of friends and create intimacy by disclosing their emotions (Howes, 2009; Maguire and Dunn, 1997).

Friendships create contexts in which basic social skills are acquired and extended (Dunn, 2004; Hartup, 1992). They give children opportunities to care about and try to understand others; and to respond to the feelings, needs and concerns of their friends (Dunn, 1993, 2004). Within friendships there are also opportunities for mutual regulation of emotion, which helps children manage their own emotions and be better at problem-solving (Maguire and Dunn, 1997).

Friends provide an opportunity to have real feedback and encounter different points of view. Interaction between friends presents more criticism of their partners and explanation of their views and opinions. Friends working together present higher levels of pro-social behaviour and share more information than when non-friends work together. This high level of disagreement and discussion leads to cognitive growth (Azmitia, 1988; Garvey, 1990; Schneider, 2000).

Making friends, maintaining friendships and fitting in is a challenging process for all children (Ladd, 2005). Having positive social experiences is important to motivate CYP with VI to want to interact socially with others.

Role of adults

Adults play an important role when interacting with young children, building relationships, modelling language and thinking, extending children's knowledge and understanding. Therefore, the quality of these interactions is crucial. Adults need to have a good understanding of what the child already knows and how to expand their knowledge and thinking (Fisher, 2016).

Fisher (2016) refers to the effectiveness of adults who quietly pay attention to children, waiting for them to initiate a conversation and how the interactions established in this way are richer and more sustained. This is due to the fact that it starts from the child's perspective rather than from the adult's agenda. Fisher (2016) also refers to the importance of independent learning and the fact that children present more interaction between them and solve problems between themselves, take more risks and make more mistakes when adults are not present.

Self-regulation is crucial to development, children need to learn to control themselves and share a toy with a peer, etc. (Silkenbeumer et al., 2016). Too much intervention (help/support) may interfere with the development of self-regulation. The focus needs to be on helping children think for themselves and on adults providing effective scaffolding to promote development.

This may present challenges for children with VI who are passive. Adults may initiate conversation to stimulate the child but in doing so they are starting from their own agenda. While there is a role in stimulating the child, it is important that children have opportunities to initiate interaction and that adults do not to break the flow of the play that the children initiate.

In fact different studies have shown that children with VI spend more time with adults and tend to control activity (Harris et al., 2014; Preisler, 1993; Roe, 1998).

Sometimes, children with VI find it hard to move on to new experiences and prefer to stick to an activity that they find enjoyable and safe. It can be challenging to encourage a child to expand their experiences while trying to take the child's lead.

During play situations in mainstream settings, adults tend to control the play activity more when interacting with children with VI who are younger or have a more severe VI. Both adults and peers tend to verbally interact with the child to request information about the child's own actions, wishes or feelings; while children with VI tend to verbally interact with others to request objects, information about localisation of objects or people or for an action (Roe, 1998).

It is crucial that adults are good observers and readers of the interests of the child, as well as those of their peers to ensure that they can promote social interaction. Often adults ask peers to play with the child with VI (Kekelis, 2006; Preisler, 1997) but this strategy is often unsuccessful. Even if it works at times, it is unlikely that this would support natural, equal status and meaningful relationships.

Adults cannot make friendship happen but they can create an environment that promotes interaction between children. By ensuring that the materials available are accessible and promote interaction, that play rules are made clear, the peer group is consistent, small and compatible (including peers with good communication skills), the physical layout is accessible and consistent, etc. (Celeste, 2007; D'Allura, 2002; Kekelis and Sacks, 1992; Ozaydin, 2015; Rettig, 1994; Webster and Roe, 1998).

Vision and social interaction

Vision plays an important role in early social interaction as young children spend long periods of time watching other children, imitating each other and giving objects. Free play is particularly difficult for children with VI as other children move around, join in and leave the group, imitate each other and communicate non-verbally (Eckerman, 1993; Preisler, 1997).

Positive social interaction and play are important experiences for children with VI to learn about other people and how to join in a group, how to direct the attention of others, initiate and sustain interactions. Whether these experiences occur at home with siblings, with friends of the family or in educational settings, the more experiences children with VI can have, the more opportunities they have to learn.

Evidence of the play and social interaction skills of children with VI is varied, with some authors referring to difficulties presented by these children and others referring to a similar range of play presented by these children (Celeste, 2007; D'Allura, 2002; Ferguson and Buultjens, 1995; Rettig, 1994; Sacks, Kekelis and Gaylord-Ross, 1992; van den Broek et al., 2017). However, it is recognised that play and social interaction can be challenging for children with VI. Those who present pro-social behaviour and positive play have developed language, play and social skills, which enable them to succeed in social interaction with peers. Pretend play can be particularly challenging and children with VI who engage more and for longer in pretend play tend to have good verbal comprehension (Ferguson and Buultjens, 1995).

Dunn (1993) refers to the correlation between experience of arguments between siblings and their success in socio–cognitive tasks. Still, many children with VI tend to play by themselves and may not learn to interact with others incidentally (Sacks and Wolffe, 2006). They may also miss out on subtle feedback from facial expressions and other people's responses to social situations and receive limited feedback on their own social behaviours.

Children with VI do not always respond to their peers' attempts to interact with them (Kekelis, 2006; Roe, 1998). For example, a girl in the home corner simply ignored her peer's questions and a blind boy in nursery seemed to ignore his peers' invitations to join in (turning his head away and upwards and not replying) and only responded after many attempts from his peers when they finally explained: "Would you like to push the pushchair with us?"

Although this is not necessarily true for all children with VI, many have fewer friends and perceive friends to be those who help them, sit next to them during tutor group or those who do not pick on them (Khadka et al., 2012; Lavoie, 2005; MacCuspie, 1992; Preisler, 1997; Sacks and Silberman, 2000). CYP with VI have fewer opportunities to practise and develop social skills and those CYP who do not master these skills are often socially isolated (Sacks et al., 1992; Salleh and Zainal, 2010; Verdier, 2016).

Joining a group can be challenging for CYP with VI, as a lot of the successful strategies are very subtle and often rely on visual information (Celeste, 2007; Verdier, 2016). A good level of social competence and determination is required to be successful at gaining entry in a group. As children develop and become more aware of their social status, it can be harder to gain group entry if equal peer relationships have not been developed and nurtured. Often those who have difficulties in this area go on to get further behind (Maguire and Dunn, 1997). Verdier (2016) mentioned that children with VI who gained access to a group and developed more equal peer relationships tend to continue developing these over time, but those who didn't had further difficulties in gaining entry to groups and developing peer relationships.

Even children who are socially competent experience a lot of rejection when attempting to join in a group. However, successful children learn a number of strategies that support group entry, such as observing and waiting before trying to join in (this provides children with information about the group activity, establishing what the group interests are and rules used, etc.), behaving in similar ways to the group (often non-verbally) or making statements that show agreement with the group's activity. Strategies that focus on the child's own wishes, feelings (drawing attention to the child trying to gain entry) rather than the group's activity and that interrupt the group's activity or play, are likely to be unsuccessful (Ely, 2014). To achieve this, children need to be aware of other people, their wishes and feelings. Children with VI may not realise that other children are rejected as well and what it takes to gain entry in a group.

Children who are socially competent are able to use successful strategies in dealing with conflict such as avoiding events or subjects that will create conflict, explain their viewpoint when they disagree with their peers and suggest alternative activities (Kekelis and Sacks, 1992).

Although this is not true for all children with vision impairment, it is important to recognise how challenging it is for many children with VI to acquire the necessary skills to be socially competent in a complex environment.

In schools, MacCuspie, (1992) found that children with VI may find it difficult to locate their friends in the playground, may not access visual information to be able to compare their own performance to that of their peers, find it hard to complete work in time to join in other activities and that they do not always receive appropriate feedback from peers due to concerns that they may be reprimanded by adults.

CYP with VI often have to put in a high level of effort to accomplish academic tasks and face challenges in high-visual activities such as sports. At times adults' concerns about the safety of CYP with VI further impact on their opportunities to socialise, e.g. not letting them outside, not letting them read (so as to not put so much effort and further deteriorate their eyesight) (Khadka et al., 2012).

Verdier (2016) found that at some stage all CYP with VI struggle with their identity and want to fit in. Often this means that they hide their visual impairment and give up using aids such as a cane or braille as they feel this makes them different to their peers. This means that teachers may find it hard to recognise the level of difficult they face.

Some CYP with VI enjoy the fact that they work one on one with a specialist teacher in a quiet environment, while others do not like this at all (Verdier, 2016). It is important to ensure that CYP with VI develop the specialist skills they require to achieve educationally, but careful consideration and planning needs to take place so as to not socially isolate CYP with VI further, particularly as limited positive interpersonal relationships may lead to low self-esteem and depression (Bailey, 2012). Equally, the views of CYP with VI need to be taken into consideration on how to best support them.

Specialist teachers have expressed concerns of having to fit in everything that needs to be done, such as ensuring access to an accessible broad curriculum, developing skills within the expanded/specialist curriculum, promoting social inclusion and ensuring CYP with VI have opportunities for self-directed activity, informal interactions with peers and time to rest. Some have observed that at times adults put so much emphasis on taking every opportunity to learn (in order to compensate for limited incidental learning) that little time is left to relax (and indeed for incidental social interaction to take place).

They have also expressed concerns about some CYP with VI who are overprotected by families and school staff or who experience over praising and/or over scaffolding, which seems to lead to limited initiative and self-determination. They refer to challenges in promoting social interaction, particularly when CYP with VI themselves do not seem motivated to interact with their peers. Sometimes the body language of CYPs with VI does not help either, e.g. keeping their head down, not facing people they are talking to etc. Overprotection can promote learned helplessness, which further limits opportunities to learn (Bailey, 2012).

Khadka et al. (2012) found that many CYP with VI spend more time inside and often spend time in their rooms after school. The same pattern was found when we interviewed CYP with VI. Some of them mentioned that they were tired after school. Specialist teachers mentioned, however, that this depended a lot on the family's capacity to provide opportunities to access extra school activities and whether they had the energy to take their CYP with VI to see friends or clubs, etc.

Views of CYP with VI

In interviews with CYP with VI they mentioned that adults tried their best to promote social interaction but often this did not work. Although they felt they needed support in class, they also felt that at times adults were providing support when they did not require it. One student mentioned that adults cannot help themselves, they want to see you doing well when in fact it is better not to intervene. He went on to give examples of adults supporting during lunch time and asking questions such as "Did you get that question right?" or "Is that nice?" which interrupted any opportunity to interact with peers.

Another issue mentioned was that they would like to have more time to chat with peers and they did not like having adults watching what they did and often interfering too much, particularly when concerned about their safety.

Some found it easier to interact and make friends in smaller primary schools, while others found it easier in secondary schools because there is less running around and more chatting to peers. Examples given of their friends were those who they felt understood their needs, sat next to them, discussed a topic with them or were interested in the equipment they used. But they could not expand on any details about these peers (what their peers are like or what their interests are). One student mentioned that he felt tolerated but did not always have real friends.

They mentioned that accessing adapted materials and keeping with the pace of work can make it harder for CYP with VI to work with others. Some also felt that independence training started too late and adults were doing too much for them. One student mentioned that it is important to experience some failure and learn to try again.

When asked about positive experiences they had, some CYP with VI could not always recall many of these. Examples given included one student who went for a sleepover with friends once and another student who felt included in a school activity, which involved peers asking questions about herself.

CYP with VI also mentioned some issues that helped them interact with others, such as accessing playground equipment that you can climb or swing on, organised support at school so that you can get on with learning, accessing peers' interests (one student used social media, which allowed her to have some understanding of what her peers liked and were interested in), opportunities to visit each other's houses and going to the garden or park.

Although CYP with VI mentioned interests that were similar to sighted young people, some of them were not able to expand on this. For example, often they were interested in music but they could not necessarily explain what type of music they liked nor name any particular bands. This limited knowledge can be a barrier to developing common interests with their peers.

Promoting inclusion and the development of social-emotional competence in educational settings

Promoting inclusion in educational settings requires a good understanding about how to create environments that facilitate interaction and the development of relationships, which lead to emotional well-being. Specialist teachers can provide information and training to professionals in educational settings to ensure that they understand the child's needs and effectively meet these. They can also contribute to the development of an inclusive ethos where differences are positively accepted.

Brown, Odom and Conroy (2001) propose a hierarchy of a continuum of interventions to support adults making decisions about how to promote young children's peer interactions and peer-related social competence. They refer to the importance of focusing on the least intrusive interventions before moving to more intensive interventions.

This hierarchy starts from classroom interventions (creating environments that promote interaction, influencing attitudes), to naturalistic interventions (incidental teaching of social behaviours, friendship activities), social integration activities where activities are planned to provide access to positive role models and explicit social skills training (Brown et al., 2001).

To promote inclusion, Buultjens and Stead (2002) refer to the importance of ensuring educational staff understand the needs of CYP with VI, support being available but discrete, having positive social interactions and friendships (for emotional well-being and protection from bullying), effective communication between everyone involved and ensuring that CYP with VI are involved in decisions that impact on them.

There is not a simple answer or a single way of promoting inclusion and social-emotional competence. It requires a flexible, reflective approach and adults play a critical role in making decisions on how best to promote the development of CYP with VI and evaluating the effectiveness of strategies and interventions used.

Next we will focus on some of the possible strategies and interventions including those that should be used incidentally. Specialist teachers can model how to sustain effective interactions, for example how to use strategies such as commenting, pondering and imagining (Fisher, 2016).

Commenting is a particularly effective strategy to provide information in a non-directive way, e.g. instead of an adult asking the child to check what another child is building (directive approach), the adult can make a comment on the activity of a peer and let the child take the initiative to find out more, ask questions or initiate interaction with the other child (indirect approach). Commenting provides an opportunity for CYP with VI to gain information they cannot access incidentally and make choices about whether to initiate interaction or not. Pondering invites the child to join in to find out more and opens their thinking. Pondering often involves asking questions such as "I wonder . . ." and "What if . . ." Imagining helps children to put themselves in someone else's position and consider different points of view.

In the early years, some CYP with VI do not engage easily in pretend play and may require a high level of scaffolding to do this. It may be useful to start with semi-structured activities, such as a simple familiar play sequence in a one-to-one situation using real objects and props, for example getting up in the morning and having breakfast. Then progressively introduce some peers or some changes in the play sequence to starting to create their own and collaborate with others with a focus on having fun. Adults need to have a good understanding of what the child already knows, what interests them and encourage them to take the lead. Children need to learn to play so that social interaction with peers can be facilitated (Celeste, 2007; Ozaydin, 2015).

Encouraging a realistic sense of themselves

The effective use of praise can help CYP with VI develop a realistic perception of themselves, which supports their sense of self-worth and self-efficacy (Bailey, 2012; Lewis and Wolffe, 2006; MacCuspie, 2006). Although praise can be seen as a way of encouraging the child, continuously providing unspecific praise does not promote a realistic sense of themselves. When interviewed, specialist teachers were very aware of the negative effects of too much praise. Effective praise can also help peers have a realistic perception of the child and support more equal relationships. The child's peers may also end up resenting them if they feel that the child with VI receives special treatment (MacCuspie, 2006). Careful consideration of when and how CYP with VI are expected to do things differently in order for them to be able to participate and access and when they should be treated the same as their peers is crucial to promote social inclusion.

In interviews, specialist teachers referred to the importance of encouraging analysis, self-evaluation and reflection on social situations that failed or succeeded, to enable CYP with VI to understand their strengths and what they are finding challenging; a point that is also supported by Sacks (2006). While being encouraging and maintaining interest and engagement, adults need to ensure children develop skills that build their resilience, allowing them to have a go, to fail and try again, encouraging them to learn about sustained effort and feel confident in their self efficacy (Silver, 2012).

Appropriate levels of scaffolding are important to ensure CYP with VI have opportunities to engage in discussions, argue and resolve conflict by themselves, which promotes cognitive gains and social competence. It is important that peers see the child with VI as an equal-status peer. Adults' overprotection interferes with the development of natural relationships and gives a message that CYP with VI are not as capable.

Silver (2012) refers to the importance of promoting autonomy in learning by providing choices, encouraging CYP with VI to try things and challenge themselves, presenting activities in the zone of proximal development, providing effective feedback (which provides specific information and is non-judgemental) and ensuring CYP with VI understand why they are learning a particular topic.

Learning to face challenges, persisting with a task and developing a growth mindset is important for all children. One of the young people with VI we interviewed, mentioned the importance of developing a mindset of becoming independent and trying again when facing challenges as he reflected on his experiences.

Learning social skills

Social skills can be taught through individual instruction, role play, peer mentoring, peer coaching, social skills training in small groups and the use of cooperative learning approaches (Erin, 2006; MacCuspie, 2006; Schneider, 2000).

Individual instruction enables CYP with VI to discuss issues, raise awareness of self and others, to plan next steps, practise skills and reflect and evaluate on their progress. Help from peers can be supportive in developing these by sharing experiences and receiving feedback. It is important that CYP with VI understand that everyone makes mistakes and needs to learn these skills. Getting things wrong, worrying about new experiences or times of transition is part of life and sighted CYP experience these as well.

Specific sessions to teach social skills have had mixed results, it can help raise awareness and provide opportunities to share ideas with peers but skills learnt are not easily transferred to more natural contexts and some studies have found they can have a negative impact on peer acceptance (Odom et al., 1999; Schneider, 2000). Specialist teachers interviewed mentioned that small group sessions can be helpful but they are only a small part of the intervention required and do not replace real experiences in natural contexts.

Cooperative learning is one of the most effective processes available to promote social inclusion and cognitive gains. It involves CYP working towards a specific learning outcome, taking individual accountability and sharing responsibility for shared goals (D'Allura, 2002; MacCuspie, 2006; Schneider, 2000). In cooperative learning CYP are not competing with each other as the focus is on group achievement and equally that each member of the group is able to answer any question, so they tend to include each other as success is dependent on everyone in the group being able to provide answers for the group.

Learning to cooperate with others is an essential skill for life, understanding group dynamics, roles and responsibilities within a group, understanding reciprocity and shared responsibilities within a group. It is crucial that young people develop the required skills to be able to collaborate with others effectively. This includes developing a theory of mind that enables them to consider the feelings of others and understand their psychological states.

Self-determination

CYP with VI need to have opportunities to develop self-determination from an early age, they need to learn to make choices, to speak for themselves in a socially appropriate way and develop confidence in communicating with others in an assertive way. They need to have an age-appropriate understanding of their own condition, how it affects them and what they need to be able to access and participate.

They may need encouragement to find out what choices are there so that they can make their individual choices and feel that they have control over these (Rosenblum, 2006). Adults need to ensure that support does not interfere with the development of self-determination. If adults tend to direct children's activities and they have little experience of making choices and taking decisions for themselves, it is harder to suddenly be expected to be able to do so in their natural contexts.

Opportunities to access out-of-school activities

It is important to support and encourage families to provide opportunities for CYP with VI to meet peers, attend clubs, extra-school activities, parties and family events. They need to be allowed to experience risk, try new experiences and meet new people, etc. These activities may also provide opportunities to meet peers with similar interests and practise social skills in a range of contexts, as well as to become independent and develop a sense of efficacy.

Families may have varying capacity to provide these opportunities as accessing these may depend on where they live, their financial situation and individual context. They may need support to ensure they feel confident in promoting their child's independence.

Supportive family environments and friendships seem to play a crucial role in increasing resilience by improving coping performance, having a positive effect on self-esteem, self-regulation and providing stress relief (van Harmelen et al., 2016).

Peer culture and peer influence

As young people develop, peers become increasingly important in their lives. Peer influence is often considered a concern as at this stage peer culture places a lot of value on becoming independent from parents' control and parents may be concerned about their child becoming involved in risky or deviant behaviours. However, to become a well-socialised individual requires that individual to be influenced by peers and to behave in a way that they find acceptable (Allen and Antonishak, 2008). Increasing the sense of engagement with their peer group can actually be a protection factor against risky behaviour (Allen and Antonishak, 2008).

CYP with VI need to understand their peer culture to support the development of friendships. This requires access to information about their peers' interests, hobbies, what music, books or TV series they enjoy, what sports they play or follow and provides themes for conversations and joint interests and activities. It also enables CYP with VI to make choices about what their own interests are and compare these to those of their peers.

Developing relationships with other people with VI provides opportunities to share experiences and strategies that support them and reduce their sense of isolation. Accessing positive role models, face to face or through media, can give a sense of what is possible and inspire CYP with VI to achieve. Again this is an important issue that has been mentioned by specialist teachers.

Learning environment

Promoting social interaction with peers requires a lot of sensitivity by adults who are more likely to be successful in promoting this by observing, standing back and listening rather than intervening directly. While standing back, they are allowing children to find their own strategies, to have a go at resolving conflict and build resilience. Adults can then create opportunities for reflection by analysing recent events and situations.

Adults have a crucial role in promoting social-emotional development when planning educational provision for CYP with VI. Creating environments that promote interaction require consideration of the physical layout, the social context, resources used and the type of activity (Brown et al., 2001; D'Allura, 2002; Rettig, 1994; Roe, 2008; Webster and Roe, 1998).

Specialist teachers can work with other educational staff to ensure effective planning and ensure learning activities take into consideration the needs of CYP with VI from the start. This involves making sure that activities are relevant, accessible, hands-on as much as possible and can be shared with sighted peers. This will ensure that right from the beginning everything is in place to enable CYP with VI to participate and any potential barriers to interaction are minimised. It also involves ensuring seating arrangements and location of equipment do not create a barrier to interaction. Having to access a power point or large pieces of equipment may leave few options about where to sit. An organised consistent physical environment enables CYP with VI to be more independent in moving around and getting resources. Planning should also involve enabling CYP with VI to work with sighted peers who have good social and language skills, providing opportunities to access good role models.

Social inclusion can be further developed by increasing peers' level of understanding of the needs of CYP with VI. This has to be done sensitively and with the involvement of CYP with VI so that they take decisions about which information they would like to share, whether they would like information provided by themselves or someone else, etc.

Conclusion

Vision impairment can impact on many areas of development. From the very beginning, social-emotional development is an area that may be at risk and it is crucial to understand the significance of relationships and consider how these are being established and nurtured throughout the lives of CYP with VI. It is also crucial that learning is not too narrowly focused on academic achievement but on a wider curriculum.

Even if certain interventions are used to support development in this area, this is not just something to be delivered at a particular point, it requires an ongoing development of relationships in order to create an environment where different people are valued, where the way language is used provides supportive messages of encouragement but also realistic feedback and opportunities for reflection, an environment that encourages CYP with VI to have a go, fail and try again rather than overprotecting and that promotes independence and leads to a positive sense of self-efficacy and well-being.

Acknowledgement

I would like to thank all the children and young people who over the years have taught me so much about their interests and how they learn and for contributing their views to develop our understanding. I would also like to thank my colleagues for our joint learning and for those who shared their views for the purpose of writing this chapter: Sue Rogers, Marion Donaldson, Clare Gordon, Nathan Meager and Amit Sadh.

References

Allen, J.P. and Antonishak, J. 2008. Adolescent peer influences: Beyond the dark side. In M.J Prinstein and K.A Dodge, *Understanding peer influences in children and adolescents*. New York: Guilford.

Andersen, E.S., Dunlea, A. and Kekelis, L. 1993. The impact of input: Language acquisition in the visually impaired. *First Language*, 13, 23–50.

Aviles, A.M., Anderson, T.R. and Davila, E.R. 2006. Child and adolescent social-emotional development within the context of school. *Child and Adolescent Mental Health*, 11(1), 32–39.

Azmitia 1988. Peer interaction and problem solving: When are two heads better than one? *Child Development*, 59, 87–96.

Bailey, G. 2012. *Emotional well-being for children with special educational needs and disabilities*. London: Sage.

Brown, W.H., Odom, S.L. and Conroy, M.A. 2001. An intervention hierarchy for promoting young children's peer interactions in natural environments. *Topics in Early Childhood Special Education*, 21(3), 162–175.

Bruce, T. 2004. *Developing learning in early childhood*. London: Sage

Buultjens, M. and Stead, J. 2002. *Promoting social inclusion of pupils with visual impairment in mainstream schools in Scotland*. Report on project funded by Scottish Executive Education Department. Edinburgh: Scottish Sensory Centre.

Celeste, M. 2007. Social skills intervention for a child who is blind. *Journal of Visual Impairment and Blindness*, 101(9), 521–533.

Celeste, M and Grum, D.K. 2010. Social integration of children with visual impairment: A developmental model. *Elementary Education Online*, 9(1), 11–22.

Coplan, R.J. and Arbeau, K.A. 2009. Peer interactions and play in early childhood. In K.H. Rubin, W.M. Bukowski and B. Laursen (eds), *Handbook of peer interactions, relationships and groups*. New York: Guilford Press.

D'Allura, T. 2002. Enhancing the social interaction skills of preschoolers with visual impairment. *Journal of Visual Impairment and Blindness*, 96(8), 576–584.

Dale, N. and Salt, A. 2008. Social identity, autism and visual impairment in the early years. *British Journal of Visual Impairment*, 26(2), 135–146.

Dowling, M. 2014. *Young children's personal, social and emotional development* (4th ed.). London: Sage.

Dunn, J. 1993. *Young children's close relationships: Beyond attachment.* London: Sage.

Dunn, J. 2004. *Children's friendships.* Oxford: Blackwell.

Eckerman, C.O. 1993. Imitation and toddler's achievement of co-ordinated action with others. In J. Nadel and L. Camioni (eds), *New perspectives in early communicative development.* London: Routledge.

Ely, M.S. 2014. Effective strategies for preschool peer group entry: Considered applications for children with visual impairments. *Journal of Visual Impairment and Blindness,* July–August, 287–297.

Erin, J.N. 2006. Teaching social skills to elementary and middle school students with visual impairment. In S.Z. Sacks and K.E. Wolfe (eds), *Teaching social skills to students with visual impairments: From theory to practice.* New York: American Foundation for the Blind.

Ferguson, R. and Buultjens, M. 1995. The play behaviour of young blind children and its relationship to developmental stages. *British Journal of Visual Impairment,* 13(3), 100–107.

Fisher, J. 2016. *Interacting or interfering? Improving interactions in the early years.* Berkshire, UK: Open University Press, McGraw-Hill Education.

Garvey, C. 1990. *Play.* Cambridge MA: Harvard University Press.

Gauvain, M. 2001. *The social context of cognitive development.* New York: Guilford Press.

Harris, J., Keil, S., Lord, C. and Lloyd, C.L. 2014. *Sight impairment at age eleven: Secondary analysis of the Millennium Cohort Survey.* London: NatCen Social Research.

Hartup, 1992. Friendships and their developmental significance. In H. McGurk (ed.), *Childhood social development.* Hove, UK: Lawrence Erlbaum.

Howes, C. 2009. Friendship in early childhood. In K.H. Rubin, W.M Bukowski and B. Laursen (eds), *Handbook of peer interactions, relationships and groups.* New York: Guilford Press.

Kekelis, L.S. 2006. A filed study of a blind preschooler. In S.Z. Sacks and K.E. Wolffe (eds), *Teaching social skills to students with visual impairment: From theory to practice.* New York: American Foundation for the Blind.

Kekelis, L.S. and Andersen, 1984. Family communication styles and language development. *Journal of Visual Impairment and Blindness,* 78(2), 54–65.

Kekelis, L.S. and Sacks, S.Z. 1992. The effects of visual impairment on children's social interactions in regular education programs. In S.Z. Sacks, L. Kekelis and R.J. Gaylord-Ross (eds), *The development of social skills by blind and visually impaired students.* New York: American Foundation for the Blind.

Khadka, J., Ryan, B., Margrain, T.H., Woodhouse, J.M. and Davies, N. 2012. Listening to the voices of children with a visual impairment: A focus group study. *British Journal of Visual Impairment,* 30(3), 82–196.

Ladd, G.W. 2005. *Children's peer relations and social competence.* New Haven, CT: Yale University Press.

LaVenture, S., Lesner, J. and Zabelski, M. 2006. A family perspective on social skills development. In S.Z. Sacks and K.E. Wolffe (eds), *Teaching social skills to students with visual impairment: From theory to practice.* New York: American Foundation for the Blind.

Lavoie, R. 2005. *Helping the child with learning disabilities find social success: It's so much work to be your friend.* New York: Touchstone.

Lewis, S. and Wolffe, K.E. 2006. Promoting and nurturing self-esteem. In S.Z. Sacks and K.E. Wolffe (eds), *Teaching social skills to students with visual impairment: From theory to practice.* New York: American Foundation for the Blind

Limbrick, P. 2017. *Early childhood intervention without tears.* Clifford, UK: Interconnections.

MacCuspie, P.A. 1992. The social acceptance and interaction of visually impaired children in integrated settings. In S.Z. Sacks, L. Kekelis and R.J. Gaylord-Ross (eds), *The development of social skills by blind and visually impaired students.* New York: American Foundation for the Blind.

MacCuspie P.A. 2006. Social skills in school and community. In S.Z. Sacks and K.E. Wolffe (eds), *Teaching social skills to students with visual impairment: From theory to practice.* New York: American Foundation for the Blind.

Maguire, M.C. and Dunn, J. 1997. Friendships in early childhood, and social understanding. *International Journal of Behavioral Development,* 21(4), 669–686.

Odom, S.L., McConnell, S.R., McEvoy, M.A., Peterson, C., Ostrosky, M., Spicuzza, R.J., Skellenger, A., Creighton, M. and Favazza, P.C. 1999. Relative effects of interventions supporting the social competence of young children with disabilities. *Topics of Early Childhood Special Education,* 19(2), 75–91.

Ozaydin, L. 2015. Teaching play skills to visually impaired preschool children: Its effect on social interaction. *Educational Sciences: Theory & Practice,* 15(4), 1021–1038.

Perez-Pereira, M. and Conti-Ramsden, G. 1999. *Language development and social interaction in blind children.* Hove, UK: Psychology Press.

Preisler, G.M. 1991. Blind infant – sighted mother: Interaction during the first year. *International Journal of Rehabilitation Research,* 14(3), 231–234.

Preisler, G.M. 1993. A descriptive study of blind children in nurseries with sighted children. *Child, Care, Health and Development*, 19(5), 295–315.

Preisler, G.M. 1997. Social and emotional development of blind children: A longitudinal study. In V. Lewis and G.M. Collis (eds), *Blindness and the psychological development in young children*. Leicester, UK: British Psychological Society Books.

Rettig, M. 1994. The play of young children with visual impairments: Characteristics and interventions. *Journal of Visual Impairment and Blindness*, 88(5), 410–420.

Roe, J. 1998. *Peer relationships, play and language of visually impaired children*. Unpublished PhD thesis. Bristol University, UK.

Roe, J. 2008. Social inclusion: Meeting the socio-emotional needs of children with vision needs. *British Journal of Visual Impairment*, 26(2), 147–158.

Rogoff, B. 1991. The joint socialization of development by young children and adults. In P. Light, S. Sheldon and M. Woodhead (eds), *Learning to think*. London: Routledge.

Rosenblum, L.P. 2006. Developing friendships and positive social relationships. In S.Z. Sacks and K.E. Wolffe (eds), *Teaching social skills to students with visual impairments: From theory to practice*. New York: American Foundation for the Blind.

Rubin, K.H., Fein, G.G. and Vanderberg, B. 1983. Play. In P.H. Mussen and E.M. Hetherington (eds), *Handbook of child psychology* (4th ed., vol. IV). New York, Wiley.

Sacks, S.Z. 2006. Teaching social skills to young children with visual impairments. In S.Z. Sacks and K.E. Wolffe (eds), *Teaching social skills to students with visual impairment: From theory to practice*. New York: American Foundation for the Blind.

Sacks, S.Z., Kekelis, L. and Gaylord-Ross, R.J. (eds). 1992. *The development of social skills by blind and visually impaired students*. New York: American Foundation for the Blind.

Sacks, S.Z. and Silberman, R.K. 2000. Social skills. In A.J. Koenig and M.C. Holbrook (eds), *Foundations of education. Volume II: Instructional strategies for teaching children and youths with visual impairments* (2nd ed.). New York: American Foundation for the Blind.

Sacks, S.Z. and Wolffe, K.E. (eds). 2006. *Teaching social skills to students with visual impairment: From theory to practice*. New York: American Foundation for the Blind.

Salleh, N.M. and Zainal, K. 2010. How and why the visually impaired students socially behave the way they do. *Procedia Social and Behavioral Sciences*, 9, 859–863

Schneider, B.H. 2000. *Friends and enemies: Peer relations in childhood*. London, Arnold.

Silkenbeumer, J., Schiller, E.-M. and Holodynski, M.K. 2016. The role of co-regulation for the development of social-emotional competence. *Journal of Self-Regulation and Regulation*, 2, 16–33

Silver, D. 2012. *Fall down 7 times get up 8: Teaching kids to succeed*, Thousand Oaks, CA: Corwin.

Squires, J.K., Waddell, M.L., Clifford, J.R., Funk, K., Hoseton, R.M. and Chen, C.-I. 2012. A psychometric study of the infant and toddler intervals of the social emotional assessment measure. *Topics in Early Childhood Special Education* 33(2), 78–90.

Sroufe, A.L. 1995. *Emotional development: The organization of emotional life in the early years*. Cambridge: Cambridge University Press

van den Broek, E.G.C., van Eijden, A.J.P.M., Overbeek, M.M., Kef, S., Sterkenburg, P.S. and Schuengel, C. 2017. A systematic review of the literature on parenting of young children with visual impairment and the adaptions for video-feedback intervention to promote positive parenting (VIPP). *Journal of Developmental Physical Disabilities*, 29, 503–545.

van Harmelen, A.-L., Gibson, J.L., St Clair, M.C., Owens, M., Brodbeck, J., Dunn, V., Lewis, G., Croudace, T., Jones, T.B., Kievit, R.A. and Goodyer, I.M. 2016. Friendships and family support reduce subsequent depressive symptoms in at-risk adolescents. *PLoS ONE*, 11(5), e0153715. doi:10.1371/journal.pone.0153715

Verdier, K. 2016. Inclusion in and out of the classroom: A longitudinal study of students with visual impairments in inclusive education. *British Journal of Visual Impairment*, 34(2), 132–142.

Vygostky, L. 1978. *Mind in society: The development of higher psychological processes*. Cambridge, MA: Harvard University Press.

Webster, A. and Roe, J. 1998. *Children with visual impairments: Social interaction, language and learning*. London, Routledge.

20

Self-esteem of people with visual impairment

Samir Qasim

Introduction

This chapter will begin with definition of self-esteem. However, to understand self-esteem, it is essential to clearly distinguish between self-concept and self-esteem. After that, I will critically discuss the notion of a self-esteem construct. It seems impossible to understand the meaning of self-esteem and how it develops and functions unless addressing different self domains. Therefore, a multidimensional hierarchical concept of self-esteem will be presented. Within this topic, I shall discuss how different domains may (or may not) impact global self-esteem. This will introduce us to the importance of self-esteem; we need to know whether, as believed by many people, high self-esteem is good and does low self-esteem leave undesired consequences on human health. Following this, I will present up-to-date studies that have addressed self-esteem of children, adolescents and young adults with visual impairment (VI). As will be made clear in the chapter, there still appears to be a contradiction as to whether this population have lower self-esteem than their sighted peers. Importantly, reasons for believing that people with VI have relatively low self-esteem will be identified and discussed. At the end of this chapter, I will present the strategies for self-esteem improvement of the general population followed by my view, based on the recent findings, regarding self-esteem improvement of people with VI.

Definition of self-esteem

Self-esteem has been extensively explored although there is a complexity and disagreement about its terminology, definition, how it functions and develops (Brown, 2014). For example, both "self-concept" and "self-esteem" have been used to define self-esteem itself although each term appears to have its own definition (Pavey, 2009). The importance of identifying differences among these two terms lies in the researcher's ability to identify very clearly which term is accurately described and thus used in their study. To avoid synonymously using terms there is a necessity to carefully differentiate among these terms and to know how the concept of each term is related to another (Berger, Pargman and Weinberg, 2002). One attempt at defining these terms was made by Fox (1997) when he distinguished between self-concept and self-esteem. For Fox (1997), self-concept means the individual as known to the individual.

This is a self-description profile based on the multitude of rules and attributes that make up our self. Self-concept answers the question "Who am I?" such as "I am a teacher" or only describes the individual "I like sports" and does not demonstrate elevation of the self (Harter, 2012). Importantly, self-concept is a multidimensional construct that contains more specific perceptions across various domains than a singular domain such as academic, social and physical (Shapiro and Martin, 2010).

Self-esteem itself, however, has also been explained differently. Brown and Marshall (2006) reported three ways the term self-esteem has been used: global self-esteem, feelings of self-worth and self-evaluations. Global self-esteem is the evaluative element of one's perception. It has been identified as a global construct that provides an overall statement of the degree to which an individual perceives himself or herself to be an "OK" person, dependent on whatever criteria that individual uses to determine "OK" (Fox, 1997). According to some researchers (Crocker and Park, 2004; Sherrill, 2004), global self-esteem is a decision about whether people feel worth about themselves. The other commonly used term, self-worth, refers to self-evaluative emotional reactions such as feeling pleased, proud or ashamed (Brown and Marshall, 2006). Lastly, self-esteem has been expressed through people's self-evaluations of their abilities.

To summarise this section, self-esteem answers the question "How do I feel about myself?" (Lindwall and Asci, 2014). This answer may be given within different life perceptions reflecting the general concept of self or self domains that have been explained previously. In other words, self-esteem is an evaluation of the person's perception of self-concept (Stanwyck, 1983) according to his/her own standards. Self-esteem is subjective evaluation of the self and does not necessarily reflect the reality (Baumeister et al., 2003). This means that a person may believe that they are intelligent regardless of IQ test results. This evaluation of self, however, may be expressed through two different dimensions; either within a general orientation towards the self or evaluating the self within one life domain such as academic, athletic and intellectual. According to Harter (2012) this distinction between global self-esteem and specific self-esteem domain enables people to address particular domains that may be more predictive of global self-esteem than the others, as will be explained next.

Construct of self-esteem

Similar to Harter's (2012) multidimensional concept of the self, self-esteem is considered as an evaluative component of each of these self-components (Byrne, 1996). For instance, a perception of being a student or a person in society is evaluated academically and socially, respectively. This means that a person can evaluate themselves highly in one domain and low in others (Lindwall and Asci, 2014). Global self-esteem, however, is a result of evaluations across these life areas. This model of a multidimensional hierarchical construct of self-esteem was proposed first over 40 years ago by Shavelson, Hubner and Stanton (1976) and has been examined by subsequent research. For example, two studies designed by Vallerand, Pelletier and Gagné (1991) aimed to investigate whether self-esteem is a unidimensional or multidimensional construct. In the first study, their aim was to examine if students with better academic performance and higher IQ score (talented students) differ from those with lower academic and IQ achievements (regular students) in actual school competence and in general self-esteem. Students (n = 173) with a mean age of 10.12 years participated in the study. They used the Perceived Competence Scale for Children (PCS). This scale is made up of four subscales: a global self-esteem subscale, the cognitive (school), physical (sports/physical activity) and a social subscale. Each subscale consists of seven items. The PCS showed high reliability and validity measures. The results showed that talented students had significant differences only in the cognitive (school) competence subscale without differences in the global self-esteem subscale. In the other study, following the same methodology and measurements, Vallerand et al. (1991) aimed to compare unidimensional with multidimensional views of self-esteem in the sports domain. Swimmers (n = 82) with a mean age of 13.32 years participated in the study. Swimmers who had achieved the national standards were qualified as talented and those who were members of swimming clubs and had not reached national standards were qualified as regular swimmers. The results showed that talented swimmers had better results only on the physical and swimming subscales whereas no significant differences were found in the global self-esteem measure.

It is not surprising therefore, to find that a multidimensional hierarchical concept of self-esteem has been widely accepted and supported later on in the literature in different psychological disciplines, particularly educational and developmental psychology, mental health research, personal research and sports and exercise psychology (Boyd and Hrycaiko, 1997; Marsh, 1990; Marsh, Craven and Martin, 2006; Sabiston, Whitehead and Eklund, 2012). Therefore, global self-esteem should be clearly distinguished from different self domains. However, it is not clear in the literature whether global self-esteem represents the sum total of different life domains (bottom–up approach) or global self-esteem influences these domains (up–bottom approach) (Suls, 2006).

Such a multidimensional hierarchical construct of self-esteem means that different types of self-esteem exist within one person across different life stages (Marsh et al., 2006). When I say life stages, I mean those aged 8 years and older, as only children from this age can comprehend they are someone who can express their feelings, distinguish among different domains of their self-esteem and value the importance of each domain (Harter, 2006). Consequently, Harter contributed to designing self-esteem measurements that include a global measure of self-esteem in addition to separate measures of the individual's perceived competence in different life domains for children (Harter, 1985), adolescents (Harter, 1988), college students (Neemann and Harter, 1986), and adults (Messer and Harter, 1986). According to these measurement scales, life domains that have been identified as closely related to global self-esteem vary according to the age stage although social, athletic, physical and intellectual domains exist across all life stages.

It has been argued that in addition to global self-esteem, children perceive the following five domains: scholastic competence, social competence, athletic competence, physical appearance and behavioural conduct (Harter, 1985). On the other hand, global self-esteem and eight domains are experienced by adolescents: scholastic competence, behavioural conduct, social acceptance, physical appearance, athletic competence, romantic, close friendship and job competence (Harter, 1988). Global self-esteem of college students and adults may be affected by the 12 and 11 domains respectively (Messer and Harter, 1986; Neemann and Harter, 1986).

Importantly, feeling competent in one domain does not seem to entail generalisation to the other domains or to global self-esteem. It may be possible for individuals to change in a certain domain without affecting global self-esteem. Indeed, global self-esteem is more stable compared to its domains (Shavelson et al., 1976). Only domains of high personal importance exert a strong effect on global self-esteem while evaluations in the domains of low personal importance do not (Brown and Marshall, 2006; Harter, 1999). Figure 20.1 demonstrates how different life domains may be related to global self-esteem according to their importance.

Figure 20.1 shows that only those self-esteem domains that are perceived to be important may affect, either positively or negatively, global self-esteem. By contrast, unimportant domains do not cause any change in global self-esteem. A question that may exist here is what would happen if a person achieves contradictory scores in two different, perceived as important, self-esteem domains? In such cases, more important domains will have a stronger

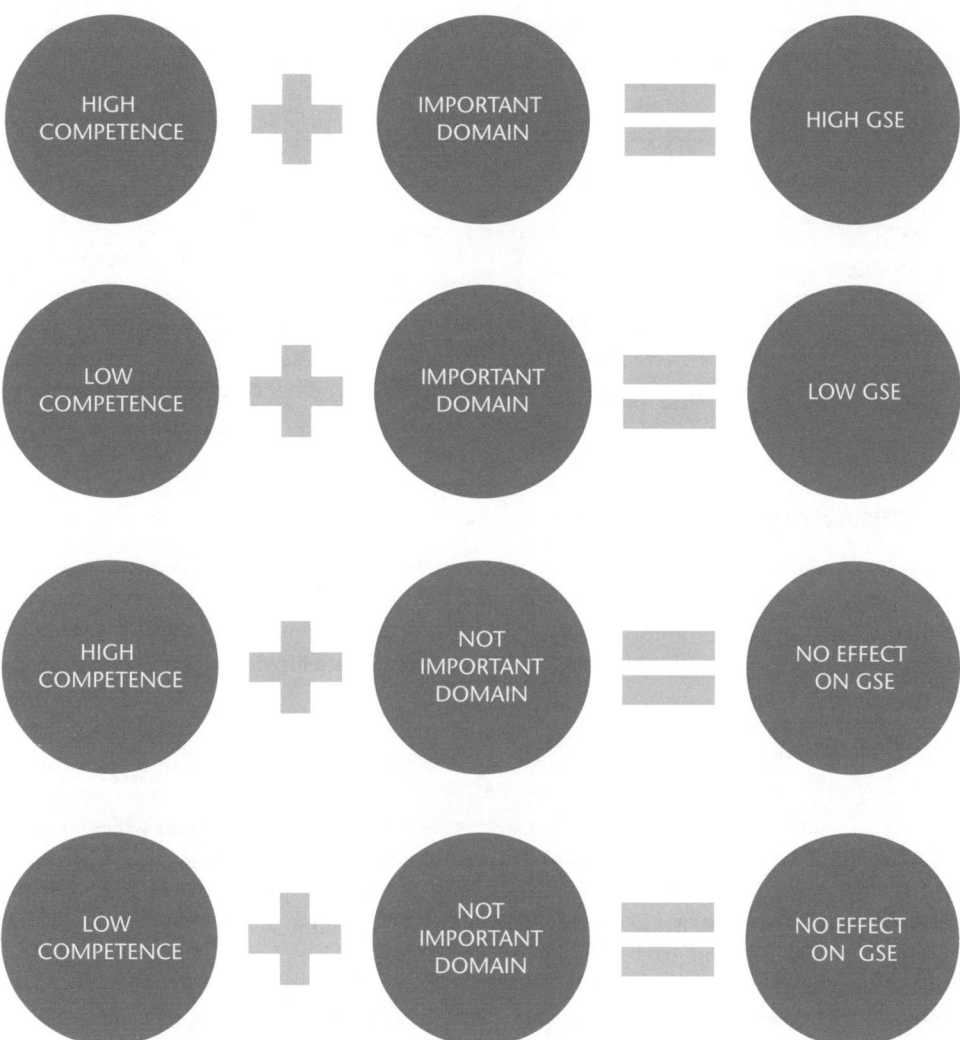

Figure 20.1 The effect of different self-esteem domains on the global self-esteem according to their importance (*GSE* = global self-esteem).

impact on global self-esteem. For example, a person may have low social but high physical self-esteem. Consequently, for the purposes of measuring global self-esteem we can use scales that were developed only for that purpose, such as Rosenberg's Self-Esteem Inventory (Rosenberg, 1965). However, these scales will not provide us with the reasons for potential low self-esteem or how to improve self-esteem. Therefore, to improve global self-esteem we need to identify domains that are perceived to be low by a person but at the same time considered as important (Harter, 1999).

As a result, in addition to the perceived competence of the self domains, a perceived importance profile (PIP) questionnaire for all age groups has been developed by Harter and colleagues (Harter 1985, 1988; Messer and Hart, 1986; Neemann and Harter, 1986). The importance of the PIP questionnaire exists in that if a person considers one domain (e.g. an athletic competence) as unimportant, then that domain score is unlikely to have a negative/positive effect on overall physical self-esteem. A discrepancy score has been recommended to be calculated differently as follows:

Discrepancy score = mean of the importance ratings – the mean of the competence scores

Fox (1990) argues that measuring perceived importance alongside self-perception is necessary to improve understanding of the mechanisms of self-esteem development. Additionally, decreasing the importance of domains with low competence is one of the strategies for avoiding low self-esteem (Harter, 2006) as will be expanded later in this chapter. Before that, however, it is necessary to identify why we should focus on boosting self-esteem and whether self-esteem (low or high) causes significant outcomes in life. Therefore, the importance of self-esteem will be addressed next.

The importance of self-esteem

People seek for success in different life domains in order to experience high self-esteem and avoid low self-esteem (Crocker, Moeller and Burson, 2010), particularly in those domains with high expectation of success. According to James' (1890) self-esteem theory, self-esteem is a result of a relationship between one's achievements and one's aspirations following a formula of:

$$Self\text{-}esteem = \frac{Success}{Pretension}$$

This formula indicates that if a person has success in his own goals then high self-esteem will ensue. Importantly, supporting the meaning of self-esteem that has been described at the beginning of this chapter, this theory also reflects subjective success as it is perceived by an individual and not objective success; which means that self-esteem becomes affected according to the individual's satisfaction and not comparing to the other.

Furthermore, teachers, parents and therapists have been extensively working on self-esteem improvement of their students, children and clients. In addition, self-esteem, namely global self-esteem, has been identified in the literature as one of the most frequently reported psychosocial measurements (Trzesniewski, Donnellan and Robins, 2003). Bleidorn et al. (2016) estimate that over 35,000 publications have addressed self-esteem. Researchers' interest to focus on self-esteem function may be due to its importance as people evaluate themselves daily and this influences their role in society. Consequently, it is important to describe how high/low self-esteem is related to different life domains and life outcomes.

Self-esteem has been identified as one of the main factors for human functioning and performance that is related to general well-being and mental health (Buckworth et al., 2013; Lindwall and Asci, 2014). Furthermore, self-esteem is a crucial component in a child's growth and development (King, 1997; Olsen, Breckler and Wiggens, 2008) since high self-esteem is positively associated with personal, mental and social health among children and adolescents (Torres, Fernandez and Maceira, 1995). High self-esteem is also linked to increased academic achievement, improved health, productive behaviour (Daglas-Pelish, 2006), happiness and life satisfaction (Harter, 1993; Lindwall and Asci, 2014).

Conversely, low self-esteem may be a precipitating factor of unhealthy behaviour (Hayes and Fors, 1990). Low self-esteem has also been identified as a possible risk factor for depression

(Harter, 1993; Peden et al., 2000) and can result in the development of behavioural disorders (Egan and Perry, 1998; Mann et al., 2004).

Although self-esteem is related to a wide range of important consequences in life; teachers, administrators and parents should be cautious and not incorrectly view low self-esteem as the cause of all negative behaviours and high self-esteem as the cause of all positive behaviours (Manning, Bear and Minke, 2006).

Self-esteem of children and adolescents with visual impairment

A relatively low number of studies have investigated self-esteem (not self-concept) levels of children and adolescents with visual impairment (VI) (those with visual impairment and blindness). This issue becomes more complicated taking into account that some studies examined general self-esteem of children and adolescents with VI (e.g. Kef, 2002) whereas others also included specific self-esteem domains (e.g. Shapiro et al., 2008). Due to such low number of studies it is difficult to distinguish between levels of global self-esteem and self-esteem domains. Consequently, I will discuss below self-esteem including global and particular self domains together.

Generally, Obiakor and Stile (1990) argued that little evidence exists that proves that children and adolescents with VI have lower self-esteem than sighted peers regardless of their age. By contrast, children with VI have greater difficulty with the development of social skills, which may decrease their self-esteem (Jindal-Snape, 2004). Moreover, Pierce and Wardle (1996) claimed that children and adolescents with VI may have lower self-esteem as children with VI are often excluded, isolated and have limited contact with their peers (Kroksmark and Nordell, 2001; Wagner, 2004). According to Tuttle and Tuttle (2004), enough evidence supports the idea that children and adolescents with VI face social exclusion. They further argue that social domain is one of the crucial factors for self-esteem as self-esteem for children and adolescents with VI emerge from their interactions with both physical and social environments. It is not surprising to find that children and adolescents with VI have limited social contact with their sighted peers, as research has found that children with impairments (including those with VI) often experience bullying (Bourke and Burgman, 2010). Moreover, Horwood et al. (2005) found that 35%–37% of people who wear glasses are more likely to be bullied compared to those who do not. Similarly, Pinquart and Pfeiffer (2011) found that adolescents with VI reported higher levels of victimisation than students without VI. Consequently, being stigmatised may lead to social exclusion, and importantly low self-esteem, since people with impairments would try to avoid discrimination. Also, studies have found that children who had a tendency to be bullied had lower self-esteem ($p = 0.001$) (Rigby and Slee, 1993), felt sad ($p < 0.0001$) (Williams et al., 1996) and were less happy in the school context (Boulton and Underwood, 1992). These findings were supported by Qasim (2015) who reported that people with VI were bullied and teased in school, which reflected negatively on their global self-esteem. One of the participants in Qasim's study said:

> At the age of seven I was at school and, erm, kids started to tease me about the way I look. Erm, they started to bully me about, you know, basically all sorts of things about my glasses, the shape of my face, and all this stuff. And it was destroying my self-esteem. And at that point in my life I had, or so I am told, I don't really remember all this, but so I am told I really just didn't want to be me, and I wanted to be other people that, that didn't look different, had their full sight, all that sort of stuff.

> *(Qasim, 2015, p. 170)*

311

Thus, it is important to understand that being physically together with sighted persons does not necessarily mean that children with VI are included (Nixon, 1989). Inclusion is based on the principle of valuing diversity, a feeling of acceptance, belonging and being supported. Although inclusion may be promoted through different forms such as social or physical, these two types of inclusion are different (Sherrill and Williams, 1996). Inclusion is important for people with VI but needs to be seen in the context of feeling valued, respected, loved and dependent. Students need to feel accepted, loved and appreciated for both what they can and cannot do (Sherrill, 2004). Social inclusion therefore has been described as a frequent pleasant interaction between the students who contribute to feelings of acceptance, respect and value (Spencer-Cavaliere and Watkinson, 2010) without stigmatising and potentially disabling (Nixon, 1989). Importantly, the love and belonging needs to involve both giving and receiving affection (Maslow, 1987), which is a precondition for achieving a satisfied level of self-esteem (Figure 20.2).

According to Maslow's hierarchical theory, unless people feel accepted and loved they will not feel a satisfaction of the self-esteem needs, such as self-confidence, self-worth, capability, adequacy and of being useful in the world. In agreement with Maslow's hierarchical theory of self-actualisation, multidimensional self-esteem scales contain a social domain across childhood, adolescence and adulthood that reflects people's need for feeling that they belong and are accepted through social satisfaction and the ability and desire to meet new people. It is

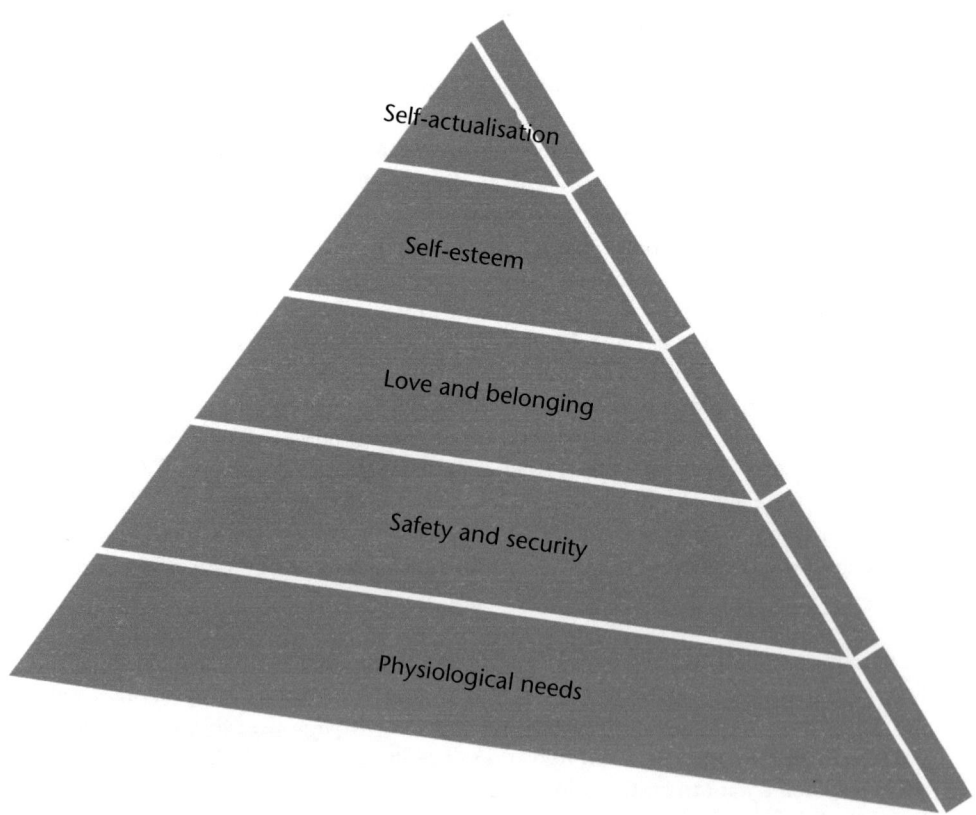

Figure 20.2 Maslow's hierarchy of human needs.

important to remember however, that self-esteem has been considered as a wider concept than the one that was proposed by Maslow. As a multidimensional construct, different domains may impact global self-esteem and not only social domain.

Regardless of these social barriers, Bigelow (2003) argued that a deficit in one domain related to the child's development (loss of sight) influences different life and personal developmental domains, such as self-esteem. This issue was expanded by Lowenfeld (1981) who described that due to their impaired vision, children with VI have a limited range and variety of experience, limited ability to move independently and limited control of the environment. Furthermore, a few people with VI reported that they faced self-esteem issues because they became visually impaired or blind and were consequently dependent. For example, Paul (pseudonym) explained his difficulties and feelings as he started becoming blind:

> It was very difficult to deal with, because most people as we're born, we are individual creatures. We like to do things by our self, and as my sight got worse, that got taken away from me and I had to depend on the other people and I'll be honest with you, I didn't like it. Because I felt myself asking more and more for help with everything from eating because I couldn't see my food anymore to writing, I couldn't write, couldn't read a book so other people would have to read for me so now I can't read or write. Couldn't see TV so people were now talking all the time telling me what's going on TV. Even when you need a toilet, you have to ask somebody to take you to the toilet. And it became too much, it's a lot to deal with, you have to be strong to deal with that.
>
> *(Qasim, 2015, p. 171)*

In fact, in the literature of self-esteem and children and adolescents with VI there appears to be a contradiction (Augestad, 2017; Datta, 2014). For example, the following five studies have used different measurements of self-esteem to investigate self-esteem levels of children and adolescents with VI: Rosenberg Self-Esteem Inventory (Garaigordobil and Bernarás, 2009; Huurre, 2000; Kef, 2002) and Coopersmith's Self-Esteem Inventory (Griffin-Shirley and Nes, 2005). All of these five studies found that participants with VI had similar levels of self-esteem as their sighted peers. Interestingly, Kef (2002) found that adolescents with VI had higher self-esteem than their sighted peers. By contrast, Gronmo and Augestad (2000) found that children and adolescents with VI have lower global self-esteem than their sighted peers.

With respect to those who have claimed that children and adolescents with VI have lower global self-esteem than their sighted peers, recent studies do not support that assumption. In fact, global self-esteem of children and adolescents with VI appears to be similar to those with normal vision. This does not mean that more research is not needed to explore specific self-esteem domains and the importance of these domains. To my knowledge, only Shapiro et al. (2008) examined global self-esteem and different self-esteem domains in addition to the importance of the self-esteem domain on children and adolescents with VI . Children in their study did not value three (athletic, social or physical competence) out of the five domains as important factors in their lives. The other two domains (behavioural conduct and scholastic competence) were not included in this study. In addition, the authors found no significant differences in global self-esteem between children with VI and those normally sighted. As it has been mentioned previously at this chapter, examining self-esteem domains is necessary to boost understanding of the mechanisms of self-esteem improvement. This helps to identify which domains need to be improved and which domains are perceived as (un)important. Furthermore, it is important to develop the importance of self domains such as those that were low in Shapiro et al.'s (2008) study. For instance, previous findings show that children with VI are less physically active than their sighted peers (Kozub and Oh, 2004). It is expected, therefore to find that children and adolescents with VI are at a higher risk of developing a sedentary lifestyle and consequently increased risk of developing several chronic diseases (Lieberman, 2011). Consequently, we need to increase the importance of the athletic domain in children and adolescents with VI, so they can be more physically active and hopefully decrease a potential risk for developing diseases. Strategies for improving the global self-esteem and specific self-esteem domains will be discussed at the end of this chapter.

Self-esteem of young adults with visual impairment

As noted above, most of the studies have focused on children and adolescents with VI, whereas previous literature paid little attention to adults, namely young adults. "Young adult" is a complex term since there is no clear definition of an age group that falls under this definition. According to Geiger and Castellino (2011) studies in clinical research define people younger than 24, 29 and up to 40 as young adults. However, to my knowledge within different categories of young adults, there is only one study (Papadopoulos, Montgomery and Chronopoulou, 2013) that included young adults to investigate the self-esteem level of people with VI. In their study, among 108 adults (M = 34.81 years, SD = 11.35 years), people with VI achieved significantly lower self-esteem scores on the Rosenberg Self-Esteem Inventory (Rosenberg, 1965) than those with normal sight (F $(2,157)$ = 10,200, p<.01).

Furthermore, a major loss (such as sight) is significantly related to the feeling of a little value or worth (Tuttle and Tuttle, 2004). Therefore, symptoms such as depression, disbelief and denying the impairment were reported by Fitzgerald (1970). Above 80% of his sample, which included 66 adults aged 21–65 years, were depressed when they realised that they became blind and about 60% of the participants reported low self-esteem. However, in Roy and MacKay's (2002) study the 20 statements test showed that participants with VI referred to themselves positively although they had gradually lost their sight.

None of the previous studies identified the self-esteem domains of young adults with VI, although self-esteem may be high/low in one domain and not in the other. Furthermore, previous literature failed to investigate whether particular intervention may improve the global self-esteem or specific self-esteem domain in people (children, adolescents and adults) with VI. But it is necessary to identify strategies for self-esteem improvement so a better understanding about designing programmes for self-esteem improvement and recognising all issues that need to be avoided should be ensured.

Strategies for self-esteem improvement of people with VI

It has been suggested that that self-esteem interventions should not focus only on global self-esteem improvement but also on the specific domain of self-esteem (Bos et al., 2006) because self-esteem is a multidimensional hierarchical construct in which an individual's global self-esteem is affected by self-esteem subdomains such as social, physical, athletic, intellectual and moral subdomains (Bracken et al., 2000; Marsh, 1990). However, as has been explained previously in this chapter, only self-esteem domains that are perceived as important for an individual may impact upon their global self-esteem level (Harter, 1999). Therefore, Buckworth et al. (2013) argue that controlled research designs based on a multidimensional and hierarchical model of self-esteem contributes to the knowledge regarding the effects of constructed interventions on self-esteem in various populations, including those with VI.

In general, supporting Fox's (1997) strategies for self-esteem improvement, Buckworth et al. (2013) claimed that two core types of strategies exist to improve self-esteem:

1   *Psychological strategies*:

    (a)   Reducing the importance of activities that do not produce positive affect or success (discounting principle) (Harter, 1996).

    (b)   Convincing others that self-esteem is high.

    (c)   Engaging in self-affirmation when the self-esteem is likely to become low.

2   *Behavioural strategies*:

    (a)   People need to choose activities that have a high probability of success or positive affect.

    (b)   People need to withdraw from activities that have a low probability of success or negative affect.

    (c)   Social support and approval need to be maximised.

Although it is not clear whether the two core strategies – psychological and behavioural – are necessary for self-esteem improvement, or if one strategy – psychological or behavioural – would be sufficient, certainly when we consider a social model of disability (society disables people with impairments by limiting their worth in society) it appears that people with VI rarely receive all three components of the behavioural strategy for their self-esteem improvement. They do not always receive maximal support. For example, children and adolescents with VI are excluded from physical activities despite their integration (George and Duquette, 2006; Place and Hodge, 2001) and do not have options to choose activities because coaches and PE teachers lack the knowledge of how to teach them either a curricular or extra-curricular activity (Stuart, Lieberman and Hand, 2006). Moreover, people with VI do not want to exercise because of a fear of failure that has been originally rooted in their own self-perception as a result from previous social negative experiences and exclusion (Brittain, 2004). In her study, Bredahl (2013) interviewed participants with physical and visual impairments aged 18–65 years. She found a significant number (13 out of 17) of negative experiences originating from physical education centred in the following three domains: (a) experiences of not being included; (b) experiences of failing; and (c) experiences of not being listened to. Also, Rankin (2012) found that people with impairments perceive themselves and beliefs of others as the main barrier of being physically active. Interestingly, personal perceptions were constructed on the previous experience in which others were involved, such as being made fun of, which impacted their confidence and self-esteem.

With respect to all self domains that are related to global self-esteem, the improvement and maintenance of self-esteem, particularly in children and adolescents, depend on the following two factors: (a) perceived competence in areas of importance and (b) the experience of social support (Harter, 1999). When studying people with VI, however, social competence is considered to be a main component of high self-esteem (Wagner, 2004).

Furthermore, to my knowledge, all previous multidimensional measurements of self-esteem contain social acceptance as one of the self-esteem domains. Sociability scales across different life stages reflect, in some way, people's satisfaction, ability and desire to meet new people and feel accepted (Harter, 1985, 1988; Messer and Harter, 1986; Neemann and Harter, 1986). This social acceptance may be a result of a contact between people with VI, which has been suggested by a contact theory developed by Allport (1954) to reduce prejudice and stereotypes (Slininger, Sherrill and Jankowski, 2000) and improve their social acceptance and comfort (Tripp, French and Sherrill, 1995; Tripp and Sherrill, 1991).

Additionally, Harter (1999) claims that if a person values one domain as important and achieves a high score, this is better than to value another domain as important and achieve a low score. In order to achieve and/or protect high self-esteem people with VI should increase the importance of those domains in which they have higher probability to perform well. At the same time, people with VI should decrease the importance of those domains in which they continuously perform badly to avoid low self-esteem. It is important, however, to focus on boosting the importance of the domains that are related to the everyday activities of people with VI. For example, if a child with VI does not consider social domain as important, we should work on increasing sighted children's knowledge about inclusion and then try to force the social domain and its importance in children with VI. This is due to the importance of the social domain and social relationships in children's everyday lives.

Furthermore, Harter's (1978) theory of competence suggests that people are motivated where their competence can be demonstrated, particularly in the areas where they feel a perception of personal control. This means that those who perceive themselves as highly competent in physical activity, for example, would be more likely to participate in such activities. By contrast, when children and adolescents with VI feel excluded due to the perception of their normally sighted peers, it is not likely that children and adolescents with VI will score well in the social domain. This also may be related to the importance of their social life. When people with VI have awareness of achieving self-potential challenging goals through mastery attempts, they will more likely receive positive support by significant others, show higher levels of perceived competence and feel a sense of internal control according to Harter's competence motivation theory. Moreover, people with VI have noted that their significant others, namely friends and family members, had changed their perception about abilities once they had acquired an impairment (Brittain, 2004). This is a consistent finding in studies, which indicates that mastery attempts and feeling valued by significant others are the most important sources of self-esteem (Twenge and Campbell, 2001). As for people without disability, recent findings show that being accepted and valued by others played an important role in self-esteem improvement (Qasim, 2015). Interviewing 12 martial artists with VI, Qasim (2015) found that because of being included (accepted, valued and respected) by their instructors and peers their social and global self-esteem have been improved. One of the participants from this study said:

> After the first week I was addicted! I couldn't wait to go back. After the second week I just kept wanting to go back, but after the second week I had made some really good judo friends, you know, in the judo club because judo's a contact sport. You have to take hold of somebody to do it. And that was teaching me communication skills that I had never known before . . . I felt part of the community, I felt part of a club which was helping my self-esteem rise because I had mates and I had mates that weren't teasing me about the way I looked. I actually started feeling good about myself for, you know, which I hadn't apparently felt for a long time.
>
> *(Qasim, 2015, p. 192)*

However, what may be challenging for researchers and practitioners is the stability of self-esteem. Previous research found that that the stability of self-esteem is lower during childhood (6–11 years) compared to adolescence (12–17 years) and adulthood (18–29 years) (Trzesniewski et al., 2003). In addition, research in this area supports the idea that self-esteem domains are more stable than global self-esteem (Marsh, Richards and Barnes, 1986). We need to identify the causes of self-esteem changes and then we should expect self-esteem improvement. According to James' theory, success or failure experiences can increase or decrease self-esteem of people even if they have relatively stable self-esteem. Additionally, a need for increasing/decreasing the expectations of domains with high/low adequacy exists. If a child with VI expects good marks in school but his real level is under his expectations than the decrease in global self-esteem can be expected. Either improving the child's performance or decreasing his/her expectations in this case becomes necessary for high self-esteem attainment.

Conclusion

Global self-esteem is a sum of evaluations across different life domains. These evaluations are personal according to the person's standards. Only those domains that are perceived to be important for a person may increase/decrease global self-esteem. It is important to have high global self-esteem due to its relation to several healthy measurements, such as mental health.

Most of the previous research agrees that children and adolescents with VI have similar global self-esteem levels as their sighted peers. However, research failed to explore in detail self-esteem domains and its relationship to global self-esteem. This becomes important considering that people with VI are often socially excluded and bullied, which may lead to low social self-esteem and likely also low global self-esteem. Future research therefore should focus on identifying causes for social barriers that socially restrict people with VI and potentially lead to health issues and investigating strategies that will find out the most efficient methods for reducing these barriers. Finally, more research should focus on self-esteem of young adults with VI as thus far only very limited studies have investigated this target group.

References

Allport, G.W. 1954. *The nature of prejudice*. Boston, MA: Addison-Wesley.

Augestad, L.B. 2017. Self-concept and self-esteem among children and young adults with visual impairment: A systematic review. *Cogent Psychology*, 4(1). www.tandfonline.com/doi/abs/10.1080/2331190 8.2017.1319652.

Baumeister, R.F., Campbell, R.F., Krueger, J.I. and Vohs, K.D. 2003. Does high self-esteem cause better performance, interpersonal success, happiness, or healthier lifestyles? *Psychological Science in the Public Interest*, 4(1), 1–44.

Berger, B.G., Pargman, D. and Weinberg, R. 2002. *Foundations of exercise psychology* (2nd ed.). Morgan Town, WV: Fitness Information Technology.

Bigelow, A.E. 2003. The development of joint attention in blind infants. *Development and Psychopathology*, 15(2), 259–275.

Bleidorn, W., Arslan, R.C., Denissen, J.J.A., Rentfrow, P.J., Gebauer, J.E., Potter, J. and Gosling, S.D. 2016. Age and gender differences in self-esteem: A cross-cultural window. *Journal of Personality and Social Psychology*, 111(3), 396–410.

Bos, A.E.R., Muris, P., Mulkens, S. and Schaalma, H.P. 2006. Changing self-esteem in children and adolescents: A roadmap for future interventions. *Netherlands Journal of Psychology*, 62(1), 26–33.

Boulton, M.J. and Underwood, K. 1992. Bully/victim problems among middle school children. *British Journal of Educational Psychology*, 62(1),73–87.

Bourke, S. and Burgman, I. 2010. Coping with bullying in Australian schools: How children with disabilities experience support from friends, parents and teachers. *Disability & Society*, 25(3), 359–371.

Boyd, K. and Hrycaiko, D. 1997. The effect of a physical activity intervention package on the self-esteem of pre-adolescent and adolescent females. *Adolescence*, 32(127), 693–708.

Bracken, B.A., Bunch, S., Keith, T.Z. and Keith, P.B. 2000. Child and adolescent multidimensional self-concept: A five-instrument factor analysis. *Psychology in the Schools*, 37(6), 483–493.

Bredahl, A.-M. 2013. Sitting and watching the others being active: The experienced difficulties in PE when having a disability. *Adapted Physical Activity Quarterly*, 30(1), 40–58.

Brittain, I. 2004. Perceptions of disability and their impact upon involvement in sport for people with disabilities at all levels. *Journal of Sport and Social Issues*, 28(4), 429–452.

Brown, J.D. 2014. Self-esteem and self-evaluation: Feeling is believing. In J. Suls (ed.), *Psychological perspectives on the self* (pp. 27–58). Oxford: Taylor & Francis.

Brown, J.D. and Marshall, M.A. 2006. The three faces of self-esteem. In M. Kernis (ed.), *Self-esteem: Issues and answers* (pp. 4–9). Hove, UK: Psychology Press.

Buckworth, J., Dishamn, R., O'Connor, P. and Tomporowski, P. 2013. *Exercise psychology* (2nd ed.). Champaign, IL: Human Kinetics.

Byrne, B.M. 1996. *Measuring self-concept across the lifespan: Issues and instrumentation.* Washington, DC: American Psychological Association.

Crocker, J., Moeller, S. and Burson, A. 2010. The costly pursuit of self-esteem. In R.H. Hoyle (ed.), *Handbook of personality and self-regulation* (pp. 403–429). Hoboken, NJ: Wiley-Blackwell.

Crocker, J. and Park, L.E. 2004. The costly pursuit of self-esteem. *Psychological Bulletin*, 130(3), 392–414.

Daglas-Pelish, P. 2006. Effects of a self-esteem intervention program on school-age children. *Pediatric Nursing*, 32(4), 341–348.

Datta, P. 2014. Self-concept and vision impairment: A review. *British Journal of Visual Impairment*, 32(3), 200–210.

Egan, S.K. and Perry, D.G. 1998. Does low self-regard invite victimization? *Developmental Psychology*, 34(2), 299–309.

Fitzgerald, R.G. 1970. Reactions to blindness: An exploratory study of adults with recent loss of sight. *Archives of General Psychiatry*, 22(4), 370–379.

Fox, K.R. 1990. *The physical self-perception profile manual.* Dekalb, IL: Northern Illinois University Press.

Fox, K.R. 1997. *The physical self: From motivation to well-being.* Champaign, IL: Human Kinetics.

Garaigordobil, M. and Bernarás, E. 2009. Self-concept, self-esteem, personality traits and psychopathological symptoms in adolescents with and without visual impairment. *Spanish Journal of Psychology*, 12(1), 149–160.

Geiger, A.M. and Castellino, S.M. 2011. Delineating the age ranges used to define adolescents and young adults. *Journal of Clinical Oncology*, 29(16), e492–e493.

George, A.L. and Duquette, C. 2006. The psychosocial experiences of a student with low vision. *Journal of Visual Impairment & Blindness*, 100(3), 152–163.

Griffin-Shirley, N. and Nes, S.L. 2005. Self-esteem and empathy in sighted and visually impaired preadolescents. *Journal of Visual Impairment & Blindness*, 99(5), 276–285.

Gronmo, S.J. and Augestad, L.B. 2000. Physical activity, self-concept, and global self-worth of blind youths in Norway and France. *Journal of Visual Impairment and Blindness*, 94(8), 522–526.

Harter, S. 1978. Effectance motivation reconsidered: Toward a developmental model. *Human Development*, 21(1), 34–64.

Harter, S. 1985. *Manual for the self-perception profile for children.* Denver, CO: University of Denver.

Harter, S. 1988. *Manual for the self-perception profile for adolescents.* Denver, CO: University of Denver.

Harter, S. 1993. Causes and consequences of low self-esteem in children and adolescents. In R. Baumeister (ed.), *Self-esteem: The puzzle of low self-regard* (pp. 87–116). New York: Plenum.

Harter, S. 1996. Historical roots of contemporary issues involving self-concept. In B.A. Bracken (ed.), *Handbook of self-concept* (pp. 1–37). Oxford: Wiley.

Harter, S. 1999. *The construction of the self* (1st ed.). New York: Guilford.

Harter, S. 2006. The development of self-esteem. In M.H. Kernis (ed.), *Self-esteem issues and answers: A sourcebook of current perspectives* (pp. 144–150). Hove, UK: Psychology Press.

Harter, S. 2012. *The construction of the self: Developmental and sociocultural foundations* (2nd ed.). New York: Guilford.

Hayes, D.M. and Fors, S.W. 1990. Self-esteem and health instruction: Challenges for Curriculum development. *Journal of School Health*, 60(5), 208–211.

Horwood, J., Waylen, A., Herrick, D., Williams, C. and Wolke, D. 2005. Common visual defects and peer victimization in children. *Investigative Ophthalmology & Visual Science*, 46(4), 1177–1181.

Huurre, T. 2000. *Psychosocial development and social support among adolescents with visual impairment.* Dissertation. University of Tampere, Finland.

James, W. 1890. *The principles of psychology.* Cambridge, MA: Harvard University Press.

Jindal-Snape, D. 2004. Generalization and maintenance of social skills of children with visual impairments: Self-evaluation and the role of feedback. *Journal of Visual Impairment & Blindness*, 98(8), 470–483.

Kef, S. 2002. Psychosocial adjustment and the meaning of social support for visually impaired adolescents. *Journal of Visual Impairment & Blindness*, 96(1), 22–37.

King, K.A. 1997. Self-concept and self-esteem: A clarification of terms. *Journal of School Health*, 67(2), 68–71.

Kozub, F.M. and Oh, H. 2004. An exploratory study of physical activity levels in children and adolescents with visual impairments. *Clinical Kinesiology*, 58(3), 1–8.

Kroksmark, U. and Nordell, K. 2001. Adolescence: The age of opportunities and obstacles for students with low vision in Sweden. *Journal of Visual Impairment & Blindness*, 95(4), 213–225.

Lieberman, L.J. 2011. Visual impairments. In J.P. Winnick (ed.), *Adapted physical education and sport* (pp. 233–249). Champaign, IL: Human Kinetics.

Lindwall, M. and Asci, H.F. 2014. Physical activity and self-esteem. In A. Clow and S. Edmunds (eds.), *Physical activity and mental health* (pp. 83–105). Champaign, IL: Human Kinetics.

Lowenfeld, B. 1981. *Berthold Lowenfeld on blindness and blind people*. New York: American Foundation for the Blind.

Mann, M.M., Hosman, C.M.H., Schaalma, H.P. and De Vries, N.K. 2004. Self-esteem in a broad-spectrum approach for mental health promotion. *Health Education Research*, 19(4), 357–372.

Manning, M., Bear, G. and Minke, K. 2006. Self-concept and self-esteem. In G. Bear and K. Minke (eds), *Children's needs III: Development, prevention, and intervention* (pp. 341–356). Bethesda, MD: National Association of School Psychologists.

Marsh, H.W. 1990. A multidimensional, hierarchical model of self-concept: Theoretical and empirical justification. *Educational Psychology Review*, 2(2), 77–172.

Marsh, H.W., Craven, R.G. and Martin, A. 2006. What is the nature of self-esteem? Unidimensional and multidimensional perspectives. In M.H. Kernis (ed.), *Self-esteem issues and answers: A sourcebook of current perspectives* (pp. 16–26). Hove, UK: Psychology Press.

Marsh, H.W., Richards, G.E. and Barnes, J. 1986. Multidimensional self-concepts: A long-term follow-up of the effect of participation in an outward bound program. *Personality and Social Psychology Bulletin*, 12(4), 475–492.

Maslow, A.H. 1987. *Motivation and personality* (3rd ed.). New York: Harper Collins.

Messer, B. and Harter, S. 1986. *Manual for the adult self-perception profile*. Denver, CO: University of Denver.

Neemann, J. and Harter, S. 1986. *Manual for the self-perception profile for college students*. Denver, CO: University of Denver.

Nixon, H.L. 1989. Integration of disabled people in mainstream sports: Case study of a partially sighted child. *Adapted Physical Activity Quarterly*, 6(1), 17–31.

Obiakor, F.E. and Stile, S.W. 1990. The self-concepts of visually impaired and normally sighted middle school children. *Journal of Psychology*, 124(2), 199–206.

Olsen, J.M., Breckler, S.J. and Wiggens, E.C. 2008. *Social psychology alive*. Belmont, CA: Thomson Nelson.

Papadopoulos, K., Montgomery, A.J. and Chronopoulou, E. 2013. The impact of visual impairments in self-esteem and locus of control. *Research in Developmental Disabilities*, 34(12), 4565–4570.

Pavey, T. 2009. *The relationship between children's psychological well-being, habitual physical activity, and sedentary behaviours*. PhD thesis. University of Exeter, UK.

Peden, A., Hall, L., Rayens, M. and Beebe, L. 2000. Negative thinking mediates the effect of self-esteem on depressive symptoms in college women. *Nursing Research*, 49(1), 201–207.

Pierce, J.W. and Wardle, J. 1996. Body size, parental appraisal, and self-esteem in blind children. *Journal of Child Psychology and Psychiatry*, 37(2), 205–212.

Pinquart, M. and Pfeiffer, J.P. 2011. Bullying in German adolescents: Attending special school for students with visual impairment. *British Journal of Visual Impairment*, 29(3), 163–176.

Place, K. and Hodge, S.R. 2001. Social inclusion of students with physical disabilities in general physical education: A behavioral analysis. *Adapted Physical Activity Quarterly*, 18(4), 389–404.

Qasim, S.H. 2015. *The effect of martial arts practice on global self-esteem in people with visual impairment and the associated mechanisms and strategies*. PhD thesis. Moray House School of Education, University of Edinburgh.

Rankin, M. 2012. *Understanding the barriers to participation in sport: Views and opinions of active and non active disabled people*. English Federation of Disability Sport. Accessed 8 April 2014. www.activity alliance.org.uk/assets/000/000/807/Understanding_the_barriers_to_participation_20120510_original. pdf?1473697192.

Rigby, K. and Slee, P.T. 1993. Dimensions of interpersonal relation among Australian children and implications for psychological well-being. *Journal of Social Psychology*, 133(1), 33–42.

Rosenberg, M. 1965. *Society and the adolescent self-image*. Princeton, NJ: Princeton University Press.

Roy, A.W.N. and MacKay, G.F. 2002. Self-perception and locus of control in visually impaired college students with different types of vision loss. *Journal of Visual Impairment & Blindness*, 96(4), 254–266.

Sabiston, C., Whitehead, J.R. and Eklund, R.C. 2012. Exercise and self-perception constructs. In G. Tenenbaum, R.C. Eklund and A. Kamata (eds), *Measurement in sport and exercise psychology* (pp. 227–238). Champaign, IL: Human Kinetics.

Shapiro, D.R. and Martin, J.J. 2010. Multidimensional physical self-concept of athletes with physical disabilities. *Adapted Physical Activity Quarterly*, 27(4), 294–307.

Shapiro, D.R., Moffett, A., Lieberman, L. and Dummer, G.M. 2008. Domain-specific ratings of importance and global self-worth of children with visual impairments. *Journal of Visual Impairment & Blindness*, 102(4), 232–244.

Shavelson, R.J., Hubner, J.J. and Stanton, G.C. 1976. Self-concept: Validation of construct interpretations. *Review of Educational Research*, 46(3), 407–441.

Sherrill, C. 2004. *Adapted physical activity, recreation, and sport: Crossdisciplinary and lifespan* (6th ed.). London: McGraw-Hill.

Sherrill, C. and Williams, T. 1996. Disability and sport: Psychosocial perspectives on inclusion, integration, and participation. *Sport Science Review*, 5(1), 42–64.

Slininger, D., Sherrill, C. and Jankowski, C.M. 2000. Children's attitudes toward peers with severe disabilities: Revisiting contact theory. *Adapted Physical Activity Quarterly*, 17(2), 176–196.

Spencer-Cavaliere, N. and Watkinson, E.J. 2010. Inclusion understood from the perspectives of children with disability. *Adapted Physical Activity Quarterly*, 27(4), 275–293.

Stanwyck, D.J. 1983. Self-esteem through the life span. *Family & Community Health*, 6(2), 11–28.

Stuart, M., Lieberman, L. and Hand, K. (2006). Beliefs about physical activity among children who are visually impaired and their parents. *Journal of Visual Impairment & Blindness*, 100(4), 223–234.

Suls, J. 2006. On the divergent and convergent validity of self-esteem. In M.H. Kernis (ed.), *Self-esteem issues and answers: A sourcebook of current perspectives* (pp. 36–43). Hove, UK: Psychology Press.

Torres, R., Fernandez, F. and Maceira, D. 1995. Self-esteem and value of health as correlates of adolescent health behavior. *Adolescence*, 30(118), 403–412.

Tripp, A., French, R. and Sherrill, C. 1995. Contact theory and attitudes of children in physical education programs toward peers with disabilities. *Adapted Physical Activity Quarterly*, 12(4), 323–332.

Tripp, A. and Sherrill, C. 1991. Attitude theories of relevance to adapted physical education. *Adapted Physical Activity Quarterly*, 8(1), 12–27.

Trzesniewski, K., Donnellan, B. and Robins, R. 2003. Stability of self-esteem across the life span. *Journal of Personality and Social Psychology*, 84(1), 205–220.

Tuttle, D.W. and Tuttle, N.R. 2004. *Self-esteem and adjusting with blindness: The process of responding to life's demands*. Springfield, IL: Charles C. Thomas.

Twenge, J.M. and Campbell, W.K. 2001. Age and birth cohort differences in self-esteem: A cross-temporal meta-analysis. *Personality and Social Psychology Review*, 5(4), 321–344.

Vallerand, R.J., Pelletier, L.G. and Gagné, F. 1991. On the multidimensional versus unidimensional perspectives of self-esteem: A test using the group-comparison approach. *Social Behavior and Personality: An International Journal*, 19(2), 121–132.

Wagner, E. 2004. Development and implementation of a curriculum to develop social competence for students with visual impairments in Germany. *Journal of Visual Impairment & Blindness*, 98(11), 703–709.

Williams, K., Chambers, M., Logan, S. and Robinson, D. 1996. Association of common health symptoms with bullying in primary school children. *British Medical Journal*, 313(7048), 17–19.

21

Human mate selection theory
Specific considerations for persons with visual impairments

Gaylen Kapperman and Stacy M. Kelly

Introduction

We wish to address the issue of individuals who are totally blind or very severely visually impaired "playing the mating game" and all of the impediments thereto attached. Research has shown that finding a mate and forming a relationship that is warm and intimate are key goals in life for most people (Reis and Downey, 1999). Of course, we contend that this same statement has equal validity in the lives of persons who are blind or severely visually impaired.

We will approach this topic from an evolutionary psychological point of view. In summary, when one reviews the literature on the topic of *Homo sapiens* finding appropriate breeding partners there are a considerable number of characteristics that both males and females take into consideration. While assessing the desirable characteristics of potential mates, there are always inevitable alterations that must be made in the array of those characteristics that one must make. The changes in one's set of desired characteristics are generally necessitated because there are very few, and most likely not any, perfect "tens" available to most people in reality (Li et al., 2002). Thus, people seeking a partner make compromises in their acceptance of certain attributes as opposed to others in consideration of the context in which the relationship exists and their goals that they hold for that relationship (Fletcher et al., 2004). We address several of these aspects of mate selection while also discussing the challenges that individuals who are blind or severely visually impaired must face given these factors.

Additionally, we address the issue of the lack of sight in the pursuit of suitable romantic partners based upon the fact that finding a suitable partner most importantly depends on being able to see the potential partner and being able to judge the suitability of the individual. Also, of course, initial communication in this activity generally hinges upon being able to communicate using visual cues in addition to judging the potential partner's suitability using sight.

We approach the topic of judging the suitability of an individual from the perspective of the gender of the pursuer. Thus, the information supplied below regarding the characteristics of potential female partners has been developed by Gaylen Kapperman, a male, and the information developed regarding the female's point of view has been developed by Stacy Kelly, a female. We address the issues involved from an evolutionary psychology point of view.

Attributes males seek in potential female partners

Facial features

There are several factors researchers have discovered that males, emanating from all regions of the planet, consider in their attempts to find an appropriate breeding partner. Two of the most important factors are the health and youth that serve as observable indicators of the fertility of potential partners (Buss, 2015; Buss et al., 2001; Symons, 1979; Williams, 1957). Health and youth can be estimated by males in numerous ways and chief among those is the appraisal of facial features of the potential partner. In short, she must have a symmetrical face. Evolutionary psychologists have generally agreed for a considerable period of time that female faces that exhibit symmetry indicate to the male of the species that she possesses good health (Malinowski, 1929). Given that the overriding reason for choosing a breeding partner, of course, is to produce healthy babies, from aeons in the past, the male of the species has depended upon the facial features of potential breeding partners to judge their ability to produce healthy babies. Diseases and injuries experienced by our ancestors over the past millennia, for example, sometimes caused asymmetries to develop that have had an impact on perceptions of attractiveness (Gangestad, Thornhill and Yeo, 1994). Thus, a female who possessed an asymmetrical face had also been deemed not to be able to produce healthy babies. We understand that there is no valid scientifically proven correlation between symmetry or lack thereof in a mother and the mother's ability to produce healthy babies. We use this point to illustrate the fact that we *Homo sapiens'* present-day attitudes have been imprinted upon us from the past.

Another important factor regarding males placing great importance upon the symmetry of potential breeding partners is that the level of attractiveness of his female partner's face, in some fashion, determines the status of the male. Put simply, the more attractive a female partner is the higher the status that is attributed to her male partner (Grammer, 1992). The factor of facial symmetry on the part of the female, then, plays an important part in the ability of a female who is blind to attract sighted males. As we elucidate in the description of each of the factors, individuals who are blind must exceed the usual level of achievement with regard to most of those factors to overcome the major disadvantage of being blind. Thus, the female who is blind must be considerably more attractive than her sighted female competitors to be able to meet this challenge. This will be a theme throughout this chapter. In short, in order to compete with sighted individuals, persons who are blind must be able to achieve at much higher levels in the arena in which they are competing in order to have an opportunity to reach success. This point will be repeated with regard to nearly every characteristic upon which we will expand.

In addition to symmetry, there are other facial features or characteristics that the male takes into consideration in his search for a suitable partner. The universally attractive female face (for men) has a relatively child-like appearance, with wide-set, large eyes, a small nose and chin, prominent cheekbones, high eyebrows, large pupils and a warm smile (Cunningham, 1986). All of these characteristics are interpreted by males that the female who exhibits these is young enough to bear children. There is, of course, very little that can be done to change the facial features of a female who does not exhibit these characteristics. However, many women are heavily invested in enhancing their facial features cosmetically. The use of make-up and plastic surgery in modern-day society are examples of this artificial enhancement of facial features that is in many ways derived from mating preferences established by our ancient ancestors (Buss, 2016).

Again, the female who is blind is at a disadvantage. Her eyes present an additional challenge in that in some persons who are blind, the eyes are seen as unattractive by sighted individuals. Blindness-related characteristics may be exhibited. For example, she may have nystagmus, the involuntary movement of the eyes. Or, she may not be able to focus her eyes on the speaker. There is a large array of eye-related behaviours that augur against the female who is blind. There is little that can be done to compensate for this challenge except to wear dark glasses. The wearing of dark glasses then presents an additional problem in that the sighted observer cannot see her eyes. She is disadvantaged if she does wear dark glasses and disadvantaged if she does not wear them. Thus, the condition of her eyes presents an additional challenge in the search for an appropriate breeding partner. It is, therefore, even more important from this perspective that females who are blind can appropriately use make-up to enhance the range of facial features that, according to this theory, males have been genetically programmed from aeons ago to seek in their breeding partners.

Hair condition

The condition of the female's hair plays a major role in the level of attractiveness as judged by potential sighted male partners. Once again, the importance of the condition of her hair has been imprinted upon modern males' judgement over the passage of aeons (Bobrow and Bailey, 2001). The condition of her hair, in some fashion, indicates the level of her health. The condition of her hair, then, reveals her potential for giving birth to healthy babies. Once again, we do not in any fashion want to leave the reader with the impression that we believe that this is true. We only wish to describe the factors from an evolutionary psychological point of view.

Waist size

The size of the female's waist in comparison to the size of her hips is of great importance to males searching for breeding partners. Researchers have found that a ratio of 70% waist-to-hip size (the size of waist is 70% of the size of the hips) is seen as the ultimate in attractiveness in females (Singh, 1993a, 1993b, 1994). The ratio of 70% is viewed as most attractive among males from all cultures and regions of the world. The assumption is that when males view females with ratios greater than 70%, they believe that the females could be pregnant (i.e. demonstrating a lack of availability for procreation) or have a condition such as hypertension or diabetes (i.e. indicating an unhealthy body). Once again, we do not assert that the modern male makes that assumption in all cases, but once again, that ideal in waist-to-hip ratio has been brought down to him for aeons. Also, it is noted that if a female has a smaller ratio of waist-to-hip size that is less than 70%, then she is viewed as unhealthy and thus may be unable to bear healthy babies.

With regard to females who are blind, the factor of waist-to-hip size is one that can be controlled to a certain degree. That is, it is possible for most average-sized females to exhibit the most attractive waist-to-hip ratio of 70%. Unlike the waist-to-hip ratio, there is no agreed upon size of breasts that is favoured by males. The only factors taken into consideration by males appears to be the symmetry of the breasts along with their shape and youthful appearance (Gangestad et al., 1994). Thus, under normal circumstances, a female who is blind may not be at a disadvantage with regard to this aspect of the feminine figure compared to her sighted rivals.

Chronological age

Age is another important factor taken into consideration by males when they are searching for potential breeding partners. Throughout the United States and all across the world results of research over the past half century have repeatedly shown that males seek mating partners younger in age than they are (Buss, 1989; Hill, 1945; Hudson and Henze, 1969; McGinnis, 1958; Symons, 1989). This is an obvious factor given that the ability of females to bear children is time-limited. Males with a higher occupational status, for example, often marry females who are decades younger because those men who can attract women who are younger than they are frequently do so (Elder, 1969; Taylor and Glenn, 1976; Udry and Eckland, 1984). Chronological age is a very important factor for males in this way from an evolutionary psychological perspective. Movie stars and professional athletes include many individuals who demonstrate this propensity for breeding with much younger women (Buss, 2016).

Education and financial resources

Males tend not to seek out females who have achieved higher levels of education than they have (Buss et al., 2001). Thus, the level of education of the male will, to a certain extent, determine the level of education of females to whom he is attracted. Generally, that is approximately his level of educational attainment.

In the past, researchers found that males did not place heavy emphasis upon the potential earning power of their female partners (Langhorne and Secord, 1955). Thus, in the past, the female who is blind who had not been involved in a career that promised to provide high earnings was not at a major disadvantage. If this factor remains valid today, then the underemployment of persons who are blind may not result in a severe disadvantage to the female who is blind. Because of the rather dated results of the research alluded to, the authors wish to express their uncertainty regarding the continued validity of this issue in the current economic environment.

Males generally search for females who are sexually generous. Obviously, this should not present a challenge for a female who is blind if she is willing to have sex as frequently as her male partner wishes. In this situation, a female who is blind is not necessarily placed at a disadvantage with regard to her rivals.

Attributes females seek in potential male partners

Reproductive biology

The gender differences related to what women seek in male partners have also been demonstrated as universal traits across cultures with evolutionary roots that go back to the beginning of sexual reproduction (Buss, 1989; Kenrick and Keefe, 1992). Women's preferences are complex. One reason for this, from an evolutionary psychological perspective, is reproductive biology. Males can replenish their supply of sex cells and reproduce a number of times that is limited only by the number of fertile females available to have sex with them (Buss, 2016). Females, however, have a fixed number of ova that cannot be replenished (Buss, 2016). Also, when pregnancy does occur, females are committed to the investment of the nine-month gestation process (Buss, 2016). Females hold exceptionally valuable and limited resources when taking these factors into account. Thus, women are highly selective in the mating process having been imprinted by evolutionary forces. For women, the stakes are extremely high in the mate selection process and, for these reasons, the responsibility for choosing a mate falls to them (Fedigan, 1992). The preferences females seek in a mate give the utmost importance to financial resources and social status as opposed to males' high-ranking preferences for signs of physical health, attractiveness and youthfulness (Feingold, 1992; Fletcher, 2002; Geary, 2010).

Financial resources

The characteristic that ranked first and foremost in the array of preferences of ancestral women was the males' ability to provide resources such as food (Conroy-Beam et al., 2015). In modern times, the ability to provide resources has been transformed into earning power. This desire for breeding partners with financial resources has been found worldwide to be valued by women far more than men. The fertilisation, nine-month gestation and child-rearing undertaken by *Homo sapien* females down through the aeons has been supported in numerous ways when their mating partners have had resources to support this expensive process (Buss, 2016).

Unfortunately, the vast majority of working-age people who are blind do not participate in the labour force (Kelly, 2013; Zuckerman, 2004). This high degree of unemployment among people who are blind exists regardless of the gender of the person who is blind. The under-employment of persons who are blind results in a severe disadvantage to the male who is blind. The vast majority of males who are blind and not in the labour force do not have the financial resources readily available for the competitive process of mate selection that, according to this longstanding theory, is driven in large part by the females' desire for mates who have financial resources to support them and their offspring. The research consistently shows that the ability of breeding partners to provide resources has been viewed by our ancestors as well as modern-day females as being of extraordinary importance (Hill, 1945; Hudson and Henze, 1969; Li et al., 2002; McGinnis, 1958). Males who are blind may have to strive more diligently to overcome this situation, which presents numerous challenges in mate selection.

Social status

Another trait that women value with a high degree of importance in terms of mate selection is social status. Social status as an "alpha" male is the second most desirable trait women want in a mate (Buss and Barnes, 1986; Hill, 1945; Hudson and Henze 1969; Langhorne and Secord 1955; McGinnis, 1958). Again, this preference has been traced back in time, aeons ago. During the hunter-gatherer period, lower-status men had malnourished children and inadequate territories that left these men, their breeding partners and their offspring languishing at the bottom of the social hierarchy (Betzig, 1986). Higher-status men had mates and offspring who were provided with more than ample food and security that enabled them to thrive (Betzig, 1986).

The female desire for "alpha" males again presents explicit challenges among men who are blind. The high unemployment of people who are blind makes it difficult for males who are blind to acquire the power and social status to enable them to occupy a high rank in the social hierarchy to which they belong. Again, men who are blind are faced with numerous obstacles to overcome not only in terms of how they are viewed by women in terms of financial prospects but also in terms of social standing among their sighted peers and social networks.

Education

The next most important characteristic that a woman seeks is that the male is slightly more intelligent than she is, by a small degree (Cashdan, 1996). There are numerous potential benefits of intelligence for the long-term well-being of couples and their offspring (Barkow, 1989). On the other hand, men who are less intelligent present many potential liabilities for women and their children that can have damaging and unhealthy consequences (Buss, 2016).

Presently, this means that the education of a woman's breeding partner is also of importance (Buss, 2016). Men who are blind and acquire a high degree of formal education can increase their attractiveness in terms of this specific characteristic. Additionally, generally, higher levels of education result in greater earning power and, thus, a substantial increase in how men who are blind are viewed by modern women with regard to long-term financial prospects and social standing.

Body size and strength

An additional set of traits that females desire has evolved from aeons ago to address the need for protection for themselves and their children. Women have a well-documented preference for males who are athletic, strong and tall with a V-shaped torso (Buss and Schmitt, 1993). From an evolutionary psychological viewpoint, males who possess these traits have the physical ability to deter threats and protect their families from harm. If the male who is blind is short, there is nothing that can be done about height. However, if a male who is blind does not exhibit athleticism, strength or a V-shaped torso, then he, in most cases, can take steps to remedy the situation.

Short-term liaisons

Researchers have found that when males are seeking short-term liaisons using dating apps such as Tinder and Hinge, they lower their standards regarding the characteristics of their potential female partners but females maintain their standards at their usual level (Semmelroth and Buss, n.d.). Thus, in this situation, a female who is blind may find more success in attracting the attention of sighted male partners for short-term liaisons. A male who is blind will likely not be able to change his level of success in attracting sighted female partners for short-term relationships. The results of a recently unpublished study (Kapperman and Kelly, 2017) that we conducted would indicate that this assumption is correct, especially for females who are blind. In the study we enlisted the aid of four sighted female graduate students who ranged in age from 23 to 27. Each posed as a sighted woman and as a blind woman on the popular dating site, Tinder, which has the reputation for fostering short-term relationships that are commonly referred to as "hook-ups".

The graduate student participants posed for pictures that were to be placed on the site. For their "sighted" poses, they wore conservative clothing and were stationed in a neutral location. For their "blind" poses, they wore sunglasses and held a white cane used in orientation and mobility by blind persons. Each of the young women wore the same clothing as they had in their "sighted" poses and the locations were the same as in their sighted poses.

We used the following process to gather data. Each participant "went online" in a predetermined order. Only one participant was "online" at a time. Each night, she "swiped" her account and counted the number of matches that she received. A total of 700 swipes were made over a 14-day period by each participant. This process was repeated by each participant using her "blind" pose also. Additionally, each participant recorded comments offered by the males who "swiped" their pictures. At the conclusion of the study, all matches for each pose were counted.

The purpose was to determine if sighted men who frequented the site would prefer sighted women over blind women. The results were equivocal. That is two of the four young women's "blind" poses receive more matches indicating interest than their comparable sighted poses (Kapperman and Kelly, 2017).

An informal assessment of the many comments offered by the male visitors also provided evidence that they were interested in short-term relationships. For example, more than one "pick-up line" stated that the visitor had always wanted to "have sex with a blind girl". We found a considerable number of comments that expressed that or similar sentiments. Based on the results of the study, we believe that females who are blind are not placed at such a dramatic disadvantage when short-term liaisons are sought by sighted males. It goes without saying that we realise that the intention of the males who find themselves in this situation is not to procreate. We believe that the females, who enter into these potentially short-term relationships, harbour the same intentions.

In a previous study by Kapperman et al. (2017) using the same dating site, Tinder, and employing the same procedures as described above, we asked two female graduate students and two male graduate students to pose as sighted and blind individuals. Thus, there were eight total poses. The poses were made available on the site for a 14-day period one at a time. That is, one "sighted" female pose was followed by a blind female pose. At the conclusion of the study, data were compiled and analysed.

In summary, there was no significant difference with regard to the visual condition of each of the female or male participants displaced in the poses. That is, no significant difference was found to exist between the sighted poses and the blind poses, leading us to conclude that with regard to short-term "hook-ups" the condition of blindness had no effect on the willingness of sighted males or sighted females to form a short-term relationship with the individual who they were attempting to contact. For the males who posed as blind, there were significantly fewer matches than there were for the females. Less than 4% of the swipes made by those who posed as blind males resulted in a "like" or a match whereas between 39% and 60% of the swipes made by those who posed as blind females resulted in a "like" or a match.

Our interpretation of these rather unclear results is that in the case of short-term relationships, sighted males are willing to form short-term liaisons with females who are blind without a significant regard to whether the individual is blind or sighted. Other studies of Tinder use among the general population have supported this theory and these findings. Sighted men have demonstrated far less regard for short-term mating partners selecting hundreds of potential sighted female partners to "swipe right" in the hope that a few of them will reciprocate. Sighted women have demonstrated much more selectivity in their use of Tinder while selecting only a few potential sighted male partners (Kuhle et al., 2016). Males relax their standards for these short-term "hook-ups" and females do not (Buss, 2016). Thus, again, in short, females who are blind do not suffer a significant disadvantage in forming short-term relationships that are not designed to produce babies. Males who are blind and seeking brief sexual encounters continue to face the high standards and specific preferences females have brought to mate selection for many millennia.

Summary of gender differences in selection of mates

There are significant gender differences in the priorities that are given to the mate selection process. Table 21.1 summarises each of the important characteristics that men and women desire to find with those they select for intimate relationships. The results of research regarding gender preferences in romantic partnerships have been well replicated by large-scale regularly occurring research studies over the past 100 years (Fletcher et al., 2013). The research that supports these gender differences has been gathered, not only throughout the United States but also across cultures worldwide (Buss 2016; Fletcher et al., 2013). The differences on the part of the two genders with regard to mate selection preferences that still impact us today have been imprinted on the *Homo sapien* species from our earliest ancestors.

Table 21.1 Overview of gender differences that impact mate selection.

What men want in a mate	What women want in a mate
High interest in finding a mate who is physically attractive	Less interest in physical attractiveness of a mate
Less interest in financial resources, social status and intelligence of a mate	High interest in finding a mate with financial resources, superior social standing and intelligence
Less interest in physical strength of mate	High interest in finding a mate who is physically strong
Less interest in taller mates	High interest in finding a mate who is taller
High interest in younger mates	Less interest in younger mates
More interest in casual sex	Less interest in casual sex

Source: Adapted from Buss (2016) and Fletcher et al. (2013).

Conclusion

A major point that we wish to make at this juncture is that we have concentrated on the issue of sighted individuals forming breeding partnerships with blind individuals. We want to emphasise that we do not in any way wish to be interpreted by the reader as denigrating the possibility of two blind individuals forming such partnerships. Based on our personal acquaintances with blind couples, we are convinced that two people who are blind or severely visually impaired can, in fact, form very successful breeding pairs. Our intention with this chapter is to elaborate on the issue of persons who are blind coupling with sighted individuals given that there are vastly more sighted individuals on the planet than blind individuals. The challenges faced by blind breeding pairs are best left for another treatise.

References

Barkow, J. 1989. *Darwin, sex, and status*. Toronto, ON: University of Toronto Press.
Betzig, L. 1986. *Despotism and differential reproduction: A Darwinian view of history*. New York: Aldine de Gruyter.
Bobrow, D. and Bailey, J.M. 2001. Is male homosexuality maintained via kin selection? *Evolution and Human Behavior*, 22(5), 361–368.
Buss, D.M. 1989. Sex differences in human mate preferences: Evolutionary hypotheses tested in 37 cultures. *Behavioral and Brain Sciences*, 12(1), 1–49.
Buss, D.M. 2015. *Evolutionary psychology: The new science of the mind* (5th ed.). Oxford: Taylor & Francis.
Buss, D.M. 2016. *The evolution of desire: Strategies of human mating*. New York: Basic Books.
Buss, D.M. and Barnes, M.F. 1986. Preferences in human mate selection. *Journal of Personality and Social Psychology*, 50(3), 559–570.
Buss, D.M. and Schmitt, D.P. 1993. Sexual strategies theory: An evolutionary perspective on human mating. *Psychological Review*, 100(2), 204–232.
Buss, D.M., Shackelford, T.K., Kirkpatrick, L.A. and Larsen, R.J. 2001. A half century of mate preferences: The cultural evolution of values. *Journal of Marriage and Family*, 63(2), 491–503.
Cashdan, E. 1996. Women's mating strategies. *Evolutionary Anthropology*, 5(4), 134–143.
Conroy-Beam, D., Buss, D.M., Pham, M.N. and Shackelford, T.K. (2015). How sexually dimorphic are human mate preferences? *Personality and Social Psychology Bulletin*, 41(8), 1082–1093.
Cunningham, M.R. 1986. Measuring the physical in physical attractiveness: Quasi-experiments on the sociobiology of female facial beauty. *Journal of Personality and Social Psychology*, 50(5), 925–935.
Elder, G.H., Jr. 1969. Appearance and education in marriage mobility. *American Sociological Review*, 34(4), 519–533.
Fedigan, L.M. 1992. *Primate paradigms, sex roles and social bonds*. Chicago, IL: University of Chicago Press.
Feingold, A. 1992. Good-looking people are not what we think. *Psychological Bulletin*, 111(2), 304–341.
Fletcher, G.J.O. 2002. *New science of intimate relationships*. Oxford: Wiley-Blackwell.
Fletcher, G.J.O., Simpson, J.A., Campbell, L. and Overall, N. 2013. *The science of intimate relationships*. Oxford: Wiley-Blackwell.

Fletcher, G.J.O., Tither, J.M., O'Loughlin, C., Frisen, M. and Overall, N. 2004. Warm and homely or cold and beautiful? Sex differences in trading off traits in mate selection. *Personality and Social Psychology Bulletin*, 30(6), 659–672.

Gangestad, S.W., Thornhill, R. and Yeo, R.A. 1994. Facial attractiveness, developmental stability, and fluctuating asymmetry. *Ethology and Sociobiology*, 15(2), 73–85.

Geary, D.C. 2010. *Male, female: The evolution of human sex differences* (2nd ed.). Washington, DC: American Psychological Association.

Grammer, K. 1992. Variations on a theme: Age dependent mate selection in humans. *Behavioral and Brain Sciences*, 15(1), 100–102.

Hill, R. 1945. Campus values in mate selection. *Journal of Home Economics*, 37(9), 554–558.

Hudson, J.W. and Henze, L.F. 1969. Campus values in mate selection: A replication. *Journal of Marriage and the Family*, 31(4), 772–775.

Kapperman, G. and Kelly, S.M. 2017. *A second look at an assessment of the Tinder mobile data application for individuals who are visually impaired*. Unpublished data. Dekalb, IL: Department of Special and Early Education, Northern Illinois University.

Kapperman, G., Kelly, S.M., Kilmer, K. and Smith, T.J. 2017. An assessment of the tinder mobile dating application for individuals who are visually impaired. *Journal of Visual Impairment & Blindness*, 111(4), 369–374.

Kelly, S.M. 2013. Labor force participation rates among working-age individuals with visual impairments. *Journal of Visual Impairment & Blindness*, 107(6), 509–513.

Kenrick, D.T. and Keefe, R.C. 1992. Accuracy and bias in the perception of the partner in a close relationship. *Journal of Personality and Social Psychology*, 80(3), 439–448.

Kuhle, B.X., Beasley, D.O., Beck, W.C., Brezinski, S.M., Cnudde, D., Lavelle, K.D., Moran, J.B., O'Connor, E.N., Piranio, A.M. and Woehrle, R.C. 2016. *To swipe left or right: Sex differences in tinder profiles*. Paper presented at the annual meeting of the Human and Behavior Evolution Society, Vancouver, Canada.

Langhorne, M.C. and Secord, P.F. 1955. Variations in marital needs with age, sex, marital status, and regional composition. *Journal of Social Psychology*, 41(1), 19–37.

Li, N.P., Bailey, J.M., Kenrick, D.T. and Linsenmeiser, J.A.W. 2002. The necessities and luxuries of mate preference: Testing the tradeoffs. *Journal of Personality and Social Psychology*, 82(6), 947–955.

McGinnis, R. 1958. Campus values in mate selection. *Social Forces*, 36(4), 368–373.

Malinowski, B. 1929. *The sexual life of saves in north-western Melanesia*. Oxford: Routledge.

Reis, H.T. and Downey, G. 1999. Social cognition in relationships: Building essential bridges between two literatures. *Social Cognition*, 17(2), 97–117.

Semmelroth, J. and Buss, D.M. n.d.. *Studies on conflict between the sexes*. Unpublished data. Ann Arbor, MI: Department of Psychology, University of Michigan.

Singh, D. 1993a. Adaptive significance of waist-to-hip ratio and female physical attractiveness. *Journal of Personality and Social Psychology*, 65(2), 293–307.

Singh, D. 1993b. Body shape and female attractiveness: Critical role of waist-to-hip ratio. *Human Nature*, 4(3), 297–321.

Singh, D. 1994. Is thin really beautiful and good? Relationship between waist-to-hip ratio and female attractiveness. *Personality and Individual Differences*, 16(1), 123–132.

Symons, D. 1979. *The evolution of human sexuality*. Oxford: Oxford University Press.

Symons, D. 1989. The psychology of human mate preferences. *Behavioral and Brain Sciences*, 12(1), 34–35.

Taylor, P.A. and Glenn, N.D. 1976. The utility of education and attractiveness for females' status attainment through marriage. *American Sociological Review*, 41(3), 484–498.

Udry, J.R. and Eckland, B.K. 1984. Benefits of being attractive: Differential payoffs for men and women. *Psychological Reports*, 54(1), 47–56.

Williams, G.C. 1957. Pleiotropy, natural selection, and the evolution of the sciences. *Evolution*, 11(4), 398–411.

Zuckerman, D.M. 2004. *Blind adults in America: Their lives and challenges*. Washington, DC: National Center for Policy Research for Women & Families.

Part VIII

Orientation, mobility, habilitation and rehabilitation

22

Modern approaches to orientation and mobility

Habilitation and rehabilitation

Karl Wall

Introduction

"Habilitation" (e.g. in the UK: Miller, Wall and Garner, 2011; Wall, 2012a, 2012b) as an approach, is based on ideas developed in the 1970s–1980s, in relation to children and young people particularly, in the UK and abroad, about how strategies for every aspect of daily living might be developed for those with a range of particular needs, including visual and multisensory needs (e.g. in the United States: Goble, 1983; Ling and Ling, 1978; Rosen, Clark and Kivitz, 1977). These often took account of physical disabilities where individual locomotion by walking (e.g. through the need to use a wheelchair) was restricted.

The chapter aims to offer starting points for those new to the field of habilitation; for those who wish to explore it more deeply in terms of current research and for those practitioners who seek further understanding of how practice might be supported and explicated by research.

Issues affecting habilitation and rehabilitation

Six dimensions inform the contents of this chapter:

1   Changes in the visual need population worldwide.
2   The UN Convention on the Rights of Persons with Disabilities (CRPD).
3   The emergence of habilitation and rehabilitation.
4   The extended core curriculum for CYPVN.
5   Technology and habilitation.
6   Prospective research, training and practice issues.

Changes in the visual need population worldwide

In mid-2017, the world population stands at around 7.6 billion (UN, 2017a): a growth of 1 billion people in the last 12 years. This represents, however, a *slowing* down. Ten years ago the world population was growing at about 1.24% per year (it is now growing at a rate of

1.1% per year). Projections around future growth suggest a further slowing down, with the world population anticipated to reach 8.6 billion in 2030.

The structure of this population, germane to understanding the extent of visual needs and the likely balance of habilitation and rehabilitation activity likely to be needed worldwide, is changing: the world population is ageing. A decline in fertility and an increase in life expectancy are apparent. These changes affect the *structure* of the population and the balance between those in the age range 15–59 (currently at 61%); those who are children – under the age 15 (26%) and those over 60 (13%). It is this older group that is growing fastest, indeed faster than the under-15 group, which is expected to stay relatively stable throughout the rest of the century (at about 2 billion).

The under-15 group forms the main population from which the CYPVN population arises, as we shall see shortly. The projections for the over-60 groups – a near doubling by 2050 – encompass the greater part of those who may need *rehabilitation* as many of the visual needs affecting this group are linked directly to aging itself (UN, 2017b).

Visual needs data can be defined in a number of different ways; from an international health perspective (e.g. WHO, 2017); or at national or regional levels in terms of "blindness" registrations or, for the younger age group, in educational terms, whether a visual need affects access to learning or not. As an example, in the UK, in the habilitation context, it is defined broadly as being: "any level of visual impairment that has an effect on education, mobility and the ability to live independently" (Miller et al., 2011, p. 6).

The definition here is intentionally non-clinical, broadly based and *functionally* focused (that is, it attends to how a person uses their available vision in everyday activities) so that it may be applicable to as many CYPVN as possible (e.g. including cerebral visual impairment (CVI), see Chapters 5, 6 and 7 in this volume).

International health data (e.g. WHO, 2017) classifies vision function into four broad categories, drawing on the International Classification of Diseases-10 descriptions (ICD, 2006):

1 Normal vision
2 Moderate vision impairment
3 Severe vision impairment
4 Blindness.

Categories (2) and (3) are often combined as "low vision", meaning that low vision and blindness taken together represent all levels of vision impairment.

Vision impairment in this sense has a number of origins: globally, recent estimates (Bourne et al., 2017) suggest that the major causes of moderate to severe vision impairment (i.e. low vision) are:

- uncorrected refractive error (53%);
- un-operated cataract (25%);
- age-related macular degeneration (4%);
- glaucoma (2%);
- diabetic retinopathy (1%).

In relation to blindness, the major causes of blindness are:

- un-operated cataract (35%);
- uncorrected refractive error (21%)
- glaucoma (8%).

In terms of the groups identified earlier in relation to population growth, the over-50 group (for which rehabilitation may be needed), constitute about 81% of all people who are blind *or* have moderate to severe vision impairment. As the population ages, more people are likely to experience visual needs due to chronic eye disease and aging, suggesting an increased need for this type of support.

Equally, the under-15 group with visual needs constitute some 19 million children – of these it is noteworthy that some 12 million children have a need linked to refractive error, which in the majority of cases can be corrected optically. However, some 1.4 million have irreversible blindness, requiring access to habilitation (Mariotti, 2010). The balance, some, 5.6 million have visual needs across moderate to severe visual needs that *also* require habilitation.

These estimates are, however, not straightforward: they draw on international and regional data (some 59 studies from 39 countries) and where these were not available, measures linked to socio-economic level (Mariotti, 2010). These imputed estimates, suggest the over-50 groups may be subject to an error of 10%: for the under 15s it may be 20%. In addition, the estimates were based on global population figures for 2010 (global population at this time being lower than currently) and not the updated data for 2017. They therefore likely represent actual *under-estimates* while maintaining the same general trend and, as noted in the introduction, do not include data for brain-related visual needs.

In terms of CYPVN, some 4% of global causes are specifically linked to childhood. In the UK this amounts to around at least 25,000 children and young people in the age range 0–18 (e.g. Keil, 2012). However, as for global data, the *actual* levels are less certain: the methods yielding the data, given their range and account of degree of impact on functional vision are themselves prone to error (usually being based on self-report, survey and observational criteria – see from the UK, D'Ardenne, Hall and McManus, 2012).

Given, the international purview of this handbook and using the WHO regional organi-sation of countries as a way of structuring the global data Mariotti (2010) suggests that the percentage of overall visual needs varies by global region (as defined by the WHO): with the most, allowing for a world figure total (T), of 285.4 million, being in China (26.5%) and the least in the Western Pacific, excluding China (5.2%) (see Mariotti, 2010, for further discussion).

Across the regions, a clinical diagnosis does not necessarily offer a clearer picture. In some cultures and settings children with visual needs may not have their need reported to the authori-ties; other types of visual need (e.g. the relatively large area of CVI may not be accepted or acknowledged as a "legitimate" diagnosis for support or funding purposes).

Research coverage by region is uneven: in this chapter, where possible, the country in which research was conducted will be emphasised (for international data, no country will be given (e.g. Mariotti, 2010). This will make apparent the arguably largely American and European centricity of much current research – new researchers from outside these two contexts will need to look to *local literature* as a starting point for their investigations.

This is definitely not to say "research" in national areas outside these two regions does not take place or exist; rather that it is published – to the extent that peer-reviewed journals are used as a publication route – in local languages (other than English) and retained in the collec-tive memory of the countries concerned in terms of its focus and findings. One insight into this is through the work of Tom Lorimer (UK) and his WhiteStick website (Lorimer, 2017) and the World Blind Union (WBU, 2017). These sites currently host expanding lists of worldwide organisations involved in visual impairment, within which mobility, orientation and independ-ence skill practice can often be found. Table 22.1 lists the current coverage.

Table 22.1 Indicative list of organisations supporting visual needs in different countries of the world in 2017.

Country	Visual need related organisations
Albania	• Albanian Blind Association
Argentina	• Argentine Federation of Institutions for Blind and Visually Impaired
Australia	• Association for the Blind of WA – Guide Dogs
	• Blind Citizens Australia
	• Royal Institute for Deaf and Blind Children
	• Royal Victorian Institute for the Blind
	• Vision Australia
Austria	• Austrian Federation of the Blind and Partially Sighted
Brazil	• Brasilian Blind Sports Association – ABDC
	• Brazilian Council for the Welfare of the Blind – CBBEC
	• Dorina Nowill Foundation
	• Benjamin Constant Institute
Belgium	• Belgium Confederation for the Blind
Canada	• Canadian Council of the Blind
	• Canadian Federation of the Blind
	• Canadian National Institute for the Blind
	• The Raj Foundation
Colombia	• National Institute for the Blind
Croatia	• Croatian Association of the Blind
Cyprus	• Pancyprian Organization of the Blind
Czech Republic	• Czech Blind United
Denmark	• Dansk Blindesamfund
Estonia	• Estonian Federation of the Blind
Europe	• European Blind Unión – EBU
Finland	• Finnish Federation of the Visually Impaired
France	• Confédération Française pour la Promotion Sociale des Aveugles et Amblyopes
	• Association Valentin Hauy – AVH
	• French Federation of Blind and Visually Impaired – FAF
Germany	• German Federation of the Blind and Partially Sighted
Hungary	• Hungarian Federation of the Blind and Partially Sighted
Iceland	• The Icelandic Organization of the Visually Impaired
India	• National Association for the Blind – NAB
Ireland	• National Council for the Blind of Ireland
Italy	• Italian Union of the Blind and Partially Sighted
Japan	• Altair for Windows – Free Japanese Screen Reader
Jordan	• Friendship Association of the Blind – FABJO
Latvia	• Latvian Society of the Blind
Lithuania	• Lithuanian Association of the Blind and Visually Handicapped.
Luxembourg	• Fondation Lëtzebuerger Blannevereenegung
Nepal	• Nepal Association for the Welfare of the Blind
	• Nepal Association of the Blind
Netherlands	• Bartimeus Institute for the Blind and Partially Sighted
	• Dutch Federation of the Blind and Partially Sighted
New Zealand	• Association of Blind Citizens of New Zealand
	• Royal New Zealand Foundation for the Blind – RNZFB
Norway	• Norwegian Association of the Blind and Partially Sighted
Pakistan	• Pakistan Assistive Technology Foundation
	• Pakistan Foundation fighting Blindness

Poland	• Polish Association of the Blind
Portugal	• Associação dos Cegos e Amblíopes de Portugal
Romania	• Asociatia Nevazatorilor din România.
Serbia	• Union of the Blind of Serbia
Slovakia	• Slovak Blind and Partially Sighted Union
Slovenia.	• Union of the Blind and Partially Sighted of Slovenia
South Africa	• Blind SA
	• League of Friends of the Blind – LOFOB
	• South African National Council for the Blind – SANCB
	• Tape Aids for the Blind
Spain	• Organizacion Nacional de Ciegos de España
Sri Lanka	• Federation of the Visually Handicapped – SLFVH
Sweden	• Swedish Association of the Visually Impaired
Switzerland	• Swiss Federation of the Blind and Visually Impaired
United Kingdom	• Royal National Institute for the Blind – RNIB
	• Habilitation VIUK
United States	• ACB Radio
	• American Foundation for the Blind
	• American Printing House for the Blind
	• Braille Institute of America
	• Freedom Scientific, Jaws Screen Reader
	• National Braille Association
	• National Federation of the Blind
	• National Federation of the Blind of New Mexico
	• Seeing Eye
	• Serotek Corporation
Uruguay	• Braille Foundation of Uruguay

Note: This information is drawn from WBU (2017) and Lorimer (2017).

UN Convention on the Rights of Persons with Disabilities (CRPD)

The United Nations Convention on the Rights of Persons with Disabilities (CRPD) (UN, 2006) had its tenth anniversary in 2016. As of 2016, 175 (89%) member states of the UN had ratified the Convention; with its Optional Protocol (OP) adopted in 2016 being ratified by 92 (47%) of UN members (UN, 2017c). The OP established a committee to oversee progress in the implementation of the CRPD. Despite overall support for the introduction of the OP only 92 (47%) UN members have adopted it so far (UN, 2017c).

Embarking on a chapter focusing on *paediatric* visual needs, it is important to address – at least initially – both habilitation *and* rehabilitation and in doing so to reference the CRPD. Of the Charter's 50 articles, some 15 articles relate directly to issues current in the field of mobility, orientation and independent living skill support across the age ranges, including technological issues.

The 15 sections of the CRPD (UN, 2006) (see Table 22.2 for details) address disabilities in general, although there are some specific references to particular visual need (VN) issues, such as braille (Articles 9 and 24). In focusing on the needs of CYPVN, the CRPD phrase "persons with disabilities" could be changed to "CYPVN" and the 15 articles would then directly address key issues in habilitation (see Table 22.2). In addition, running through many of these is a need for state bodies to focus on *technological* changes and how they must be accessible, for those in the current context, with visual needs. Article 26, Habilitation and Rehabilitation specifically captures these issues (see Table 22.2).

Table 22.2 Summary of key articles of the UN CRPD (and Optional Protocol) relating to habilitation.

Article number	Title	Focus	Page no.
2	Definitions	Reasonable accommodation	4
3	General principles	Universal design	5
		(h) [E]volving capacities of children with disabilities . . . for the right of children with disabilities to preserve their identities	
4	General obligations	(1f) [U]ndertake or promote research and development of universally designed goods, services, equipment and facilities . . . minimum possible adaptation . . . least cost to meet the specific needs of a person with disabilities . . . promote their availability . . . promote universal design	6
		(1g) [U]ndertake . . . promote research and development of . . . the availability . . . use of new technologies, including: information communications technologies, mobility aids, devices and assistive technologies, suitable for persons with disabilities, giving priority to . . . affordable cost	
		(1h) [P]rovide accessible information to persons with disabilities about mobility aids, devices . . . assistive technologies . . . new technologies . . . other forms of assistance, support services and facilities	
		(1i) [P]romote the training of professionals and staff working with persons with disabilities in the rights recognized in the present Convention so as to better provide the assistance . . . services guaranteed by those rights	
6	Women with disabilities	(1) [R]ecognize that women and girls with disabilities are subject to multiple discrimination, and in this regard shall take measures . . . guaranteeing them the exercise and enjoyment of the human rights . . . and fundamental freedoms	7
7	Children with disabilities	(1) [A]ll necessary measures to ensure the full enjoyment by children with disabilities of all human rights and fundamental freedoms	7
		(2) [A]ll actions concerning children with disabilities, the best interests of the child shall be a primary consideration	
		(3) [S]hall ensure that children with disabilities have the right to express their views freely on all matters affecting them, their views being given due weight . . . their age and maturity . . . an equal basis with other children . . . provided with disability and age-appropriate assistance to realize that right.	
8	Awareness-raising	(2iii) To promote recognition of the skills, merits and abilities of persons with disabilities . . . their contributions to the workplace and the labour market	8
		(2b) Fostering . . . all levels of the education system, including in all children from an early age . . . attitude of respect for the rights of persons with disabilities	

9	Accessibility	(1) [E]nable persons with disabilities . . . [to] live independently . . . participate fully in all aspects of life . . . take appropriate measures to ensure persons with disabilities access . . . [on an] equal basis with others . . . physical environment, to transportation, to information and communications . . . information and communications technologies . . . systems . . . other facilities . . . services open . . . provided to the public, . . . in urban . . . in rural areas . . . include . . . identification . . . elimination of obstacles . . . barriers to accessibility, shall apply	9–10
		(a) Buildings, roads, transportation and other indoor and outdoor facilities . . . schools, housing, medical facilities . . . workplaces	
		(b) Information, communications . . . other services, . . . electronic services . . . emergency services	
		(2) [S]hall also take appropriate measures [to]:	
		(a) develop, promulgate . . . monitor the implementation of minimum standards . . . guidelines . . . accessibility of facilities and services open or provided to the public	
		(b) ensure that private entities . . . offer facilities . . . services . . . open or provided . . . public take . . . account all aspects of accessibility . . . persons with disabilities	
		(c) provide training for stakeholders . . . accessibility issues persons with disabilities	
		(d) provide in buildings . . . other facilities open to the public signage in braille . . . easy to read . . . understand forms	
		(e) provide forms of live assistance and intermediaries, . . . guides, readers . . . professional sign language interpreters, . . . facilitate accessibility to buildings . . . other facilities open to the public	
		(f) promote . . . appropriate forms of assistance . . . support to persons with disabilities . . . ensure . . . access to information	
		(g) promote access . . . persons with disabilities . . . new information . . . communications technologies . . . systems . . . the Internet	
		(h) promote . . . design, development, production . . . distribution of accessible information . . . communications technologies . . . systems at an early stage . . . that these technologies and systems become accessible at minimum cost	
19	Living independently and being included in the community	[T]he equal right of all persons with disabilities . . . live . . . community . . . choices equal to others . . . shall take effective . . . appropriate measures . . . facilitate full enjoyment . . . persons with . . . this right . . . their full inclusion . . . participation . . . community . . . ensuring that:	13
		(a) Persons with disabilities . . . opportunity . . . choose . . . place of residence . . . where . . . with whom they live . . . equal basis with others . . . not obliged to live . . . particular living arrangement	
		(b) Persons with disabilities . . . access to a range of in-home, residential . . . community support services . . . personal assistance necessary to support living . . . inclusion in . . . community . . . prevent isolation or segregation from the community	

(continued)

Table 22.2 (continued)

Article number	Title	Focus	Page no.
20	Personal mobility	[S]hall take effective measures . . . ensure personal mobility . . . greatest possible independence for persons with disabilities . . . by: (a) facilitating . . . personal mobility . . . persons with disabilities . . . manner . . . time of their choice . . . affordable cost (b) facilitating access by persons with disabilities . . . quality mobility aids, devices, assistive technology . . . forms of live assistance . . . intermediaries . . . making them available . . . affordable cost (c) providing training in mobility skills . . . persons with disabilities . . . to specialist staff working . . . persons with disabilities (d) encouraging entities that produce mobility aids, devices . . . assistive technologies . . . aspects of mobility for persons with disabilities	14
24	Education	[R]ecognize . . . right of persons with disabilities to education . . . without discrimination . . . basis of equal opportunity . . . ensure an inclusive education system at all levels and lifelong learning directed to: (1b) the development by persons with disabilities . . . personality, talents and creativity . . . their mental . . physical abilities . . fullest potential (1c) enabling persons with disabilities . . . participate effectively . . . free society (2) [S]hall ensure that: (a) persons with disabilities are not excluded . . . general education system on the basis of disability . . . children with disabilities are not excluded from free . . . compulsory primary education, or . . . secondary education, on the basis of disability (b) persons with disabilities . . . access . . . inclusive, quality . . . free primary education . . . secondary education on an equal basis . . . others in the communities . . . they live (c) reasonable accommodation . . . individual's requirements . . . provided (d) persons with disabilities receive . . . support required, within . . . general education system . . . facilitate . . . effective education (e) effective individualized support measures . . . provided in environments . . . maximize academic . . . social development, consistent . . . goal . . . full inclusion (3) [S]hall enable persons with disabilities . . . learn life . . . social development skills . . . facilitate . . . full and equal participation . . . education . . . members of the community . . . shall take appropriate measures, including: (a) braille, alternative script, augmentative . . . alternative modes, means . . formats of communication . . . orientation . . . mobility skills, . . . facilitating peer support and mentoring (b) facilitating the learning of sign language . . . promotion . . . linguistic identity . . . deaf community (c) ensuring . . . education of persons . . . in particular children . . . blind, deaf or deafblind . . . delivered . . . most appropriate languages . . . modes . . . means of communication for the individual, . . . in environments . . . maximize academic and social development	16–18

		(4) [H]elp ensure the realization of this right . . . shall take appropriate measures . . . employ teachers . . . teachers with disabilities . . . qualified in sign language and/or braille . . . train professionals and staff who work at all levels of education . . . training shall incorporate disability awareness . . . use of appropriate augmentative . . . alternative modes, means . . . formats . . . communication, educational techniques . . . materials . . . support persons with disabilities	18
		(5) [E]nsure . . . persons with disabilities . . . able to access general tertiary education, vocational training, adult education . . . lifelong learning without . . . an equal basis with others . . . shall ensure that reasonable accommodation is provided . . . persons with disabilities	
25	Health	(b) [P]rovide those health services needed by persons with disabilities specifically because of their disabilities . . . early identification . . . intervention as appropriate . . . services designed to minimize . . . prevent further disabilities, . . . among children and older persons	19
26	Habilitation and rehabilitation	[S]hall take effective . . . appropriate measures . . . through peer support . . . enable persons with disabilities . . . attain . . . maintain *maximum independence*, full physical, mental, social and vocational ability . . . full inclusion and participation in all aspects of life . . . *shall organize, strengthen and extend comprehensive habilitation . . . rehabilitation services . . . programmes . . . the areas of health, employment, education . . . social services . . .* these services and programmes:	
		(a) *earliest possible stage* . . . based on . . . multidisciplinary assessment . . . individual needs . . . strengths	
		(b) support *participation . . . inclusion . . . community . . . all aspects of society . . . voluntary . . .* available to persons with disabilities . . . close as possible . . . their own communities, including . . . rural areas	
		(2) [S]hall promote . . . development of initial . . . *continuing training for professionals* . . . staff working in habilitation . . . rehabilitation services	
		(3) [S]hall promote . . . availability, knowledge . . . use of *assistive devices and technologies*, designed for persons with disabilities . . . habilitation and rehabilitation	
27	Work and employment	(d) [E]nable persons with disabilities . . . effective access . . . general technical . . . vocational guidance programmes, placement services . . . vocational . . . continuing training	20
		(k) [P]romote vocational . . . professional rehabilitation, job retention . . . return-to-work programmes . . . persons with disabilities	

(continued)

Table 22.2 (continued)

Article number	Title	Focus	Page no.
29	Participation in political and public life	[S]hall guarantee . . . persons with disabilities political rights . . . opportunity to enjoy them . . . equal basis with others . . . (a) [E]nsure that persons with disabilities . . . effectively . . . fully participate . . . political . . . public life . . . equal basis with others, directly or through freely chosen representatives . . . right . . . opportunity for persons with disabilities to vote . . . be elected	21
30	Participation in cultural life, recreation, leisure and sport	[R]ecognize the right of persons with disabilities . . . take part on an equal basis with others in cultural life, ... take all appropriate measures (5) [T]o enable persons with disabilities to participate . . . an equal basis with others . . . recreational, leisure . . . sporting activities (a) [E]ncourage . . . promote . . . participation . . . fullest extent possible, . . . persons with disabilities in mainstream sporting activities . . . all levels (b) [E]nsure . . . persons with disabilities . . . opportunity . . . organize, develop . . . participate . . . disability-specific sporting . . . recreational activities . . . encourage . . . provision . . . an equal basis with others . . . appropriate instruction, training . . . resources (c) [T]o ensure . . . persons with disabilities . . . access . . . sporting, recreational . . . tourism venues (d) [T]o ensure . . . children with disabilities . . . equal access . . . other children . . . participation . . . play, recreation . . . leisure . . . porting activities, including . . . activities in the school system (e) [E]nsure that persons with disabilities . . . access . . . services . . . those involved in the organization of recreational, tourism, leisure . . . sporting activities	23

Note: The Charter has 50 articles: the optional protocol (recognising the UN Committee on the Rights of Persons with Disabilities) has 18 articles. Only those with a direct relevance to the education, health, social/mental well-being and careers and employment of children and young people in relation to habilitation (mobility, orientation and independent living skills) have been identified above.

Table 22.3 Five key compendious sources to access research and practice informing contemporary habilitation.

Foundations of Education, Volume I: History and Theory of Teaching Children and Youths with Visual Impairments (3rd ed.)	Foundations of Education, Volume II: Instructional Strategies for Teaching Children and Youths with Visual Impairments (3rd ed.)	Foundations of Orientation and Mobility, Volume 1: History and Theory (2nd ed.)	Foundations of Orientation and Mobility, Volume 2: Instructional Strategies and Practical Applications (2nd ed.)	Orientation and Mobility Techniques: A Guide for the Practitioner (2nd ed.)
Cay Holbrook et al. (2017a)	Cay Holbrook et al. (2017b)	Wiener, Welsh, and Blasch (2010a)	Wiener, Welsh, and Blasch (2010b)	Fazzi and Barlow (2017)

Cay Holbrook et al. (2017a)

Part I:
History and theory
1 Historical perspectives
2 Visual impairment: terminology, demographics, society
3 The visual system
4 Growth and development of young children
5 Growth and development in middle childhood and adolescence
6 Psychosocial needs of children and youths
7 Children and youths with visual impairments and other exceptionalities
8 Diversity and its implications
9 Educational programming
10 Professional practice
Part II:
Connecting to the broader context
11 Applying general education theory to visual impairment
12 Motivation

Cay Holbrook et al. (2017b)

Part I:
Ensuring high-quality instruction
1 Creating and nurturing effective educational teams
2 Overview of assessment
3 Assessment techniques
4 Specialized assessments
5 Moving from assessment to instruction
6 Planning Instruction in unique skills
7 Supporting differentiated instruction and inclusion in general education
8 Educating groups about students with visual impairments
Part II:
Modifying and designing instruction
9 Early childhood interventions
10 Students with visual impairments and additional disabilities
11 Compensatory skills

Wiener, Welsh, and Blasch (2010a)

Part I:
Human systems
1 Perceiving to move and moving to perceive: control of locomotion by students with vision loss
2 Establishing and maintaining orientation for mobility
3 Low vision for orientation and mobility
4 Audition for students with vision loss
5 Kinesiology and sensorimotor functioning for students with vision loss
6 Psychosocial dimensions of orientation and mobility
7 Learning theories and teaching methodologies for orientation and mobility

Wiener, Welsh, and Blasch (2010b)

Part II:
Sensory use and psychosocial function
1 Improving perception for orientation and mobility
2 Improving orientation for students with vision loss
3 Improving the use of low vision for orientation and mobility
4 Improving the use of hearing for orientation and mobility
5 Improving sensorimotor functioning for orientation and mobility
6 Improving psychosocial functioning for orientation and mobility
Part II:
Age-related instruction
7 Teaching orientation and mobility for the early childhood years
8 Teaching orientation and mobility to school-age children
9 Teaching orientation and mobility to adults
10 Teaching orientation and mobility to older adults

Fazzi and Barlow (2017)

Introduction
1 Basic teaching principles
2 Orientation for mobility
3 Guide techniques
4 Hand trailing and protective techniques
5 Cane techniques
6 Block travel
7 Street crossings
8 Transportation systems
9 Special situations
10 Travel techniques for learners who have low vision

(continued)

Table 22.3 (continued)

Foundations of Education, Volume I: History and Theory of Teaching Children and Youths with Visual Impairments (3rd ed.)	Foundations of Education, Volume II: Instructional Strategies for Teaching Children and Youths with Visual Impairments (3rd ed.)	Foundations of Orientation and Mobility, Volume 1: History and Theory (2nd ed.)	Foundations of Orientation and Mobility, Volume 2: Instructional Strategies and Practical Applications (2nd ed.)	Orientation and Mobility Techniques: A Guide for the Practitioner (2nd ed.)
13 Augmentative and alternative communication	12 Literacy skills	**Part II:** **Mobility systems and adaptations**	**Part III:** **Adapted tools and complex environments**	
14 Consultation and collaboration	13 Social studies	8 Adaptive technology for orientation and mobility	11 Teaching the use of orientation aids for orientation and mobility	
15 The changing landscapes of rural education	14 Science	9 Dog guides for orientation and mobility	12. Teaching travel at complex intersections	
16 Tiered models of behavioral and instructional support	15 Mathematics	10 Orientation aids for students with vision loss	13 Teaching the use of transportation systems for orientation and mobility	
17 Reading and interpreting research	16 Arts education	11 Environmental accessibility for students with vision loss	14 Teaching the use of electronic travel aids and electronic orientation aids for orientation and mobility	
18 Transition planning for young adults with disabilities	17 Physical education and health	12 Administration, assessment, and programme planning for orientation and mobility services	15 Orientation and mobility for adverse weather conditions	
19 Problem solving and critical thinking	18 Sensory efficiency: assessment and instructional strategies	**Part III:** **The profession of orientation and mobility and its development**	16 Dog guides and the orientation and mobility specialist	
20 Social and emotional learning: recent research and practical strategies for educators	19 Assistive technology	13 The originators of orientation and mobility training	**Part IV** **Orientation and mobility and different disabilities**	
	20 Orientation and mobility	14 The history and progression of the profession of orientation and mobility	17 Teaching orientation and mobility to students with vision and hearing loss	
	21 Independent living skills	15 The development of the profession of orientation and mobility around the world	18 Teaching orientation and mobility to learners with visual, physical, and health impairments	
	22 Social skills	16 Research and the orientation and mobility specialist	19 Teaching orientation and mobility to students with cognitive impairments and vision loss	
	23 Recreation and leisure		20 Teaching orientation and mobility to students with cortical visual impairment	
	24 Career education		21 Travel instruction for individuals with nonvisual disabilities	
	25 Self-determination			

Note: Details for these sources and their contents taken from AFB (2017).

Many of the issues identified in the CRPD, taken as starting points for research and practice, can be married up to research and practice issues contained in the compendium of references listed in Table 22.3. These five sources represent important starting points for research (and practice) in this area. Each chapter is a specialist and contemporary review in the area concerned: for VN education in general: Cay Holbrook et al. (2017a, 2017b); for mobility, orientation and independence in general (Wiener, Welsh and Blasch, 2010a, 2010b). Fazzi and Barlow (2017) address mobility, orientation and independence from a practitioner's and skills perspective but from a more US focused perspective than the other volumes. All five sources constitute a widely used starting point for investigating the issues identified in the current chapter, for both younger or older people.

The emergence of habilitation and rehabilitation

Those who work with CYPVN will describe the main areas of practice in this area as "mobility, orientation and independent living" (MOI): someone supporting adults will likely say, "orientation, mobility and independent living (OMI). This reflects more than the ordering of the three words. Those who take the MOI perspective would identify their work as "habilitation" while those who take the OMI perspective would describe it as "rehabilitation". A difference captured in Article 26 (Habilitation and Rehabilitation) in the CRPD (UN, 2006).

The "MOI" of habilitation also captures the fact that habilitation addresses the needs of CYPVN from a *developmental* approach and so focuses on the three key areas framing them as they occur, in what children actually do as they develop (e.g. as in the legislation relating to special educational needs and disability – the Code of Practice in England (DoH/DfE, 2015) and in the Quality Standards underpinning habilitation practice in the UK (Miller et al., 2011). In both cases there is a focus on ages 0–25, allowing for intellectual needs that might reflect an earlier developmental stage than indicated by chronological age alone. This view is grounded in how children develop from birth, through early childhood, adolescence and into early adulthood, both typically and atypically (in the UK, Herbert, 2002; see also in relation to visual needs, Warren, 1984, 1994) and in terms of disability more generally (e.g. in the UK, Lewis, 2002).

In terms of the CRPD, a child is defined in terms of a particular state's view and definition of, "childhood" – this varies dramatically around the world and within countries for specific aspects of provision and legislation. Researchers need to be clear about the arrangements in specific countries of interest to them; cross-country comparisons are therefore not straightforward and need to be assayed with caution (in large multi-state countries like the United States, these also vary state by state). Where participant ages are reported this should be as their chronological age (and/or their developmental age, which may be different) and not some proxy for age such as "K2" (as in the United States).

This issue is significant because states often structure their provision – where it exists – according to users' chronological ages (this is also reflected in how research and practice is viewed, e.g. in Wiener et al., 2010b, pt 2). In the UK, for example, special needs and disability (including VN) support in terms of legislation, drawing on education, health and social care inputs cover the age range 0–25 years (DoH/DfE, 2015), however in VN terms a "child" is viewed as being in the age range 0–19 years – thereafter they become "young adults" and are supported by adults', as opposed to children's, services.

The developmental approach informing habilitation frames much of the approach and rationale for habilitation *in practice* (e.g. in the United States, Fazzi and Barlow, 2017). Within a holistic overview, there is a need to consider children's typical *and atypical* developmental processes: physical, motor, sensory and more broadly, psychologically, if the implications and impacts of VN are to be understood and addressed. Research reviewed by Gori et al. (2016), for example, suggests that a lack of vision from an early age affects spatial and social skills in children, this being associated with a range of other sensory and motor issues.

Development underpinning habilitation

Prior to birth, development in the womb lays the foundation for post-birth activity. (Cay Holbrook et al., 2017a; Piek, 2006). At birth, the baby experiences the full effects of gravity for the first time and must bear its own weight, initially on its back and tummy and then, as the baby rolls over more often on to its tummy, increasingly through its developing back and abdominal muscle systems. In time the baby is able to raise its head allowing its various senses, largely concentrated in the head, to fully access the surrounding environment. Detecting interesting objects in its immediate environment motivates the typically developing baby to seek to move toward that stimulus. Moving more and more in the environment, baby begins to orientate toward features that attract its interest. People, moving objects, differences represented in shape, colour, contrast, sound (as distal stimuli) smell and taste, texture and touch (as more proximal stimuli) attract its attention: mobility is the priority, followed by orientation, hence the emphasis on MOI rather than OMI.

Mobility, permitting orientation, progresses through crawling, bottom sliding in a seated position, cruising (holding on to objects to raise itself up and then move) and finally walking, then running. These changes do not all have to occur – some babies move from crawling, straight to walking for example (Largo, Kunda and Thun-Hohenstein, 1993, UK) but they do usually follow a similar sequence – at least in Western societies using the same milestones in similar cultural contexts. Warren (1984, 1994, UK) has noted that among children with visual needs, development follows a similar course to that of typically developing children but either more slowly or via alternative avenues. Parenting approaches can have an impact as well as cultural practices such as toileting strategies (Herbert, 2002, UK).

Thus, from a "typical child", developmental perspective, the first goal of the developing child is movement and mobility, second, orientation and navigation. This also allows time for the incompletely developed visual system and its neural pathways to mature after birth to a functional and useable level. Whether sensory stimulus leads to movement or vice versa, is however, contested (see Wiener et al., 2010a, ch. 1)

The visual system (e.g. Cay Holbrook et al., 2017a, ch. 3) is one of the last to fully develop: as internal muscle systems, in and around the eye mature, so does focusing and accommodation. The visual system will achieve its basic extent at around the age of 7: it will then be relatively stable through childhood and into young adulthood, deteriorating with increasing age through the life course. Balance develops last as it is dependent on integrating body position in space with movement under the influence of gravity along with visual inputs. Understanding the role of balance in locomotion – for all children – is key for habilitation specialists in their practice (see Piek, 2006, pp. 85–100 and Wiener et al., 2010a, ch. 5).

As the child ages it becomes more independent, through the teaching and training of its parents (its first and, for the typical child, principal habilitation specialist – but consider for example the impact of a grandparent caring for the child as a proxy for parental input). Wider societal modelling provides other models but most early skill development occurs in and around the home, usually by direct and repeated observation by the child of others and their activity, via incidental learning; the developing child thus becomes more able to perform self-care and maintenance in washing, teeth brushing, dressing and feeding – some of the initial independent living skills needed throughout life. A learning route denied to those who are blind or have limited vision.

As personal mobility and orientation progresses during childhood, adolescence and into early adulthood (see Fazzi and Barlow, 2017; Wiener et al., 2010b, ch. 7–9), the young person establishes many of the independence skills it will use throughout its life. This process of development including the mastering of language and communication skills, social skills (e.g. Cay Holbrook et al., 2017a, ch. 20), a sense of self, of motivation (Cay Holbrook et al., 2017a, ch. 12), of interests and empathy (e.g. Cay Holbrook et al., 2017a, ch. 20) for others, continues into young adulthood.

However, for the child with a VN, a different prospect is likely without the intervention of professionals. Not being able to see may remove the motivation for movement – sound, although useful, as a distal stimulus is limited because when it ceases, it disappears, its information value, even its location, are lost (see Fazzi and Barlow, 2017; Wiener et al., 2010b, ch. 17 and 18). Vision allows stimuli to remain in a person's view, even if their attention is directed elsewhere and so can motivate exploration. However, person-initiated sound and attention to its reflections (echolocation) *can* be used to access important features of the environment and this forms a useful tool in the habilitation specialist's armoury and as a strategy for CYPVN (e.g. Kish and WAFB, 2017; Johnson and Louchart, 2012).

It is thus important from an habilitation point of view to take account of both typical development and development affected by visual loss whatever its nature: it is *not enough* to only view CYPVN as having a visual need – they also need to be viewed as developing children and young people as well. The impact of additional comorbid sensory and physical needs will also have to be taken account of.

Historical aspects of habilitation and rehabilitation

The impact of war on combatants is not a new issue even as it is a contemporary news item: indeed it arguably fuelled the development of rehabilitation and then habilitation provision in many countries following the Second World War and in the case of the United States, after the Korean war (see Cay Holbrook et al., 2017a, ch. 1; Wiener et al., 2010a, pt 3, ch. 13–16). Returning combatants needed rehabilitation because of the extensive vision-related damage (among other forms such as limb loss, internal injuries and psychological damage) they were experiencing.

The United States began to develop rehabilitative approaches; these became established among practitioners by the 1960s, including the introduction of the long cane and the Perkins brailler: the lessons learned from adult rehabilitation were then applied to CYPVN in the 1980s forming the beginnings of habilitation practice, although at this stage, it was still strongly grounded in rehabilitative perspectives (e.g. dressing skills for children in the seminal work, in the United States, of Klein, 1995; more recently in Australia: Johnston, Flavel and Lunn, 2002).

These practices, both in rehabilitation and habilitation, were disseminated to countries around the world, partly through the publication of an increasing body of research and practice evidence with the American Foundation for the Blind (AFB] playing a key role. This disseminated work (e.g. Wiener et al., 2010a, pt 3, ch. 15), included training programmes supported by those experienced in the American system (this can be accessed via the websites of the organisations listed in Table 22.1 and the sources shown in Table 22.3).

Where training had not existed its development was informed and developed by taking account of local family composition and organisation; child-rearing practices for CYPVN, the provision of training and support services (especially for adults) and their organisation, criteria for entitlement to access the services provided and their organisation and funding (see Table 22.1, which offers more locally nuanced sources than the aggregated historical accounts in some sources, such as Wiener et al., 2010a, ch. 15; Fazzi and Barlow, 2017, intro.).

Equally, attention had to be paid to the variations in transport system layout, the use of street and road furniture, signage and accepted behaviours on roads and at intersections. The use and provision of public transport and attitudes and practices towards accessibility in home, educational, employment and public spaces (e.g. for objects on the "pavement" (in the UK)/"sidewalk"; in the United States, e.g. Fazzi and Barlow, 2017; Wiener et al., 2010b, ch. 12) have also to be considered.

Habilitation or rehabilitation for CYPVN?

The distinction between habilitation and rehabilitation still lacks clarity in many jurisdictions: for the purposes of this chapter, the CRPD differentiation is accepted and used. This different perspective does have practical ramifications, particularly on which service, in a particular juris-diction, provides support services for CYPVN and who coordinates those services – education, health or social care – and who leads on their provision. In the case of the CRPD, much attention is focused on Article 26, which identifies the need for child- and adult-focused work as distinctive provision, and crucially, that this requires appropriate *training of the trainers* for each group. More broadly, the other CRPD articles identified earlier in Table 22.2, emphasise the educative- and ultimately employment-focused need for effective habilitation (see Table 22.2)

How then do habilitation and rehabilitation differ? Clearly from this perspective, habilitation is a learning focused field informed by an understanding of child development: its consequences for and connections to, learning, in a range of domains: academic/cognitive social and personal. It is clearly not a therapy, health or social care intervention per se but it may, especially where other needs are comorbid, involve crucial inputs from these areas by other practitioners (e.g. Wiener et al., 2010b, ch. 17 and 18). Habilitation must necessarily address the home, educa-tional and public spaces and how they work and the transitions, spatial, temporal and social between these settings (Miller et al., 2016).

In contrast, those who emphasise OMI are arguably viewing the issues from the perspec-tive of working with adults. Here the issues are rather different however (see Ponchillia and Ponchillia, 1996; for the cross-over aspects of both habilitation and rehabilitation see Cay Holbrook et al., 2017a, ch. 18; Wiener et al., 2010b, ch. 9 and 10).

The majority of adults receiving *rehabilitation* in the Western world are largely doing so having had sight for part of their lives (elsewhere it may be as a result of a sight loss due to infection). Sight loss can occur for a number of reasons: trauma (e.g. a car accident or sporting accident) or illness e.g. from diabetes, infectious diseases, parasitic infections and malnutrition. In some instances, an inher-ited condition can be present but not expressed until young adulthood and later life. Overall those receiving rehabilitation support have had a typical childhood, have effective communication skills and an extensive working knowledge of the world and its contents. They have likely developed decision-making skills, self-identity and have lived independently, often with a partner/family.

The "re-" of *re*-habilitation in a sense focuses on supporting such persons as they come to terms with their sudden or progressive sight loss, often during late middle age and for the over 60s, and its impact on their daily living (and that of their partner/family), their employment and social life, through the introduction of alternative strategies for completing tasks that once they would have done through sight-informed strategies alone.

Developing habilitation in the UK: an example

In the case of England and Wales (as devolved countries within the UK), practice was incoher-ent, inconsistent and highly variable: training then provided in MOI for children and young people was significantly underdeveloped. Informed by the work of Pavey et al. (2002), Olga Miller and Karl Wall sought funding for a substantial research and development project, the "Mobility21Project" (M21) (Wall, 2010), to address this confusion in provision.

The M21 project was tasked, during the period 2007–2010, with (1), a systematic review of current research and practice in MOI and to write, (2) a set of Quality Standards for MOI conceived as "habilitation", in collaboration with key stake holders including existing related practitioners, carers, CYPVN, providers of visual needs education and a range of national, regional and local government organisations. These standards (subsequently published as Miller et al., 2011) would necessarily embrace working practices, service organisation and individual professional competencies, knowledge, skills, training and understanding. The standards were also to form the basis of (3) a new training programme at graduate level, balancing academic and practical skills at what is now UCL-IOE, in London, specifically adapted for the UK setting.

Ably supported by the Mobility and Independence Specialists in Education (MISE) organisation – now called HabilitationVIUK (2017) – and in particular: Mary Pullen, Angie Bisson, Linda Bain, initially, and, subsequently, Sue Mort, Alison Hollands and Joyce Allinson and other members, Wall (2007, 2008a, 2008b, 2010) created and had validated, the resulting Graduate Diploma in Habilitation Studies for Visual Impairment course. Specially created video materials drawing on key background areas in ophthalmology, typical and atypical child development, vision sciences, physiotherapy and MOI practical skills were also developed as resources for the programme.

The new programme started in September 2009 and is still running to this day. In its collaborative approach it was an early example of knowledge mobilisation between researchers and practitioners (e.g. Wall and Hayton, 2017). Delivered in London, Edinburgh and Wakefield, it has trained some 160 new practitioners from across the UK: these currently work across the four devolved countries of the UK, in Ireland and in Australia and New Zealand. It is now the only direct route into habilitation practice in the UK.

Based on the same Quality Standards and working with the newly re-named Habilitation VIUK (the voluntary professional body for habilitation practitioners in the UK) a further training route was established. This was for rehabilitation-trained practitioners to enhance their previously adult-focused practice and was introduced at the City University, Birmingham (BCU, 2017) in 2016.

In 2007 there were just under 70 habilitation/rehabilitation practitioners working with children in the UK. Of these, some 30% were about to retire. As of 2017, there are now some 280 practitioners. This history will not be found in the compendious sources cited earlier in Table 22.1: it will be found via the websites of key organisations such as Habilitation VIUK (2017), which hosts the downloadable current Register of Qualified Habilitation Practitioners. Thereby illustrating the need, noted earlier, to use published accounts as starting points, but to look closely at contemporary and increasingly web-based resources.

The extended core curriculum for CYPVN

Habilitation with CYPVN in the UK is usually, but not exclusively, through education-focused services and to a lesser extent, health and social care. In other jurisdictions, particularly where there are federal/national and state/regional/devolved nation systems co-occurring in the same country (as in UK (devolved nations), Canada, India, the United States and Australia (federal and state systems) this may be arranged differently. Overall, habilitation and rehabilitation service provision here is often publically funded but may then be largely supported, supplemented by or effectively delegated to, charitable organisations of various types, size and national reach.

Provision of habilitation outside of core education and/or health provision can be further complicated by situations where countries mix both national, state and public responsibilities with privately funded provision, usually through insurance arrangements (e.g. in the United States).

The development of the Quality Standards in the UK (Miller et al., 2011; Wall and Hayton, 2017) involved creating a curriculum that drew, in the first instance on international practice (e.g. the sources shown in Table 22.2), extant UK research and curriculum proposals (e.g. Pavey et al., 2002) and adapting them for the UK context. Influential here were the ideas behind the extended core curriculum (ECC) (e.g. Huebner et al., 2004), which suggested that the standard curriculum was appropriate for those with visual needs in the absence of any additional cognitive need but, by virtue of their visual need, that additional learning opportunities would be required.

The ECC has nine domains that address the additional learning opportunities needed by those with visual needs: (1) compensatory or functional academic skills, including communication modes; (2) orientation and mobility; (3) social interaction skills; (4) independent living skills; (5) recreation and leisure skills; (6) career education; (7) use of assistive technology; (8) sensory efficiency skills and (9) self-determination (Allman and Lewis, 2014; Sacks and Zatta, 2016)

In the UK some of these skills are addressed by habilitation practitioners' (e.g. domains 1, 2, 3, 4, 5, 7, 8 and 9 while other vision-related professionals, particularly qualified specialist teachers of the visually impaired (QTVIs) focus on the main academic-related skills in an educational context (domains 1, 3, 6, 7, and 9). Together the two types of professionals support a variant of the ECC adapted to the UK context.

Unfortunately this *notional* ECC in the UK context is not widely recognised and is not statutory or necessarily accepted by those who run mainstream provision, although it is an integral part, generally, of special provision. Herein lies one of the main tensions for practitioners in the UK setting: that habilitation is recognised as an activity in the UK (and is identified in legislation) but its role in extending the curriculum for the CYPVN is not necessarily accepted, permitted and supported in practice, to the same degree as the core curriculum. This same issue may well apply in other jurisdictions.

This issue is not restricted to the UK – it is apparent in the information passing through the various national organisations shown in Table 22.1 and even in parts of the United States. Only when the *right* to access habilitation along with the rest of the ECC curriculum as an integral part of the entitlement of CYPVN to a curriculum that meets *their* needs is accepted as legitimate and achievable, will the situation – and thus the tension – be relieved.

In addition, for CYPVN and their trainers, fitting the demanding work of habilitation around the normal school day and core curriculum study is very challenging, exhausting and hard work – but crucial: CYPVN, it seems, are expected to work much harder than their sighted peers to even be in a position to compete with them on an equitable basis.

The right to an education that meets the needs of CYPVN should be beyond question: preparation for independent living as an employed person needs to embrace preparation for everyday living as much as for the gaining of academic qualifications. This is arguably more challenging in mainstream/public settings than in special school provision. It is still a right asserted but not fulfilled.

One organisation actively promoting this right – and so the importance of an integrated and effective extended core curriculum – is the International Council for the Education of the Visually Impaired (ICEVI, 2017). The ICEVI takes a lifelong learning view of education and training and is a useful starting point for contact to access the particular circumstances of provision in a particular region or country. ICEVI has representatives in many parts of the world who act as a hub for local national/regional information, statistical and practice information.

As a result of these localisations of rehabilitation and habilitation practice (still significantly informed by the compendious publications of the ARB (see Table 22.3) and the dissemination of research and practice through the pages of the *Journal of Visual Impairment and Blindness* (JVIB, 2017), US developed insights and practices have been disseminated to many countries: more broadly, a number of other peer-reviewed journals have developed in parallel, reflecting particular national perspectives and have also become increasingly international in their nature (e.g. the *British Journal of Visual Impairment*, BJVI, 2017). Over time, new journals such as the *International Journal of Orientation and Mobility* (IJOM, 2017) have also emerged.

Technology and habilitation

Technologies have always been part of how visual needs have been supported – a stick, a long cane; a Brailler; an acoustic cane, a guide dog, all represent different forms of assistive technology. As the twenty-first century has developed more and more diverse forms of technology, particularly in electronics, computing systems, materials (including fabrics) and their interconnectivity continue to be created.

To report particular examples in this chapter would be to report on what was instantly out of date, such is the rate of change. The sources cited in Table 22.3 offer many substantive starting points (see Cay Holbrook et al., 2017a, ch. 13; Cay Holbrook et al., 2017b, ch. 19; Fazzi and Barlow, 2017; Wiener et al., 2010a, ch. 8 and 10; Wiener et al., 2010b, ch. 11, 14, 17, 18, 19, 20, and 21).

Different commercially produced computing platforms compete with each other and open source materials are also becoming more prevalent (e.g. see Lorimer, 2017). Tablets, phones and ultra-thin computers, the development of wireless inter-device communications and task-specific mini-applications (programmes or "apps") offer many opportunities for the user with visual needs. National VN organisations now frequently host specialist teams (e.g. RNIB in the UK (RNIB, 2017) and user groups who test materials aimed at a wider public and more VN-specific materials. Good design works well for those with sight and without sight as noted in the CRDP (UN, 2017c).

In a review in 2016, Gori et al. (2016) looked at the issue from a different and arguably more useful perspective. They asked, why are such technological advances *not generally taken up* by adults and children with visual needs, many of whom still rely on a long cane or dog? In answering this question, Gori et al. (2016) also addressed some fundamental issues around the utility, in practice, of much of the proposed technology. They argue that technological devices have been broadly of two types: those that compensate for the absence of sight by substituting inputs from a different sensory modality, such as sound and touch; and, second, where an additional strategy is proposed to circumvent a visual need (Gori et al., 2016). The former will be focused on here as it forms by far the largest focus of technological development in relation to those with visual needs.

Among the former, sensory substitution devices (SSD) (Gori et al., 2016, p. 82) convert a visual stimulus into one accessible to the person with VN, usually via an audio or haptic signal. Gori et al. (2016) list some 22 devices of this type (pp. 83–84, table 2) including the original, video-based signal conversion to a tongue-received, "haptic image" stimulus (Bach-y-Rita et al., 1969; Bach-y-Rita and Kercel, 2003); through the sonic guide (Kay, 2000, 2001); iGlasses, for assisted navigation (Rempel, 2012); stimulation of the middle part of the sole contained in a shoe-based vibro-tactile interface called the "shoe-integrated-tactile display" (Velázquez, 2010); refreshable braille displays (e.g. Yobas et al., 2003); a further tongue-based interface, the Brainport Vision device (Arnoldussen and Fletcher, 2012; Nau et al., 2015); the KNFB reader that converts images and documents on "the go" (LCC, 2016); and for touch phones, VoiceOver and Talking Tap Twice (TTT) (Apple, 2017; Central, 2014). This demonstrates the range of what can be crudely divided into (a) devices that substitute for vision, (b) those that aid navigation and (c) those that aid reading or the accessing of text including braille text. But why are these and the other devices, not used more often?

Gori et al. (2016) suggest a number of reasons: many of the devices, even when miniaturised, remain bulky and intrusive to the person; they require extensive training for what may seem relatively little practical advantage on a day-to-day basis; they mark a user out as different to their peers (a particular issue for younger teenagers). The majority of the devices are laboratory based; were trialled with a very small number of individuals and so, because of the heterogeneity issues noted earlier around VN, may be less applicable to those outside of the initial test group. These are seldom scaled up to larger numbers, evaluated beyond their initial use or examined, through user-group trials, in extended everyday use. This series of issues *not* addressed forms a needed improvement agenda for future research in this area.

Many of these SSD devices work as ideas but are perceived perhaps as non-translatable and not usable in everyday life by VN users. There are also subtler reasons why they may not be more widely used: their use often blocks a sensory route while it is being used for the device: e.g. the tongue when used as an interface, cannot be used for taste detection or eating; an ear connection occupies one (or both) ear(s), via an ear piece, which reduces access to environmental sounds; their bulk may lead to bodily imbalance, which in turns affects gait and assured movement.

From a habilitation point of view virtually none of the devices mentioned in the Gori et al. (2016) review have been trailed with children – they were developed for adults. Arguably, given the plasticity of the child's developing neurosystem, developing applications for children might be more fruitful.

Another, subtler issue, which may mitigate their use with children, is concerns about the cognitive load they impose on the user when they already have to deal with substantial amounts of processing when engaging with the environment. Such loading may be reduced for experimental purposes in the controlled conditions of a laboratory but needs to be taken account of when the device is used in less controlled and constrained public settings. This can only be achieved with extensive user trials, which sadly are seldom undertaken when new SSD devices are developed. For children, cognitive load would be a particular issue, depending on their age, as it is not clear whether or to what extent multi-channel processing is effective in younger children: the close link between perception and action, fundamental to much habilitation practice and experientially crucial for CYPVN work, may be missing from some of these devices. Indeed there is a view that there is no perception *without* action of some sort (e.g. Lenay et al., 2003).

Linked to this is the issue of whether or not the incoming sensory experience afforded by the device can be integrated into the broader multi-sensory experience of CYPVN (work by Gori and colleagues in Italy (Gori, 2015) suggests that before the age of 10 years, children do not show much evidence of multi-sensory integration across modalities).

The remaining issue is one of clinical validation. Once developed, larger-scale trials with a range of users are not usually undertaken. This means that potential users may know of a device but it may not be accessible to them, not being manufactured or clinically validated as an intervention or "prescribed" in support systems, where clinical validation is required in order to access a device.

Gori et al (2016) argue that developers need to consider the needs of children and young people as distinct from those of adults (consistent with the CRPD; UN, 2017c) and take into account their developmental and in particular, *neuro*-developmental characteristics. These authors note the potential significance of devices that mobilise social interaction opportunities for CYPVN – the development of speech-accessed and speech-producing devices offers such a route although not specifically developed for those with visual needs. Where these are in the form of software "apps" many of the objections noted earlier for other SSDs disappear as the "apps" in question are hosted on ubiquitous smartphones; often enthusiastically embraced by CYP and adults with and without visual needs (in relation to persons with visual needs across the age range, see Griffin-Shirley et al., 2017).

However, others have sounded a warning in relation to the extent that braille is being used: braille offers access to a distinct world of knowledge, through braille *literacy*. However it takes much practice, is hard work and potentially isolating in classroom contexts, even with modern braille input devices/keyboards. The National Federation of the Blind in the United States reported in the 1950s that about half of blind children could read braille (Gori et al., 2016, p. 85). More recent figures suggest a dramatic drop in such usage (Abboud et al., 2014) to about 10%. Tobin and Hill (2015), however, note that braille, as a tactile-based code has potential to work with touch-based technologies, thus maintaining braille's usefulness as a route into literacy. The use of "apps" (e.g. "iOS VoiceOver" for Apple (2017) and for Android platforms, "TalkBack" Central (2014)), including the use of haptic feedback to the user via the screen of a device, make smartphone interaction easier and requires little or no training or practice, and for young people, smartphones are something that everyone uses, so using them would not make them appear "different" from their peers.

National VN groups are increasingly taking an evaluative and advisory role for VN members via their online presence (see Table 22.1). These groups, via active and frequently updated websites and discussion groups, offer an extensive and comprehensive window into technological developments. They also frequently campaign for wider public trials and the active involvement of those with visual needs in trialling and developing technological solutions. Here the key word is "online": access to the web is increasingly viewed as a requirement for modern living and in some respects, a "right".

People with visual needs can now access online environments and everything they contain (not withstanding that they are presented visually) directly by speech, typing and gesture. The visual nature of the web brings with it an increasing tendency to construe information visually, but to be accessible this needs to be companied by audio or video description. Increasing the amount, extent and quality of audio description is a key campaigning issue for many national VN organisations around educational, cinematic, video and workplace materials and training materials/resources (e.g. in the United States, AFB, 2017; in the UK, RNIB, 2017).

Access to the web, including its increasing number of social media platforms and apps offers the person with VN access to new social contact contexts. User research is needed to assess technological impacts and the utility of particular technologies and their drawbacks. Here the very social nature of messaging, access to discussion groups and social media sites offers a potential research route to evaluating particular technologies, particularly for those with VN. Here habilitation (and rehabilitation) practitioners should be encouraging discerning and critical/evaluative skills among those with visual needs – as among all such users – as well as making sure that training keeps up with and develops an understanding of, any such new technologies, not least by seeking their students' views of what is needed (e.g. see Ajuwon et al., 2016).

The rise of "fake news" and apparent interference with distributed public information is a warning that all that appears online may not be true. The vulnerabilities those with VN have in using the web are actively being discussed across national organisations: CYPVN attract additional concerns around child protection, exposure to traumatising behaviours such as bullying and politically motivated and abusive grooming. Here, as with older users in the financial context, the training of those using the web is vital and, again, habilitation and rehabilitation specialists clearly have a role – potentially compromised by the need for such professionals to be trained *themselves* and to keep up to date.

Prospective research, training and practice issues

Rehabilitation and habilitation practice (still significantly informed by the compendious publications of the ARB (see Table 22.3) is disseminated through research journals and practitioner organisations and VN organisations (e.g. see Table 22.1).

The five key and compendious starting points for work in this field (see Table 22.3), showcase much of the common understanding of habilitative (and to some extent rehabilitative) research and practice. Strikingly however, a detailed reading of these resources reveals the enormous gaps in research in validating *particular* habilitation practices in different contexts and for different groups of potential service uses.

In his seminal writings on visual impairments relating to CYPVN, although now comparatively old, Warren (1984, 1994), still captures many of the methodological and research issues for those working in this field. The regular statistical and method elements discussed in journals such as JVIB and BJVI serve to remind researchers of the significant impact on possible methodologies (and on choices of statistical analysis) that the very high heterogeneity of visual needs may have, and will need to take account of, even among those with the same notional diagnosis and of the same age, sex and circumstance. This is particularly so for neural function-related aspects of blindness or visual needs (e.g. CVI, see Chapter 5 in this volume).

Combined with the low incidence of many CYPVN conditions and their associated needs, these two factors – complex heterogeneity and low incidence – demarcate the two biggest issues that limit and to some extent compromise systematic large-scale research in this area. Not surprisingly perhaps, coupled with a widespread lack of funding and research training opportunities at doctoral level in many countries, such research that is available shows a preponderance of single-case studies (often single-person, controlled, experimental studies); multiple case study work and rather fewer longitudinal studies or large-scale sample studies.

In the case of habilitation, very little is known about the *efficacy over time* of interventions, their timeliness for particular CYPVN, long-term efficacy and impact. Although the "what works and why" agenda (e.g. GovUK, 2017; WCC, 2017 in the United States) apparent in many fields relating to educational, health and care practice has gained ground in recent years, its influence in the VI literature in this context is apparently very limited, as is the use of meta-analysis, which has had a noteworthy impact on educational research in general (e.g. the "visible learning" approach of Hattie, 2008; Hattie, Masters and Birch, 2015) and on aspects of VN work (e.g. in relation to the use of tactile maps and models, e.g. Wright, Harris and Stricken, 2010).

The limited longitudinal studies that are available (e.g. VICTAR, 2017 in the UK) illustrates the potential power and utility such studies offer, but also the difficulties in sustaining funding over such the long term, while maintaining a large enough and representative sample.

A number of practices, apparent in research in this area, arguably create as many problems as they seek to address. These include:

- Use of *mixed-age samples* within a specific or closely related group of diagnosis defined needs. Here a sample of older and younger adults (and sometimes adolescents) is aggregated to constitute a single sample, often without acknowledging the different rehabilitative, habilitative and developmental experiences of the individuals concerned.
- *Age of onset of visual need* is seldom reported.
- Lack of *follow-up assessment* of the impact or longevity of an intervention, its use in actual daily practice or its longer-term efficacy.
- Lack of *repetition of studies*.
- Inconsistent use of *effect sizes*, whether overall or on an element-by-element basis within a study (often linked to a *lack of power analysis* informing the study).
- Lack of use of recognised guidelines to *maximise robustness in qualitative* research strategies.
- *Multiple and inconsistently used definitions of particular VN populations.*
- *Definitions of what constitutes a visual need* in a particular piece of work. This is important because habilitation draws on many different fields, as illustrated in the wide range of disciplinary sources used in this chapter.
- *Identifying the national context of particular studies* (as done in this chapter) is important given the very different legislative, jurisdictional, cultural, social, economic and service provision contexts and approaches of different countries worldwide.
- Equally, as age – chronological and/or developmental age is particularly important in any CYPVN related work, *giving the actual age of the participants* (rather than a proxy term such as a key stage, year group or phase) is both necessary and important analytically.

The issue of a lack of research opportunity availability could be significantly supported by encouraging existing practitioners (both in habilitation and rehabilitation contexts) to engage in action research into their own and colleagues' practices: here the various national professional bodies (mandatory or voluntary as in the UK) have a significant role to play. Professionals working with researchers, taking account of the economic costs of *not* providing habilitation and rehabilitation, how we evaluate research, where it exists and the role of CYPVN and professionals in those processes are themselves urgently needed areas of research (e.g. see Labbett, 2018).

Training and continuing professional development providers at various levels of provision also have a key role to play. As practice should wherever possible be research-informed, evidence-based and evidence-led, such courses must provide trainees with the means to access research literature and to understand and critically evaluate such research. Being able to engage with and understand published research needs more than simply *reading* research: it needs specific opportunities to undertake research itself, suggesting an element to be actively incorporated into habilitation training (as it is in the UK). However, the changing and challenging nature, of teaching roles (e.g. in Australia, Brown and Beamish, 2012); of the provision of mobility and orientation services (e.g. in South Africa, Maguvhe, Dzapasi and Sabeya, 2012) and service provision (e.g. in the Asia-Pacific region, Ern Lim et al., 2014; in China, Marinoff and Heiberger, 2017) needs also to be examined and acknowledged.

Finally, the incipient retirement of longstanding researchers and practitioners and an apparent shortage of middle-career practitioners in many jurisdictions is a further issue for action. At the same time, similar concerns are being voiced among other professionals whose work informs habilitation and rehabilitation practice in many states: colleagues working in physical therapy, physiotherapy, speech and language therapy and occupational therapy seem to be declining in numbers. Specialist teachers and trainers of the visually impaired (and in overlapping needs, e.g. deafblindness), in various jurisdictions around the world, also seem to be declining on the basis of national, web-based sources.

These shortages (e.g. in the United States, see Pogrund, 2017) reflect a lack of funding availability and uncertainties in national priorities: an increasing focus on joint working to support those with visual needs (e.g. in the United States, Szabo and Panikkar, 2017) that impacts on professional time are also causes for rising concern, even though they should be promoted in terms of service effectiveness, particularly given the likely increase in numbers of those with visual needs, especially among older persons, as populations age, health care improves and greater longevity becomes significant. A key issue underpinning much of what is linked to habilitation and rehabilitation is the largely unexamined area of the economic costs – direct and indirect – for the individual and for societies as a whole, of *not* providing habilitation or rehabilitation.

Conclusion

This chapter has looked back over recent decades and, first, identified the origins of "habilitation" as an approach being more than "mobility and orientation" practices; it has looked at habilitation in comparison to rehabilitation and explored the rationale for its use in relation to children and young people. The chapter has cautioned against relying on the compendious publications that summarise much of the current literature around children and young people's habilitation needs, alerting the reader to the need to explore national literatures (often web-based); national VN organisations and journals less accessible for being in languages other than English. The potential of technology to inform subsequent developments in supporting those with visual needs has been discussed, the need to involve users much more in the trialling and deployment of new technologies has been noted, as has a proposed agenda for researchers working in and entering the field, as much as for professionals and their practice. This has been located more broadly in the need to consider the impact –particularly economically and socially – of *not* addressing the habilitation needs of CYPVN in coming decades.

References

Abboud, S., Hanassy, S., Levy-Tzedek, S., Maidenbaum, S. and Amedi, A. 2014. EyeMusic: Introducing a colourful experience for the blind using audiosensory substitution. *Restorative Neurology and Neuroscience*, 32(2), 247–257.

AFB. 2017. American Foundation for the Blind. Accessed December 2017. www.afb.org/default.aspx.

Ajuwon, P.M., Kalene Meeks, M., Griffin-Shirley, N. and Okungu, P.A. 2016. Reflections of visually impaired students on their assistive technology competencies. *JVIB*, 110(2) 128–134.

Allman, C.B. and Lewis, S. 2014. *ECC essentials: Teaching the expanded core curriculum to students with visual impairments*. New York: AFB.

Apple. 2017. *VoiceOver and Talking Tap Twice [TTT]* [e-resource]. Accessed December 2017. https://support.apple.com/en-sg/HT202362.

Arnoldussen, A. and Fletcher, D.C. 2012. Visual perception for the blind: The BrainPortvision device. *Retinal Physician*, 9(Jan./Feb.), 32–34.

Bach-y-Rita, P., Collins, C.C., Saunders, F.A., White, B. and Scadden, L. 1969. Vision substitution by tactile image projection. *Nature*, 221(5184), 963–964.

Bach-y-Rita, P. and Kercel, S.W. 2003. Sensory substitution and the human–machine interface. *Trends in Cognitative Science*, 7(12), 541–546.

BCU. 2017. *Habilitation work: Working with children and young people* [e-publication]. Accessed December 2017. www.bcu.ac.uk/courses/habilitation-work-visual-impairment-top-up.

BJVI. 2017 *British Journal of Visual Impairment.* Accessed December 2017. http://journals.sagepub.com/home/jvi.

Bourne, R.R.A., Flaxman, S.R., Braithwaite, T., Cicinelli, M.V., Das, A., Jonas, J.B., Keefe, J., Kempen, J. H., Leasher, J., Limburg, H., Naidoo, K., Pesudovs, K., Resnikoff, S., Silvester, A., Stevens, G.A. Tahhan, N., Wong, T.Y., Taylor, H.R. and the Vision Loss Expert Group. 2017. Magnitude, temporal trends, and projections of the global prevalence of blindness and distance and near vision impairment: A systematic review and meta-analysis. *Lancet Global Health*, 5(9), 888–897.

Brown, E.J. and Beamish, W. 2012. The changing role and practice of teachers of students with visual impairments: Practitioners' views from Australia. *Journal of Visual Impairment and Blindness*, 106(2), 81–92.

Cay Holbrook, M., McCarthy, T.S., Kamei-Hannan, C. and Zebehazy, K.T. 2017a. *Foundations of education. Volume I: History and theory of teaching children and youths with visual impairments* (3rd ed.). New York: AFB.

Cay Holbrook, M., McCarthy, T.S., Kamei-Hannan, C. and Zebehazy, K.T. 2017b. *Foundations of education. Volume II: Instructional strategies for teaching children and youths with visual impairments.* New York: AFB.

Central, A., 2014. *What is Google Talk Back?* [e-resource]. Accessed December 2017. www.androidcentral.com/what-google-talk-back.

D'Ardenne, J., Hall, M. and McManus, S. 2012. *Measurement of visual impairment in national surveys: A review of available data sources.* London: Thomas Pocklington Trust/NatCen.

DoH/DfE. 2015. *Special educational needs and disability code of practice: 0 to 25 years.* London: DoH/DfE/HMSO.

Ern Lim, Y., Vukicevic, M., Koklanis, K. and Boyle, J. 2014. Low vision services in the Asia-Pacific region: Models of low vision service delivery and barriers to access. *Journal of Visual Impairment and Blindness*, 108(4), 311–322.

Fazzi, D.L. and Barlow, J.M. 2017. *Orientation and mobility techniques: A guide for the practitioner* (2nd ed.). New York: AFB.

Goble, J.L. 1983. *Visual disorders in the handicapped child* (ed. Alfred. L. Schezer). Paediatric Habilitation. New York: Marcel Dekker.

Gori, M. 2015. Multisensory integration and calibration in children and adults with and without sensory and motor disabilities. *Multisensory Research*, 28(1), 71–99.

Gori, M., Cappagli, G., Tonelli, A., Baud-Bovy, G. and Finocchietti, S. 2016. Devices for visually impaired people: High technological devices with low user acceptance and no adaptability for children. *Neuroscience and Biobehavioral Reviews*, 69, 79–88.

GovUK. 2017. *What works network* [e-publication]. Accessed December 2017. www.gov.uk/guidance/what-works-network.

Griffin-Shirely, N., Banda, D.R., Ajuwon, P.M., Cheon, J., Lee, J., Ran Park, H. and Lyngdoh, S.N. 2017. A survey on the use of mobile applications for people who are visually impaired. *Journal of Visual Impairment and Blindness*, 111(4), 307–323.

HabilitationVIUK. 2017. Accessed December 2017. https://habilitationviuk.org.uk.

Hattie, J. 2008. *Visible learning.* London: Routledge.

Hattie, J., Masters, D. and Birch, K. 2015. *Visible learning into action: International case studies of impact.* London: Routledge.

Herbert, M. 2002. *Typical and atypical development: From conception to adolescence.* Oxford: Blackwell.

Huebner, K., Merk-Adam, B., Stryker, D. and Wolf, K. 2004, revised. *The national agenda for the education of children and youths with visual impairments, including those with multiple disabilities.* New York: AFB.

ICD. 2006. *International Classification of Diseases-10* [e-resource]. Accessed December 2017. http://apps.who.int/classifications/apps/icd/icd10online2006.

ICEVI. 2017. International Council for the Education of the Visually Impaired. Accessed December 2017. http://icevi.org.

IJOM. 2017. *International Journal of Orientation and Mobility.* Accessed December 2017. www.ijorientationandmobility.com.

Johnson, T. and Louchart, J. 2012. *Beginner's guide to echolocation for the blind and visually impaired: Learning to see with your ears.* CreateSpace Independent Publishing Platform.

Johnston, C., Flavel, R. and Lunn, H. 2002. *Do it yourself: Encouraging independence in children who are blind.* Sydney, Australia: Vision Australia Foundation/University of Sydney.

JVIB. 2017. *Journal of Visual Impairment and Blindness.* Accessed December 2017. www.afb.org/info/publications/jvib/12.

Kay, L. 2000. Auditory perception of objects by blind persons, using a bioacoustic high-resolution air sonar. *Journal of the Acoustical Society of America*, 107(6), 3266–3275.

Kay, L. 2001. Bioacoustic spatial perception by humans: A controlled laboratory measurement of spatial resolution without distil clues. *Journal of the Acoustical Society of America*, 109(2). 803–808.

Keil, S. 2012. *RNIB survey of VI services in England and Wales 2012: Report for England.* London: RNIB.

Kish, D. and WAFB. 2017. *World access for the blind: Our vision is sound.* Accessed December 2017. http://waftb.net.

Klein, M.D. 1995. *Pre-dressing skills: Revised.* Tuscon, AZ: Elsevier Health Sciences.

Labbett, S. 2018. Invited editorial comment. *British Journal of Visual Impairment*, 36(2), 107–109.

Largo, R.H., Kunda, S. and Thun-Hohenstein, L. 1993. Early motor development in term and pre-term children. In A.F. Kalverboer, B. Hopkins and R. Geuze (eds), *Motor development in early and later childhood: Longitudinal approaches* (p. 247–265). Cambridge: Cambridge University Press.

LCC, K.R. 2016. KNFB reader [e-publication]. Accessed December 2017. www.knfbreader.com.

Lenay, C., Gapenne, O., Hanneton, S., Marque, C. and Genouelle, C. 2003. Sensory substitution: Limits and perspectives. In *Touching for knowing: Cognitive psychology of haptic manual perception* (pp. 275–292). Amsterdam: John Benjamins.

Lewis, V. 2002. *Development and disability.* Oxford: Wiley.

Ling, D. and Ling, H.A. 1978. *Aural habilitation-the foundations of verbal learning in hearing-impaired children.* Washington, DC: AGB Association for the Deaf.

Lorimer, T. 2017. The WhiteStick. Accessed December 2017. www.whitestick.co.uk.

Mariotti, S.P. 2010. *Global data on visual impairments 2010* (WHO/NMH/PBD/12.01). WHO. Accessed December 2017. www.who.int/blindness/GLOBALDATAFINALforweb.pdf

Maguvhe, M.O., Dzapasi, A. and Sabeya, P. 2012. Orientation and mobility services for persons with visual impairments: South African orientation and mobility practitioners' eye view. *Journal of Visual Impairment and Blindness*, 106(11) 750–755.

Marinoff, R. and Heiberger, M.H. 2017. Lessons learned from the creation of a center of excellence in low vision and vision rehabilitation in Wenzhou, China. *Journal of Visual Impairment and Blindness*, 111(5), 453–464.

Miller, O., Wall, K.R. and Garner, M. 2011. *Quality standards: Delivery of habilitation training (mobility and independent living skills) for children and young people with visual impairment.* London: IOE/RNIB/DCSF

Nau, A.C., Pintar, C., Arnoldussen, A. and Fisher, C. 2015. Acquisition of visual perception in blind adults using the BrainPort artificial vision device. *American Journal of Occupational Therapy*, 69(1), 1–8. www.ncbi.nlm.nih.gov/pmc/articles/PMC4281706.

Pavey, S., Douglas, G., Mccall, S., McLinden, M. and Arter, C. 2002. *Steps to independence: The mobility and independence needs of children with a visual impairment.* London: VICTAR (RNIB/Guide Dogs / OPSIS/Des.

Piek, J.P. 2006. *Infant motor development.* Champaign, IL: Human Kinetics.

Pogrund, R.L. 2017. Is personnel preparation in the field of visual impairment keeping up with the realities of the 21st century? *Journal of Visual Impairment and Blindness*, 111(6) 585–587.

Ponchillia, P.E. and Ponchillia, S.V. 1996. *Foundations of rehabilitation teaching with persons who are blind or visually impaired.* New York: AFB.

Rempel, J. 2012. Glasses that alert travelers to objects through vibration? An evaluation of iGlasses by RNIB and AmbuTech. *AFB AccessWorld MagazineTechnology*. News Foundation for the Blind. Accessed December 2017. https://ambutech.com/shop-online/iglasses%E2%84%A2-ultrasonic-mobility-aid.

RNIB. 2017. Royal National Institute of Blind People. Accessed December 2017. www.rnib.org.uk.

Rosen, M., Clark, G.R. and Kivitz, M.S. 1977. *Habilitation and the handicapped.* Baltimore, ML: University Park Press.

Sacks, S.Z. and Zatta, M.C. 2016. *Keys to educational success: Teaching students with visual impairments and multiple disabilities.* New York: AFB.

Szabo, J. and Panikkar, R.K. 2017. Bridging the gap between physical therapy and orientation and mobility in schools: Using a collaborative team approach for students with visual impairments. *Journal of Visual Impairment and Blindness*, 111(6) 495–510.

Tobin, M.J. and Hill, E.W. 2015. Is literacy for blind people under threat? Does braille have a future? *British Journal of Visual Impairment*, 33(3), 161–166.

UN. 2006. *UN convention on the rights of persons with disabilities* [e-publication]. Accessed December 2017. www.un.org/disabilities/convention/conventionfull.shtml.

UN. 2017a. *2017 revision of world population prospects.* UN/DESA Population Division. Accessed 7 January 2019. www.un.org/development/desa/publications/world-population-prospects-the-2017-revision.html.

UN. 2017b. *World population prospects 2017: Data booklet* (ST/ESA/SER.A/401- revised December 2017) UN/DESA Population Division [e-publication]. Accessed December 2017. https://esa.un.org/unpd/wpp/Publications/Files/WPP2017_DataBooklet.pdf.

UN. 2017c. *UN convention on the rights of persons with disabilities: Updated 2016* [e-publication]. Accessed December 2017. www.un.org/development/desa/disabilities/convention-on-the-rights-of-persons-with-disabilities.html.

Velázquez, R. 2010. Wearable assistive devices for the blind. In A. Lay-Ekuakille and S.C. Mukhopadhyay (eds), *Wearable and autonomous biomedical devices and systems for smart environment.* Lecture notes in electrical engineering, 75 (pp. 331–349). Berlin: Springer.

VICTAR. 2017. *Vision impairment centre for teaching and research (VICTAR)* [e-publication]. Accessed December 2017. www.birmingham.ac.uk/schools/education/research/victar/index.aspx.

Wall, K.R. 2007. *Mobility and independent living: Developing the workforce.* Liverpool: MISE Annual Conference.

Wall, K.R. 2008a. *Developing habilitation standards: Initial consultations.* Liverpool: MISE Annual Conference.

Wall, K.R. 2008b. *The Mobiltiy21 project.* Birmingham: Heads of Sensory Services Annual Conference.

Wall, K.R. 2010. *End of project report on the Mobiltiy21 project.* London: IOE/DCSF.

Wall, K.R. 2012a. Developing national habilitation (mobility, orientation and independence skills) standards and training for children and young people with visual needs in the UK. *Proceedings of the Research in Education and Rehabilitation Sciences, 8th International Scientific Conference.* Zagreb: Edukacijski fakultet, Sveuciliste u Zaagrebu.

Wall, K.R. 2012b. Establishing standards for the habilitation training (mobility, orientation and independence skills) of specialists, working with children and young people (CYP) with visual needs: the UK National Quality Standards. *Proceedings of the Research in Education and Rehabilitation Sciences, 8th International Scientific Conference.* Zagreb: Edukacijski fakultet,Sveuciliste u Zaagrebu.

Wall, K.R. and Hayton, J. 2017. Researcher and practitioner inputs into knowledge exchange 1: Children's visual needs, habilitation and the training of habilitation specialists. In Symposium 3694588: K. Wall, C. Carroll, G. Brackenbury and A. Roberts. *Putting researcher and practitioner inputs into knowledge exchange in practice in aspects of inclusive education: Four cases studies and a general model* (pp. 23–24). Brighton: BERA Annual Conference.

Warren, D.H. 1984. *Blindness and early childhood development* (2nd ed.). Cambridge: Cambridge University Press.

Warren, D.H. 1994. *Blindness and children: An individual differences approach.* Cambridge: Cambridge University Press.

WBU. 2017. World Blind Union. Accessed December 2017. www.worldblindunion.org/English/Pages/default.aspx.

WHO. 2017. *World report on vision* [e-publication]. Accessed December 2017 www.who.int/blindness/vision-report/en.

Wiener, W.R., Welsh, R.L. and Blasch, B.B. 2010a. *Foundations of orientation and mobility. Volume 1: History and theory* (2nd ed.). New York: AFB.

Wiener, W.R., Welsh, R.L. and Blasch, B.B. 2010b. *Foundations of orientation and mobility. Volume 2: Instructional strategies and practical applications* (2nd ed.). New York: AFB.

Wright, T., Harris, B. and Stricken, E. 2010. A best evidence synthesis of research on orientation and mobility involving tactile maps and models. *Journal of Visual Impairment and Blindness,* 104 (2) 95–106.

WWC. 2017. *What Works Clearinghouse* [e-publication]. Accessed December 2017.

Yobas, L., Durand, D.M., Skebe, G.G., Lisy, F.J. and Huff, M.A. 2003. A novel integrable microvalve for refreshable braille display system. *Journal of Microelectromechanical Systems,* 12(3), 252–263.

23

Measuring vision, orientation and mobility in the wild

Lil Deverell

Introduction

During my initial training as an O&M specialist, I was part way down the stairs with my hand on the rail when I paused, transfixed. I was blindfolded, but forgot about my long cane and explored with my fingertips and palm. I knew the rail was hard, but it felt surprisingly soft and satiny, perfectly smooth when I stroked up or down. I sighed with pleasure. Feeling around the tubular curve was different somehow – gripping was less satisfying than stroking, but still good. The moment held me in a private pleasure bubble, the highlight of my day.

I went back later to have a look, and found that the rail was made of stainless steel, with the same dull, utilitarian sheen as my cooking pots and kitchen sink – nothing special to look at. My bubble burst.

Years later, I do not remember the travel route I was supposed to be learning that day, but the stair-rail incident is still clear in my mind. The transforming thing was realising how much I miss, if I only think about orientation and mobility (O&M) in terms of deficits, compensatory skills and utility. I learned there are moments of bliss that are only accessible *without* vision. Having experienced this once, I knew it could happen again. Blindfold travel became something that held promise of innate delight, not just effort, or a sense of satisfied achievement upon arrival.

O&M practice involves many such learning moments, but how do these moments impact everyday travel with low vision or blindness, and how do we measure the outcomes?

This chapter explores the challenges of assessing and measuring functional vision and mobility "in the wild" (Wang and Belongie, 2010) – the untamed places beyond the eye clinic where lighting, weather and the events that transpire cannot be controlled by the assessor.

Orientation and mobility embraces any whole-body action we undertake from the time we get up in the morning, until going to bed at night. It includes intentional route travel and incidental mobility, the foot-shuffling and side-stepping that links and facilitates activities throughout the day. Of particular interest is functional vision for mobility – the ways that vision becomes useful as "we live and move and have our being" (Holy Bible, Acts 17:28).

It is estimated that 10% of people with visual impairment are blind (Access Economics, 2010), but many people with low vision experience transient functional blindness and some who have been diagnosed blind show surprisingly visual behaviours. O&M studies have shown repeatedly that clinical vision measures do not predict a person's functional competence (Lepri, 2009). Relationships between vision, orientation and mobility are irreducibly complex (Marron and Bailey, 1982) with O&M combined being greater or other than the sum of its parts (Urry, 2006). Capturing this complexity in the wild requires a fresh approach to measuring functional outcomes, so we need to consider the nature of O&M knowledge.

Tacit knowledge and threshold concepts

Everyday travel with low vision or blindness is imbued with *tacit knowledge* about the non-visual world that is difficult to articulate (Polanyi, 1966/2009). It can take time to work out what has been important about an experience and realise the implications, by which time we have already moved on. Petrie (2014) recommends that anyone undertaking low vision research do some O&M training to gain insight into the non-visual world.

Those who practise long enough to become competent non-visual travellers embody *threshold concepts* that are shared with other O&M insiders, but that remain obscure to O&M outsiders who have not yet learned these travel skills (Bartunek and Louis, 1996; Mettler, 2008). Meyer and Land (2003) define threshold concepts as difficult knowledge, counter-intuitive, but nevertheless transformational. Threshold concepts work like a port-key to a new place that we cannot otherwise access. They change the way we perceive everything, and we cannot return to unknowing. A trainee O&M specialist learns to recognise sensory cues that trigger a response in the client, to choose and sequence relevant training opportunities, to appreciate timeliness in dynamic places, to step back out of the way and to recognise and work with the learning moment.

Measurement challenges

O&M assessment, which includes functional vision assessment, is essentially a qualitative process comprising interview and observed travel. The O&M specialist works with the client to interpret observed behaviours and clarify assumptions, gaining a more complete understanding of the client's capabilities than is possible without collaboration. The O&M profession has never had an efficient, satisfactory way to *quantify* a client's functional vision or mobility skills. In a culture of evidence-based practice, measurement becomes important because numbers facilitate easy comparisons.

Woolf (2008) suggested that translational research should be regarded as a two-part process, with clinical trials showing that an intervention works effectively, and subsequent research showing how the intervention impacts everyday life. We know that O&M training can improve a client's confidence and travel capability, but how much change can we expect, and how do we measure and compare the lifestyle benefits that clients gain?

Frytak (2000) observed that good measurement requires both conceptualisation and operationalisation: first identifying what to measure, then deciding how best to go about it. Good measurement also involves finding the sweet spot between standardisation, precision and feasibility. Standardisation underpins measurement and helps to reduce unwieldy qualitative data to comparable numbers. However, meaning is always lost as data are reduced and quantified (Richards, 2009). In functional vision assessment, precision helps to fan out subtle differences in capability, but comprehensively detailed checklists can become infeasible to implement.

Instead of comprehensive, I reasoned, how about universal? In O&M assessment, is there anything universally relevant to our clients of all ages and abilities that will provide a stable foundation for measurement? I used grounded theory methodology to identify the universal elements of pedestrian travel.

Choosing what to measure

Grounded theory methodology is an approach to research that develops new theory or models from a live data set including participants' stories and experiences, rather than testing hypotheses that are derived from the peer-reviewed literature (Charmaz, 2014). This qualitative approach is particularly useful when a new research field needs scoping, or when an old field of inquiry has become stuck. This is the case in O&M outcomes research where limited measures used for over 30 years still do not capture the functional benefits that clients say they gain from intervention (Virgili and Rubin, 2010).

New theories about O&M and functional vision in this chapter are grounded in a series of O&M studies undertaken in Melbourne, Australia between 2010 and 2016. The first studies explored scooter travel. O&M specialists in Australia and New Zealand (n = 41) discussed their readiness to work with low vision clients who use a motorised mobility scooter (Deverell, 2011a, 2011c). Then O&M specialists (n = 4) tested different low vision simulators while driving a scooter on a 1 km urban route to discover how much vision is needed for safe travel (Deverell and Ong, 2011). These studies prompted scalar thinking about functional vision for mobility and informed development of the O&M Environmental Complexity Scale (Deverell, 2011b).

Next, a doctoral study (Deverell, 2016) investigated perceptions of effective mobility with O&M specialists and clients resulting in the Effective Mobility Framework (Deverell et al., 2015). Guide dog mobility instructors and teachers identified visual behaviours that can be evident in people who are diagnosed "blind". Adults (n = 40) who had advanced retinitis pigmentosa undertook a day-long research session including clinical vision tests, interviews, semi-standardised O&M tasks and activities of daily living to help develop a bionic vision research protocol (Fenwick et al., 2016; Finger et al., 2016; Finger et al., 2014). Then the protocol was implemented with three people who had a prototype retinal implant (Ayton et al., 2014). The project identified viable measurement scales and flagged aspects of functional vision and O&M that mattered to participants, which weren't yet measured.

Lastly, interviews with guide dog clients (n = 51) provided a context to pilot two new co-rated measures of functional vision and mobility (Deverell and Meyer, 2016). These two assessment tools, called VROOM and OMO, will be described later in this chapter.

Clinical and functional phenomena

O&M parlance distinguishes between clinical and functional performance. Clinicians tend to interpret functional performance as any action or activity that patients show they *can do* (e.g. Chung et al., 2017), whereas O&M specialists reserve "functional" to mean what a client *chooses to do in everyday life.*

Hybrid O&M studies that combine clinical and functional characteristics without clear priorities, result in methodological incongruity and poor-quality data (Virgili and Rubin, 2010), whereas robust O&M research falls into one of two groups. *Clinical O&M research* (e.g. CONSORT group, 2010) can be undertaken to investigate selected aspects of O&M such as veering at road crossings instead of crossing straight (Guth, 1991; Kallie, Schrater and Legge, 2007) or scanning for traffic before crossing (Geruschat et al., 2006). This approach strips away confounding variables to distil precise information about the selected behaviours of interest.

Conversely, *functional O&M research* needs to embrace rather than reduce the complexity of resources and options available to clients in the wild.

Analysis of tensions that arose in a hybrid O&M study distilled six defining characteristics of functional inquiry: authenticity, embodiment, community, integration, diversity and learning

(Deverell, 2016). From an O&M perspective, *functional measures* rate things that matter to clients in their own "communities of practice" (Wenger, 1998), according to their own priorities, drawing on multiple sources from multiple contexts, expecting a client to try different responses to events that transpire.

The O&M profession needs functional measures for use in ordinary O&M assessment to benchmark the client's everyday competence and quantify programme outcomes, without standardising tasks or venues or compromising the client's natural responses (Shaw et al., 2009).

Functional vision

Comprehensive assessment of functional vision incorporates vision for reading and near tasks as well as vision for mobility (Figure 23.1) Eye care professionals and educators are likely to approach functional vision assessment from the perspective of reading and watching because gold standard eye tests use optotype recognition, and formal learning is dependent on literacy. Functional vision assessment can move naturally from optotypes to a range of everyday reading

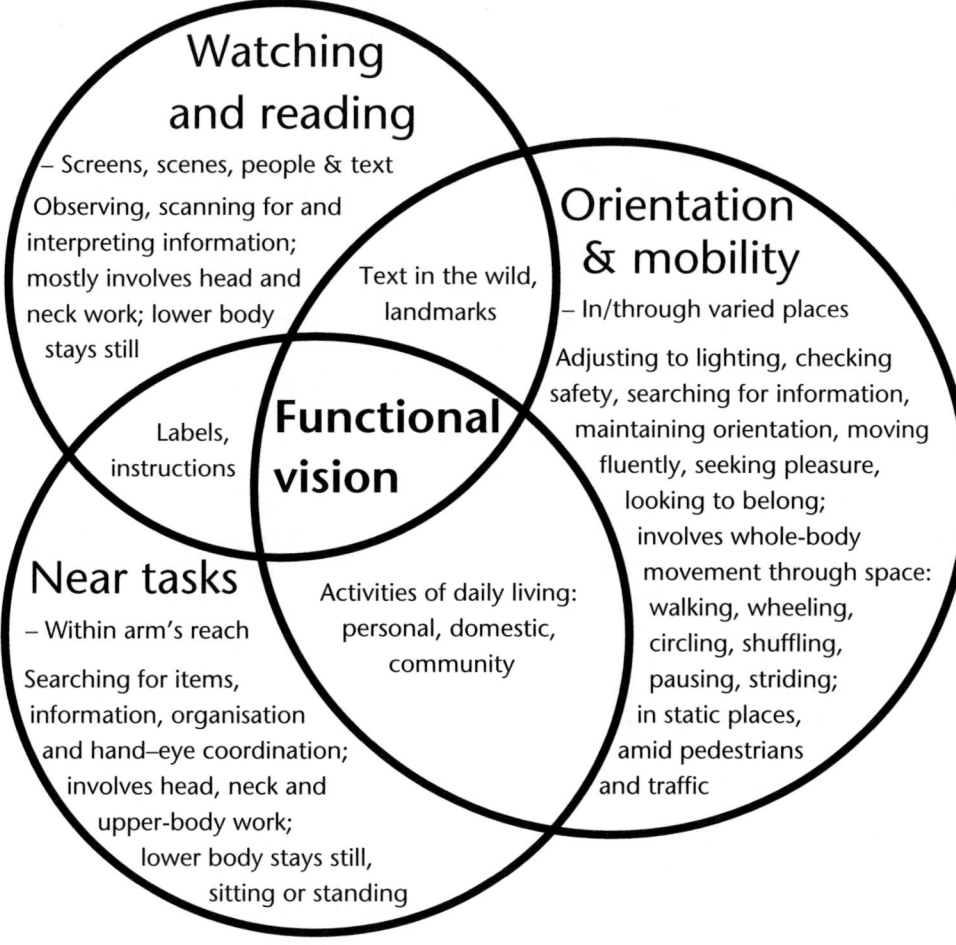

Figure 23.1   Three manifestations of functional vision.

materials, experimenting with font sizes, lighting, viewing distances and postures (Lueck, 2004). The assessor explores visual fluctuations and discovers what conditions enable the reader to gain best access, and sustainable access to different texts, also investigating scanning strategies for watching – whether television, a sports match, a play, a sunset or a conversation partner's face.

An occupational therapist is likely to approach functional vision assessment from the perspective of near tasks like making a sandwich or managing medications. *Arm's reach* helps to define a person's body space, and frames an ergonomic range of movement. Near tasks can require high visual acuity and a range of scanning strategies, but people soon settle into visual routines that involve selective attention to some visual information while filtering out other details (Hayhoe, 2000). An assessor observing vision for near tasks considers whether the client can organise the necessary equipment to find things sequentially and efficiently to complete the task.

Reading, watching and near tasks involve upper-body work, with emphasis on visual details, interpretation and hand–eye coordination, so functional vision assessment might begin in controlled conditions but at some point, it needs to move into the wild. O&M necessitates whole-body movement from one place to the next, maintaining orientation while dealing with changes and unexpected events in dynamic places. Dodds (1988) suggests that assessment of functional vision for mobility should encompass the widest possible range of conditions with varied lighting, indoors and outside, also considering psychosocial factors like anxiety, social awareness, confidence and tension.

Functional mobility

Grounded theory methodology has identified five functions that are universal to any travel experience, whether intentional or incidental: getting your bearings, checking groundplane, wayfinding, recognising moving parts and finding things (Deverell, 2016). During functional assessment, the O&M specialist considers (1) how competently the client achieves each function and (2) how vision supports the process. These functions introduce some standardisation to professional observations without standardising tasks, venues or the client's travel choices.

Getting your bearings

Before setting out, a traveller needs to confirm their position in space and choose which direction to go, then update orientation in transit. A vision-assisted traveller might scope the scene at a glance, identify and triangulate familiar visual landmarks, or piece together visual fragments to gain a sense of the bigger picture. A non-visual traveller needs to rely on auditory or tactile landmarks to gain and maintain orientation. GPS technology can provide real-time updates on location and direction.

Checking groundplane

Whether consciously or unconsciously, a traveller checks the ground surface before stepping out, alert to hazardous features like steps, ramps and platform edges, or loose materials like gravel that might cause slips, trips or falls. A primary mobility aid (long cane, dog or human guide) can check the near groundplane for safety, freeing low vision to scope the path ahead.

Wayfinding

A traveller looks for a clear, continuous path of travel, identifying fixed structures and estimating the spaces between them. A wall or path edge can provide a shoreline to follow. A long cane can provide more environmental information than a guide dog, because the cane contacts obstacles, whereas a dog avoids them.

Recognising moving parts

Moving parts have a different imperative than static environmental features, requiring a timely response that can prompt anxiety. A traveller notices action, people, animals, traffic and potential missiles, interpreting their trajectory and distance, gauging time to contact, choosing to engage or to avoid collision. There are social and safety implications as a traveller navigates crowds, crosses roads or plays ball sports.

Finding things

O&M is usually purposeful, but searching for things like missing items, dropped objects, known landmarks or an address can be time consuming with little or no vision. Effective search strategies, contrast and familiarity can speed the process, and social assistance, audio cues, GPS and beacon technology can help to narrow the search.

Visual purposes in O&M

When low vision is frustrating, unreliable or slow to interpret, it can be easier to travel with eyes closed. This prompts the question: What makes competent non-visual travellers bother to open their eyes? Grounded theory methodology identified six common visual purposes that motivate looking during O&M: safety, information, orientation, fluency, belonging and pleasure (Deverell, 2016). Their relative importance can change in response to task requirements, travel skills, personal priorities, level of vision, familiarity, recollections and unexpected events.

Safety: real risk and safety neurosis

Safety is a dominant social theme today, as multimedia bring catastrophes and incidents from faraway places into our immediate sphere of attention (Cairns, 2008). A pervasive safety neurosis seems to evolve if people accumulate safety concerns without evaluating real risks.

In the study involving adults with retinitis pigmentosa, participants were ambivalent about bumping into things, although several said they did not want to fall (Finger et al., 2016). In the guide dog study (Deverell and Meyer, 2016), participants cared about safety, but there were no universal safety concerns: 41% were cautious about traffic, 28% mentioned risk of falling, 24% felt vulnerable using public transport and 20% wanted to know who was around. Rowdy or erratic behaviour was worrying; it could just be natural exuberance, or related to drugs or alcohol or some kind of psychotic episode. Only 14% were concerned about collisions, while 16% were worried about getting lost.

Perceptions of risk and judgements about safety in O&M are relative, so walking unknowingly on to the road in front of a car *might* constitute unsafe mobility for some, but not for all clients – it depends on travel speed, reaction time and how the driver and the client both respond when they realise. Similarly, clients feel differently about social safety – some want to avoid public embarrassment at all costs, while others do not care how they appear to onlookers.

When assessing functional vision, O&M specialists encourage clients to explore the boundaries of safety and risk in ways that seem incredible to other professionals, and challenge conservative thinking about occupational health and safety. When the client veers into the path of oncoming traffic, the O&M specialist must time intervention perfectly to manage risk *and* capture the learning moment. The client who learns to cope with risky situations under supervision becomes equipped to deal with unexpected events when travelling solo, whereas the client who is repeatedly rescued during O&M training just becomes skilled at being rescued.

Dignity of risk is important – people need to roam, to establish their own boundaries and to live dangerously if they so choose (Cairns, 2008; Schloss, Alper and Jayne, 1993). However, skills for self-determination cannot be assumed. They need to be built into O&M programmes and education for people with low vision or blindness (American Foundation for the Blind, 2014). These skills are needed to counter the learned helplessness and reduced life-space that too often result from prescribed, limited expectations and cloistered blindness services. Scott (1969) proposed that the disability of blindness is socially ascribed and has little to do with visual status.

Information: text in the wild

Assessment of functional vision for reading might begin in static settings, but "text in the wild" (Li et al., 2014) provides a crossover into community travel (Figure 23.1). Static signage is abundant in the built environment on buildings, footpaths, gantries, poles and letterboxes, then in shops with prices, sale signs and packaging that lists ingredients, instructions and use-by dates. Text in the wild is dynamic too, seen on number plates and the sides of moving vehicles, fluttering banners, skywriting and branding on the carrier bags and clothes of passers-by.

The logical flow of language and the structure of text can enable a print reader to access meaning even when it is difficult to see individual letters or words. The promise of meaning gives text in the wild a seductive visual interest that is different to, and arguably more powerful than other visible features in the travel environment. Thus, text in the wild becomes a useful resource for assessing functional vision during travel: What text catches the client's eye? What meaning does the client derive? What difference does lighting or time of day make to accessibility? Can the text be used to inform or confirm travel decisions? Is its usefulness consistent as a landmark, or variable as a clue, in supporting navigation?

Since the advent of computers, the notion of literacy has expanded such that "multiliteracies" include linguistic, audio, spatial, gestural and visual elements of design (New London Group, 1996). This extends reading to include environmental and social literacy as the traveller interprets environmental features and social behaviour during O&M. Multiliteracies are good for people with low vision or blindness: mainstream technologies include zoom and voiceover functions, so O&M clients can access the same information as fully sighted people, with braille becoming optional, reducing segregation. We found that 92% of guide dog clients travelled with a smartphone, and synchronised platforms enabled clients to carry fewer assistive devices (Deverell and Meyer, 2016).

Orientation: ambient vision

Light perception only can be useful for orientation, but its usefulness depends on (1) familiarity and (2) spatial cognition. People with ultra-low vision see isolated visual elements like tiny patches of colour, contrast, light intensity, movement or specular reflections that, on their own, are too small or generic to identify an object. When these fragments are placed accurately into a traveller's mental map, the traveller can make rapid, accurate spatial inferences and maintain surprisingly confident travel fluency with ultra-low vision, even in unfamiliar places. I call this facility *ambient vision*.

Dodds and Davis (1989) observed that motion parallax facilitates edge detection during travel. But our room self-orientation task (Finger et al., 2016) showed that ambient vision was only available to people with strong mental mapping skills: 85% of the cohort. These travellers could combine motion parallax and an awareness of likely objects in the environment, with mental mapping skills and spatial memory to integrate visual fragments into a bigger picture. In contrast, people with ultra-low vision and limited spatial cognition had no ambient vision: 15% of the cohort. Visual fragments remained spatially unrelated and meaningless to them, prompting no visual response.

Fluency: flinches, glances and flow

Graceful fluency is the epitome of competent O&M performance (Hill and Ponder, 1976). Graceful travellers anticipate. They preview the environment to cut corners and walk within an inch of static or moving features without collision. If they do make unexpected contact, they respond fluidly and keep moving.

Encounters with sensory stimuli in the travel environment can prompt a flinch or a glance response. A flinch arrests progress; it breaks mental flow and demands attention requiring time and mental effort to get back on track. The experience might range in intensity from mild distraction to a sense of assault. Cumulative flinches increase body tension and can invoke dread of the next encounter, making travel exhausting. In contrast, a glance might involve a brief change of pace that is benign or even reassuring, confirming that events are proceeding according to plan. A glance demands little physical or mental effort, so it doesn't compound fatigue.

Consideration of mental effort is important in O&M assessment. Cognitively, flow is "a subjective state that people report when they are completely involved in something to the point of forgetting time, fatigue and everything else but the activity itself" (Csikszentmihalyi, Abuhamdeh and Nakamura, 2007, p. 600). This deep involvement facilitates learning and transformation (Laevers, 2003). Flow fosters development of O&M skills and confidence to look ahead, anticipate and move more fluently, whereas travel that is fragmented by flinches and frustration soon feels too daunting to undertake.

Belonging: not just arriving or fitting in

Vision provides a quick way for people to recognise the familiar, especially from a distance. Familiarity with people, places and culture breeds a sense of belonging that is fundamental to well-being (Savage, Bagnall and Longhurst, 2005). During functional assessment, an O&M specialist evaluates the quality of social encounters and looks for evidence of belonging. Familiarity with a place shows in relaxed gait and fluent travel, but travelling confidently to a place is different to navigating social complexities. Adults with advanced retinitis pigmentosa spoke about their difficulty working a room; they valued vision for (1) locating people, (2) recognising people, (3) reading facial expressions, (4) knowing when a conversation partner has departed and (5) self-monitoring their own appearance and behaviour in relation to others (Deverell, 2016).

Rudman et al. (2016) found that elders with vision impairment were concerned about social embarrassment, and responded to their deteriorating vision by either (1) scaling back their participation to stick with the familiar, (2) acting with caution or (3) changing the way they did things. Scaling back is particularly concerning because a reduced life-space and associated loss of relationships are associated with depression (Horowitz, 2004; McCarthy, 2009).

Vision is important for learning "cultural capital" (Bourdieu, 1986/2010) and there is often a disjunct between what people say with their words and with their bodies. Sighted people can develop social insight as they sift and test possible meanings inherent in the behaviours they see. A person who has never watched social behaviour can function socially like someone with autism, missing clues that indicate mixed messages, and taking another person's words too literally (Kaiser and Shiffrar, 2012). The loss of visual certainty as vision deteriorates can also raise the suspicion of "tricking", highlighting a chronic power imbalance between people with and without visual access to social information (Deverell, 2016).

Cultural capital equips a person to make informed choices about social conformity. Fitting in can seem particularly important when first impressions count, such as starting at a new school or attending a job interview. However, Brown (2012) suggests that fitting in can ultimately obstruct belonging because it means submitting to others' expectations and judgements, with pressure to behave inauthentically. In contrast, belonging requires us to be vulnerable and genuine – to be seen for who we really are – providing an authentic foundation for human relationships.

Pleasure: immediate and vicarious

Disability studies often focus on deficits, difficulties, limitations and utility as they explore barriers to participation (e.g. Massof et al., 2005; Turano et al., 1999). Vision is valuable for the things it helps us to achieve, but seeing can also be innately delightful, bringing enormous pleasure (Figure 23.2). This raises an interesting tension between visual utility and aesthetics.

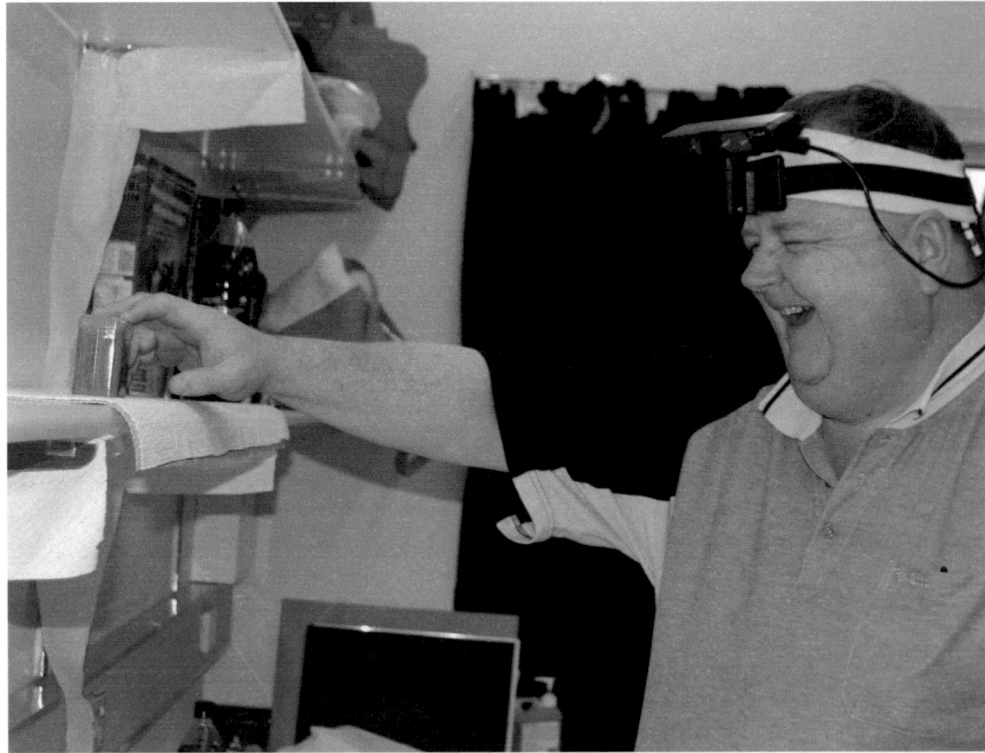

Figure 23.2 Prototype retinal implant being trialled. After ten years with light perception only, Wayne trialled a prototype retinal implant from Bionic Vision Australia. He was amazed and delighted to find he could use "phosphene vision" – just spots of light – to identify and accurately grasp a little tin of curry powder amidst other pantry items on the shelf. Used with permission.

Research into visual appeal tends to be located in the arts, design (Fleming, 2014), marketing (Clement, Kristensen and Grønhaug, 2013), neuroscience (Cela-Conde et al., 2004) and sexuality (Sabatinelli et al., 2007). Stepping into the wild, Kaplan (1987) considered what makes a landscape aesthetically appealing. Beauty? Novelty? Surprisingness? Content? He found that people preferred natural scenes over urban landscapes, and the most appealing scenes invited the viewer to move deeper into the setting, such as a winding path disappearing from view, promising more. This sense of mystery and hopefulness resonates with Metz' (2000) suggestion that any mobility incorporates "potential travel – knowing that a trip could be made, even if not actually undertaken" (p. 150). Thus, vision and mobility can both inspire the pleasure of possibility thinking.

Scene recognition matters to some O&M clients, while others care to see people or things. Perhaps it is less important to know what causes visual pleasure than to recognise the importance of visual pleasure in people's lives, and to acknowledge grief when any hope of visual pleasure has waned.

Having explored the phenomenon of functional vision for mobility, we now consider how it might be measured.

How to measure functional vision for O&M

Ordinary O&M assessment provides an obvious context for measuring functional vision for mobility, but good research clarifies ontology (notions of being), epistemology (theories of knowledge) and theoretical frameworks before jumping into methodologies and measurement (Hamilton and Ravenscroft, 2018)

Constructivism and embedded mixed methods

How do we regard people?

Ordinary O&M assessment values different people and their opinions equally (Orientation and Mobility Association of Australasia, 2013). *Person-centred* means focusing on the priorities, needs and concerns of individual clients in their own context, rather than expecting the client to fit into standardised, norm-referenced expectations (Dodds, 1988).

How do we know what we know?

An O&M specialist does not take the client's opinion at face value (subjectivity), or observe from a distance presuming the client's actions have a singular meaning (objectivity). Rather, we explore environments with the client, ask questions, discuss observations and consider multiple interpretations. This process of building strong, substantiated knowledge together is called constructivism (Charmaz, 2014).

What theories inform our approach?

Complexity theory provides a useful theoretical framework because effective O&M is a "complex adaptive system" (Braithwaite et al., 2017, p. vii) with many interrelated components, including vision. O&M specialists approach functional assessment whole-to-parts, aware that any human behaviour can have numerous influences and interpretations (Robson, 2011).

What are embedded mixed methods?

Mixed methods research has at least one qualitative and one quantitative data stream, analysed together (Creswell and Plano Clark, 2011). *Embedded* means that both data streams are generated in the same context with a clear priority on words or numbers. Embedded words and numbers are more precise than words and numbers generated in sequential events, because functional vision fluctuates such that vision described today might be different to vision measured tomorrow.

A clinical mixed methods O&M study is likely to have a QUAN/qual priority (Creswell and Plano Clark, 2011) with standardised measurement practices supplemented by participants' opinions. A functional O&M study requires a QUAL/quan priority, with collaboration creating a relevant, meaningful context for person-centred measurement.

What qualitative methodologies shape data generation?

Hermeneutical phenomenology (van Manen, 2006) explores and interprets learning and meanings inherent in complex human activities like O&M. *Heuristic inquiry* is a congruent research methodology used to articulate tacit knowledge that shapes decision-making (Hiles, 2008).

How do we transform qualitative data into numbers?

Grounded theory methodology (Charmaz, 2014) has identified relevant constructs to be measured using ordinal scales. Behaviourally anchored rating scales (Atkin and Conlon, 1978) are more precise than Likert scales – performance indicators for each number take the guesswork out of co-rating and prevent drift in meaning from one scale to the next, resulting in more reliable measures. In the research literature, it is uncommon to measure shared opinions, but during a co-rating conversation the client and assessor discuss, confirm and contest different opinions to arrive at shared ratings.

The VROOM and OMO tools

Using these principles and processes, two new functional assessment tools were developed. The VROOM (Vision-Related Outcomes in O&M) tool measures functional vision for mobility, and the OMO (O&M Outcomes) tool measures a person's travel competence regardless of vision. Each is a suite of behaviourally anchored ordinal scales that are co-rated by the O&M specialist, the client and any other stakeholders (e.g. family member, carer, teacher) present during ordinary O&M assessment (Deverell et al., 2017).

The tools use the same measurement template, with Part A rating observed travel, scored out of 30, and Part B assessing five relevant aspects of well-being, scored out of 20. The scales in each tool aggregate to a score out of 50 on the spot so that results can be discussed with the client. Comments noted next to ratings provide contextual details, capturing different opinions, while warranting the relevance of measurement data to the individual client.

The VROOM and OMO tools use multiple disciplines of qualitative research to generate strong data: rapport, collaboration, multiplicity, triangulation, member-checking, resonance and reflexivity (Curtin and Fossey, 2007; Tracy, 2010). They facilitate intra-personal comparisons between vision and mobility, functional fluctuations, different timepoints and skills pre-post intervention, as well as comparisons between different people and places.

Why are these functional measures significant?

The VROOM and OMO tools represent a new person-centred approach to measuring functional outcomes in O&M practice, founded on constructivist knowledge, not objectivity. Constructivist (qualitative) research methods abound, but there is little evidence in the peer-reviewed literature of robust, meaningful measurement data generated on the spot from qualitative inquiry.

The VROOM and OMO tools address multiple issues in vision-related research.

A persistent assumption that vision predicts travel capability

Loss of driver's licence because of low vision can significantly restrict a person's life-space, and this loss is associated with depression (McCarthy, 2009). It is easy to assume that as vision deteriorates further, mobility will too, but this is not the case. The decision to measure functional vision and O&M skills separately was justified in the guide dog pilot study when it became apparent that, equipped with the right mobility aid, two blind participants (VROOM 0/50) were the most capable travellers (OMO 49/50 and 50/50) (Deverell and Meyer, 2016). Loss of driver's licence because of low vision has prompted an uneasiness about use of a motorised mobility scooter with low vision. O&M specialists can use the VROOM and OMO tools to generate measurable evidence of competent scooter travel with low vision to inform fair, inclusive attitudes and scooter policies.

Funding frameworks

The advent of the government-funded National Disability Insurance Scheme (NDIS), with its strong focus on person-centred practice and self-determination for clients, is revolutionising the disability sector in Australia. The NDIS welcomes outcome measures like the VROOM and OMO tools that are person-centred, co-designed and co-rated with clients (NDIS, 2017).

Assistive technologies

Specialist technologies like the bionic eye are slow and costly to develop, whereas phone apps that use mainstream platforms are quicker and cheaper to develop. In either case, functional outcome measures are needed to show that these new technologies meet real needs and that ongoing investment is warranted.

Definitions of blindness

The current WHO guidelines for interpreting visual acuity have three categories of blindness, such that anyone with acuity less than 3/60 (1/20) is blinded by definition (WHO, 2016). The common understanding of blindness is what you can see with your eyes closed. Yet, it is possible to walk around quite safely without a mobility aid with 3/60 vision, so a diagnosis of blindness with 3/60 acuity seems unnecessarily jarring and confusing. Scott (1969) showed that vision professionals and blindness services too often reinforce the very disability they are trying to alleviate, which is a confronting notion for professionals who are committed to do no harm. The VROOM and OMO tools can show that visual acuity less than 3/60 is useful vision, also providing language to reframe professional thinking about functional capability so that these WHO categories of ultra-low vision can be more accurately named.

Conclusion

Functional vision and O&M skills evaluated during ordinary O&M assessment are different phenomena than have typically been investigated in peer-reviewed outcome studies to date. O&M in the wild is irreducibly complex, greater and other than the sum of its parts, and it includes constructs like pleasure that have not previously been measured in O&M studies. Functional outcome measures need to embrace rather than simplify this complexity.

With a shift towards person-centred O&M practice, a suite of person-centred measures is needed to generate evidence about the everyday impact of O&M training, mobility aids, assistive devices and vision-related policies on clients' lives.

The VROOM and OMO tools are constructivist measures that represent a fresh approach to measuring functional vision and O&M. They do not account for all aspects of functional vision and mobility, but they do measure universally relevant elements that matter to clients, also providing a template for development of other functional measures.

Over time, the VROOM and OMO tools, used in ordinary professional practice as well as formal research, promise to generate a rich body of evidence about the functional capability of people with low vision or blindness. This evidence can be used to design and review relevant services, address discrimination, shape policies, warrant funding claims and develop assistive technologies that can improve quality of life for O&M clients.

References

Access Economics. 2010. *Clear focus: The economic impact of vision loss in Australia in 2009* [e-publication]. Accessed August 2018. www.vision2020australia.org.au/uploads/resource/85/v2020aus_report_clear_focus_overview_jun10.pdf.

American Foundation for the Blind. 2014. The expanded core curriculum for blind and visually impaired children and youths [e-publication]. Accessed August 2018. www.afb.org/info/programs-and-services/professional-development/teachers/expanded-core-curriculum/the-expanded-core-curriculum/12345.

Atkin, R. S. and Conlon, E. J. 1978. Behaviorally anchored rating scales: Some theoretical issues. *Academy of Management Review*, 3(1), 119–128.

Ayton, L.N., Blamey, P.J., Guymer, R.H., Luu, C.D., Nayagam, D.A., Sinclair, N.C., Shivdasani, M.N., Yeoh, J., McCombe, M.F., Briggs, R.J., Opie, N.L., Villalobos, J., Dimitrov, P.N., Varsamidis, M., Petoe, M.A., McCarthy, C.D., Walker, J.G., Barnes, N., Burkitt, A.N., Williams, C.E., Shepherd, R.K., Allen, P.J. and the Bionic Vision Australia Research Consortium. 2014. First-in-human trial of a novel suprachoroidal retinal prosthesis. *PLoS One*, 9(12), e115239. http://dx.doi.org/10.1371/journal.pone.0115239

Bartunek, J.M. and Louis, M.R. 1996. *Insider/outsider team research* (vol. 40). London: Sage.

Bourdieu, P. (1986/2010). The forms of capital. In I. Szeman and K. Timothy (eds), *Cultural theory: An anthology* (pp. 81–93). Oxford: Wiley-Blackwell.

Braithwaite, J., Churruca, K., Ellis, L.A., Long, J., Clay-Williams, R., Damen, N., Herkes, J., Pomare, C. and Ludlow, K. 2017. *Complexity science in healthcare – aspirations, approaches, applications and accomplishments: A white paper* [e-publication]. Accessed 13 August 2018. www.researchgate.net/publication/319643112_Complexity_Science_in_Healthcare_Aspirations_Approaches_Applications_and_Accomplishments_A_White_Paper.

Brown, B. 2012. *The power of vulnerability: Teachings on authenticity, connection, and courage* [audiobook]. Louisville, CO: Sounds True (Producer).

Cairns, W. 2008. *How to live dangerously: Why we should all stop worrying and start living*. Basingstoke, UK: Macmillan.

Cela-Conde, C.J., Marty, G., Maestú, F., Ortiz, T., Munar, E., Fernández, A., Roca, M., Rosselló, J. and Quesney, F. 2004. Activation of the prefrontal cortex in the human visual aesthetic perception. *Proceedings of the National Academy of Sciences of the United States of America*, 101(16), 6321–6325. http://dx.doi.org/10.1073/pnas.0401427101

Charmaz, K. 2014. *Constructing grounded theory* (2nd ed.). London: Sage.

Chung, D.C., McCague, S., Yu, Z.-F., Thill, S., DiStefano-Pappas, J., Bennett, J. and High, K.A. 2017. Novel mobility test to assess functional vision in patients with inherited retinal dystrophies. *Clinical & Experimental Ophthalmology*, 46(3), 247–259. http://dx.doi.org/10.1111/ceo.13022

Clement, J., Kristensen, T. and Grønhaug, K. 2013. Understanding consumers' in-store visual perception: The influence of package design features on visual attention. *Journal of Retailing and Consumer Services*, 20(2), 234–239. http://dx.doi.org/10.1016/j.jretconser.2013.01.003

CONSORT group. 2010. CONSORT: Transparent reporting of trials [e-publication]. Accessed August 2018. www.consort-statement.org/downloads/consort-statement.

Creswell, J.W. and Plano Clark, V.L. 2011. *Designing and conducting mixed methods research* (2nd ed.). London: Sage.

Curtin, M. and Fossey, E. 2007. Appraising the trustworthiness of qualitative studies: Guidelines for occupational therapists. *Australian Occupational Therapy Journal*, 54(2), 88–94. http://dx.doi.org/10.1111/j.1440-1630.2007.00661.x

Csikszentmihalyi, M., Abuhamdeh, S. and Nakamura, J. 2007. Flow. In A.J. Elliot and C.S. Dweck (eds), *Handbook of competence and motivation* (pp. 598–608). London: Guilford Press.

Deverell, E.A.L. 2016. *Functional vision research: Measuring vision-related outcomes in orientation and mobility – VROOM*. PhD thesis. University of Melbourne, Australia.

Deverell, L. 2011a. *Equipping orientation and mobility specialists for low vision scooter work*. Master's thesis. Monash University, Melbourne, Australia.

Deverell, L. 2011b. O&M environmental complexity scale. *International Journal of Orientation & Mobility*, 4(1), 64–77.

Deverell, L. 2011c. Orientation and mobility involvement with scooter travel in Australasia. *International Journal of Orientation & Mobility*, 4(1), 32–47.

Deverell, L., Bentley, S.A., Ayton, L.N., Delany, C. and Keeffe, J.E. 2015. Effective mobility framework: A tool for designing comprehensive O&M outcomes research *International Journal of Orientation & Mobility*, 7(1), 74–86.

Deverell, L. and Meyer, D. 2016. *Benefits of guide dog mobility*. Kew, Australia: Guide Dogs Victoria.

Deverell, L., Meyer, D., Lau, B.T., Al Mahmud, A., Sukunesan, S., Bhowmik, J., Chai, A., McCarthy, C., Zheng, P., Pipingas, A. and Islam, F.A. 2017. Optimising technology to measure functional vision, mobility, and service outcomes for people with low vision or blindness: Protocol for a prospective cohort study in Australia and Malaysia. *BMJ Open*, 7(12), e018140. http://dx.doi.org/10.1136/bmjopen-2017-018140

Deverell, L. and Ong, D. 2011. Removing the blinkers on scooter use with low vision. *Independent Living*, 27(4), 22–25.

Dodds, A.G. 1988. *Mobility training for visually handicapped people: A person-centred approach*. London: Croom Helm.

Dodds, A.G. and Davis, D.P. 1989. Assessment and training of low vision clients for mobility. *Journal of Visual Impairment & Blindness*, 83(9), 439–446.

Fenwick, E.K., O'Hare, F., Deverell, L., Ayton, L.N., Luu, C.D., McSweeney, S.C., Bentley, S.A., Guymer, R.H. and Finger, R.P. 2016. Rasch analysis of the independent mobility questionnaire. *Optometry and Vision Science*, 93(2), 181–187. http://dx.doi.org/10.1097/OPX.0000000000000787

Finger, R.P., Ayton, L.N., Deverell, L., O'Hare, F., McSweeney, S.C., Luu, C.D, Keeffe, J.E., Guymer, R.H. and Bentley, S.A. 2016. Developing a very low vision orientation & mobility test battery (O&M-VLV). *Optometry and Vision Science*, 93(9), 1127–1136. http://dx.doi.org/10.1097/OPX.0000000000000891

Finger, R.P., McSweeney, S.C., Deverell, L., O'Hare, F., Bentley, S.A., Luu, C.D., Guymer, R.H. and Ayton, L.N. 2014. Developing an instrumental activities of daily living tool as part of the low vision assessment of daily activities (LoVADA) protocol. *Investigative Ophthalmology and Visual Science*, 55(12), 8458–8466. http://dx.doi.org/10.1167/iovs.14-14732

Fleming, R.W. 2014. Visual perception of materials and their properties. *Vision Research*, 94(Supplement C), 62–75. http://dx.doi.org/10.1016/j.visres.2013.11.004

Frytak, J. 2000. Measurement. *Journal of Rehabilitation Outcomes Measurement*, 4(1), 15–31.

Geruschat, D.R., Hassan, S.E., Turano, K.A., Quigley, H.A. and Congdon, N.G. 2006. Gaze behavior of the visually impaired during street crossing. *Optometry and Vision Science*, 83(8), 550–558. http://dx.doi.org/1040-5488/06/8308-0550/0

Guth, D. 1991. Tendency or pattern: The nature of veering among blind pedestrians. *Bulletin of the Psychonomic Society*, 29(6), 489–489.

Hamilton, L. and Ravenscroft, J. 2018. *Building research design in education: Theoretically informed advanced methods*. London: Bloomsbury.

Hayhoe, M. 2000. Vision using routines: A functional account of vision. *Visual Cognition*, 7(1–3), 43–64. http://dx.doi.org/10.1080/135062800394676

Hiles, D.R. 2008. Heuristic inquiry. *The SAGE encyclopedia of qualitative research methods* (pp. 390–393). London: Sage.

Hill, E. and Ponder, P. 1976. *Orientation and mobility techniques: A guide for the practitioner*. New York: American Foundation for the Blind.

Horowitz, A. 2004. The prevalence and consequences of vision impairment in later life. *Topics in Geriatric Rehabilitation*, 20(3), 185–195.

Kaiser, M.D. and Shiffrar, M. 2012. Variability in the visual perception of human motion as a function of the observer's autistic traits. In K. Johnson and M. Shiffrar (eds), *People watching: Social, perceptual, and neurophysiological studies of body perception* (pp. 159–178). Oxford: Oxford University Press.

Kallie, C.S., Schrater, P.R. and Legge, G.E. 2007. Variability in stepping direction explains the veering behavior of blind walkers. *Journal of Experimental Psychology: Human Perception and Performance*, 33(1), 183–200. http://dx.doi.org/10.1037/0096-1523.33.1.183

Kaplan, S. 1987. Aesthetics, affect, and cognition. *Environment and Behavior*, 19(1), 3–32. http://dx.doi.org/10.1177/0013916587191001

Laevers, F. 2003. Experiential education: Making care and education more effective through well-being and involvement. In F. Laevers and L. Heylen (eds), *Involvement of children and teacher style: Insights from an international study on experiential education* (Studia Paedagogical, vol. 35, pp. 13–24). Leuven, Belgium: Leuven University Press.

Lepri, B.P. 2009. Is acuity enough? Other considerations in clinical investigations of visual prostheses. *Journal of Neural Engineering*, 6(3), 1–4. http://dx.doi.org/10.1088/1741-2560/6/3/035003

Li, Y., Jia, W., Shen, C. and van den Hengel, A. 2014. Characterness: An indicator of text in the wild. *IEEE Transactions on Image Processing*, 23(4), 1666–1677.

Lueck, A.H. (ed.) 2004. *Functional vision: A practitioner's guide to evaluation and intervention*. New York: AFB Press.

McCarthy, D. P. 2009. Preface: Transitioning from driver to passenger. *Topics in Geriatric Rehabilitation: Transitioning from Driver to Passenger*, 25(1), 2. http://dx.doi.org/10.1097/01.TGR.0000351748.47169.1d

Marron, J.A. and Bailey, I.L. 1982. Visual factors and orientation–mobility performance. *American Journal of Optometry and Physiological Optics*, 59(5), 413–426. http://dx.doi.org/10.1097/00006324-198205000-00009

Massof, R.W., Hsu, C.T., Baker, F.H., Barnett, G.D., Park, W.L., Deremeik, J.T., Rainey, C. and Epstein, C. 2005. Visual disability variables II: The difficulty of tasks for a sample of low-vision patients. *Archives of Physical Medicine and Rehabilitation*, 86(5), 954–967. http://dx.doi.org/10.1016/j.apmr.2004.09.017

Mettler, R. 2008. *Cognitive learning theory and cane travel instructions: A new paradigm* (2nd ed.). Lincoln, NE: Nebraska Commission for the Blind and Visually Impaired.

Metz, D. 2000. Mobility of older people and their quality of life. *Transport Policy*, 7(2), 149–152. http://dx.doi.org/10.1016/S0967-070X(00)00004-4

Meyer, J. and Land, R. 2003. *Threshold concepts and troublesome knowledge: Linkages to ways of thinking and practising within the disciplines* [e-resource]. Accessed August 2018. www.etl.tla.ed.ac.uk//docs/ETLreport4.pdf.

NDIS. 2017. What help can I get? [e-resource]. Accessed August 2018. www.ndis.gov.au/people-disability/what-help-can-i-get.

New London Group. 1996. A pedagogy of multiliteracies: Designing social futures. *Harvard Educational Review*, 66(1), 60–92.

Orientation and Mobility Association of Australasia. 2013. *O&M code of ethics* [e-resource]. Accessed August 2018. https://omaaustralasia.com/about-us/quality-framework.

Petrie, H. 2014. *Technological developments for visually impaired people: recent successes, future needs*. Paper presented at the The 11th International Conference on Low Vision, Melbourne, Australia. Accessed August 2018. http://vision2014.org/conference_abstracts.html.

Polanyi, M. 1966/2009. *The tacit dimension*. Chicago, IL: University of Chicago Press.

Richards, L. 2009. *Handling qualitative data: A practical guide* (2nd ed.). London: Sage.

Robson, C. 2011. *Real world research* (3rd ed.). Chichester, UK: John Wiley & Sons.

Rudman, D.L., Gold, D., McGrath, C., Zuvela, B., Spafford, M.M. and Renwick, R. 2016. "Why would I want to go out?" Age-related vision loss and social participation. *Canadian Journal on Aging*, 35(4), 465–478. http://dx.doi.org/10.1017/S0714980816000490

Sabatinelli, D., Bradley, M.M., Lang, P.J., Costa, V.D. and Versace, F. 2007. Pleasure rather than salience activates human nucleus accumbens and medial prefrontal cortex. *Journal of Neurophysiology*, 98(3), 1374–1379. http://dx.doi.org/10.1152/jn.00230.2007

Savage, M., Bagnall, G. and Longhurst, B.J. 2005. *Globalization and belonging*. London: Sage.

Schloss, P.J., Alper, S. and Jayne, D. 1993. Self-determination for persons with disabilities: Choice, risk, and dignity. *Exceptional Children*, 60(3), 215–225. http://dx.doi.org/10.1177/001440299406000303

Scott, R.A. 1969. *The making of blind men: A study of adult socialization*. New York: Russell Sage.

Shaw, R., Russotti, J., Strauss-Schwartz, J., Vail, H. and Kahn, R. 2009. The need for a uniform method of recording and reporting functional vision assessments. *Journal of Visual Impairment and Blindness*, 103(6), 367–371.

Tracy, S.J. 2010. Qualitative quality: Eight "big-tent"criteria for excellent qualitative research. *Qualitative Inquiry*, 16(10), 837–851. http://dx.doi.org/10.1177/1077800410383121

Turano, K.A., Geruschat, D.R., Stahl, J.W. and Massof, R.W. 1999. Perceived visual ability for independent mobility in persons with retinitis pigmentosa. *Investigative Ophthalmology & Visual Science*, 40(5), 865–877.

Urry, J. 2006. Complexity. *Theory, Culture and Society*, 23(2–3), 111–117.

van Manen, M. 2006. *Researching lived experience: Human science for an action sensitive pedagogy*. London, ON: Althouse Press.

Virgili, G. and Rubin, G. 2010. Orientation and mobility training for adults with low vision. *Cochrane Database of Systematic Reviews*, 5(CD003925). doi: 10.1002/14651858.CD003925.pub3

Wang, K. and Belongie, S. 2010. *Word spotting in the wild*. Paper presented at the 11th European Conference on Computer Vision, Computer Vision, Heraklion, Crete, Greece. ECCV 2010 Proceedings, Part I. Accessed August 2018. http://vision.ucsd.edu/~kai/pubs/wang_eccv2010.pdf.

Wenger, E. 1998. *Communities of practice: Learning, meaning, and identity*. Cambridge: Cambridge University Press.

Woolf, S.H. 2008. The meaning of translational research and why it matters. *Journal of the American Medical Association*, 299(2), 211–213. http://dx.doi.org/10.1001/jama.2007.26

World Health Organization. 2016. *International statistical classification of diseases and related health problems 10th Revision (ICD-10): WHO version for 2016 chapter VII diseases of the eye and adnexa (H00–H59), visual disturbances and blindness (H53–H54). H54.9 Unspecified visual impairment* [e-publication]. Accessed August 2018. http://apps.who.int/classifications/icd10/browse/2016/en#/H53-H54.

Part IX

Recent advances in "eye" research and sensory substitution devices

24

An overview of human pluripotent stem cell applications for the understanding and treatment of blindness

Louise A. Rooney, Duncan E. Crombie, Grace E. Lidgerwood, Maciej Daniszewski and Alice Pébay

Introduction

When the eye is subjected to trauma or disease, repair mechanisms are required to rehabilitate damaged tissues to a functional state and thus restore vision. Lower vertebrates, such as *Danio sp.* and *Xenopus sp*, are capable of cellular regeneration of many ocular structures after significant trauma, such as lens, optic nerve and retina (Sherpa et al., 2008; Yoshii et al., 2007). The human eye, however, lacks extensive regenerative capacity, hence insults or diseases affecting the viability of cells involved in visual processing can result in permanent visual impairment or loss of vision. Animal models and cell cultures can provide insight into loss of vision mechanisms, and are subsequently an avenue for therapy. The limited availability of post-mortem ocular tissues and the biological variability between individual donors restricts the practicality of *ex vivo* human samples as a source of experimental cells. These samples are, however, invaluable for treatments such as corneal transplants. To address this need for a reliable and reproducible source of ocular cells, human pluripotent stem cells (hPSCs) have been employed. Inherent to hPSCs, is their potential to be differentiated into all cell types of the eye, given the appropriate differentiation signals. Importantly, hPSCs can be indefinitely maintained in an undifferentiated state and thus provide an unlimited source of undifferentiated progeny for use. There are two main types of hPSCs: human embryonic stem cells (hESCs) and induced pluripotent stem cells (iPSCs). hESCs are derived from the inner cell mass of pre-implantation embryos (Reubinoff et al., 2000; Thomson et al., 1998), while human iPSCs are obtained by the reprogramming of somatic cells into pluripotent cells using a combination of transcription factors involved in the maintenance of pluripotency (Park et al., 2008; Takahashi et al., 2007; Yu et al., 2007). Importantly, iPSCs can be generated from a person's own somatic cells, typically fibroblasts cultured from a simple skin punch biopsy. It is theoretically possible, given efficient stem cell differentiation protocols, to generate any cell type from any person, which could then be used for autologous cell-replacement therapy. Further, iPSCs can be readily generated from patients with genetic disease or even genetic predispositions to disease, which is valuable for understanding the pathogenesis of ophthalmic diseases and retinal development *in vitro* (Garcia et al., 2015; Golestaneh et al., 2016; Lukovic et al., 2015; Phillips et al., 2014; Saini et al., 2017; Singh et al., 2013; Tucker et al., 2014; Yoshida et al., 2014). Together, these aspects of iPSC research have established the potential for personalised medicine through both drug discovery and cell-based therapeutics. Other sources of stem cells are also available for ocular cell generation. In this chapter, we will concentrate on the use of hPSCs as a source of ocular cells. For information pertaining to the use of adult stem cells for disease modelling and regeneration of ocular tissue, please see (Jones et al., 2017) and (Rao, Dedania and Johnson, 2017).

Differentiation of hPSCs

The simplest method of hPSC differentiation is commonly referred to as spontaneous differentiation. Using either adherent or suspension culture methodologies, hPSCs differentiate into cell types of each germ layer: ectoderm, endoderm and mesoderm. For many cell lineages, this form of differentiation and growth is inefficient for generation of cells for research. Currently, these protocols are predominantly used for confirming pluripotency of hPSCs, or as a first stage in guided differentiations. Research, usually based on developmental signalling pathways learnt from embryology, has allowed for the development of a multitude of directed differentiation techniques. These can involve co-cultures and/or conditioned media, specific growth factors, small molecules and cell culture medium formulations designed to drive differentiation towards a certain lineage or cell type. More recent methodologies involve the formation of three-dimensional organoids, which show some levels of organisation of the human retina (Ader and Tanaka, 2014). Much work has been undertaken employing these techniques and protocols to differentiate hPSCs to retinal cells.

Retinal pigment epithelium

The retinal pigment epithelium (RPE) cells are a polarised monolayer of polygonal pigmented epithelial cells. The RPE has many functions including light absorption, epithelial transport and homeostatic support of the underlying photoreceptors. Dysfunction of the RPE is associated with various conditions, including age-related macular degeneration (AMD), retinitis pigmentosa and other rare retinal dystrophies such as Best disease, Doyne honeycombe retinal dystrophy and Sorsby's fundus dystrophy.

Development of retinal cells can be mimicked *in vitro*, and many protocols have been published on the differentiation of hPSCs into RPE cells. RPE differentiation can been achieved with harvesting and expanding RPE cells from spontaneously differentiating hPSCs, but the major drawback of this method is the long differentiation period, often over 4–6 months (Buchholz et al., 2009; Buchholz et al., 2013; Vaajasaari et al., 2011; Zahabi et al., 2012). Guided differentiation methods have proven to be great alternatives, as they are more reproducible and faster. Various molecules have been described as efficient for the generation of RPE cells, including basic fibroblast growth factor (bFGF), Noggin, Dickkopf-1 (DKK1), Insulin Growth Factor 1 (IGF1), nicotinamide, casein kinase I inhibitor 7, the ALK4 inhibitor SB-431542 and the Rho-associated kinase inhibitor Y-27632 (Buchholz et al., 2013; Idelson et al., 2009; Kuwahara et al., 2015; Lidgerwood et al., 2016; Osakada et al., 2009; Reichman et al., 2014). An enrichment of retinal cells prior to RPE isolation and expansion can also be used (Cho et al., 2012; Lamba et al., 2006; Lamba et al., 2010; Nakano et al., 2012; Reichman et al., 2014; Sluch et al., 2015; Zhu et al., 2013).

Retinal ganglion cells

Retinal ganglion cells (RGCs) transfer visual information between the retina and brain via the optic nerve (Sanes and Masland, 2015). Degeneration of these cells in the course of several optic neuropathies including glaucoma leads to irreversible vision loss and blindness (Coleman, 1999; Quigley, 1999). Because of its slow and asymptomatic progression, glaucoma diagnosis at early stages is challenging, and accounts for a high percentage of patients who are unaware of their condition (Weinreb, Aung and Medeiros, 2014). It is estimated that by 2020 there will be nearly 80 million of people affected worldwide with more than 11 million bilaterally blind (Quigley and Broman, 2006). According to the World health Organization, it is estimated that around 80% of blindness is either avertible or treatable (Thylefors, 1998), so new means of screening are required to identify individuals at risk of developing glaucoma (Weinreb and Khaw, 2004).

Presently, research on optic neuropathies is hampered by paucity of both readily available RGCs from living patients and *in vitro* RGC models. However, these issues may be addressed by use of hPSCs (Chamling, Sluch and Zack, 2016; Riazifar et al., 2014). Various protocols have been established for the generation of RGCs from stem cells (reviewed in Gill et al., 2014). Multiple groups, including ours, have focused on developing efficient and robust hPSC-derived RGC differentiation protocols (Gill et al., 2016; Huang et al., 2017; Reichman et al., 2014; Riazifar et al., 2014; Sluch et al., 2015). Differentiation protocols typically rely on modulation of several cellular signalling pathways known to be involved in embryogenesis and early eye development in order to obtain retinal progenitor cells, RGCs and then enrichment of RGCs by cell sorting (Gill et al., 2016; Sluch et al., 2015). Those RGC populations show functionality and marker profiles with close resemblance to native RGCs (Gill et al., 2016; Sluch et al., 2015). Single cell RNA sequencing analysis of RGCs differentiated and enriched by selection with the sensory neuron marker THY1 through our method has revealed three main subpopulations within the hPSC-derived RGCs (Daniszewski et al., 2018).

Optic cup/neural retina

Many diseases affect multiple cell types and cellular interactions are likely fundamental to normal function and pathogenesis. These are not recapitulated in conventional cell cultures. Recent advances now enable the generation of neural retinas that efficiently replicate the structures that exist in higher organisms (Eiraku et al., 2011; Nakano et al., 2012; Volkner et al., 2016; Zhong et al., 2014). Organised neural retina, or optic cups, can be obtained from the differentiation of hPSCs, giving rise to structures containing stratified layers of retinal cells with RPE, retinal neurons including RGCs, photoreceptors, amacrine cells, horizontal cells and Müller cells (Nakano et al., 2012). By tracing the formation of these organoids in real time, one can gather knowledge on fundamental processes involved in retinogenesis, while simultaneously generating models that more accurately mimic the native eye. Given the inter-relatedness of the cells within the eye, it is important that such models exist, building a more complete picture of developmental processes and disease pathogenesis. Important limitations of the current optic cups are lack of vasculature, microglia and lens placode.

There is currently no efficient protocol to generate homogenous cultures of functional mature photoreceptors from hPSCs. This is significant as many conditions are likely to start with photoreceptor degeneration. Hence, there is a need to obtain photoreceptors for disease modelling and cellular transplantation (Jayakody et al., 2015). Immature photoreceptor differentiation has been reported from hPSCs using a staged-differentiation into self-organising neuroepithelium followed by a maturation of photoreceptor precursors with addition of retinoic acid, FGFs, Tau and Sonic hedgehog (Boucherie et al., 2013). The most typical method of obtaining photoreceptors is through the differentiation of hPSCs into optic cups. The process of differentiation into photoreceptors is long and maturity remains an issue, with mature and functional photoreceptors observed around at least six months of differentiation (Reichman et al., 2017). In those settings, the interactions of photoreceptors with the other layers of the retina can be studied. The main limitation of this method is that it does not allow assessment of photoreceptors in isolation. This could potentially be overcome by harvesting of photoreceptors from optic cups (Nakano et al., 2012) by selection with specific progenitor or photoreceptor markers such as CD73 (Koso et al., 2009; Lidgerwood et al., 2018; Santos-Ferreira et al., 2016; Reichman et al., 2017). Obviously, this method could be applied to all cell types present within the optic cup.

Lens differentiation

The lens of the eye is a transparent avascular disk structure that focuses light on to the retina. Disruption to healthy lens functions can result in protein aggregation in the lens and subsequently opacity and cataract – an increasingly common eye disease, which is the leading cause of blindness worldwide.

To date, researchers have elucidated the requirement of the signal transduction pathways FGF, Bone Morphogenetic Protein (BMP), Notch, Wingless Integration Site (Wnt) and Tumour Growth Factor beta (TGFβ) for lens cell formation from hPSCs (Yang et al., 2010). Yang and colleagues successfully differentiated hESCs into lens progenitor-like cells and lentoid bodies (Yang et al., 2010). This process involved a three-stage growth factor treatment, which first produced neuroectoderm (Noggin), followed by lens progenitor cells (FGF and BMPs), then lens epithelial and lens fibre cells (FGF and Wnt). It led to generation of heterogeneous mix of lens progenitor-like and non-lens cells. Lens cells were produced by this methodology, but in a heterogeneous mix of other cells.

To obtain a homogenous population of lens epithelial cells, Mengarelli and Barberi (2013) cultured hESCs in a serum-free medium supplemented with insulin, transferrin and selenium. This differentiation method resulted in a heterogeneous cell population of mesodermal, non-neural ectoderm and neural ectoderm cells. A complex fluorescence-activated cell sorting (FACS) method was subsequently employed to purify the cell population to target lens cells, using c-Met/HGFR and CD44 lens cell surface markers for selection. However, this method was ineffective and resulted in a mixed population of lens and non-lens cells. More recently, research into the development of iPSCs from urinary cells and subsequent differentiation into lentoid bodies has been conducted (Fu et al., 2017). iPSCs were differentiated to neuroectoderm using Noggin. After mechanical isolation of differentiating hPSCs, colonies were treated with BMP4 and BMP7, which were then replaced with Wnt3a for subsequent differentiation of lens epithelial cells into lens fibre cells. This protocol reportedly generates functional lentoid bodies that express lens-specific markers, possess transparent lens-like structures and exhibit ocular characteristics.

Corneal cells

The cornea is the avascular and transparent outermost layer of the eye, which, in conjunction with the lens, refracts light to the back of the eye. Five layers constitute the human cornea; the corneal epithelium, Bowman's membrane, the corneal stroma, Descemet's membrane and the corneal endothelium. The corneal endothelium is largely responsible for the maintenance of corneal transparency as it facilitates transport of necessary solutes and ions to and from other layers of the cornea. Dysfunction of the corneal endothelium can result in corneal blindness, a condition that has predominantly been treated by healthy donor tissue transplantation. However, there is an immense demand for cadaveric human cornea and limited supply, particularly in countries in which eye bank systems are not well established. This necessitates alternative endothelia generation techniques, such as isolation and culture of corneal endothelia cells and generation of corneal cells from hPSCs, for the transplantation and therapy of corneal diseases.

McCabe et al. (2015) described a two-step methodology for the generation of corneal endothelium from hESCs. First, neural crest and central nervous system progenitors were generated by the treatment of hESCs with SB431542 and Noggin. Following this, neural crest cells were differentiated to corneal epithelium by the addition of platelet-derived growth factor B (PDGFB), DKK2 and bFGF. This approach produces large quantities of corneal endothelial cells, similar to adult corneal endothelial cells, characterised by morphology, gene expression and protein expression. Other work has been undertaken to generate hPSC-derived corneal organoids for the investigation of cornea development and disease modelling (Foster et al., 2017). Through sequential differentiation protocols, retinal, and at later stages, corneal organoids were generated comprising the cell types of the cornea. This induction was achieved by forced aggregation of single cell dissociated iPSCs, followed by treatment with neural induction medium and later DMEM/F12 supplemented with B27, a neural cell culture supplement, fetal bovine serum (FBS) and retinoic acid to induce retinal maturation and corneal generation. The cornea organoids expressed markers of the epithelium (Keratin 14), stroma (Keratocan, Collagen types I and V, and Lumican) and endothelium (Collagen Type VIII Alpha Chain 1 and F11 Receptor (endothelial tight junction protein)) and notably extracellular matrix collagens and stromal matrix proteins. This work provides a platform to investigate corneal disease phenotypes, including interactions of different cell types, over long periods of time.

Trabecular meshwork

The trabecular meshwork is a small area of cells surrounded by extracellular matrix, located at the base of the cornea, close to the ciliary body. Functioning as the drainage system of the eye, the trabecular meshwork actively redistributes fluid from the anterior chamber of the eye to Schlemm's canal to maintain intraocular pressure. Additionally, the trabecular meshwork phagocytoses debris, an important feature of the maintenance of healthy aqueous humor and its clearance system. If the trabecular meshwork is inoperable or poorly functioning and regular homeostatic regulation is lost, intraocular pressure rises, which can result in damage to the optic nerve. Therefore, defective functionality of the trabecular meshwork is thought to result in open-angle glaucoma, the most common form of glaucoma. Ding et al. (2014) co-cultured mouse iPSCs with immortalised human trabecular meshwork cells. This technique induces distinct morphological changes and generates iPSC-trabecular meshwork cells that resemble trabecular meshwork cells as described in the literature. Importantly, these cells also exhibit phagocytic functionality, a key feature of trabecular meshwork. hPSCs have been differentiated to trabecular meshwork-like cells by generation of embryoid bodies on trabecular meshwork extracellular matrix in a medium conditioned with meshwork (Abu-Hassan et al., 2015). Trabecular meshwork cells have been then transplanted into animal models of glaucoma, effectively restoring intraocular pressure and improving aqueous humor outflow facility (Abu-Hassan et al., 2015; Zhu et al., 2016; Zhu et al., 2017).

Ophthalmic disease modelling

Modelling of human diseases using hPSCs has proven to be very powerful. Some key examples of modelling are described below.

In the case of complex diseases such as AMD, iPSCs have been generated from patients with high-risk genetic variants to understand the influence these genetic variants have on the RPE to contribute to the pathogenesis of AMD. Such an approach has already proven successful in modelling aspects of AMD *in vitro*. Indeed, Yang et al. (2014) reprogrammed fibroblasts from individuals with an AMD-protective haplotype for both *CFH* and *ARMS2/HTRA1* and from patients with an AMD-risk haplotype for both *CFH* and *ARMS2/HTRA1* and assessed biological functions in differentiated RPE cells, which an increased susceptibility to oxidative stress. Further, AMD-patient (*ARMS2/HTRA1*) iPSC-derived RPE cells also showed increased inflammatory and complement factors that could be rescued with the addition of nicotinamide (Saini et al., 2017).

Interestingly, the presence of drusen in a dish was recently reported in iPSC-derived RPE cells (Galloway et al., 2017). The study demonstrates that RPE cells generated from patients suffering from various maculopathies (Sorsby's fundus dystrophy, Doyne honeycomb retinal dystrophy and autosomal dominant radial drusen) are responsible for the formation of drusen-like deposits underneath the epithelium, which was accompanied by an increased expression of complement factor pathway genes. Similarly, the retinal dystrophy Best disease (BD) was modelled using patient specific iPSCs. Once differentiated to RPE cells, those showed functional defects, including a delayed degradation of photoreceptor outer segments and increased oxidative stress following chronic photoreceptor outer segment feeding (Singh et al., 2015; Singh et al., 2013).

Likewise, studying patient iPSC-derived RGCs has proven useful to the description of pathogenic events in neuropathies. For instance, iPSC-derived RGCs from Leber hereditary optic neuropathy patients have an increased basal susceptibility to apoptosis (Wong et al., 2017). This data can now potentially serve as a platform for drug screening. Interestingly, iPSC differentiation to RGCs was proven to be less efficient when performed from glaucoma patient iPSCs with a SIX6 risk allele (Teotia et al., 2017). Whether or not this has implication for adulthood remains to be described.

In cases of monogenic diseases of the eye, gene editing is now commonly used to either introduce or correct mutations of interest (Hung et al., 2016). Correction of genetic mutations in diseased hPSCs is an important procedure for modelling diseases *in vitro* but also has potential for future clinical application. Corrected cell lines, sharing the rest of the genetic background with the diseased lines, provide the ideal basis for comparison of healthy versus diseases phenotypes without the confounding genetic influences of using hPSCs from related or unrelated individuals.

Retinal organoids (optic cups) are also very useful for disease modelling as they can be used for phenotypic screening in retinal dystrophies and optic neuropathies, to interrogate interactions between RPE, photoreceptors or RGCs, providing a model to study interactions of the various cell layers within the neural retina. Hence, it can be used as a tool to model development and degenerative diseases of the retina and optic nerve. Once key phenotypes will have been identified, those can become a screening outcome in the search of treatments to counteract these pathological processes. The potential of optic cups for disease modelling and screening of novel therapies was recently described in (Parfitt et al., 2016). Researchers demonstrated that the common mutation CEP290 responsible for Leber congenital amaurosis induced a cilia defect in photoreceptors within the optic cup obtained from patient-derived iPSCs, and described how treating optic cups with an antisense nucleotide restored CEP290 and cilia functions in the photoreceptors.

Cell therapies using hPSCs and derivatives

The science

The eye is an attractive target for stem cell replacement therapies, in part due to its accessibility, small size (requiring less cells for replacement), distinct organisation protecting it from the immune system (thereby minimising the risk of rejection) and its ability to be closely monitored for functionality, owing to the array of clinical assessments available to clinicians to evaluate the effectiveness of treatment (Davidson et al., 2014). Indeed, hPSC-derived RPE cells have been reported to be effective at maintaining vision when transplanted into the Royal College of Surgeons rat model for AMD. In this model, RPE derived from human ESCs and iPSCs were capable of forming a monolayer between surviving rat host RPE layers and phagocytosing degenerating photoreceptor cells, a necessary function of the RPE to maintain photoreceptor health (Krohne et al., 2012; Song et al., 2015).

A current phase II clinical trial for Stargardt disease and AMD has shown that hESC-derived RPE cells in suspension safely integrate in the human eye following submacular transplantation (Schwartz et al., 2012; Schwartz et al., 2015). However, recent reports from the trial have indicated that despite the repopulation of RPE at the macula, coverage is often patchy (Schwartz et al., 2012; Schwartz et al., 2015). A second clinical trial using iPSCs to treat AMD was briefly interrupted following changes to Japanese regulations governing clinical trials. It resumed in 2016, and the individual receiving the iPSC-derived RPE is apparently progressing satisfactorily, and her vision has stopped deteriorating; however, the experimental procedure was not performed on any further individuals after serious spontaneous mutations were identified in the iPSCs of the second patient due to receive the treatment (Mandai et al., 2017). As a consequence, Japan now requires iPSCs to be used as allogeneic rather than autologous transplants.

Clinical trials for hPSC-derived RPE transplantation requires immune suppression in patients receiving the transplants, however concerns about immune rejection of hPSC-derived RPE have been allayed by research in humanised mice, showing an immune response is mounted against iPSC-derived smooth muscle cells but not iPSC-derived RPE, suggesting that iPSC derivatives may vary in their immunogenicity, and potentially the site of transplantation (Zhao et al., 2015).

Words of caution

Before being used in transplantation, safety and regulatory issues of stem cell therapies must be addressed to ensure safe and efficacious treatment of patients. First, any cells to be used in stem cell transplant therapies must be highly characterised by surface markers and cytogenetic tests to confirm the desired transplantation cell karyotype. A number of clinically compliant stem cell lines have been generated, some of which have been retrospectively assessed, substantiating them for clinical usage. Second, differentiation protocols need to be employed for efficient selection and purification of the desired cell type(s) for transplantation. This is particularly important for hPSC-derived cells as transplantation of any undifferentiated hPSCs could lead to teratoma formation in the recipient. Both stem cell characterisation and differentiation protocols must comply with relevant current good manufacturing practice and regulatory body requirements. Third, all therapies should be supported by robust and peer-reviewed pre-clinical and clinical trials to ensure treatments have suitable efficacy and minimal adverse effects.

The procedures and regulations described above and subsequently the establishment of stem cell transplantation as legitimate therapeutic options for patients can take years or decades.

Consequently, few stem cell transplant therapies are available in most developed countries where rigorous safety regulations are in place. This extensive timeline of therapy development, coupled with often sensationalist reports in the media regarding treatments, has provided inaccurate impressions regarding the availability and promise of current treatments. While many trials for stem cell therapies are underway, many are in the early stages of clinical translation and are focused on patient safety. According to the Australian National Health and Medical Research Council, the only well-established stem cell treatment in Australia is bone marrow transplants for the treatment of blood and immune system diseases (see "NHMRC Public Consultation", https://consultations.nhmrc.gov.au). As such, some patients have sought untested, unproven and unpublished stem cell treatments in countries where regulatory requirements are less rigorous. Additionally, even where tight regulatory practices are in place, stem cell clinics have been established that exploit laws designed to allow surgeons some degree of flexibility for medical innovation for patient treatment, again to practice unproven therapies (Lindvall and Hyun, 2009).

To distinguish these issues from the broader problem of medical tourism, the term "stem cell tourism" was coined to describe occasions in which patients pay large sums of money to travel to such countries to receive stem cell treatments that have not necessarily been proven safe or effective (Barclay, 2009; MacReady, 2009). Treatments are advertised to treat conditions such as multiple sclerosis, motor neuron disease, cerebral palsy, optic nerve damage, ataxia, spinal cord injury and the effects of stroke. Clinics offering stem cell therapies often employ direct-to-consumer advertising with the promise of great therapeutic benefit and no risk. These marketing ploys often have emphasis on patient testimonials rather than scientific data to support treatments. Consumers to which this advertising appeals are often suffering from chronic or terminal illness and may have exhausted all other treatment options in their home country. Therefore, the decision to undertake these journeys and associated risks is usually based upon false hope, optimism and misinformation such as promise of efficacious treatment that has not been sufficiently researched and proven. It is not just health consumers that the optimism of stem cell therapies has affected – patient advocates and service providers who are finding ways to service the growing demand for these treatments are also influenced, promoting the employment of sceptical therapies.

It is critical that specialists and clinicians have an up-to-date understanding of the current state of cellular therapies, especially stem cell therapies in their given fields, in order to correctly advise patients of the dangers of unproven cellular therapies. The international Society for Stem Cell Research has released a *Patient Handbook on Stem Cell Therapies* and a website called "Closer Look at Stem Cell Treatments" (www.closerlookatstemcells.org) to help inform health consumers and patient advocates about the safety and efficacy of stem cell therapies.

Conclusion

There is a pressing need for human disease models to improve our understanding of neurodegeneration. hPSC-derived ocular cells are powerful and relevant tools for understanding pathophysiology of ophthalmic diseases and the development of drug therapies. Merging recent technological advances with the flexibility of stem cells may generate entirely new means of treatment. For instance, the ability to precisely edit genes using CRISPR methodologies could allow the prevention of cellular degeneration. Similarly, the ability to directly reprogramme cells intrinsically as a way to replace dying layers of the eye could allow for targeted approaches without the need for cell replacement. Those technologies require extensive additional research and optimisation before therapeutic potential can be claimed; however, if successful, their implementation could revolutionise personalised medicine for the treatment of blindness, allowing a panel of therapeutical options to be considered depending on the progression of individuals' respective condition.

Acknowledgements

GEL and MD are supported by postgraduate award scholarships from the University of Melbourne and AP by an Australian Research Council Future Fellowship (FT140100047). CERA receives operational infrastructure support from the Victorian Government.

References

Abu-Hassan, D.W., Li, X., Ryan, E.I., Acott, T.S. and Kelley, M.J. 2015. Induced pluripotent stem cells restore function in a human cell loss model of open-angle glaucoma. *Stem Cells*, 33(3), 751–761.

Ader, M. and Tanaka, E.M. 2014. Modeling human development in 3D culture. *Current Opinion in Cell Biology*, 31, 23–28.

Barclay, E. 2009. Stem-cell experts raise concerns about medical tourism. *Lancet*, 373(9667), 883–884.

Boucherie, C., Mukherjee, S., Henckaerts, E., Thrasher, A.J., Sowden, J.C. and Ali, R. R. 2013. Brief report: Self-organizing neuroepithelium from human pluripotent stem cells facilitates derivation of photoreceptors. *Stem Cells*, 31(2), 408–414.

Buchholz, D.E., Hikita, S.T., Rowland, T.J., Friedrich, A.M., Hinman, C.R., Johnson, L.V. and Clegg, D.O. 2009. Derivation of functional retinal pigmented epithelium from induced pluripotent stem cells. *Stem Cells*, 27(10), 2427–2434.

Buchholz, D.E., Pennington, B.O., Croze, R.H., Hinman, C.R., Coffey, P.J. and Clegg, D.O. 2013. Rapid and efficient directed differentiation of human pluripotent stem cells into retinal pigmented epithelium. *Stem Cells Translational Medicine*, 2(5), 384–393.

Chamling, X., Sluch, V.M. and Zack, D.J. 2016. The potential of human stem cells for the study and treatment of glaucoma. *Investigative Ophthalmology & Visual Science*, 57(5), ORSFi1-6.

Cho, M.S., Kim, S.J., Ku, S.-Y., Park, J.H., Lee, H., Yoo, D.H., Park, U.C., Song, S. A., Choi, Y.M. and Yu, H.G. 2012. Generation of retinal pigment epithelial cells from human embryonic stem cell-derived spherical neural masses. *Stem Cell Research*, 9(2), 101–109.

Coleman, A. L. 1999. Glaucoma. *Lancet*, 354(9192), 1803–1810.

Daniszewski, M., Senabouth, A., Nguyen, Q.H., Crombie, D.E., Lukowski, S.W., Kulkarni, T., Sluch, V.M., Jabbari, J.S., Chamling, X., Zack, D.J., Pébay, A., Powell. J.E. and Hewitt, A.W. 2018. Single cell RNA sequencing of stem cell-derived retinal ganglion cells. *Scientific Data*, 5, 180013.

Davidson, K.C., Guymer, R.H., Pera, M.F. and Pebay, A. 2014. Human pluripotent stem cell strategies for age-related macular degeneration. *Optometry and Vision Science*, 91(8), 887–893.

Ding, Q.J., Zhu, W., Cook, A.C., Anfinson, K.R., Tucker, B.A. and Kuehn, M.H. 2014. Induction of trabecular meshwork cells from induced pluripotent stem cells. *Investigative Ophthalmology & Visual Science*, 55(11), 7065–7072.

Eiraku, M., Takata, N., Ishibashi, H., Kawada, M., Sakakura, E., Okuda, S., Sekiguchi, K., Adachi, T. and Sasai, Y. 2011. Self-organizing optic-cup morphogenesis in three-dimensional culture. *Nature*, 472(7341), 51–56.

Foster, J.W., Wahlin, K., Adams, S.M., Birk, D.E., Zack, D.J. and Chakravarti, S. 2017. Cornea organoids from human induced pluripotent stem cells. *Science Reports*, 7, 41286.

Fu, Q., Qin, Z., Jin, X., Zhang, L., Chen, Z., He, J., Ji, J. and Yao, K. 2017. Generation of functional lentoid bodies from human induced pluripotent stem cells derived from urinary cells. *Investigative Ophthalmology & Visual Science*, 58(1), 517–527.

Galloway, C.A., Dalvi, S., Hung, S.S.C., Macdonald, L.A., Latchney, L.R., Wong, R. C.B., Guymer, R.H., Mackey, D.A., Williams, D.S., Chung, M.M., Gamm, D.M., Pebay, A., Hewitt, A.W. and Singh, R. 2017. Drusen in patient-derived hiPSC-RPE models of macular dystrophies. *Proceedings of the National Academy of Sciences of the United States of America*, 114(39), E8214–E8223.

Garcia, T.Y., Gutierrez, M., Reynolds, J. and Lamba, D.A. 2015. Modeling the dynamic AMD-associated chronic oxidative stress changes in human ESC and iPSC-derived RPE cells. *Investigative Ophthalmology & Visual Science*, 56(12), 7480–7488.

Gill, K.P., Hewitt, A.W., Davidson, K.C., Pebay, A. and Wong, R.C. 2014. Methods of retinal ganglion cell differentiation from pluripotent stem cells. *Translational Vision Science and Technology*, 3(4), 7.

Gill, K.P., Hung, S.S., Sharov, A., Lo, C.Y., Needham, K., Lidgerwood, G.E., Jackson, S., Crombie, D.E., Nayagam, B.A., Cook, A.L., Hewitt, A.W., Pebay, A. and Wong, R.C. 2016. Enriched retinal ganglion cells derived from human embryonic stem cells. *Scientific Reports*, 6, 30552.

Golestaneh, N., Chu, Y., Cheng, S.K., Cao, H., Poliakov, E. and Berinstein, D.M. 2016. Repressed SIRT1/PGC-1alpha pathway and mitochondrial disintegration in iPSC-derived RPE disease model of age-related macular degeneration. *Journal of Translational Medicine*, 14(1), 344.

Huang, L., Chen, M., Zhang, W., Sun, X., Liu, B. and Ge, J. 2017. Retinoid acid and taurine promote NeuroD1-induced differentiation of induced pluripotent stem cells into retinal ganglion cells. *Molecular and Cellular Biochemistry*, 438(1–2), 67–76.

Hung, S.S.C., Mccaughey, T., Swann, O., Pebay, A. and Hewitt, A.W. 2016. Genome engineering in ophthalmology: Application of CRISPR/Cas to the treatment of eye disease. *Progress in Retinal and Eye Research*, July, 531–520.

Idelson, M., Alper, R., Obolensky, A., Ben-Shushan, E., Hemo, I., Yachimovich-Cohen, N., Khaner, H., Smith, Y., Wiser, O., Gropp, M., Cohen, M.A., Even-Ram, S., Berman-Zaken, Y., Matzrafi, L., Rechavi, G., Banin, E. and Reubinoff, B. 2009. Directed differentiation of human embryonic stem cells into functional retinal pigment epithelium cells. *Cell Stem Cell*, 5(4), 396–408.

Jayakody, S.A., Gonzalez-Cordero, A., Ali, R.R. and Pearson, R.A. 2015. Cellular strategies for retinal repair by photoreceptor replacement. *Progress in Retinal and Eye Research*, 46, 31–66.

Jones, M.K., Lu, B., Girman, S. and Wang, S. 2017. Cell-based therapeutic strategies for replacement and preservation in retinal degenerative diseases. *Progress in Retinal and Eye Research*, 58, 1–27.

Koso, H., Minami, C., Tabata, Y., Inoue, M., Sasaki, E., Satoh, S. and Watanabe, S. 2009. CD73: A novel cell surface antigen that characterizes retinal photoreceptor precursor cells. *Investigative Ophthalmology & Visual Science*, 50(11), 5411–5418.

Krohne, T.U., Westenskow, P.D., Kurihara, T., Friedlander, D.F., Lehmann, M., Dorsey, A.L., Li, W.L., Zhu, S.Y., Schultz, A., Wang, J.H., Siuzdak, G., Ding, S. and Friedlander, M. 2012. Generation of retinal pigment epithelial cells from small molecules and OCT4 reprogrammed human induced pluripotent stem cells. *Stem Cells Translational Medicine*, 1(2), 96–109.

Kuwahara, A., Ozone, C., Nakano, T., Saito, K., Eiraku, M. and Sasai, Y. 2015. Generation of a ciliary margin-like stem cell niche from self-organizing human retinal tissue. *Nature Communications*, 6, 66286.

Lamba, D.A., Karl, M.O., Ware, C.B. and Reh, T.A. 2006. Efficient generation of retinal progenitor cells from human embryonic stem cells. *Proceedings of the National Academy of Sciences of the United States of America*, 103(34), 12769–12774.

Lamba, D.A., McUsic, A., Hirata, R.K., Wang, P.R., Russell, D. and Reh, T.A. 2010. Generation, purification and transplantation of photoreceptors derived from human induced pluripotent stem cells. *PLoS One*, 5(1), e8763.

Lidgerwood, G.E., Lim, S.Y., Crombie, D.E., Ali, R., Gill, K.P., Hernandez, D., Kie, J., Conquest, A., Waugh, H.S., Wong, R C., Liang, H.H., Hewitt, A.W., Davidson, K.C. and Pebay, A. 2016. Defined medium conditions for the induction and expansion of human pluripotent stem cell-derived retinal pigment epithelium. *Stem Cell Review*, 12(2), 179–188.

Lidgerwood, G.E., Morris, A.J., Conquest, A., Daniszewski, M., Rooney, L.A., Lim, S.Y., Hernandez, D., Liang, H.H., Allen, P., Connell, P.P., Guymer, R.H., Hewitt, A.W. and Pebay, A. 2018. Role of lysophosphatidic acid in the retinal pigment epithelium and photoreceptors. *Biochimica et Biophysica Acta*, 1863(7), 750–761.

Lindvall, O. and Hyun, I. 2009. Medical innovation versus stem cell tourism. *Science*, 324(5935), 1664–1665.

Lukovic, D., Artero Castro, A., Delgado, A.B., Bernal Mde, L., Luna Pelaez, N., Diez Lloret, A., Perez Espejo, R., Kamenarova, K., Fernandez Sanchez, L., Cuenca, N., Corton, M., Avila Fernandez, A., Sorkio, A., Skottman, H., Ayuso, C., Erceg, S. and Bhattacharya, S.S. 2015. Human iPSC derived disease model of MERTK-associated retinitis pigmentosa. *Scientific Reports*, 5, 12910.

McCabe, K.L., Kunzevitzky, N.J., Chiswell, B.P., Xia, X., Goldberg, J.L. and Lanza, R. 2015. Efficient generation of human embryonic stem cell-derived corneal endothelial cells by directed differentiation. *PLoS One*, 10(12), e0145266.

Macready, N. 2009. The murky ethics of stem-cell tourism. *Lancet Oncology*, 10(4), 317–318.

Mandai, M., Watanabe, A., Kurimoto, Y., Hirami, Y., Morinaga, C., Daimon, T., Fujihara, M., Akimaru, H., Sakai, N., Shibata, Y., Terada, M., Nomiya, Y., Tanishima, S., Nakamura, M., Kamao, H., Sugita, S., Onishi, A., Ito, T., Fujita, K., Kawamata, S., Go, M.J., Shinohara, C., Hata, K.-I., Sawada, M.,

Yamamoto, M., Ohta, S., Ohara, Y., Yoshida, K., Kuwahara, J., Kitano, Y., Amano, N., Umekage, M., Kitaoka, F., Tanaka, A., Okada, C., Takasu, N., Ogawa, S., Yamanaka, S. and Takahashi, M. 2017. Autologous induced stem cell-derived retinal cells for macular degeneration. *New England Journal of Medicine*, 376(11), 1038–1046.

Mengarelli, I. and Barberi, T. 2013. Derivation of multiple cranial tissues and isolation of lens epithelium-like cells from human embryonic stem cells. *Stem Cells Translational Medicine*, 2(2), 94–106.

Nakano, T., Ando, S., Takata, N., Kawada, M., Muguruma, K., Sekiguchi, K., Saito, K., Yonemura, S., Eiraku, M. and Sasai, Y. 2012. Self-formation of optic cups and storable stratified neural retina from human ESCs. *Cell Stem Cell*, 10(6), 771–785.

Osakada, F., Jin, Z.-B., Hirami, Y., Ikeda, H., Danjyo, T., Watanabe, K., Sasai, Y. and Takahashi, M. 2009. In vitro differentiation of retinal cells from human pluripotent stem cells by small-molecule induction. *Journal of Cell Science*, 122(17), 3169–3179.

Parfitt, D.A., Lane, A., Ramsden, C.M., Carr, A.J., Munro, P.M., Jovanovic, K., Schwarz, N., Kanuga, N., Muthiah, M.N., Hull, S., Gallo, J.M., Da Cruz, L., Moore, A.T., Hardcastle, A.J., Coffey, P.J. and Cheetham, M.E. 2016. Identification and correction of mechanisms underlying inherited blindness in human iPSC-derived optic cups. *Cell Stem Cell*, 18(6), 769–781.

Park, I.H., Zhao, R., West, J.A., Yabuuchi, A., Huo, H., Ince, T.A., Lerou, P.H., Lensch, M.W. and Daley, G.Q. 2008. Reprogramming of human somatic cells to pluripotency with defined factors. *Nature*, 451(7175), 141–146.

Phillips, M.J., Perez, E.T., Martin, J.M., Reshel, S.T., Wallace, K.A., Capowski, E.E., Singh, R., Wright, L.S., Clark, E.M., Barney, P.M., Stewart, R., Dickerson, S.J., Miller, M.J., Percin, E.F., Thomson, J.A. and Gamm, D.M. 2014. Modeling human retinal development with patient-specific induced pluripotent stem cells reveals multiple roles for visual system Homeobox 2. *Stem Cells*, 32(6), 1480–1492.

Quigley, H.A. 1999. Neuronal death in glaucoma. *Progress in Retinal and Eye Research*, 18(1), 39–57.

Quigley, H.A. and Broman, A.T. 2006. The number of people with glaucoma worldwide in 2010 and 2020. *British Journal of Ophthalmology*, 90(3), 262–267.

Rao, R.C., Dedania, V.S. and Johnson, M.W. 2017. Stem cells for retinal disease: A perspective on the promise and perils. *American Journal of Ophthalmology*, 179, 32–38.

Reichman, S., Slembrouck, A., Gagliardi, G., Chaffiol, A., Terray, A., Nanteau, C., Potey, A., Belle, M., Rabesandratana, O., Duebel, J., Orieux, G., Nandrot, E.F., Sahel, J.A. and Goureau, O. 2017. Generation of storable retinal organoids and retinal pigmented epithelium from adherent human iPS cells in xeno-free and feeder-free conditions. *Stem Cells*, 35(5), 1176–1188.

Reichman, S., Terray, A., Slembrouck, A., Nanteau, C., Orieux, G., Habeler, W., Nandrot, E.F., Sahel, J.-A., Monville, C. and Goureau, O. 2014. From confluent human iPS cells to self-forming neural retina and retinal pigmented epithelium. *Proceedings of the National Academy of Sciences of the United States of America*, 111(23), 8518–8523.

Reubinoff, B.E., Pera, M.F., Fong, C.Y., Trounson, A. and Bongso, A. 2000. Embryonic stem cell lines from human blastocysts: Somatic differentiation in vitro. *Nature Biotechnology*, 18(4), 399–404.

Riazifar, H., Jia, Y., Chen, J., Lynch, G. and Huang, T. 2014. Chemically induced specification of retinal ganglion cells from human embryonic and induced pluripotent stem cells. *Stem Cells Translational Medicine*, 3(4), 424–432.

Saini, J.S., Corneo, B., Miller, J.D., Kiehl, T.R., Wang, Q., Boles, N.C., Blenkinsop, T.A., Stern, J.H. and Temple, S. 2017. Nicotinamide ameliorates disease phenotypes in a human iPSC model of age-related macular degeneration. *Cell Stem Cell*, 20(5), 635–647.e7.

Sanes, J.R. and Masland, R.H. 2015. The types of retinal ganglion cells: current status and implications for neuronal classification. *Annual Review Neuroscience*, 38, 221–246.

Santos-Ferreira, T., Volkner, M., Borsch, O., Haas, J., Cimalla, P., Vasudevan, P., Carmeliet, P., Corbeil, D., Michalakis, S., Koch, E., Karl, M.O. and Ader, M. 2016. Stem cell-derived photoreceptor transplants differentially integrate into mouse models of cone-rod dystrophy. *Investigative Ophthalmology & Visual Science*, 57(7), 3509–3520.

Schwartz, S.D., Hubschman, J.P., Heilwell, G., Franco-Cardenas, V., Pan, C.K., Ostrick, R.M., Mickunas, E., Gay, R., Klimanskaya, I. and Lanza, R. 2012. Embryonic stem cell trials for macular degeneration: a preliminary report. *Lancet*, 379(9817), 713–720.

Schwartz, S.D., Regillo, C.D., Lam, B.L., Eliott, D., Rosenfeld, P.J., Gregori, N.Z., Hubschman, J.P., Davis, J.L., Heilwell, G., Spirn, M., Maguire, J., Gay, R., Bateman, J., Ostrick, R.M., Morris, D., Vincent, M., Anglade, E., Del Priore, L. V. and Lanza, R. 2015. Human embryonic stem cell-derived retinal pigment epithelium in patients with age-related macular degeneration and Stargardt's macular dystrophy: Follow-up of two open-label phase 1/2 studies. *Lancet*, 385(9967), 509–516.

Sherpa, T., Fimbel, S.M., Mallory, D.E., Maaswinkel, H., Spritzer, S.D., Sand, J.A., Li, L., Hyde, D.R. and Stenkamp, D. L. 2008. Ganglion cell regeneration following whole-retina destruction in zebrafish. *Developmental Neurobiology*, 68(2), 166–181.

Singh, R., Kuai, D., Guziewicz, K.E., Meyer, J., Wilson, M., Lu, J., Smith, M., Clark, E., Verhoeven, A., Aguirre, G.D. and Gamm, D.M. 2015. Pharmacological modulation of photoreceptor outer segment degradation in a human iPS cell model of inherited macular degeneration. *Molecular Therapy*, 23(11), 1700–1711.

Singh, R., Shen, W., Kuai, D., Martin, J.M., Guo, X., Smith, M.A., Perez, E.T., Phillips, M.J., Simonett, J.M., Wallace, K.A., Verhoeven, A.D., Capowski, E.E., Zhang, X., Yin, Y., Halbach, P.J., Fishman, G.A., Wright, L.S., Pattnaik, B.R. and Gamm, D.M. 2013. iPS cell modeling of Best disease: Insights into the pathophysiology of an inherited macular degeneration. *Human Molecular Genetics*, 22(3), 593–607.

Sluch, V.M., Davis, C.H., Ranganathan, V., Kerr, J.M., Krick, K., Martin, R., Berlinicke, C.A., Marsh-Armstrong, N., Diamond, J.S., Mao, H.Q. and Zack, D.J. 2015. Differentiation of human ESCs to retinal ganglion cells using a CRISPR engineered reporter cell line. *Scientific Reports*, 5, 16595.

Song, W.K., Park, K.M., Kim, H.J., Lee, J.H., Choi, J., Chong, S.Y., Shim, S.H., Del Priore, L.V. and Lanza, R. 2015. Treatment of macular degeneration using embryonic stem cell-derived retinal pigment epithelium: Preliminary results in Asian patients. *Stem Cell Reports*, 4(5), 860–872.

Takahashi, K., Tanabe, K., Ohnuki, M., Narita, M., Ichisaka, T., Tomoda, K. and Yamanaka, S. 2007. Induction of pluripotent stem cells from adult human fibroblasts by defined factors. *Cell*, 131(5), 861–872.

Teotia, P., Hook, M.J.V., Wichman, C.S., Allingham, R.R., Hauser, M.A. and Ahmad, I. 2017. Modeling glaucoma: Retinal ganglion cells generated from induced pluripotent stem cells of patients with SIX6 risk allele show developmental abnormalities. *Stem Cells*, 35(11), 2239–2252.

Thomson, J.A., Itskovitz-Eldor, J., Shapiro, S.S., Waknitz, M.A., Swiergiel, J.J., Marshall, V.S. and Jones, J.M. 1998. Embryonic stem cell lines derived from human blastocysts. *Science*, 282(5391), 1145–1147.

Thylefors, B. 1998. A global initiative for the elimination of avoidable blindness. *American Journal of Ophthalmology*, 125(1), 90–93.

Tucker, B.A., Solivan-Timpe, F., Roos, B.R., Anfinson, K.R., Robin, A.L., Wiley, L. A., Mullins, R.F. and Fingert, J.H. 2014. Duplication of TBK1 stimulates autophagy in iPSC-derived retinal cells from a patient with normal tension glaucoma. *Journal of Stem Cell Research & Therapy*, 3(5), 161.

Vaajasaari, H., Ilmarinen, T., Juuti-Uusitalo, K., Rajala, K., Onnela, N., Narkilahti, S., Suuronen, R., Hyttinen, J., Uusitalo, H. and Skottman, H. 2011. Toward the defined and xeno-free differentiation of functional human pluripotent stem cell-derived retinal pigment epithelial cells. *Molecular Vision*, 17, 558–575.

Volkner, M., Zschatzsch, M., Rostovskaya, M., Overall, R.W., Busskamp, V., Anastassiadis, K. and Karl, M.O. 2016. Retinal organoids from pluripotent stem cells efficiently recapitulate retinogenesis. *Stem Cell Reports*, 6(4), 525–538.

Weinreb, R.N., Aung, T. and Medeiros, F.A. 2014. The pathophysiology and treatment of glaucoma: A review. *JAMA*, 311(18), 1901–1911.

Weinreb, R.N. and Khaw, P.T. 2004. Primary open-angle glaucoma. *Lancet*, 363(9422), 1711–1720.

Wong, R.C.B., Lim, S.Y., Hung, S.S.C., Jackson, S., Khan, S., Van Bergen, N.J., De Smit, E., Liang, H.H., Kearns, L.S., Clarke, L., Mackey, D.A., Hewitt, A.W., Trounce, I.A. and Pebay, A. 2017. Mitochondrial replacement in an iPSC model of Leber's hereditary optic neuropathy. *Aging (Albany NY)*, 9(4), 1341–1350.

Yang, C., Yang, Y., Brennan, L., Bouhassira, E.E., Kantorow, M. and Cvekl, A. 2010. Efficient generation of lens progenitor cells and lentoid bodies from human embryonic stem cells in chemically defined conditions. *FASEB Journal*, 24(9), 3274–3283.

Yang, J., Li, Y., Chan, L., Tsai, Y. T., Wu, W.H., Nguyen, H.V., Hsu, C.W., Li, X., Brown, L.M., Egli, D., Sparrow, J.R. and Tsang, S.H. 2014. Validation of genome-wide association study (GWAS)-identified disease risk alleles with patient-specific stem cell lines. *Human Molecular Genetics*, 23(13), 3445–3455.

Yoshida, T., Ozawa, Y., Suzuki, K., Yuki, K., Ohyama, M., Akamatsu, W., Matsuzaki, Y., Shimmura, S., Mitani, K., Tsubota, K. and Okano, H. 2014. The use of induced pluripotent stem cells to reveal pathogenic gene mutations and explore treatments for retinitis pigmentosa. *Molecular Brain*, 7, 45.

Yoshii, C., Ueda, Y., Okamoto, M. and Araki, M. 2007. Neural retinal regeneration in the anuran amphibian Xenopus laevis post-metamorphosis: Transdifferentiation of retinal pigmented epithelium regenerates the neural retina. *Developmental Biology*, 303(1), 45–56.

Yu, J., Vodyanik, M.A., Smuga-Otto, K., Antosiewicz-Bourget, J., Frane, J.L., Tian, S., Nie, J., Jonsdottir, G. A., Ruotti, V., Stewart, R., Slukvin, I.I. and Thomson, J.A. 2007. Induced pluripotent stem cell lines derived from human somatic cells. *Science*, 318(5858), 1917–1920.

Zahabi, A., Shahbazi, E., Ahmadieh, H., Hassani, S.N., Totonchi, M., Taei, A., Masoudi, N., Ebrahimi, M., Aghdami, N., Seifinejad, A., Mehrnejad, F., Daftarian, N., Salekdeh, G.H. and Baharvand, H. 2012. A new efficient protocol for directed differentiation of retinal pigmented epithelial cells from normal and retinal disease induced pluripotent stem cells. *Stem Cells and Development*, 21(12), 2262–2272.

Zhao, T.B., Zhang, Z.N., Westenskow, P.D., Todorova, D., Hu, Z., Lin, T.X., Rong, Z.L., Kim, J., He, J.J., Wang, M.Y., Clegg, D.O., Yang, Y.G., Zhang, K., Friedlander, M. and Xu, Y. 2015. Humanized mice reveal differential immunogenicity of cells derived from autologous induced pluripotent stem cells. *Cell Stem Cell*, 17(3), 353–359.

Zhong, X., Gutierrez, C., Xue, T., Hampton, C., Vergara, M.N., Cao, L.H., Peters, A., Park, T.S., Zambidis, E.T., Meyer, J.S., Gamm, D.M., Yau, K.W. and Canto-Soler, M.V. 2014. Generation of three-dimensional retinal tissue with functional photoreceptors from human iPSCs. *Nature Communications*, 5, 54047.

Zhu, W., Gramlich, O.W., Laboissonniere, L., Jain, A., Sheffield, V.C., Trimarchi, J.M., Tucker, B.A. and Kuehn, M.H. 2016. Transplantation of iPSC-derived TM cells rescues glaucoma phenotypes in vivo. *Proceedings of the National Academy of Sciences of the United States of America*, 113(25), E3492–E3500.

Zhu, W., Jain, A., Gramlich, O.W., Tucker, B.A., Sheffield, V.C. and Kuehn, M.H. 2017. Restoration of aqueous humor outflow following transplantation of iPSC-Derived trabecular meshwork cells in a transgenic mouse model of glaucoma. *Investigative Ophthalmology Visual Science*, 58(4), 2054–2062.

Zhu, Y., Carido, M., Meinhardt, A., Kurth, T., Karl, M.O., Ader, M. and Tanaka, E.M. 2013. Three-dimensional neuroepithelial culture from human embryonic stem cells and its use for quantitative conversion to retinal pigment epithelium. *PLoS One*, 8(1), e54552.

25

Technologies for vision impairment

Bionic eyes and sensory substitution devices

Lauren N. Ayton, Penelope J. Allen, Carla J. Abbott and Matthew A. Petoe

Introduction

Despite medical interventions being available for some forms of low vision, such as cataracts or uncorrected refractive error, there remains a significant proportion of vision loss that currently has no cure. As such, research programmes are investigating a number of avenues to develop novel treatment options, including pharmaceuticals, cell-based therapies, gene therapies and medical devices. This chapter provides an update on two current medical device options for low vision: vision prostheses (also known as "bionic eyes") and sensory substitution devices.

Vision prostheses (bionic eyes)

Background

Vision prostheses, or bionic eyes, are implantable devices that use electrical currents to stimulate the residual healthy components of a damaged visual pathway. The technology is analogous to cochlear implants, which use electrical stimulation of the cochlea in the hearing impaired, and have now restored hearing to over 325,000 people worldwide. However, as the eye is anatomically more complex than the ear, the technological challenges are significant in the quest to develop a high-resolution vision prosthesis.

To understand how a vision prosthesis works, it is beneficial to review how natural human vision works. In a healthy eye, light is transmitted through the clear cornea at the front, focused through the intraocular crystalline lens, and then directed on to the retina, which lines the back of the eye. The photoreceptor cells (which are located at the posterior retinal layers) translate the light energy to electrical signals, which pass back through the neural pathways in the retina and are transmitted via the optic nerve back to the brain (via the lateral geniculate nucleus). Final processing of the signal occurs in the visual cortex, which results in a complex image with colour, spatial, temporal, edge and motion information.

A vision prosthesis replaces part of this visual pathway, which has become damaged due to disease or trauma. Prostheses can either use electrodes or photodiodes, which utilise electrical current and light energy respectively, for neural stimulation. Most electronic vision prostheses, such as the Argus II epiretinal implant, have a similar overall design; a video camera captures the visual scene, which is then converted to electrical signals via an external processing unit. The electrical signals are then transmitted to the implanted electrodes, which stimulate the residual visual pathway to provide artificial vision (Figure 25.1). One of the advantages with a camera–based prosthesis is that it allows manipulation of the image through external vision processing, which can optimise the signals sent to the electrode to highlight particular areas of interest in the environment.

Photovoltaic prostheses such as in the Retina Implant AG Alpha AMS subretinal implant (Stingl et al., 2017), do not require a video camera, as they use the incident light from the visual scene. Other photovoltaic prostheses such as the Pixium subretinal implant (Lorach et al., 2015), use a camera and processing unit near the eye to convert the visual scene into infrared light to operate the photovoltaic implant.

The ideal location of the prosthetic implant varies depends on the cause of vision loss. For example, if the photoreceptors are lost or damaged (as in the hereditary eye disease, retinitis pigmentosa), then the prosthesis could be implanted within the eye to stimulate the inner retinal neurons and produce a visual percept. This is ideal in order to utilise the visual processing power of the inner retina. On the other hand, if the eye itself was non-functional or missing (for example, after trauma), then a prosthesis could be implanted in the lateral geniculate nucleus, or

The bionic eye – how it works

First prototype: wide-view neurostimulator

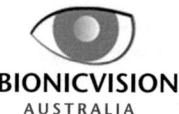

BIONICVISION
AUSTRALIA

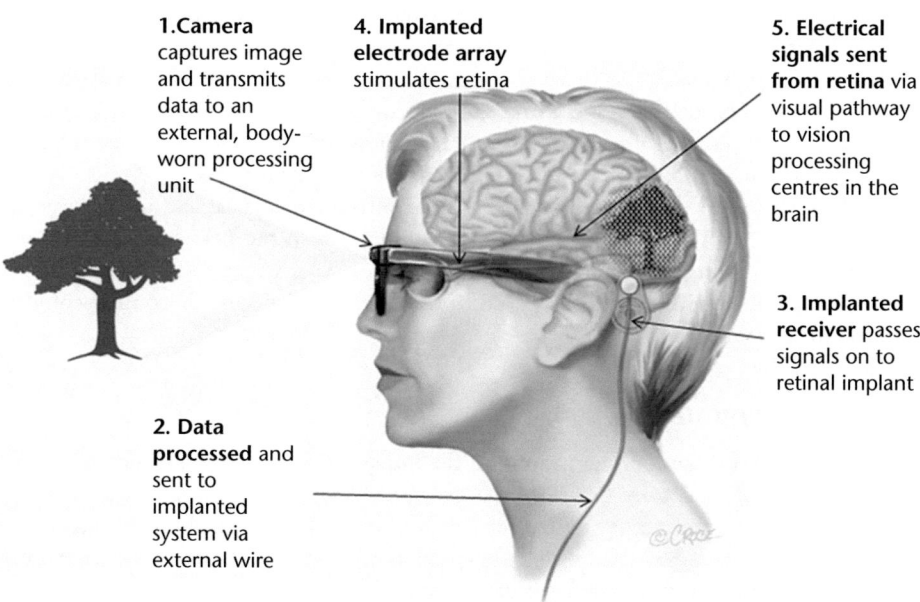

1.Camera captures image and transmits data to an external, body-worn processing unit

4. Implanted electrode array stimulates retina

5. Electrical signals sent from retina via visual pathway to vision processing centres in the brain

3. Implanted receiver passes signals on to retinal implant

2. Data processed and sent to implanted system via external wire

Figure 25.1 General schematic of a camera-based vision prosthesis system.

Source: Image courtesy of Bionic Vision Australia.

directly into the visual cortex. These are technically more challenging and none are currently commercially available. It is important to note that the neural stimulation from visual prostheses is markedly different from normal neural signalling because the electrodes or photodiodes, being relatively large, are non-specific in the cell types they stimulate. For this reason, prosthetic vision is very different to natural vision and significant post-implant visual rehabilitation is required.

History

Preliminary investigations into the use of cortical stimulation for vision restoration has been attributed to the German ophthalmologist Carl Foerster, who showed that direct application of current to the visual cortex enabled a blind patient to see spots of light, and that the light moved when different parts of the cortex were stimulated (Foerster, 1929). Krause and Schum (1931) then showed that it was possible to generate visual phosphenes through cortical stimulation in a man who had been blind for eight years (following a gunshot injury), confirming that it was possible to restore visual percepts even after a period of vision loss.

Several decades later, Brindley and Dobelle investigated the use of cortically implanted electronics to produce phosphenes (Brindley and Lewin, 1968; Dobelle et al., 1976). The work of Dobelle, in particular, continued for another 20 years (Dobelle, 2000). However, these early devices had poor resolution, implemented basic technology (due to the limitations of the era) and often resulted in serious adverse events, both medical (Margalit et al., 2002) and psychological (Lane, 2012). Advances in technology and clinical trial protocols since this time have led to improved outcomes, which will be discussed further in this chapter.

The first investigations into retinal prostheses began in the 1950s, with an Australian engineer named Graham Tassicker patenting a photosensitive array that could be implanted either within or behind the retinal layers (Tassicker, 1956). However, it was a number of decades before larger-scale clinical trials commenced, with the work of Alan and Vincent Chow (Optobionics) and Mark Humayun, Jim Weiland and Robert Greenberg (Second Sight). The success of this work led to approximately 20 groups worldwide developing their own retinal prostheses. A smaller number of groups have also worked to develop optic nerve and lateral geniculate nucleus devices. Although cortical prostheses were the first type of prostheses to be tested in humans, currently only retinal prostheses have developed to the standard required for regulatory approval.

To date, there have been human clinical trials of retinal, cortical and optic nerve devices, all which have shown the ability to restore basic visual percepts to people with very low vision (see the section "clinical trials and participant outcomes" later in the chapter for more details).

As of 2018, these clinical trials have led to three retinal prostheses becoming commercially available for patients.

Type of vision prostheses

There are four main anatomical locations for the implantation of a vision prosthesis: intraocular, optic nerve, lateral geniculate nucleus or visual cortex (Figure 25.2). In general, the intraocular locations (within or around the retina) tend to benefit from the retinal processing and residual visual pathway, but are restricted to people who have lost sight from retinal degenerations such as retinitis pigmentosa, choroideremia or macular degeneration. This restricted indication is because retinal implants require a working inner retina and optic nerve, so that the transmission of the electrical signal to the brain is viable. In these outer retinal degenerations, the inner retina and optic nerve are relatively intact (Kim et al., 2002; Santos et al., 1997), although they are disorganised and altered both anatomically and physiologically (Jones et al., 2016).

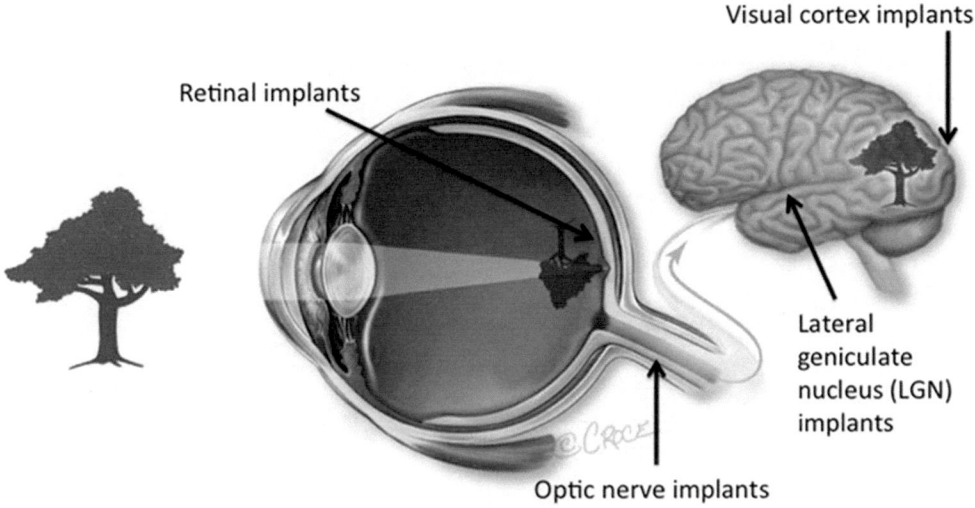

Figure 25.2 Schematic of the human visual pathway, indicating the possible implantation sites for vision prostheses.

Source: Image adapted from Bionic Vision Australia.

On the other hand, cortical implants have increased surgical complexity, but are intended to be used by people with a much broader range of vision loss conditions. As the electrodes are implanted directly within the lateral geniculate nucleus (Vurro, Crowell and Pezaris, 2014) or the cortex (Kane et al., 2013), they do not require a retina or optic nerve to function, and hence could be a treatment option for people with conditions such as glaucoma, traumatic injury and diabetic retinopathy (Lewis et al., 2016). However, it is presumed that interpretation of prosthetic vision requires a developed visual cortex (Beyeler et al., 2017), and therefore congenital blindness has not yet been considered as a suitable indication for any implantable vision prosthesis.

Within intraocular prostheses, there are four further subtypes of implant (Figure 25.3):

(a) *Epiretinal*: on the anterior surface of the retina.
(b) *Subretinal*: below the retina, above the vascular blood supply (the choroid).
(c) *Suprachoroidal*: below the choroid, next to the white outer layer of the eye (the sclera).
(d) *Intrascleral*: within the sclera.

Again, each retinal location has advantages and disadvantages. Generally, it is thought that devices closer to the anterior surface of the retina (i.e. epiretinal and subretinal implants) will be more proximal to target cells and therefore require less energy to cause a visual sensation, and also generate smaller percepts that should help with resolution. The three regulatory approved devices are all in these locations; two in the epiretinal space (da Cruz et al., 2016; Velikay-Parel et al., 2013), and one subretinal (Stingl et al., 2015).

The more posterior locations (suprachoroidal and intrascleral) tend to be easier to access surgically, with less inherent risk of surgical complications to the retina, and provide a more stable "pocket" for implantation. However, they are further away from the neurons that they are attempting to stimulate. More energy is required to cause a visual sensation, and the percepts from neighbouring electrodes have a tendency to overlap (Sinclair et al., 2016). However, it

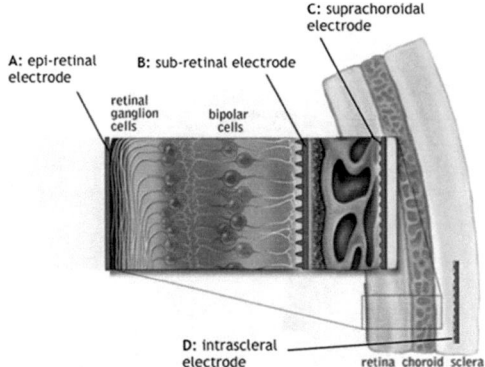

Figure 25.3 Implant locations for retinal implants: (a) epiretinal, (b) subretinal, (c) suprachoroidal and (d) intrascleral.

Source: Image adapted from Bionic Vision Australia.

has been shown that both suprachoroidal (Ayton et al., 2014) and intrascleral (Fujikado et al., 2016) implants can provide useful visual phosphenes to recipients, within safe stimulation limits.

Clinical trials and participant outcomes

It is important to note that the visual sensations produced by current prosthetic implants are not like normal human vision. The devices produce "phosphenes", which are spots of light in the visual field. These spots are generally white, but may have colour characteristics, and can have various spatial and temporal properties (Sinclair et al., 2016). The aim of a vision prosthesis is to use these spots to map out the visual scene, to allow people to identify objects and navigate. A simulated representation of phosphene vision is shown in Figure 25.4 but in reality the images

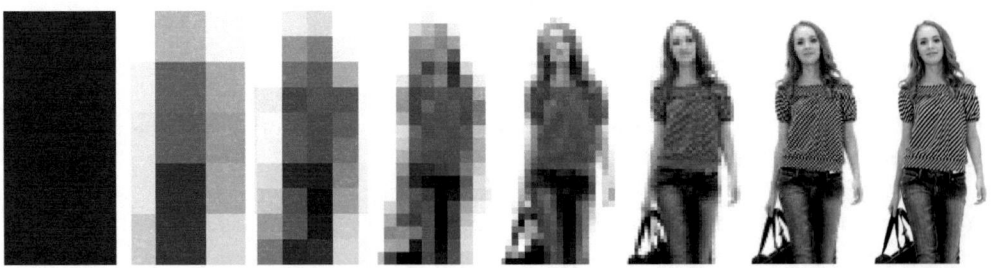

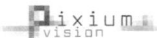

Figure 25.4 A simulated representation of phosphene vision.

Source: Image courtesy of Pixium Vision SA, France.

Table 25.1 Summary of the modern vision prosthesis clinical trials, from 2000 (in alphabetical order).

Name of company/ research group	Name of device	Implant location	Number of electrodes	Summary of results	References
Bionic Vision Australia, Australia	24-channel percutaneous connector device	Suprachoroidal	20	Phase I clinical trial in three participants showed improvements in grating visual acuity and functional vision over a two-year study period. No retinal damage	(Ayton et al., 2014; Petoe et al., 2017)
EpiRET GmbH, Germany	EPI-RET3	Epiretinal	25	Devices were implanted for four weeks, and allowed participants to perceive phosphenes, but there was significant variability in thresholds. Removal was possible in all cases. Five years later, five participants were reviewed; all showed retinal gliosis at the site of tack implantation, but no other damage to the retina	(Menzel-Severing et al., 2012; Roessler et al., 2009; Schimitzek, Roessler and Walter, 2016)
Intelligent Medical Implants AG, Germany	Learning retinal implant	Epiretinal	50	Technology has been licensed by the Pixium Vision SA group, and is currently undergoing clinical testing	(Eckmiller, 1997; Hornig et al., 2007)
Optobionics, USA	Artificial silicon retina (ASR)	Subretinal	5000 photodiodes	Phase II clinical trials showed that incident light was not sufficient for reliable device activation. However, improvements in retinal function away from the implant were noted, suggesting a possible neuroprotective effect	(Chow et al., 2010; Chow et al., 2004)
Osaka University, Japan	Suprachoroidal-transretinal stimulation (STS)	Intrascleral	49	Improvements in both lab-based vision function tests and mobility assessments	(Fujikado et al., 2016; Fujikado et al., 2011)

(continued)

Table 25.1 (continued)

Name of company/ research group	Name of device	Implant location	Number of electrodes	Summary of results	References
Pixium Vision SA	IRIS	Epiretinal	150	Was commercially available (CE mark approval), but has been discontinued as Pixium will commence clinical trials of a new, more advanced, PRIMA subretinal device in 2018	(Kitiratschky et al., 2015; Stingl et al., 2013; Stingl et al., 2015)
Retina Implant AG	Alpha IMS	Subretinal	1500 photodiodes	Was commercially available (CE mark approval), but has been replaced by the second-generation Alpha AMS (below)	(Kitiratschky et al., 2015; Stingl et al., 2013; Stingl et al., 2015)
Retina Implant AG	Alpha AMS	Subretinal	1600 photodiodes	Now commercially available (CE mark approval)	(Edwards et al., 2017; Stingl et al., 2017; Zrenner et al., 2017)
Second Sight Medical Products, USA	Argus I	Epiretinal	16	Improvements in object detection and motion detection. These promising results led to the development of the second-generation Argus II device (60 electrodes), which is now regulatory approved	(Humayun et al., 2003; Weiland et al., 2004)
Second Sight Medical Products, USA	Argus II	Epiretinal	60	Now commercially available (both FDA and CE mark approval)	(da Cruz et al., 2016; Dagnelie et al., 2017; Duncan et al., 2017)
Université Cathlolique de Louvain, Belgium	Optic nerve visual prosthesis (ONVP)	Optic nerve cuff	4 or 8	Recipients were able to localise and discriminate basic objects and had basic pattern recognition ability	(Brelen et al., 2005; Duret et al., 2006; Veraart et al., 2003)

are dynamic and are affected by factors such as phosphene fading (Stingl et al., 2013) and variations in phosphene appearance (Sinclair et al., 2016).

At present, devices are only capable of providing a relatively low number of phosphenes, which means the outcomes are restricted to gross visual abilities, such as obstacle avoidance, navigation and recognition of large objects. However, the devices tested in clinical trials to date have shown that these performance indicators are possible in the majority of recipients (Ayton et al., 2014; da Cruz et al., 2016; Fujikado et al., 2016; Stingl et al., 2013).

The regulatory approved devices are detailed below (see the section entitled "commercially available technologies"). In addition to these three implants, a number of clinical trials have been completed since the early work of Dobelle and Brindley. A summary of these modern-era implant trials is provided in Table 25.1 While outside the scope of this chapter, full clinical results of these trials can be obtained from the references provided within the table. A semi-regularly updated list of developments in electronic visual prosthetics is also available at www.eye-tuebingen.de/zrenner/retimplantlist.

Another important aspect of these trials, which is relevant to any medical intervention, is the appropriate screening and management of participant mental health and emotional well-being (Lane et al., 2016). It is vital that participants understand the current early nature of the devices, and have realistic expectations about the potential outcomes. As such, the majority of research groups and companies work closely with psychologists, psychiatrists and other low vision trained personnel to ensure that this is achieved.

Testing of participant outcomes in vision prosthesis clinical trials can be challenging, due to the very low vision of participants at baseline and the complex nature of functional vision. Hence an international consensus was developed to try to gain consistency in testing and reporting methods (Rizzo and Ayton, 2014). The Harmonisation of Outcomes and Vision Endpoints in Vision Restoration Trials (HOVER) Taskforce will shortly publish guidelines for the field, which will be available at www.artificialvision.org. These guidelines also provide easy access to a number of low vision tests that have been developed specifically for the assessment of vision prostheses, such as the Basic Assessment of Light and Motion, BaLM (Bach et al., 2010), the Functional Low-Vision Observer Rated Assessment, FLORA (Geruschat et al., 2015) and the Low Vision Assessment of Daily Activities, LoVADA (Finger et al., 2014). As is evident from these tools, the assessment of activities of daily living and orientation and mobility are key in vision prosthesis trials, and provide a broad overview of the utility of the device for recipients' everyday lives.

Commercially available technologies

The field has now progressed to the stage where three retinal prostheses have been approved by the regulatory authorities for commercial sale (see Figure 25.5):

1 *The Argus II epiretinal implant*, by Second Sight Medical Products USA, has both FDA and CE mark approval (da Cruz et al., 2016). The device consists of 60 platinum microelectrodes on a silicone-based epiretinal array that is held in place with an epiretinal tack. This device has had the greatest number of implanted participants, with over 100 recipients to date and over five years of data on the original 30 clinical trial recipients (da Cruz et al., 2016; Ghodasra et al., 2016). In addition, Second Sight has published data on the long-term safety and stability data of their first-generation device, the Argus I, which has been implanted in some participants for over ten years (Yue et al., 2015). Second Sight is now developing a cortical implant (the Orion), and conducting clinical trials with participants with age-related macular degeneration (Stanga et al., 2017).

2   *The Alpha AMS subretinal implant*, by Retina Implant AG Germany, has CE mark approval (Stingl et al., 2017). The device has 1,600 micro-photodiodes, and hence does not require an external video or image processing unit and also benefits from utilising the natural eye movements of the recipient (Hafed et al., 2016). The original Alpha IMS showed significant improvements in visual function (Stingl et al., 2015) and a clinically acceptable safety profile (Kitiratschky et al., 2015), but had poor longevity. The second-generation Alpha AMS has improved materials and design and has been predicted from laboratory aging tests to have a median lifetime of 4.7 years, compared with the clinical median lifetime of the Alpha IMS at 0.6 years (Daschner et al., 2017).

3   *The IRIS II epiretinal implant*, by Pixium Vision SA France, has CE mark approval (Keseru et al., 2012), and is a 150-electrode photovoltaic epiretinal implant. A clinical trial of the IRIS II is currently underway and an improvement in functional vision at six months has been reported in most participants (Muqit et al., 2017). Pixium are now working towards a clinical trial of a subretinal implant, the PRIMA, which is being developed in conjunction with Stanford University (Lorach et al., 2015).

Future potentials

Significant work is currently underway into the advanced technology and stimulation strategies required to make a high-resolution vision prosthesis. While the currently available devices have been shown to improve the quality of life and functional outcomes for recipients, they are not yet at the level that would allow people to read small text, drive or recognise faces. It is expected that such a device would require at least 1,000 electrodes (Cha, Horch and Normann, 1992; Dagnelie, 2008). The challenges for this include fabrication limitations, the fact that smaller electrodes require higher levels of electrical input (as they have higher impedances) and also evidence from implanted subjects that the phosphenes that they perceive tend to overlap (Sinclair et al., 2016), so 1,000 electrodes will probably not provide 1,000 individual phosphenes.

It will also require more than simply increasing the number of electrodes to provide high-resolution vision. Vision processing algorithms, which can enhance and optimise the translation of video image to electrical stimulation (Barnes et al., 2016), will likely become more and more important as the technology improves. These algorithms are designed to utilise certain features of the visual scene, such as depth cues (McCarthy et al., 2015), face recognition (Irons et al., 2017) and text optimisation (Wang, Li and Barnes, 2012). Additionally, current steering (Dumm et al., 2014) and current focusing (Jepson et al., 2014) techniques may also be important in producing phosphenes with less overlap.

Another exciting future potential for vision prostheses is their use for neuroprotection. As mentioned in Table 25.1, early subretinal prosthesis trials with the Optobionics ASR device discovered that peripheral areas of retina, which were not directly stimulated by the device, showed improvement in function during the trial (Chow et al., 2004). Further work investigated the neuroprotective effects of subretinal devices (Pardue et al., 2006; Pardue et al., 2005), which has also been noted in cochlear implants (Pettingill et al., 2007; Wise et al., 2011). Research is now underway to investigate whether electrical stimulation of the eye at earlier disease stages can be beneficial in slowing down the progression of degeneration (Schatz et al., 2017), and is commercially available in the OkuStim device by Retina Implant AG.

Currently, vision prostheses have only been tested in subjects who were born with their sight, and lost it later in life. This is to ensure that some visual pathway development occurred prior to the loss of sight. However, there is interest in the field as to whether this is essential, or whether a prosthesis may be able to be implanted in a congenitally blind person. It is possible

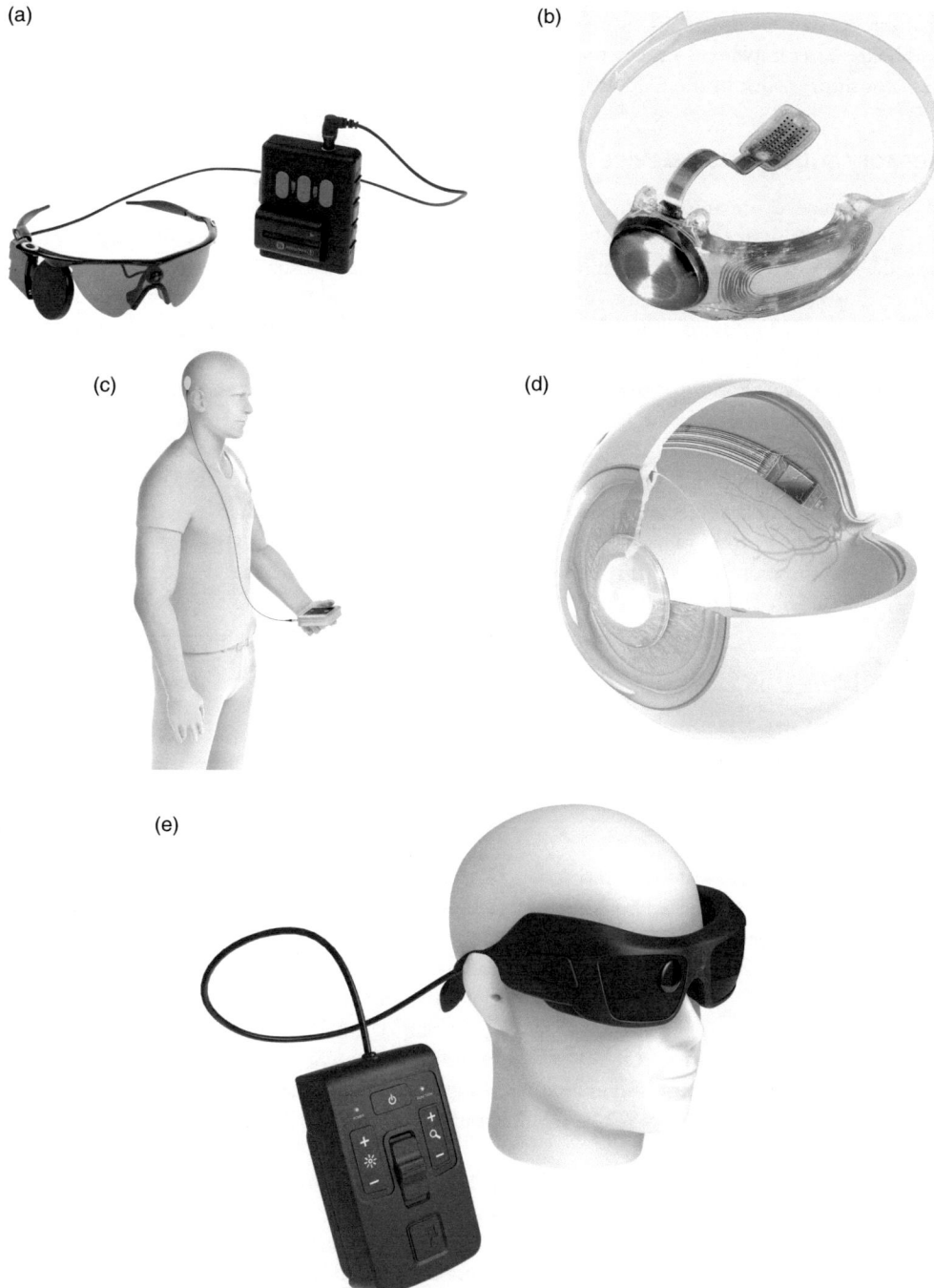

Figure 25.5 Images of the Second Sight Argus II epiretinal device (a and b), Retina Implant AG Alpha AMS subretinal device and (c and d) and the Pixium Vision IRIS epiretinal device (e). Each panel shows both the external components (glasses and external controller) and the intraocular prosthesis.

Source: Images courtesy of the manufacturing companies.

that this may be advantageous, as neuroplasticity is highest in early childhood (Dagnelie, 2008), and hence early implantation may provide better adaptation for the recipient. This will form the basis for future work in the field of vision prostheses.

Sensory substitution devices

While bionic eyes are an exciting prospect, there are many individuals who will not be suitable for, or may not wish to have, an electronic implant for vision improvement. Sensory substitution devices offer a non-surgical approach that may enhance "visual" potential for people, by converting visual information into another sensory domain (e.g. sound). They can be suitable for people with profound vision loss, and also for those with residual sight, as an additional sensory input.

The most well-known example of sensory substitution is braille, which translates visual information into tactile output. Braille has been widely used since its invention in 1821 by Louis Braille (Braille, 1839), but is now becoming superseded by more advanced technological solutions. The sensory substitution field advanced significantly with Paul Bach-Y-Rita's pioneering work with blind subjects utilising a vision substitution system (Bach-y-Rita et al., 1969), signifying the beginning of viable low vision technologies employing sensory substitution. An overview of some of the resulting technologies in this field follows, but is not exhaustive as new interventions and devices are being developed at a rapid rate.

Vision-to-auditory sensory substitution devices

These devices translate a visual input (either from a camera or through a computer system) into an audible output. Examples are detailed below.

Screen readers

Probably one of the most common forms of sensory substitution used today, screen readers are able to convert text on a visual display (such as a computer or smartphone), and read it out audibly to the user. A popular choice, for Microsoft Windows™ computers, is JAWS ("Job Access With Speech", Freedom Scientific, Florida, USA). The JAWS program provides synthesised text-to-speech of text, menus and dialog boxes, and implements keyboard shortcuts with spoken feedback. The software is actively developed, with recent new features supporting optical character recognition (OCR) of text within pictures (e.g. from a flatbed scanner, or the manufacturer's own PEARL® document reading camera). A free, open-source, alternative is NonVisual Desktop Access (NVDA), manufactured by the Australian charitable institution, NV Access (Queensland, Australia).

The Macintosh and iOS (iPhone, iPod, iPad) operating systems include a built-in screen reader called VoiceOver (Apple Inc., Cupertino, CA, USA). The capabilities are more ubiquitous than the JAWS program, as the software is deeply embedded into the operating system. For example, VoiceOver not only accepts keyboard shortcuts, but also includes support for finger gestural control via the trackpad or iPhone touchscreen. Screen readers are also present in modern web-based applications, such as social media platforms. Facebook (Menlo Park, CA, USA) includes the Navigation Assistant to provide audible menus for navigating Facebook. Additionally, Facebook has launched the Automatic Alternative Text tool that uses object recognition technology to generate descriptions of photos on Facebook. Arising from a recognised need for blind people to interact with visual content on social media (Voykinska et al., 2016), the system has been trained on the many millions of photos that Facebook has on its servers, and can provide text descriptions such as "image may contain three people, smiling, outdoors".

Video-camera readers

The PEARL® document reading camera (Freedom Scientific, Florida, USA) is an example of a desktop system that can capture a photograph of text, perform optical-character recognition (OCR), and read aloud the text content to the user via text-to-speech voice synthesis. The camera is mounted on a stand, pointing downwards at a book. This enables low vision users the ability to "read" printed material without necessitating an audiobook version.

The same OCR technology has now become portable, with the introduction in 2014 of the Eye-Pal Ace (Freedom Scientific, Florida, USA) video magnifier. This device (Figure 25.6) is a hand-held digital camera that can take a detailed photo of a page of a book, enlarge the text and present it on the 10-inch LCD screen. If the user presses the appropriate button, the device will read the text aloud. According to the manufacturer, the Eye-Pal Ace can assist with everyday text reading, such as restaurant menus, forms and even the fine text of medicine bottle labels. The user has the option of connecting a braille display via USB, allowing automatic conversion of text to braille.

OCR systems are continually improving and miniaturising; an example being the ultra-portable OrCam MyEye (OrCam Technologies Ltd, Jerusalem, Israel). Version 1 of this system

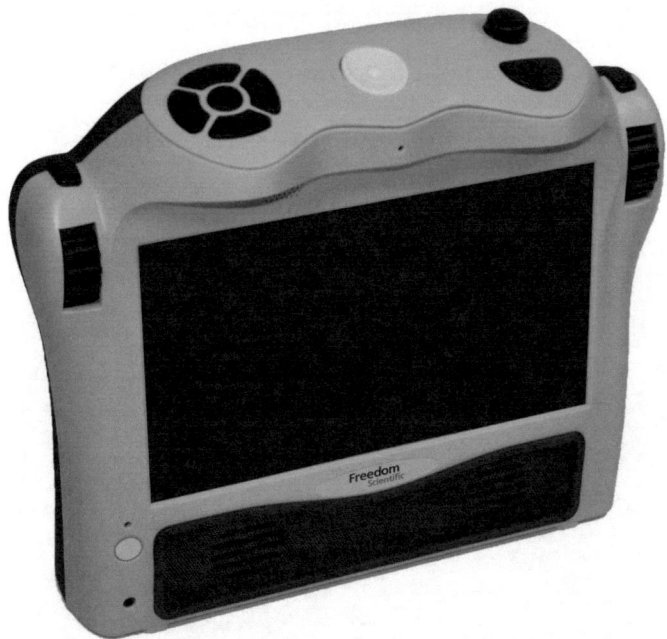

Figure 25.6   The Eye-Pal Ace portable OCR device.

Source: Freedom Scientific, Inc. www.freedomscientific.com/content/Documents/Manuals/Eye-Pal/Eye-Pal-Ace-User-Guide.pdf.

consists of a discrete video camera worn on the side of glasses, a bone conduction earpiece and a pocket processor). The system can detect the action of finger-pointing to initiate text-to-speech reading of a pointed target, or can be configured to automatically speak whenever text is detected. Importantly, the device can be programmed to recognise people's faces, pre-trained objects and identify the value written on bank notes, in a response time significantly faster than would usually be possible for people with low vision (Moisseiev and Mannis, 2016). An updated version of this device, the MyEye 2.0 (see www.orcam.com/en/myeye2) was released in late 2017 and further miniaturises the device to incorporate the former pocket processor into the glasses frame.

Seeing with sound

Aside from the specific application of text-to-speech, auditory information can also be used to describe the visual scene more holistically. In visual-to-auditory prostheses, such as the vOICe (Meijer, 1992) (Figure 25.7) users are trained to "see with sound". Sounding similar to sonar, images from a glasses-mounted camera are converted into a "soundscape", with a consistent mapping between visual location and auditory information. The stereo soundscape is heard moving from left ear to right ear, with high- and low-pitched sounds indicating the presence of an object in the upper or lower visual field respectively. The soundscape is detailed enough to convey localisation information, with users reporting an ability to navigate, recognise and locate objects, and perform standardised acuity assessments with an upper performance limit of around 20/400 (Haigh et al., 2013; Levy-Tzedek, Riemer and Amedi, 2014). Similar to studies of human echolocation (Kolarik et al., 2014), visual-to-auditory devices can result in an "acquired synaesthesia" – causing activation of the relevant visual areas while using the device (Ward and Meijer, 2010).

Two other examples of visual-to-auditory devices are EyeMusic (Abboud et al., 2014) and the lesser-known Synaestheatre (Hamilton-Fletcher et al., 2016). EyeMusic is a re-imagining of the vOICe system, but using sounds of orchestral instruments to encode the visual image. Piano and marimba sounds, among others, sonify the 24 x 40 pixel image, with one musical

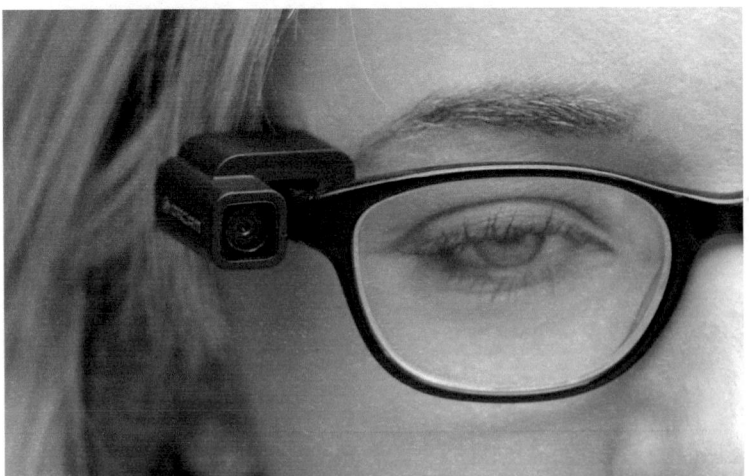

Figure 25.7   The vOICe system.

Source: www.seeingwithsound.com.

timbre assigned to each colour in the image. Studies comparing healthy vision to blindfolded healthy participants using EyeMusic reported no significant difference between vision and the blindfolded EyeMusic trials in participants' movement time, peak speed and path length, indicating that EyeMusic's encoding could inform participants' motor movements (Levy-Tzedek et al., 2012). The average error when using EyeMusic to touch each target was less than 0.5 cm (poorer than with natural vision, but unlikely to be clinically significant).

In order to provide spatial resolution through stereo sound, both the vOICe system and EyeMusic must compromise on temporal resolution and immediacy of information (Hamilton-Fletcher et al., 2016). Therefore, the last example in this section is Synaestheatre (Hamilton-Fletcher et al., 2016), which was conceived to prioritise temporal resolution over spatial resolution. The Synaestheatre algorithm represents the visual field as a grid of independent sound oscillations, each having a different frequency and panning location in the stereo soundscape. When an object is sensed in the camera image, the pitch and stereo location of the sound oscillations will indicate the objects location, distance and direction of travel. A user-experience study of ten blind and visually impaired participants reported that this system provided an instantly intuitive perception of spatial information, but was lacking in an ability to represent shape and object outlines (Hamilton-Fletcher et al., 2016).

Vision-to-tactile sensory substitution devices

These devices take the visual input from a camera and translate it into a tactile display. Devices have been trialled on various body parts, but Paul Bach-Y-Rita and colleagues identified that the tongue was a well-suited location due to its sensitivity and spatial discrimination (Bach-y-Rita et al., 1998). The obvious disadvantage is that when the device is being implemented, the user is not able to speak, eat or drink.

BrainPort 1000

The BrainPort 1000 device (Wicab Inc., WI, USA), consists of a glasses-mounted camera, which converts visual images to electrical signals that stimulate a 400-electro-tactile array placed on the tongue (Nau, Pintar et al., 2015). The electrodes are made from stainless steel, and are spaced 558 μm apart from edge to edge (Grant et al., 2016). When activated, the electrodes stimulate touch receptors on the tongue, which is felt as vibrations or "tingling sensations akin to champagne bubbles" (Grant et al., 2016). There is a one-to-one spatial correspondence between the pixels in the image and the stimulated electrodes, and luminance is translated into the intensity of stimulation.

The device has been trialled extensively, especially in returned servicemen and women who have lost their sight from trauma in war zones. The device can produce form vision perception, allowing users to identify letters or numbers, or avoid obstacles when navigating (Grant et al., 2016; Stronks et al., 2016). Of particular interest is the fact that when the device is being used, the visual cortex is activated, providing further evidence for neuroplasticity within the visual system (Lee et al., 2014; Nau, Murphy and Chan, 2015).

An advantage with the system over an implanted artificial vision device (such as a vision prosthesis) is that there have been no device-related serious adverse events reported (Grant et al., 2016). Some recipients have reported a tingling sensation in the mouth, or a metallic taste, but these were mild and quickly resolved (Stronks et al., 2016).

The BrainPort V100 system was granted CE mark approval in 2013, and FDA approval for sale in the USA in 2015. Wicab Inc., is currently in the process of applying for regulatory approval for the next-generation device, the BrainPort V200.

Vibrotactile systems

Aside from encoding the visual scene, some sensory substitution devices are directed specifically towards mobility and navigation. Safe navigation through a crowded environment can be achieved with the use of multiple vibrotacile motors worn on a belt (Johnson and Higgins, 2006), back-worn grid (Stronks et al., 2017), or hand-held device (Maidenbaum et al., 2014). These systems elicit a tactile sensation at specific points on the body to convey the location of a potential obstacle hazard, allowing the user to safely navigate around it. The hand-held EyeCane system uses multiple narrow-beam sensors to simultaneously enable both detection of near-ground-level obstacles and waist-level obstacles several metres ahead (Maidenbaum et al., 2014). Similar vibrotactile systems have been shown to improve tabletop reaching-and-grabbing tasks when the sensing nodes are worn on the user's wrists, as in the Wearable Virtual Cane Network (Gao et al., 2015). Lastly, the vibration can be used as a positive instruction – if the system connects to a mobile phone via Bluetooth, GPS and terrain information can be conveyed as directional vibrations (Elliott et al., 2010).

Vision augmentation

Last in this section are the Royal National Institute of Blind People (UK) RNIB Smart Glasses (www.rnib.org.uk/knowledge-and-research-hub-research-reports/technology-and-television-research/smartglasses), which provide visual augmentation to people with some remaining sight. Rather than substituting vision for another sense, the RNIB Smart Glasses convert the visual scene into a high-contrast representation. The distance from the wearer to nearby objects is represented by increasing levels of brightness, determined by a special depth-sensing camera (Hicks et al., 2013).

A series of studies using the RNIB Smart Glasses was conducted by RNIB throughout 2015–2016 and reported a measurable benefit for some (21%) of the 221 visually impaired participants (retinal degeneration, glaucoma, cataract and optic nerve damage) taking part in supervised testing of object identification and obstacle avoidance (Alexander et al., 2016). Although promising, the usability study concluded that further work is required to make the glasses more comfortable and intuitive for daily use (Alexander et al., 2016).

Conclusion

The devices discussed in this chapter can be broadly considered "artificial vision" systems. While they do not replace normal human vision, they provide other visual, auditory or tactile cues to improve function in daily life in people with ultra and very low vision. It is clear that while progress in these fields has been rapid, and outcomes promising, there is still work to be done.

The technologies are still in their relative infancy, and large improvements in design and manufacture are likely in the years to come. Over 20 research teams are currently working on a number of new vision prosthesis devices, for all locations (cortical, lateral geniculate nucleus, optic nerve and retina). It is likely that different device designs will be suited to people who have lost vision from different causes, and so this diversity in development is essential at this time.

One of the most important aspects to the field of artificial vision is the multi-disciplinary nature of the research teams (Ayton et al., 2013). To design, manufacture, test and implant these devices, a team of scientists and clinicians from many fields is required, including engineers, surgeons, low vision rehabilitation experts, ophthalmologists and optometrists, material scientists and computer vision specialists. This diversity has led to the invention of numerous novel interventions and methodologies to date, and will continue to produce benefits to the community in the future.

References

Abboud, S., Hanassy, S., Levy-Tzedek, S., Maidenbaum, S. and Amedi, A. 2014. Eyemusic: Introducing a "visual" colorful experience for the blind using auditory sensory substitution. *Restorative Neurology and Neuroscience*, 32(2), 247–257.

Alexander, T., Arthur, J., Chandrakanthan, R., Croxford, S. and Di Bon Conyers, L. 2016. *Smart Glasses final report*. Peterborough, UK: Royal National Institute of Blind People (UK).

Ayton, L.N., Blamey, P.J., Guymer, R.H., Luu, C.D., Nayagam, D.A., Sinclair, N.C., Shivdasani, M.N., Yeoh, J., Mccombe, M.F., Briggs, R.J., Opie, N.L., Villalobos, J., Dimitrov, P.N., Varsamidis, M., Petoe, M.A., Mccarthy, C.D., Walker, J.G., Barnes, N., Burkitt, A.N., Williams, C.E., Shepherd, R.K., Allen, P.J. and Bionic Vision Australia Research. 2014. First-in-human trial of a novel suprachoroidal retinal prosthesis. *PLoS One*, 9(12), e115239.

Ayton, L.N., Luu, C.D., Allen, P.J. and Guymer, R.H. 2013. The importance of multi-disciplinary collaborations in the future of bionic vision. *Expert Review of Ophthalmology*, 8(1), 9–11.

Bach-Y-Rita, P., Collins, C.C., Saunders, F.A., White, B. and Scadden, L. (1969). Vision substitution by tactile image projection. *Nature*, 221(5184), 963–964.

Bach-Y-Rita, P., Kaczmarek, K.A., Tyler, M.E. and Garcia-Lara, J. 1998. Form perception with a 49-point electrotactile stimulus array on the tongue: A technical note. *Journal of Rehabilitation Research & Development*, 35(4), 427–430.

Bach, M., Wilke, M., Wilhelm, B., Zrenner, E. and Wilke, R. 2010. Basic quantitative assessment of visual performance in patients with very low vision. *Investigative Ophthalmology and Vision Science*, 51(2), 1255–1260.

Barnes, N., Scott, A.F., Lieby, P., Petoe, M.A., Mccarthy, C., Stacey, A., Ayton, L. N., Sinclair, N.C., Shivdasani, M.N., Lovell, N.H., Mcdermott, H.J. and Walker, J.G. 2016. Vision function testing for a suprachoroidal retinal prosthesis: Effects of image filtering. *Journal of Neural Engineering*, 13(3), 036013.

Beyeler, M., Rokem, A., Boynton, G.M. and Fine, I. 2017. Learning to see again: Biological constraints on cortical plasticity and the implications for sight restoration technologies. *Journal of Neural Engineering*, 14(5), 051003.

Braille, L. 1839. *New method for representing by dots the form of letters, maps, geometric figures, musical symbols, etc., for use by the blind*. Paris, France: Institution royale des jeunes aveugles.

Brelen, M.E., Duret, F., Gerard, B., Delbeke, J. and Veraart, C. 2005. Creating a meaningful visual perception in blind volunteers by optic nerve stimulation. *Journal of Neural Engineering*, 2(1), S22–S228.

Brindley, G.S. and Lewin, W.S. 1968. The sensations produced by electrical stimulation of the visual cortex. *Journal of Physiology*, 196(2), 479–493.

Cha, K., Horch, K. and Normann, R.A. 1992. Simulation of a phosphene-based visual field: Visual acuity in a pixelized vision system. *Annals of Biomedical Engineering*, 20(4), 439–449.

Chow, A.Y., Bittner, A.K. and Pardue, M.T. 2010. The artificial silicon retina in retinitis pigmentosa patients (an American Ophthalmological Association Thesis). *Transactions of the American Ophthalmoogical Society*, 108, 120–154.

Chow, A.Y., Chow, V.Y., Packo, K.H., Pollack, J.S., Peyman, G.A. and Schuchard, R. 2004. The artificial silicon retina microchip for the treatment of vision loss from retinitis pigmentosa. *Archives of Ophthalmology*, 122(4), 460–469.

Da Cruz, L., Dorn, J.D., Humayun, M.S., Dagnelie, G., Handa, J., Barale, P.O., Sahel, J.A., Stanga, P.E., Hafezi, F., Safran, A.B., Salzmann, J., Santos, A., Birch, D., Spencer, R., Cideciyan, A.V., De Juan, E., Duncan, J.L., Eliott, D., Fawzi, A., Olmos De Koo, L.C., Ho, A.C., Brown, G., Haller, J., Regillo, C., Del Priore, L.V., Arditi, A., Greenberg, R.J. and Argus, I.I.S.G. 2016. Five-year safety and performance results from the Argus II retinal prosthesis system clinical trial. *Ophthalmology*, 123(10), 2248–2254.

Dagnelie, G. 2008. Psychophysical evaluation for visual prosthesis. *Annual Review of Biomedical Engineering*, 339–368.

Dagnelie, G., Christopher, P., Arditi, A., Da Cruz, L., Duncan, J.L., Ho, A.C., Olmos De Koo, L.C., Sahel, J.A., Stanga, P.E., Thumann, G., Wang, Y., Arsiero, M., Dorn, J.D., Greenberg, R.J. and Argus, I.I.S.G. 2017. Performance of real-world functional vision tasks by blind subjects improves after implantation with the Argus$^{(R)}$ II retinal prosthesis system. *Clinical and Experimental Ophthalmology*, 45(2), 152–159.

Daschner, R., Greppmaier, U., Kokelmann, M., Rudorf, S., Rudorf, R., Schleehauf, S. and Wrobel, W.G. 2017. Laboratory and clinical reliability of conformally coated subretinal implants. *Biomedical Microdevices*, 19(1), 7.

Dobelle, W.H. 2000. Artificial vision for the blind by connecting a television camera to the visual cortex. *ASAIO Journal*, 46(1), 3–9.

Dobelle, W.H., Mladejovsky, M.G., Evans, J.R., Roberts, T.S. and Girvin, J.P. 1976. "Braille" reading by a blind volunteer by visual cortex stimulation. *Nature*, 259 (5539), 111–112.

Dumm, G., Fallon, J.B., Williams, C.E. and Shivdasani, M.N. 2014. Virtual electrodes by current steering in retinal prostheses. *Investigative Ophthalmology and Vision Science*, 55(12), 8077–8085.

Duncan, J.L., Richards, T.P., Arditi, A., Da Cruz, L., Dagnelie, G., Dorn, J.D., Ho, A.C., Olmos De Koo, L.C., Barale, P.O., Stanga, P.E., Thumann, G., Wang, Y. and Greenberg, R.J. 2017. Improvements in vision-related quality of life in blind patients implanted with the Argus Ii epiretinal prosthesis. *Clinical and Experimental Optometry*, 100(2), 144–150.

Duret, F., Brelen, M.E., Lambert, V., Gerard, B., Delbeke, J. and Veraart, C. 2006. Object localization, discrimination, and grasping with the optic nerve visual prosthesis. *Restorative Neurology and Neuroscience*, 24(1), 31–40.

Eckmiller, R. 1997. Learning retina implants with epiretinal contacts. *Ophthalmic Research*, 29(5), 281–289.

Edwards, T.L., Cottriall, C.L., Xue, K., Simunovic, M.P., Ramsden, J.D., Zrenner, E. and Maclaren, R.E. 2017. Assessment of the electronic retinal implant alpha ams in restoring vision to blind patients with end-stage retinitis pigmentosa. *Ophthalmology*, 125(3), 432–443.

Elliott, L.R., Erp, J.V., Redden, E.S. and Duistermaat, M. 2010. Field-based validation of a tactile navigation device. *IEEE Transactions on Haptics*, 3(2), 78–87.

Finger, R.P., Mcsweeney, S.C., Deverell, L., O'hare, F., Bentley, S.A., Luu, C.D., Guymer, R.H. and Ayton, L.N. 2014. Developing an instrumental activities of daily living tool as part of the low vision assessment of daily activities protocol. *Investigative Ophthalmology and Vision Science*, 55(12), 8458–8466.

Foerster, O. 1929. Contributions to the pathophysiology of the visual pathway and visual sphere. *Journal of Psychology and Neurology*, 39, 435–463.

Fujikado, T., Kamei, M., Sakaguchi, H., Kanda, H., Endo, T., Hirota, M., Morimoto, T., Nishida, K., Kishima, H., Terasawa, Y., Oosawa, K., Ozawa, M. and Nishida, K. 2016. One-year outcome of 49-channel suprachoroidal-transretinal stimulation prosthesis in patients with advanced retinitis pigmentosa. *Investigative Ophthalmology and Vision Science*, 57(14), 6147–6157.

Fujikado, T., Kamei, M., Sakaguchi, H., Kanda, H., Morimoto, T., Ikuno, Y., Nishida, K., Kishima, H., Maruo, T., Konoma, K., Ozawa, M. and Nishida, K. 2011. Testing of semichronically implanted retinal prosthesis by suprachoroidal-transretinal stimulation in patients with retinitis pigmentosa. *Investigative Ophthalmology and Vision Science*, 52(7), 4726–4733.

Gao, Y., Chandrawanshi, R., Nau, A.C. and Tse, Z.T. 2015. Wearable virtual white cane network for navigating people with visual impairment. *Proceedings of the Institute of Mechanical Engineers: Part H*, 229(9), 681–688.

Geruschat, D.R., Flax, M., Tanna, N., Bianchi, M., Fisher, A., Goldschmidt, M., Fisher, L., Dagnelie, G., Deremeik, J., Smith, A., Anaflous, F. and Dorn, J. 2015. Flora: Phase I development of a functional vision assessment for prosthetic vision users. *Clinical and Experimental Optometry*, 98(4), 342–347.

Ghodasra, D.H., Chen, A., Arevalo, J.F., Birch, D.G., Branham, K., Coley, B., Dagnelie, G., De Juan, E., Devenyi, R.G., Dorn, J.D., Fisher, A., Geruschat, D.R., Gregori, N.Z., Greenberg, R.J., Hahn, P., Ho, A.C., Howson, A., Huang, S.S., Iezzi, R., Khan, N., Lam, B.L., Lim, J.I., Locke, K.G., Markowitz, M., Ripley, A. M., Rankin, M., Schimitzek, H., Tripp, F., Weiland, J.D., Yan, J., Zacks, D.N. and Jayasundera, K.T. 2016. Worldwide Argus II implantation: Recommendations to optimize patient outcomes. *BMC Ophthalmology*, 16, 52.

Grant, P., Spencer, L., Arnoldussen, A., Hogle, R., Nau, A., Szlyk, J., Nussdorf, J., Fletcher, D.C., Gordon, K. and Weiple, W. 2016. The functional performance of the Brainport® V100 device in persons who are profoundly blind. *Journal of Visual Impairment and Blindness*, 110(2), 77–88.

Hafed, Z.M., Stingl, K., Bartz-Schmidt, K.U., Gekeler, F. and Zrenner, E. 2016. Oculomotor behavior of blind patients seeing with a subretinal visual implant. *Vision Research*, 118, 119–131.

Haigh, A., Brown, D.J., Meijer, P. and Proulx, M.J. 2013. How well do you see what you hear? The acuity of visual-to-auditory sensory substitution. *Frontiers of Psychology*, 4, 330.

Hamilton-Fletcher, G., Obrist, M., Watten, P., Mengucci, M. and Ward, J. 2016. "I always wanted to see the night sky": Blind user preferences for sensory substitution devices. *Proceedings of the 2016 CHI Conference on Human Factors in Computing Systems* (pp. 2162–2174). San Jose, CA: ACM.

Hicks, S.L., Wilson, I., Muhammed, L., Worsfold, J., Downes, S.M. and Kennard, C. 2013. A depth-based head-mounted visual display to aid navigation in partially sighted individuals. *PLOS ONE*, 8(7), e67695.

Hornig, R., Zehnder, T., Velikay-Parel, M. and Richard, G. 2007. The IMI retinal implant system. In M. Humayun, J. Weiland, G.J. Chader and E. Greenbaum (eds), *Artificial vision: Basic research, biomedical engineering and clinical advances* (pp. 111–128). New York: Springer.

Humayun, M.S., Weiland, J.D., Fujii, G.Y., Greenberg, R., Williamson, R., Little, J., Mech, B., Cimmarusti, V., Van Boemel, G., Dagnelie, G. and De Juan, E. 2003. Visual perception in a blind subject with a chronic microelectronic retinal prosthesis. *Vision Research*, 43(24), 2573–2581.

Irons, J.L., Gradden, T., Zhang, A., He, X., Barnes, N., Scott, A.F. and Mckone, E. 2017. Face identity recognition in simulated prosthetic vision is poorer than previously reported and can be improved by caricaturing. *Vision Research*, 137, 61–79.

Jepson, L.H., Hottowy, P., Mathieson, K., Gunning, D.E., Dabrowski, W., Litke, A. M. and Chichilnisky, E.J. 2014. Spatially patterned electrical stimulation to enhance resolution of retinal prostheses. *Journal of Neuroscience*, 34(14), 4871–4881.

Johnson, L.A. and Higgins, C.M. A Navigation aid for the blind using tactile-visual sensory substitution. 2006. *2006 International Conference of the IEEE Engineering in Medicine and Biology Society*, Aug. 30–Sept. 3, 6289–6292.

Jones, B.W., Pfeiffer, R.L., Ferrell, W.D., Watt, C.B., Marmor, M. and Marc, R.E. 2016. Retinal remodeling in human retinitis pigmentosa. *Experimental Eye Research*, 149–65.

Kane, S.R., Cogan, S.F., Ehrlich, J., Plante, T.D., Mccreery, D.B. and Troyk, P.R. 2013. Electrical performance of penetrating microelectrodes chronically implanted in cat cortex. *IEEE Transactions on Biomedical Engineering*, 60(8), 2153–2160.

Keseru, M., Feucht, M., Bornfeld, N., Laube, T., Walter, P., Rossler, G., Velikay-Parel, M., Hornig, R. and Richard, G. 2012. Acute electrical stimulation of the human retina with an epiretinal electrode array. *Acta Ophthalmology*, 90(1), e1–e8.

Kim, S.Y., Sadda, S., Humayun, M.S., De Juan, E., Jr., Melia, B.M. and Green, W.R. 2002. Morphometric analysis of the macula in eyes with geographic atrophy due to age-related macular degeneration. *Retina*, 22(4), 464–470.

Kitiratschky, V.B., Stingl, K., Wilhelm, B., Peters, T., Besch, D., Sachs, H., Gekeler, F., Bartz-Schmidt, K.U. and Zrenner, E. 2015. Safety evaluation of "Retina Implant Alpha IMS": A prospective clinical trial. *Graefes Arch Clinical and Experimental Ophthalmology*, 253(3), 381–387.

Kolarik, A.J., Cirstea, S., Pardhan, S. and Moore, B.C. 2014. A summary of research investigating echolocation abilities of blind and sighted humans. *Hear Research*, 310, 60–68.

Krause, F. and Schum, H. 1931. *Neue Deutsche Chirurgie*. Stuttgart, Germany: Enke.

Lane, F.J. 2012. Methods and results from interviews of eleven recipients of a visual cortex implant: An analysis of their experiences. *The eye and the chip: World Congress on Artificial Vision*. Detroit, MI.

Lane, F.J., Nitsch, K., Huyck, M., Troyk, P. and Schug, K. 2016. Perspectives of optic nerve prostheses. *Disability and Rehabilitation: Assistive Technology*, 11(4), 301–309.

Lee, V.K., Nau, A.C., Laymon, C., Chan, K.C., Rosario, B.L. and Fisher, C. 2014. Successful tactile based visual sensory substitution use functions independently of visual pathway integrity. *Frontiers of Human Neuroscience*, 8, 291.

Levy-Tzedek, S., Hanassy, S., Abboud, S., Maidenbaum, S. and Amedi, A. 2012. Fast, accurate reaching movements with a visual-to-auditory sensory substitution device. *Restorative Neurology and Neuroscience*, 30(4), 313–323.

Levy-Tzedek, S., Riemer, D. and Amedi, A. 2014. Color improves "visual" acuity via sound. *Frontiers in Neuroscience*, 8, 358.

Lewis, P.M., Ayton, L.N., Guymer, R.H., Lowery, A.J., Blamey, P.J., Allen, P.J., Luu, C.D. and Rosenfeld, J.V. 2016. Advances in implantable bionic devices for blindness: A review. *ANZ Journal of Surgery*, 86(9), 654–659.

Lorach, H., Goetz, G., Smith, R., Lei, X., Mandel, Y., Kamins, T., Mathieson, K., Huie, P., Harris, J., Sher, A. and Palanker, D. 2015. Photovoltaic restoration of sight with high visual acuity. *Nature Medicine*, 21(5), 476–482.

Maidenbaum, S., Hanassy, S., Abboud, S., Buchs, G., Chebat, D.R., Levy-Tzedek, S. and Amedi, A. 2014. The "eyecane", a new electronic travel aid for the blind: Technology, behavior and swift learning. *Restorative Neurology and Neuroscience*, 32(6), 813–824.

Margalit, E., Maia, M., Weiland, J.D., Greenberg, R.J., Fujii, G.Y., Torres, G., Piyathaisere, D.V., O'hearn, T.M., Liu, W., Lazzi, G., Dagnelie, G., Scribner, D. A., De Juan, E., Jr. and Humayun, M.S. 2002. Retinal prosthesis for the blind. *Surv Ophthalmol*, 47(4), 335–356.

Mccarthy, C., Walker, J.G., Lieby, P., Scott, A. and Barnes, N. 2015. Mobility and low contrast trip hazard avoidance using augmented depth. *Journal of Neural Engineering*, 12(1), 016003.

Meijer, P.B. (1992). An experimental system for auditory image representations. *IEEE Transactions on Biomedical Engineering*, 39(2), 112–121.

Menzel-Severing, J., Laube, T., Brockmann, C., Bornfeld, N., Mokwa, W., Mazinani, B., Walter, P. and Roessler, G. 2012. Implantation and explantation of an active epiretinal visual prosthesis: 2-year follow-up data from the Epiret3 prospective clinical trial. *Eye (Lond)*, 26(4), 501–509.

Moisseiev, E. and Mannis, M.J. 2016. Evaluation of a portable artificial vision device among patients with low vision. *JAMA Ophthalmology*, 134(7), 748–752.

Muqit, M., Lemer, Y., De Rothschild, A., Velikay-Parel, M., Weber, M., Dupeyron, G., Audemard, D. and Corcostegui, B. 2017. Compensation for blindness with the Intelligent Retinal Implant System (Iris Ii) in patients with retinal dystrophy: Six-month interim results. *The Eye and the Chip World Congress*. Detroit, MI.

Nau, A.C., Murphy, M.C. and Chan, K.C. 2015. Use of sensory substitution devices as a model system for investigating cross-modal neuroplasticity in humans. *Neural Regeneration Research*, 10(11), 1717–1719.

Nau, A.C., Pintar, C., Arnoldussen, A. and Fisher, C. 2015. Acquisition of visual perception in blind adults using the brainport artificial vision device. *American Journal of Occupational Therapy*, 69(1), 6901290010p1–6901290010p8.

Pardue, M.T., Phillips, M.J., Hanzlicek, B., Yin, H., Chow, A.Y. and Ball, S.L. 2006. Neuroprotection of photoreceptors in the Rcs rat after implantation of a subretinal implant in the superior or inferior retina. *Advances in Experimental Medicine and Biology*, 572, 321–326.

Pardue, M.T., Phillips, M.J., Yin, H., Sippy, B.D., Webb-Wood, S., Chow, A.Y. and Ball, S.L. 2005. Neuroprotective effect of subretinal implants in the Rcs rat. *Investigative Ophthalmology and Vision Science*, 46(2), 674–682.

Petoe, M.A., Mccarthy, C.D., Shivdasani, M.N., Sinclair, N.C., Scott, A.F., Ayton, L.N., Barnes, N.M., Guymer, R.H., Allen, P.J., Blamey, P.J. and Bionic Vision Australia, C. 2017. Determining the contribution of retinotopic discrimination to localization performance with a suprachoroidal retinal prosthesis. *Investigative Ophthalmology and Vision Science*, 58(7), 3231–3239.

Pettingill, L.N., Richardson, R.T., Wise, A.K., O'Leary, S.J. and Shepherd, R.K. 2007. Neurotrophic factors and neural prostheses: Potential clinical applications based upon findings in the auditory system. *IEEE Transactions on Biomedical Engineering*, 54(6 Pt 1), 1138–1148.

Rizzo, J.F., III and Ayton, L.N. 2014. Psychophysical testing of visual prosthetic devices: A call to establish a multi-national joint task force. *Journal of Neural Engineering*, 11(2), 020301.

Roessler, G., Laube, T., Brockmann, C., Kirschkamp, T., Mazinani, B., Goertz, M., Koch, C., Krisch, I., Sellhaus, B., Trieu, H.K., Weis, J., Bornfeld, N., Rothgen, H., Messner, A., Mokwa, W. and Walter, P. 2009. Implantation and explantation of a wireless epiretinal retina implant device: observations during the Epiret3 prospective clinical trial. *Investigative Ophthalmology and Vision Science*, 50(6), 3003–3008.

Santos, A., Humayun, M.S., De Juan, E., Jr., Greenburg, R.J., Marsh, M.J., Klock, I.B. and Milam, A.H. 1997. Preservation of the inner retina in retinitis pigmentosa: A morphometric analysis. *Archives of Ophthalmology*, 115(4), 511–515.

Schatz, A., Pach, J., Gosheva, M., Naycheva, L., Willmann, G., Wilhelm, B., Peters, T., Bartz-Schmidt, K.U., Zrenner, E., Messias, A. and Gekeler, F. 2017. Transcorneal electrical stimulation for patients with retinitis pigmentosa: A prospective, randomized, sham-controlled follow-up study over 1 year. *Investigative Ophthalmology and Vision Science*, 58(1), 257–269.

Schimitzek, H., Roessler, G. and Walter, P. 2016. Clinical results after implantation of epiretinal visual prostheses. *Klin Monbl Augenheilkd*, 233(11), 1227–1232.

Sinclair, N.C., Shivdasani, M.N., Perera, T., Gillespie, L.N., Mcdermott, H.J., Ayton, L.N., Blamey, P.J. and Bionic Vision Australia, C. 2016. The appearance of phosphenes elicited using a suprachoroidal retinal prosthesis. *Investigative Ophthalmology and Vision Science*, 57(11), 4948–4961.

Stanga, P.E., Tsamis, E., Dorn, J.D., Jalil, A., Ch'ng, S., Stringa, F., Greenberg, R.J. and McGuire, W. 2017. Argus® Ii electronic epiretinal prosthesis in advanced dry age-related macular degeneration:

Safety and feasibility study – 1st year functional and structural results. *Investigative Ophthalmology and Vision Science*, 58(8), 4265–4265.

Stingl, K., Bartz-Schmidt, K.U., Besch, D., Braun, A., Bruckmann, A., Gekeler, F., Greppmaier, U., Hipp, S., Hortdorfer, G., Kernstock, C., Koitschev, A., Kusnyerik, A., Sachs, H., Schatz, A., Stingl, K.T., Peters, T., Wilhelm, B. and Zrenner, E. 2013. Artificial vision with wirelessly powered subretinal electronic implant Alpha-Ims. *Proceedings of the Royal Society B: Biological Sciences*, 280(1757), 20130077.

Stingl, K., Bartz-Schmidt, K.U., Besch, D., Chee, C.K., Cottriall, C.L., Gekeler, F., Groppe, M., Jackson, T.L., Maclaren, R.E., Koitschev, A., Kusnyerik, A., Neffendorf, J., Nemeth, J., Naeem, M.A., Peters, T., Ramsden, J.D., Sachs, H., Simpson, A., Singh, M.S., Wilhelm, B., Wong, D. and Zrenner, E. 2015. Subretinal visual implant Alpha Ims: Clinical trial interim report. *Vision Research*, 111(Pt B), 149–160.

Stingl, K., Schippert, R., Bartz-Schmidt, K.U., Besch, D., Cottriall, C.L., Edwards, T. L., Gekeler, F., Greppmaier, U., Kiel, K., Koitschev, A., Kuhlewein, L., Maclaren, R.E., Ramsden, J.D., Roider, J., Rothermel, A., Sachs, H., Schroder, G.S., Tode, J., Troelenberg, N. and Zrenner, E. 2017. Interim results of a multicenter trial with the new electronic subretinal implant Alpha Ams in 15 patients blind from inherited retinal degenerations. *Front Neurosciences*, 11, 445.

Stronks, H.C., Mitchell, E.B., Nau, A.C. and Barnes, N. 2016. Visual task performance in the blind with the Brainport V100 Vision Aid. *Expert Review Medical Devices*, 13(10), 919–931.

Stronks, H.C., Walker, J., Parker, D.J. and Barnes, N. 2017. Training improves vibrotactile spatial acuity and intensity discrimination on the lower back using coin motors. *Artifical Organs*, 41(11), 1059–1070.

Tassicker, G.E. 1956. Preliminary report on a retinal stimulator. *British Journal of Physiological Optics*, 13(2), 102–105.

Velikay-Parel, M., Ivastinovic, D., Georgi, T., Richard, G. and Hornig, R. 2013. A test method for quantification of stimulus-induced depression effects on perceptual threshold in epiretinal prosthesis. *Acta Ophthalmology*, 91(8), e595–602.

Veraart, C., Wanet-Defalque, M.C., Gerard, B., Vanlierde, A. and Delbeke, J. 2003. Pattern recognition with the optic nerve visual prosthesis. *Artificial Organs*, 27(11), 996–1004.

Voykinska, V., Azenkot, S., Wu, S. and Leshed, G. 2016. How blind people interact with visual content on social networking services. *Proceedings of the 19th ACM Conference on Computer-Supported Cooperative Work and Social Computing.* (pp. 1584–1595). San Jose, CA: ACM.

Vurro, M., Crowell, A.M. and Pezaris, J.S. 2014. Simulation of thalamic prosthetic vision: Reading accuracy, speed, and acuity in sighted humans. *Frontiers of Human Neuroscience*, 8, 816.

Wang, S., Li, Y. and Barnes, N. 2012. Text image processing for visual prostheses. *Conference Proceedings of the IEEE Engineering in Medicine and Biology Society*, 2977–2980.

Ward, J. and Meijer, P. 2010. Visual experiences in the blind induced by an auditory sensory substitution device. *Conscious Cognition*, 19(1), 492–500.

Weiland, J.D., Yanai, D., Mahadevappa, M., Williamson, R., Mech, B.V., Fujii, G. Y., Little, J., Greenberg, R.J., De Juan, E., Jr. and Humayun, M.S. 2004. Visual task performance in blind humans with retinal prosthetic implants. *Conference Proceedings of the IEEE Engineering in Medicine and Biology Society*, 6, 4172–4173.

Wise, A.K., Fallon, J.B., Neil, A.J., Pettingill, L.N., Geaney, M.S., Skinner, S.J. and Shepherd, R.K. 2011. Combining cell-based therapies and neural prostheses to promote neural survival. *Neurotherapeutics*, 8(4), 774–787.

Yue, L., Falabella, P., Christopher, P., Wuyyuru, V., Dorn, J., Schor, P., Greenberg, R.J., Weiland, J.D. and Humayun, M.S. 2015. Ten-year follow-up of a blind patient chronically implanted with epiretinal prosthesis Argus I. *Ophthalmology*, 122(12), 2545–2552 e1.

Zrenner, E., Bartz Schmidt, K.U., Besch, D., Gekeler, F., Koitschev, A., Sachs, H.G. and Stingl, K. 2017. The subretinal implant alpha: implantation and functional results. In P. Gabel (ed.), *Artificial vision: A clinical guide* (pp. 65–83). Switzerland: Springer.

Part X
Aging and adulthood

26

Employment and visual impairment

Issues in adulthood

Natalie Martiniello and Walter Wittich

Introduction

Gainful employment is the key to financial independence and remains the primary objective for many adults who pursue vision rehabilitation services (Ponchillia and Ponchillia, 1996). It enables adults with visual impairments (that is, those who are blind or who have low vision) to live independently, make their own choices, pursue meaningful interests and contribute to society in meaningful ways (Jo, Chen and Kosciulek, 2010). Despite advancements in civil rights and the introduction of anti-discrimination legislation and vocational rehabilitation programmes throughout the latter part of the twentieth century, the employment rates for people with visual impairments in developed countries continues to hover between 25% and 40%, with 70% of adults with visual impairments either unemployed or underemployed, working in positions that do not reflect their qualifications (O'Day, 1999). There has been an upsurge in research devoted to understanding the variables that either facilitate or impede the labour force participation of adults who are blind or who have low vision in recent decades (Goetz et al., 2010). Personal factors, such as age, onset and severity of visual impairment and degree of independent living skills (Wolffe, 1996), as well as environmental factors, such as workplace accessibility and the attitudes of employers (Crudden et al., 1998; Lepofsky and Graham, 2009; O'Day, 1999), contribute to the obstacles faced by adults with visual impairments who seek employment. Neglecting these environmental and sociocultural variables leads to the over-simplified assumption that vision status alone functions as the primary determinant of employment in the lives of people with visual impairments. In Chapter 11 of this volume Karen Wolffe highlighted the importance of ensuring early career education and skill development for children and youth with visual impairments. We will continue this story by summarising what is known about the experiences of adults with visual impairments who seek employment, and the facilitators and barriers they encounter along the way.

A lifespan perspective

In 1999, the American Foundation for the Blind (AFB) published a report on employment and visual impairment from a lifespan perspective, based on the 1994 and 1995 National Health

Interview Survey conducted by the National Centre for Health Statistics. The authors argued that little attention had often been paid to the critical influence of age, age of onset and career stage, and that a lifespan analysis would provide essential context for understanding different employment issues for subgroups of the blind and low vision population (Kirchner, Schmeidler and Todorv, 1999). For example, adults with acquired vision loss will likely be in mid-to-late careers and will confront difficulties associated with adjusting to vision loss as well as barriers related to maintaining prior employment or transitioning to a new career at an advanced working age (Caprani, O'Connor and Gurrin, 2012). This is especially relevant for those who want to maintain employment into what is considered traditional retirement age, as the number of older adults above the age of 65 is expected to double by 2050, along with the prevalence of those with age-related vision loss (Varma, Vajaranant and Burkemper, 2016).

While barriers to employment do persist, notable progress has also been made and current gaps illuminate where future efforts are needed. Understanding the current state of visual impairment and employment will help to ameliorate future service delivery, social policy and programming in these areas. This chapter will therefore provide an overview of the current state of employment for working-age adults with visual impairment, with an emphasis on those who acquire vision loss later in life.

Historical context

Employment opportunities for people with visual impairments have shifted alongside slowly changing perceptions and improved civil rights throughout the industrialised world, but only in recent decades have the unique needs of adults with vision loss gained greater consideration in programme and service delivery. Blind children were not formally educated prior to the late 1700s, when Valentin Hauy pioneered the first school for the blind in 1784 (Lorimer, 2000). It was the hope of such early educators that blind pupils with appropriate instruction could support themselves without the need to rely on family or government intervention. Though only formally adopted after his death, the braille system, invented by Louis Braille, a pupil at the school, made the distribution of information and knowledge among the blind possible, enabling both reading and writing for the first time and for talents to be explored in new ways (Lorimer, 2000). For more on these early educational initiatives, see Chapter 8 in this volume, by Lueck and Goodrich. Nonetheless, the curricula in these early schools for the blind focused on vocational training in limited manual trades perceived by the sighted to be appropriate for the blind, such as knitting, chair caning, basket weaving, broom making or alternatively, careers in music instruction (Koestler, 2004). In fact, the emphasis on such vocational training was of such central importance within the curricula of early schools for the blind that decisions about the geographic location of such institutions were at times based upon the extent to which they would support success in these endeavours. Samuel Gridley Howe, founder of the Perkins School for the Blind, for instance, commented on what he felt to be an ill choice for the location for what became known as the W. Ross School for the Blind in Brantford, Ontario, Canada, stating: "Bare in mind that one half of your pupils will try to find a livelihood in teaching music and that in order to be a good teacher of music one must live in a musical atmosphere" (Herie, 2005, p. 26), equating the blind in the small town of Brandford to "sailors in an inland town as musicians in a village" (p. 27). Unfortunately, many graduates of these schools were unable to find employment in these trades despite their vocational training, often due to the inability to sway public perceptions of the abilities of blind and visually impaired persons.

Sheltered workshops

The difficulties in securing gainful employment led to the development of separate, segregated, private "sheltered workshops" to provide more permanent, if restrictive, employment to blind adults who were unable to find work elsewhere because they were viewed as unemployable. The first sheltered workshop for blind adults in the United States was established in New York in 1850, and focused on the same trades encouraged at sheltered workshops in schools for the blind (Koestler, 2004). By 1938, US federal legislation (the Wagner-O'Day Act) mandated that the government purchase items such as brooms and mops from sheltered workshops for the blind to support the work done by blind adults within such facilities. In Canada, such work-shops were established in the 1870s by the Maritime Association for the Blind in the maritime provinces (Pearce, 2012), and became a significant part of the Canadian National Institute for the Blind's pan-Canadian operations from its inception through to the final shuttering of its catering operation (Caterplan) in 2010. In the UK, the rise of the sheltered workshop began in the early to mid-nineteenth century, and by 1930, 3,000 blind people were placed in workshops in England and Wales. This still accounted for a relatively small proportion of the blind com-munity, however: 250 of those workshop spaces were in London, where approximately 3,500 working-age blind people lived (French, 2017).

Such establishments, which provide segregated work for adults with disabilities who are perceived as incapable of competing in the open labour market (WHO, 2011), have been the subject of great controversy and debate. These specialised work environments are often author-ised by government to pay sub-minimum wages and are exempted from various employee pro-tection schemes, limiting the benefits of being employed and arguably infringing the dignity of the individual workers by essentially operating under a charity model (Visier, 1998). They also have the effect of segregating and marginalising people with disabilities, rather than encourag-ing integration, inclusion and cooperation. A 1973 inquiry in Toronto, Canada, having heard from sheltered workers in CNIB's workshops, concluded that most "physically handicapped" people in the city "if they are working at all (often in sheltered workshops) are doing so at a level which insults their potential" (Greenland, 1976). Sheltered workshops are no longer the norm for blind persons in many countries, but are still actively used in some locales for people with disabilities living in Switzerland, New Zealand and France (WHO, 2011, p. 243) where regular pay and full social security coverage is provided to people with one-third or less capac-ity loss. Other European countries have been working to transition traditional workshops into self-sustaining social enterprises or firms (Visier, 1998).

There is considerable inter-country variability in the definition and stated purpose of shel-tered employment programmes. At one end of the spectrum, sheltered employment may pro-vide real-world job readiness training and act as a stepping stone to further, more advanced opportunities, therefore functioning as vocational training grounds for adults (Galer, 2014, p. 73). In other instances, it may be permanent but largely symbolic employment, which may or may not serve therapeutic purposes for the individual with a disability (Visier, 1998). Regardless, studies indicate today that there is a low rate of transfer from sheltered workshop environments to regular employment situations, ranging from as low as 1%–2% in France, Spain, Belgium, Switzerland and Scotland to as high as 11% in Norway (Visier, 1998, p. 353).

The development of vocational rehabilitation services

The two World Wars in the first half of the twentieth century are largely credited with spurring the creation, development and proliferation of rehabilitation services for blind adults. As veterans who had been blinded on the battlefield returned home, they needed a means to support themselves and their families. At the same time, government needed workers capable of supporting the war effort from home (Koestler, 2004). In several countries, blinded adults were instrumental in the development of these services and in changing perceptions about the contributions the blind could make. For example, five of the seven adults who led the development of the Canadian National Institute for the Blind in 1918 were blind themselves (Herie, 2005). Blind Veterans UK, established in 1915 in the UK shortly after the outbreak of the First World War, was similarly founded by veterans to provide rehabilitation, training and lifelong support to those blinded by war. Institutions throughout the UK such as St Dunstan's Hostel for Blinded Soldiers and Sailors aimed to rehabilitate returning veterans by both training them for new careers and providing them with adaptive tools and strategies. A UK network of special villages was built for ex-servicemen and their families, but despite these advancements, most blind veterans could not find work after the Second World War unless it was in sheltered workshops (Historic England, n.d.).

Legislation and regulation

Over the years, a number of jurisdictions have adopted legislation and regulations intended to provide financial support and protect employment opportunities for the blind. In many cases, this has occurred as part of the larger civil rights movement, as persons with disabilities (and the organisations that support them) campaign for greater equality and inclusion in education and employment. In the United States, the Smith–Fess Act (also known as the Civilian Rehabilitation Act) was adopted in 1920, establishing one of the true first federal initiatives to invest government funding in programmes to train people with disabilities to become employable. The blind were not initially included in these early programmes, until the passage of the Randolph-Sheppard Act in 1936, which recognised the employment potential of the blind and permitted states to license qualified blind persons to operate vending stands in federal government buildings. In the 1970s, lobbying by the National Federation of the Blind resulted in this being expanded to food-line operations, which led to a number of blind individuals earning their living managing cafeterias in federal buildings (Koestler, 2004). The implementation in 1973 of the Rehabilitation Act prohibited discrimination on the basis of disability within federal government employment and the passage of the Individuals with Disabilities Education Act ("IDEA") in 1975 led to the eventual placement of blind students in mainstream classrooms (Ajuwon and Oyinlade, 2008). These philosophical shifts placed greater emphasis on viewing individuals who were blind on an equal footing, and extended opportunities to pursue post-secondary education for blind adults. The Americans with Disabilities Act (1990) offers further protections for blind employees, but its impact on actual employment rates for the blind is difficult to determine.

In Canada, employment and education-related rights, as they pertain to individuals who are blind, are protected through a patchwork of overlapping and interrelated provincial and federal "human rights" legislation, largely developed and instituted between 1962 and 1984. The Canadian Human Rights Code and the Charter of Rights and Freedoms aim to protect against discrimination by government and federally regulated enterprises, while provincial human rights legislation is primarily responsible for regulation of private enterprise (Clement, Silver and Trottier, 2012). These schemes prohibit discrimination and allow for affirmative action programmes, but do not mandate inclusion or inclusive practices per se. While these legislation schemes have undoubtedly precluded blatant discrimination against blind employees, the employment outcomes (which, as will be discussed, have not markedly changed in decades) would suggest that there are more systemic barriers to employment.

On an international stage, the United Nations Convention on the Rights of Persons with Disabilities (UNCRPD)

> recognizes the right of persons with disabilities to work, on an equal basis with others; this includes the opportunity to gain a living by work freely chosen or accepted in a labour market and work environment that is open, inclusive and accessible to persons with disabilities.
>
> *(WHO, 2011, p. 235)*

Among its provisions, this international treaty prohibits all forms of employment discrimination, promotes access to vocational training and requires reasonable accommodations in the workplace. A complaints and inquiry procedure is available to individuals within countries that ratify the treaty including its optional protocol. Currently, the UNCRPD has been ratified in 160 countries (United Nations, n.d.). The thoroughness of the convention as well as the accompanying World Report on Disability underscores the environmental and social factors that are often responsible for determining the employment experiences of persons with disabilities, and calls on societies and governments to address these societal barriers through inclusive practices.

Career prospects

The massive changes in industry, technology and a shift to a largely knowledge-based economy have drastically altered the available employment opportunities for individuals who are visually impaired. A 1926 report from the American Foundation for the Blind examined the current state of employment for the visually impaired from three perspectives: employment in mainstream occupations; employment in independent, self-employment endeavours; and employment through industries and workshops fostered by institutions for the blind. Surveys distributed through federal, state and local organisations for the blind resulted in responses from 1,141 individuals, including 185 independent businessmen, 171 factory workers, 170 salesmen, 153 professionals, 93 piano and organ tuners, 80 handicraft workers, 49 clerical workers, 49 household workers and 191 others (Koestler, 2004).

In the UK in 2016, a survey of occupations performed by individuals with visual impairments revealed a representation typical of large society, although individuals with visual impairments were more likely to be found in associate professional and technical occupations (15.9% vs 14.1% in the mainstream), administrative and secretarial occupations (11.1% vs 10.4% in the mainstream), sales and customer service occupations (11.9% vs 7.9% in the mainstream) and elementary occupations (13% vs 11% in the mainstream) (Hewett and Keil, 2016).

In some countries, particular occupations throughout the twentieth century have either been prioritised for the blind through legislation or have become de facto traditional roles. In Japan, for example, it has been traditional for persons who are blind to pursue massage therapy, musical performance and storytelling and find employment in such careers (Mochizuki, 2013, p. 6). In Spain, almost all blind persons are gainfully and successfully employed by the Organización Nacional de Ciegos Españoles, a national organisation for the blind that, in the 1930s, was granted an exclusive monopoly to sell lottery tickets thereby alleviating the perceived responsibility of the government (Garvia, 1996). In Italy, legal protection and quotas are utilised to prioritise hiring of blind individuals as switchboard operators, masseurs-physiotherapists, teachers and in public administration (Rodolfo, 2009). While these programmes foster employment, critics have pointed out that they also prevent the blind from moving outside these fields or pursuing other interests.

The changing nature of employment for the blind

The technological revolution that has been experienced since the advent of modern computers in the 1960s, and continuing modernisation and automation, has fundamentally altered the career landscape for the blind. Advancements in mainstream accessible technologies have provided previously unparalleled access to information and computer interfaces. Screen readers and optical character recognition technology make it possible for the blind to access information in electronic and print formats (Presley and D'Andrea, 2009). In an economy that is increasingly driven by the flow of information, these advancements would seem to be advantageous to the blind, and in many ways, this is true. In fact, initiatives by several organisations in the United States in the early days of such technological advancements provided targeted training to groups of blind adults throughout the 1960s and 1970s to pursue careers in computer programming and related fields (Visier, 1998). However, notwithstanding these technological advantages, the blind remain underrepresented in the science, technology, engineering and math fields, representing less than 5% of the US "STEM" workforce (Villaneuva and Di Stefano, 2017). On the other hand, occupations that were traditionally thought to be suitable for the blind (e.g. switchboard operator) are now virtually defunct and unnecessary – or have themselves become inaccessible through the proliferation of touchscreen interfaces (Rodolfo, 2009). Moreover, the typical entry-level career path (with summer and part-time employment) is often unsuitable for youth who are blind due to accessibility barriers. While access to careers that require higher education is to be applauded, proponents also raise the concern of how to best meet the needs of clients who have additional disabilities or for whom higher education may not be appropriate (Wolffe, 1996). This raises an interesting point about existing employment statistics in that they say little about whether adults with visual impairments are employed in their fields of choice, or the degree to which upward mobility has been possible.

A secondary challenge relates to the aging population. Many older individuals are likely to experience vision loss later in life (Varma et al., 2016). Such previously sighted adults may not only face the challenge of adjusting to vision loss, but also the prospect of transitioning to new careers or considering the option of early retirement (Kirchner et al., 1999; Wolffe, 1996). The needs of this population are decidedly different from children, youth and young adults with visual impairments. Vocational and rehabilitation professionals who work with the visually impaired now must consider not only the needs of congenitally blind adults, but also how to meet the needs of those losing their vision partially or completely later in life.

Employment rates and statistics

A note about definitions

Complexities abound when attempting to make any comparative assessments of statistics relating to the employment outcomes of individuals with visual impairments, on at least three levels. At the methodological level, while there are some population-based surveys, more often than not data have been collected through convenience samples that may or may not be representative of the population from which they were derived. At the measurement level, "blindness" and "low vision" have highly inconsistent definitions. In the UK, United States and Canada, "blindness" is often linked to the *legal* definition of blindness, that is, an individual with best-corrected acuity less than 20/200 or less than 20 degrees of vision (Kirchner et al., 1999, p. 44), but some studies rely on descriptors linked to activities of daily living or self-reported data, which may lead to under-reporting. Moreover, defining employment (and related terms such as "unemployment") is itself complex, as these terms can have drastically different meanings depending on the country and cultural context. Efforts at standardising these terms (including collection of data in accordance with the International Labour Office's resolution on the International Classification of Status in Employment) have been made, but in many countries, data on disability and employment are limited or completely non-existent (WHO, 2011, pp. 236–238). At the interpretive level, definitions of employment success, poverty level or low-income cut-offs, differing currencies, widely varying costs of living and the limited availability of data from differing time periods make inter-country comparisons difficult at best. Despite these methodological challenges, statistics do exist that provide enough of a snapshot of the current situation. Notably, these statistics demonstrate that even on the international stage, the employment rate of individuals with visual impairments remains significantly below that of the general population, hovering between 25% and 40% in many jurisdictions despite advancements in services and legislation.

For our purposes, where calculations have been required in order to present concordant statistics, *employment* measures the percentage of individuals with visual impairments who are working outside the home in remunerative positions, on either a part-time (<30hr/wk) or full-time (>30hr/wk) basis. *Unemployment* measures the percentage of individuals with visual impairments who are not currently working, but who wish to work and are actively seeking employment. *Underemployment* refers to situations wherein an individual is employed, but in a capacity that does not make use of their education, qualifications or certifications (such as an individual with a PhD working in a telemarketing capacity) (WHO, 2011).

Employment rates

The employment rates of individuals with visual impairments, of people with disabilities generally and of the baseline population for Australia (Australian Bureau of Statistics, 2016a, 2016b; Deloitte Access Economics Pty Ltd, 2016), Canada (Statistics Canada, 2016a, 2016; Turcotte, 2014), New Zealand (La Grow, 2004), the UK (Slade, Smith and White, 2017; Smith, 2016) and the United States (Centers for Disease Control and Prevention, 2016) are shown in Table 26.1. These figures are very consistent with earlier research that has reported employment rates among adults with visual impairments of 25%–30%, compared to 32%–50% for people with disabilities generally and 78%–80% for individuals without a disability (La Grow, 2004; Lee and Park, 2008).

There are pronounced differences in the employment rate of individuals with visual impairments across the different life stages, as illustrated by Figure 26.1. In the United States, individuals in the middle-aged groups have profoundly lower employment rates than those in the

Table 26.1 Employment rates for selected countries for the general population, adults with disabilities and adults with vision impairments.

Country	Employment rates		
	General population (%)	Adults with disabilities (%)	Adults with vision impairment (%)
Australia	84.3	51.3	36
Canada	79	49	37.6
New Zealand	70	40	39
United Kingdom	81.8	49	26
United States	63.9	35.6	34.8

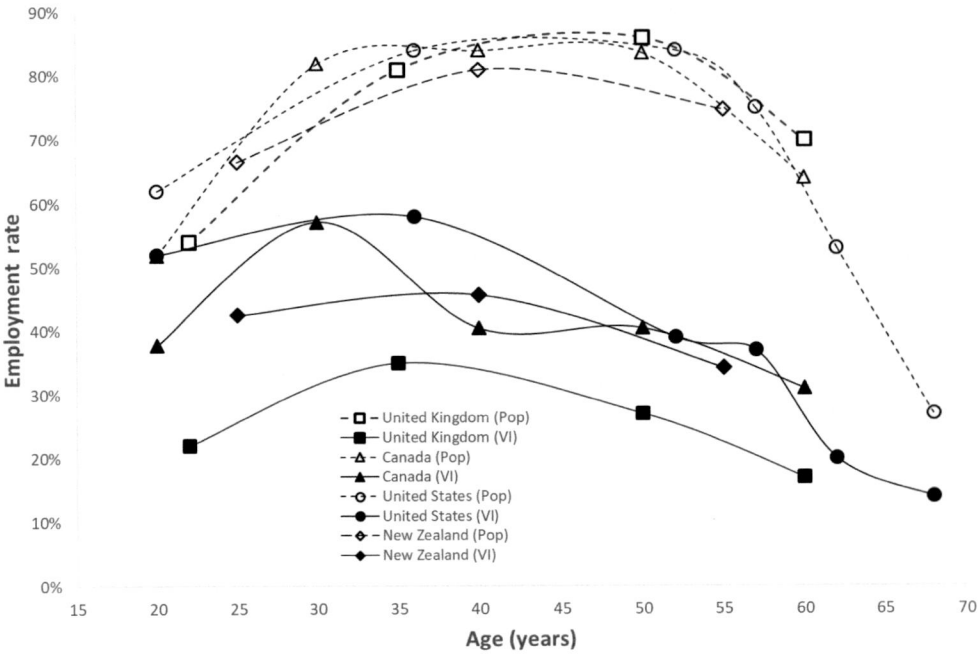

Figure 26.1   Employment rates at the population level (pop) versus for individuals with a visual impairment (VI) across four countries as a function of age.

younger and older groups (Kirchner et al., 1999). In Canada (Statistics Canada, 2016a, 2016b), the UK (Slade et al., 2017) and New Zealand (La Grow, 2004; Stats NZ, 2016) the employment gap appears to increase with age, shrinking only in the oldest individuals. However, it is evident that as adults age, they encounter additional barriers to employment.

Earnings

As shown in Table 26.2, in Canada (Arim, 2015; Statistics Canada, 2016a, 2016b) and the United States (Centers for Disease Control and Prevention, 2016; Erickson, Lee and von Schrader, 2017), people with disabilities have markedly lower earnings than individuals in the general population. When compared to people with disabilities generally, persons with visual impairments have even lower levels of income than others. Exacerbating lower income levels is the reality that individuals with visual impairments also face higher than average expenses on account of their disability (Hill et al., 2015). Even in jurisdictions where supports are available,

Table 26.2 Median annual incomes in selected countries for the general population, adults with disabilities and adults with vision impairments.

Country	Median income		
	General population	Adults with disabilities	Adults with vision impairment
Canada	C$31,160	C$20,420	C$17,700
United States	US$45,100	US$41,600	US$37,600

restrictions on who is eligible for coverage may preclude assistance for those who are only beginning to lose their vision, who are older or who are not yet working or studying (WHO, 2011).

Finally, it should be noted that there are additional factors and intersecting circumstances that can significantly alter earning outcomes. The onset, duration and severity of the impairment, as well as gender, level of education and pre-disability income levels, are important factors that influence earning potential. Statistics Canada (2016a) reported (based on 2011 data) that, of Canadians without disabilities aged 25–64 with a university degree, men earned on average \$92,681 and women \$68,041. By comparison, men with disabilities aged 25–64 with a university degree earned only \$69,197 and women \$64,503 – both statistically significant from the reference group (Turcotte, 2014, p. 8). In the United States, while employment rates are roughly equivalent across genders, women who are blind earn on average \$10,000 less than men (Bell and Mino, 2015).

The relationship between employment and poverty

While available statistics provide useful context, there is no internationally accepted conception of "poverty" that may be defined in either absolute terms (referring to the ability to access bare necessities such as food, shelter or clothing) or in relative terms, placing one's level of income or consumption within the social and economic context in which people live (Wong and Wong, 2004). Since what constitutes "bare necessities" depends greatly on social context, some countries such as Canada do not attempt to estimate the rate of poverty. Instead, a low-income cutoff is used, "set at the point where a family spends on average at least 20 percentage points more of its income than the average family on food, clothing and shelter" (Collin, 2008).

Regardless of how broadly or narrowly poverty is defined, persons with disabilities are universally disadvantaged in educational and labour market participation and are more likely to experience poverty than those without disabilities (WHO, 2011, pp. 39–40). The causal relationship between disability and poverty is such that disability itself – including visual impairment – can instigate poverty as it can impede education and employment and is attached to additional expenditures such as medical and assistive devices (Hill et al., 2015), and those who are poor can acquire disabilities due to insufficient access to services and supports (WHO, 2011, p. 10). A 2009 OCED study, for instance, indicates that working-age people with disabilities have higher poverty rates than those without disabilities in all but 3 of 21 upper-middle and high-income countries (WHO, 2011, p. 39). A study in the UK found that income and employment rates fall with the onset of disability and duration of disability, indicating that as people acquire disabilities, they tend to earn less or leave the workforce entirely (Jenkins and Rigg, 2003). Of particular relevance is that, when the additional costs associated with having a disability are taken into account, individuals with disabilities are often poorer than those without disabilities who have comparable incomes, and therefore the minimum salary they are willing to accept to enter into the employment market may be higher. Social security programmes are in place in many jurisdictions to address high unemployment and poverty but if working risks losing entitlement to the attendant benefits, this may discourage employment-seeking behaviours (WHO, 2011).

A multifaceted perspective

While the above statistics point to an association between visual impairment and lower employment, they do not tell the whole story. The tendency to emphasise impairment (in this case, visual impairment) as the primary driver of the comparatively low employment outcomes among the blind and visually impaired is centred in the medical model of disability

(Barnes, Mercer and Shakespeare, 1999, p. 27). To increase social inclusion and participation, the medical model would advocate rehabilitating the impaired person and addressing the limitations of the impairment through medical interventions or specialised technologies to compensate for lack of sight. On the other hand, the social model of disability, advanced by disability advocates beginning during the civil rights movement in the UK (UPIAS, 1976), posits that, while impairment may be attached to certain limitations, many external barriers (such as employer attitudes and inaccessibility in the workplace) greatly influence the experiences of people with visual impairments and work to maintain the disabling conditions experienced by certain groups. Disability in this model is defined as "the disadvantage or restriction of activity caused by contemporary organisation which takes no or little account of people who have physical impairments" (UPIAS, 1976, p. 14), while "impairment" is limited to the more physical manifestations (the inability to see). For example, computer software may be inaccessible to screen reader users, but in this case, it is the inaccessible design of the software rather than the impairment of the individual that gives rise to that barrier. If software is designed to be more accessible and inclusive from the start, proponents of the social model would argue that the disabling experiences encountered by many would be minimised or eliminated. Viewing employment outcomes through the social model lens would inherently involve accounting for other influencing factors above and beyond the individual.

In the present day, a blending of both the medical and social model of disability has led clinicians who provide vocational and blindness rehabilitation services to be more acutely aware of the external factors, in addition to visual impairment, which may impact upon employment outcomes. For example, the International Classification of Functioning, Disability and Health model advanced by the World Health Organization places the person at the centre of these overlapping and interrelated personal, environmental and social factors that influence their experiences as they progress through life and encounter disabling conditions (WHO, 2001). A perspective that recognises the role of visual impairment but also contextualises this with personal, environmental and social influencers, provides clinicians with the ability to more responsively address clients' unmet needs.

Against this backdrop, the discussion that follows is organised around themes that originate from this lifespan, multifaceted perspective and that emerge from the literature regarding the perceived facilitators and barriers to full employment. It is important to bear in mind, however, that in many instances, these factors are more continuous than dichotomous; that is, a single element may be either a facilitator or a barrier, depending on the personal, environmental and social circumstances of the individual.

Employment facilitators and barriers

Personal characteristics

Employment and job-seeking outcomes are significantly influenced by characteristics, attitudes and self-perceptions that are unique to each individual. Some of the characteristics that have been linked to employment outcomes are inherent to the individual and cannot be altered, including the degree of vision loss, age of onset or the presence or absence of additional impairments (Duquette and Baril, 2013). Many other factors are more attitudinal in nature and are subject to influence through appropriate social, educational, psychological and rehabilitative supports. At a base level, the psychological well-being of the individual and their degree of acceptance of, and adjustment to, their visual impairment are significantly associated with employment and job-seeking outcomes (Hagenmoser, 1996; Jo et al., 2010; Nijhuis, van Lierop and van de

Toren, 2008). Individuals who continue to hold on to unrealistic hopes of regaining their vision are known to be more dependent, less involved in rehabilitation efforts and suffer from higher rates of depression (Keegan, Ash and Greenough, 1976). This has a cascading, negative impact on many of the other personality traits and characteristics that influence ultimate employment outcomes, including assertiveness; conscientiousness, confidence and self-efficacy; self-esteem; unemployment negativity; employment commitment; and effective job-search skills.

A majority of studies indicate that, excluding other compounding variables, people with low vision are often more likely to have worked already in the past and to be currently employed, compared to those who are blind (Goetz et al., 2010; La Grow, 2004; Lee and Park, 2008; Shaw, Gold and Wolffe, 2007). A study by Wright et al. (1999) provides an alternative finding, suggesting that people with low vision encounter greater employment challenges, but the nature of these challenges is often quite different. For example, Shaw et al. (2007) found that participants with low vision were more likely to express on-the-job challenges (often related to employer attitudes) than those who were blind, despite the fact that they experienced higher employment rates. The sometimes invisible nature of low vision (particularly if the individual in question does not use a mobility aid such as a white cane or guide dog) means that it is not always apparent to prospective employers and colleagues. People with less severe visual impairments might therefore grapple with whether and how to disclose a visual impairment to employers and colleagues, especially if that visual condition fluctuates or is ambiguous to understand (Santuzzi et al., 2014).

While it is true that functionally blind job seekers are at risk of experiencing discrimination from the outset, once employed, blindness is arguably easier for others to comprehend than limitless degrees of low vision. People who are in the early stages of vision loss, particularly if that vision loss is mostly invisible, may also confront feelings of stigma and may prefer to "pass" as sighted as a consequence (Southall and Wittich, 2012). The issue of how to best disclose a disability during the job interview and how to discuss a visual impairment in a way that highlights the prospective employee's strengths and alternative methods for performing certain tasks is an important component to vocational rehabilitation training. A variety of online resources, such as the Career Connect database from the American Foundation for the Blind, provides recommendations and advice to help develop these self-advocacy skills and to anticipate potential questions that employers may have (American Foundation for the Blind, n.d.). These themes are especially pertinent for clinicians who work with clients diagnosed with age-related eye conditions, as many of these older individuals may be closer to the start of their vision loss journey and still coming to terms with the diagnosis.

Assertiveness, which refers to the ability to express both positive and negative feelings in a manner that is appropriate for a given social context to avoid being taken advantage of by others, has been found to be significantly lower among some adults with visual impairment (Hersen et al., 1995). In the context of job-seeking and employment, assertiveness has been found to be important among the general population (Schmit, Amel and Ryan, 1993), but becomes especially so as the blind or visually impaired individual will almost certainly need to explain their individual accommodation needs, their abilities and means by which they will accomplish the job at hand, both to potential employers and, ultimately, their co-workers (Bjorkmann, 2008; Crudden et al., 1998; Dixon, 1983; Joseph and Robinson, 2012). In fact, employers have indicated that they *expect* an employee with a visual impairment to assume primary responsibility for ameliorating awkwardness with co-workers by being "a diplomat and an ambassador of blindness, even though it's exhausting" (Golub, 2006, pp. 722–723).

Individuals who display conscientiousness tend to be purposeful, determined, well-organised, set intrinsically motivating goals for themselves and hold adaptive, pro-social values (Hartman and Betz, 2007; Wanberg, Watt and Rumsey, 1996). These behaviours are likewise associated

425

with greater self-efficacy in job searching, interviewing, networking and career exploration activities (Thoms, Moore and Scott, 1996). While these characteristics are to some degree determined by one's underlying personality traits, it is certainly possible to learn the skills necessary to confidently engage in those activities that will create and demonstrate to potential and actual employers an inherent sense of purposeful intent.

Related to self-confidence is the need for individuals with vision impairment to have some reasonable belief that employment is a viable possibility and, indeed, a desirable objective. Unemployment negativity (how negative, depressed or upset an individual feels about being unemployed) can be a motivator and is positively correlated with appropriate and desirable job-seeking behaviours (Feather and O'Brien, 1987), but excessively long periods of unemployment may also lead to individuals losing hope and ambition and leaving the labour force altogether (Slade and Simkiss, 2008). Job-seeking behaviours and outcomes are similarly mediated by the degree to which an individual attaches importance to work. For example, an individual with a very high employment commitment would continue working even after winning the lottery (Wanberg et al., 1996), but internalised attitudes of learned helplessness and the availability of government-funded income replacement programmes may serve to undermine or disincentivise this commitment to employment (Crudden et al., 1998, p. 21; O'Day, 1999).

A significant limitation and barrier to employment for many who are blind or have a visual impairment are effective job-seeking skills themselves. Job seekers with visual impairments have flagged the need for improved services related to the development of job search strategies (Schriner and Roessler, 1991), but research continues to suggest that blind and visually impaired job seekers do not necessarily have effective job-seeking skills. For example, in a Canadian study of younger adults (under the age of 30) with visual impairment, Shaw et al. (2007) found that 78% of those who reported they were "actively looking for work" were spending less than one hour per day on the task, and 26% of those had not submitted *any* job applications within the prior year. This minimal involvement may be explained by a lack of understanding of the nature of intensive job-seeking activities, or frustration and despondency with participants' employment prospects.

In devising intervention plans for individuals seeking employment or re-employment, rehabilitation professionals must bear in mind and appropriately address the personal factors that influence employment outcomes. While some demographic factors are outside of the individual's control, many personality traits and characteristics can be learned and trained to improve employment outcomes. Structured assertiveness training protocols have been developed to teach these skills to individuals of all ages (Donohue et al., 1995, p. 65). Self-esteem and self-confidence may be developed through vocational rehabilitation programmes that teach individuals to focus and reflect upon their abilities and capacities rather than their disabilities (Jo et al., 2010; Tuttle and Tuttle, 2004). Mentorship and career exploration activities with supported employment and employment integration programmes can likewise be utilised to provide insight to individuals about the possibilities that are open to them (Slade and Simkiss, 2008). Implementing these strategies in tandem will provide blind and visually impaired job seekers with the best opportunities to find and maintain gainful employment.

Ultimately, it is essential to acknowledge the psychological aspect of job-seeking in adulthood. Adults often consider "working" or "being employed" as an integral component of their identities (Kirchner et al., 1999), and the absence or loss of this may be distressing to adults who are unemployed but wishing to work. Clients with congenital impairments who have attempted to secure employment for a long time may feel despondent or discouraged, while adults with acquired vision loss may feel overwhelmed at the complexity of returning to work. The importance of interdisciplinary supports such as counselling and providing tangible examples of successful blind people (discussed more later) is important. Such an approach rec-ognises that quite apart from acquiring tangible employment skills, there is a need to understand how psychological emotions attached to finding employment may manifest differently accord-ing to age, career stage and age of onset.

Education

Level of educational attainment is a significant predictor of employment among the general population, but this is even more true for adults with visual impairments (Capella-McDonnall, 2005; Duquette and Baril, 2013; Kirchner et al., 1999; Kirchner and Smith, 2005; Shaw et al., 2007; Slade et al., 2017). Bell and Mino (2013) found that adults with visual impairments in the United States with a post-secondary degree are twice as likely to be employed than those without a post-secondary degree. In particular, the disparity in employment rates between adults with and without visual impairments decreases considerably at each higher level of education obtained by the visually impaired (Kirchner et al., 1999; Kirchner and Smith, 2005; Lacey and Crosby, 2004).

In a study analysing data from 181 recipients of vocational rehabilitation services, Capella-McDonnall (2005) found that completion of a degree or certificate programme as a part of that rehabilitation process increased the odds of a successful employment outcome by a factor of more than 9. On the other hand, education and training that was completed but did not lead to the granting of a recognisable degree or certificate actually *decreased* the likelihood of a successful employment outcome. This may be in part because higher levels of education provide people with visual impairments with skills and knowledge that lead to greater career options, but also because educational degrees and certificates provide prospective employers who may have res-ervations or concerns with tangible examples of what visually impaired people can accomplish.

Despite the obvious benefit of education, a closer look at findings reveals that personal and sociocultural factors (such as age, onset of vision loss, gender and ethnicity) may impede adults with visual impairments from achieving these requisite higher levels of education. It is well established that the minimum educational level required by most employers has increased over the decades, tracking societal trends toward increased enrolment in post-secondary education (Brown, 2001). Individuals with visual impairments experience a number of unique barriers in post-secondary education, including challenges in accessing information from print and elec-tronic sources, inaccessible e-learning and online learning management platforms and limited availability of on-campus access technologies (Fichten, Asuncion and Scapin, 2014). Students with visual impairments may devote so much energy to school work and overcoming the chal-lenges posed by inaccessible content and systems that they do not have the time for many of the extra-curricular activities (and volunteer opportunities) that would later serve as demonstrable evidence of their employability (Kirchner and Smith, 2005).

For older individuals with adventitious vision loss, the education milieu may pose a particular challenge. Their original career may not have required advanced levels of educational attain-ment, and they may have a more limited educational background as a result. Retraining can be difficult, because they may not have the time, resources or flexibility to easily return to a full-time education programme (Crudden, Sansing and Butler, 2005), and their fundamental tech-nology skills may be significantly more limited than those of the younger generations. Learning a new career as an older adult is likely to be exceptionally challenging, particularly since the lecture and rote memorisation methodologies used in most post-secondary educational envi-ronments are not necessarily optimal for older learners who thrive in more constructivist and participatory environments (Chu and Tsai, 2009). Older learners will also lack the work/study habits that could otherwise facilitate their educational experience (Clarke, 1980). Finally, the independent living, orientation and mobility and technology skills (discussed above), which are essential to successful employment after vision loss, are equally necessary for success in education and must be mastered before attempting advanced educational programmes.

Prior employment experiences and career stage

Despite the importance of education, research on employment and visual impairment clearly indicates that education on its own, without employment or employment-like experiences, is a poor contributor to employment outcomes (Joseph and Robinson, 2012; Kirchner et al., 1999; Kirchner and Smith, 2005; Wolffe, 2008). Work experiences, whether of a voluntary, internship or paid modality, provide concrete evidence of capabilities, and provide opportunities for job seekers with visual impairments to develop the skills, self-confidence, strategies and self-advocacy skills that will be required for success in the workplace. For adults with congenital visual impairments, early career exploration opportunities will help guide the individual toward realistic, attainable career goals. Galer (2014) recounts how several interview participants expressed significant appreciation for the early part-time employment opportunities provided to them by the CNIB, which ultimately led to full-time employment with the CNIB and eventually successful public service careers at various levels of government. Among those with adventitious vision loss who have prior work experience, these are opportunities not to prove a capability to work in a particular job, but to prove that one has learned and mastered the adaptive techniques required for accomplishing everyday workplace tasks.

For older individuals who have more established careers, the path forward will depend upon the nature of their existing line of work. If they were a lawyer, accountant, pastor or secretary, for example, it is likely that, given sufficient time to develop compensatory adaptive technology skills, they will be able to return to the same or similar line of work. Such was the case for the ten case studies (of individuals who retained competitive employment after vision loss) profiled by Crudden and Fireison (1997), many of whom were able to retain their job with their existing employer, albeit in a slightly different role. Especially for established professionals well advanced in their career, the prospect of "starting over" and accepting entry-level work in another field may be discouraging, disheartening and highly unmotivating (Crudden et al., 2005). Unfortunately, in some cases, where the loss of sight prohibits continued employment in their chosen field (e.g. truck drivers, heavy machinery operators, etc.), radical changes and re-training may be unavoidable.

Older adults with visual impairments are also subject to the same sociocultural forces that influence the employment outcomes of other older adults. There is a significant body of literature, for example, that explores the impact of ageism – "a process of systematic stereotyping of and discrimination against people because they are old, just as racism and sexism accomplish this for skin colour and gender" (Loretto, Duncan and White, 2000, p. 280) – on the employment experiences of older adults. The concept of ageism gained prominence in Britain and other Western countries in the 1990s due to concerns in the labour market about the early withdrawal of older workers. While this may happen through retirement (voluntary or otherwise), older adults who are terminated or dismissed have a disproportionately difficult time re-acquiring employment (Campbell, 1999). Among other things, employers perceive older workers as being less productive, having deficient skill sets (particularly where technology is concerned), resistant to change and prone to greater absenteeism (Loretto et al., 2000). While the reality is that age has been found to be a poor predictor of on-the-job performance (Doering, Rhodes and Schuster, 1983), older adults with visual impairments are not excluded from these societal forces. Prior experience, an up-to-date education, a demonstrable ability to learn or specialised skill sets could help to overcome these inherent prejudices.

Employer attitudes

Misconceptions about the capabilities of people with visual impairments play a significant role in the employment barriers faced by adults who are blind or who have low vision (WHO, 2011). Such stereotypes may lead to the belief among prospective employers that individuals with visual impairments will be less productive than their sighted colleagues, and may raise concerns about their ability to perform work-related tasks (WHO, 2011). Individuals with visual impairments often perceive the attitude of employers toward the hiring of a person with a visual impairment as a barrier to employment (Slade and Edwards, 2015, p. 26). Kirchner, Johnson and Harkins (1997) found that among both working and employment-seeking participants, the biggest problem in finding jobs were "employer attitudes" and employer discrimination. A study of 150 working-age members of the Royal New Zealand Foundation of the Blind found "employer attitudes" to be the second most common barrier to employment (La Grow and Daye, 2005).

While there is limited objective, empirical evidence on the attitudes that employers hold toward people with vision loss, Capella-McDonnall (2013) developed a scale intended to measure just that. The pilot study revealed that many employers did in fact have negative attitudes toward blind and visually impaired employees, but that this was largely balanced out by employers who had more positive viewpoints. Very few expressed *extremely* negative viewpoints, with only 6.5% scoring more than 1.5 standard deviations below the mean. Interestingly, employers who had hired a person who was blind or visually impaired in the past held statistically significantly more positive views than those who had not.

There is considerable evidence, including from employers themselves, that these attitudes are at least in part the result of ignorance and a lack of awareness about the abilities of people with visual impairments, rather than any overt intention to discriminate. A qualitative study by Golub (2006) focusing on the perceptions of employers integrating individuals with visual impairment into the workplace provides some insight into the employer mindset. The respondent employers acknowledged that for integration to be successful, social and cultural structures must be flexible and able to accommodate the integration of the new employees. Diversity must be seen within the workplace as an intrinsically valuable commodity and a strength rather than an accommodation. For example, the employer (and co-workers) must understand that there is not necessarily a single way of accomplishing a given task; that accommodations may need to be made to the way in which work is completed; necessary tools and equipment must be provided to facilitate the work that is to be done; and that efforts must be made to provide all workplace documentation, policies and procedures in an accessible format.

Other studies have highlighted the need for greater education and information to be provided to potential employers. One respondent to the RNIB's 2015 study of the work experiences of the blind and visually impaired in the UK noted that, "there seems to be a . . . lack of knowledge on the support you get and the duties of employer to provide this" (Slade and Edwards, 2015, p. 24). O'Day (1999) describes several negative experiences that visually impaired job seekers recounted in a qualitative study of 20 current recipients of social security benefits, including one who was not hired "because an employer did not think he could get to the bathroom or the cafeteria independently" and another who was denied the opportunity to volunteer at a community folk festival because the volunteer coordinator could not "think of something a blind person can do". Employers themselves have indicated that they would benefit greatly from having information about how a blind employee would use office technologies or communicate information, and appear to believe that specialised assistance or instruction is required in relation to otherwise routine human resource matters, such as the provision of insurance coverage or the handling of potentially negative performance reviews (Kirchner et al., 1997).

Multiple pathways have been advanced through which such education could be undertaken. Participants in the New Zealand study identified proactive vocational training and placement services as the first line of offence against "reluctant or ignorant employers", as this would allow candidates to prove themselves on the job (La Grow and Daye, 2005). Taking a different tact, the German Federation of the Blind and Partially Sighted established a Network for Vocational Participation, the goal of which is to specifically educate employers on the potential of individuals with vision loss (Reymann, 2008). In the UK, the Employers' Forum on Disability (EFD) has developed an innovative approach by making it easier for employers to employ and do business with people with disabilities, pioneering approaches in targeted recruitment and developing leaders among the disability community that work closely as advisors and ambassadors to employers worldwide (WHO, 2011, pp. 249–250). Similarly, a public utility (electricity) company in Rio de Janeiro, Brazil, takes such pride in their accomplishments that each invoice contains a picture of a wheelchair and a statement, "At Light, the number of workers with disabilities is greater than that required by law. The reason is simple – for us, the most important thing is to have valuable people" (WHO, 2011, p. 249).

The lack of awareness within the employer community about the abilities of blind and visually impaired employees and the techniques they might use to perform their jobs highlights the need for supported employment opportunities, in which transitional integration assistance is provided by professionals with specific knowledge in these areas. Even for individuals with established careers who lose their vision later in life, supportive employment circumstances may be helpful to demonstrate to both the employer and the employee that, with appropriate accommodations, the individual can continue working or begin working in a new field. Financial incentives, such as tax deductions, government funding for employment and workplace accommodations, temporary transition wage subsidy programmes and dedicated external support resources may help to assuage employer reluctance to commit to hiring employees with visual impairments (WHO, 2011, p. 242).

Environmental and workplace accessibility

Above and beyond employer attitudes, adults with visual impairments frequently cite environmental and workplace accessibility as barriers to either securing employment or to fully participating in workplace culture (Crudden et al., 1998; O'Day, 1999; Slade et al., 2017). Reflecting results from similar studies, O'Day (1999) interviewed 20 unemployed adults with visual impairments who highlighted the limited availability, reliability or scheduling of public transportation as a significant barrier to employment. Slade and Edwards (2015) likewise found (through interviews of more than 1,200 participants across the UK) that transportation was a concern among 35% of respondents, and limited the potential for working, for example, in jobs that require odd-hour shiftwork. In a similar manner, access to information both for job-search purposes and within the workplace (including the accessibility of workplace software, forms and other systems) is also frequently cited (Golub, 2006; Shaw et al., 2007).

At a broader level, however, disability activists in recent years have argued for a philosophical shift in discourse that tackles societal and environmental barriers in proactive rather than reactive ways. The concept of "universal design" is based on the notion that designing with accessibility and inclusion in mind from the *start* responds to the diverse needs of all users, without the need for a myriad of one-off special accommodations (Mueller, 1999). In technological contexts, principles of universal design have led to the widespread use of mainstream touch-screen devices such as the Apple iPhone and iPad, which incorporate built-in accessibility features for users with vision, hearing, motor and learning difficulties. These same features that increase usability for people with disabilities (such as Siri and voice-dictation) are almost always adopted by non-disabled users as well. These same principles can be extended to the workplace as a means to establish a more inclusive work culture and to minimise the need for additional accommodations. For example, forwarding inbound telephone messages to their intended recipients by email (rather than with small slips of paper left on their desk) would eliminate information access barriers *and* provide out-of-office employees with immediate access to the information. Such changes often make economic sense for the employer, as they help to keep more people productive at work in spite of changing physical and functional abilities (Mueller, 1999).

Independence and blindness skills and vocational rehabilitation

Success in employment generally requires that the prospective employee has a sufficient grasp of basic blindness and independence skills needed to function within the workplace, including the ability to independently carry out activities of daily living, orientation and mobility skills, and suitable proficiency with communication and technological aids (Shaw et al., 2007). Of these skill sets, technological proficiency, orientation and mobility, and knowledge of braille appear to be of particular importance. Capella-McDonnall and Crudden (2009), for example, showed that after participating in a vocational rehabilitation programme, 91% of those proficient with technological aids held a job, compared to 25% of those who could not use them. Mobility skills are similarly positively associated with work participation, with Bell and Mino (2013) finding a 66% employment rate among users of long white canes compared with a 34% employment rate among those not using a cane at all. Ryles (1996) found significantly increased employment rates among congenitally legally blind adults who extensively used braille and acquired braille reading skills in life. Bell and Mino (2015) likewise found that those who read braille were statistically significantly more likely to be employed (58% vs 44% of non-braille readers) and reported statistically significantly greater earnings ($45,947 vs $34,826 for non-braille readers).

Among those who are congenitally blind, these skills will hopefully have been developed as a natural progression of their general education programming and college/university transition activities (see Chapter 11 by Karen Wolffe for more information); however, gaps may remain. For those who lose significant amounts of vision as an adult, a much longer period of vocational rehabilitation may be required to acquire these skills and gain sufficient proficiency to apply them in a workplace environment.

This skills requirement may seem self-evident, but as the examples cited by Crudden et al. (2005) demonstrate, addressing these needs can become complex. Adjustment to vision loss requires significant psychosocial adaptation, and many clients may avoid participating in otherwise available rehabilitation services due to initial denial and the stigma attached to labels such as "blindness" (Adam and Pickering, 2009; Overbury, Wittich and Ferraresi, 2008; Southall and Wittich, 2012). This is especially true of individuals with low vision who may be able to "pass" or carry out most activities independently, but who might truly benefit from the use of a mobility aid such as a white cane or guide dog that would inherently disclose their impairment (Southall and Wittich, 2012). For example, in a ten-person case study of individuals who successfully maintained employment after vision loss, Mr Sanchez, a pastor of a church in a small western town (who also moonlighted as a computer salesmen and technician) admitted that he, "wasted a lot of years because of fear and laziness and just procrastination . . . That was a big pride trip with me at the time and I probably should have been learning braille and beginning to do more preparation" (Crudden and Fireison, 1997, p. 64). At the same time, some may be under significant pressure (owing to financial, psychological, familial or bureaucratic circumstances) to return to work before they are truly comfortable with adaptive techniques. In other cases, well-educated and previously "successful" individuals who acquire significant vision loss later in life may be unwilling to take entry-level positions, but lack the sophisticated adaptive skills, emotional adjustment to visual impairment or technology training to make them truly competitive in the marketplace (Crudden et al., 2005).

The infrastructure and mechanisms through which vocational rehabilitation services are delivered vary significantly from one jurisdiction to the next. In the United States, a coordinated federal–state vocational rehabilitation system exists that delivers services to all individuals with disabilities, including those who are blind or who have low vision. Current and former military personnel may also receive benefits and rehabilitation services through the Department of Veterans Affairs. In most parts of Canada, vocational rehabilitation services are primarily delivered through CNIB (formerly the Canadian National Institute for the Blind), a private charitable foundation that relies largely on donations from the general public to fund its operations (Ponchillia and Ponchillia, 1996). In the province of Quebec, services are delivered through a complex network of government agencies with partly overlapping mandates, sometimes delineated along the French–English linguistic lines (Wittich et al., 2013).

Notwithstanding these differences in administrative structures, the general vocational rehabilitation process typically consists of initial eligibility screening; preliminary vision and ophthalmic assessments to ascertain visual functioning and capabilities; planning a rehabilitation programme; providing rehabilitation instruction on the use of communication and assistive technologies, activities of daily living and orientation and mobility skills (often in parallel); and the provision of vocational training services including career prospect identification (aptitude assessment), simulated job situations, job-specific training, job-seeking skills, short-term work or internship placements and, ultimately, placement and transition to gainful employment (Ponchillia and Ponchillia, 1996; Wittich et al., 2013, p. 485). Pre- and post-training appraisals of employment readiness may be made using the validated and standardised CNIB Tool to Assess Preparedness for Employment (TAPE) measure (Shaw and Gold, 2011), which evaluates an individual's self-judgment on ten factors known to be associated with employment success, such as perceived knowledge and skills on computers and adaptive technology (Wittich et al., 2013, p. 488). Though still rarely used systematically, measures such as the TAPE would allow for comparison of employment readiness training across sites, programmes, service providers and countries, thereby helping the field of vocational rehabilitation improve outcomes by learning from each other.

One component of blind and low vision vocational rehabilitation programmes that has not been extensively studied is the incorporation of mentoring programmes, which connect career hopefuls with individuals who are blind or who have low vision and who are already working in a particular field. Such programmes have shown improvements in transition outcomes in youth and young adults, including increased optimism, self-efficacy in career decision-making and assertiveness in job hunting (Bell, 2012; O'Mally and Antonelli, 2016), but little is yet known about the potential application of these tools to older adults with adventitious vision loss. In a recently reported study of college graduates, Antonelli, Steverson and O'Mally (2018) found that students provided with a mentoring opportunity were significantly more likely than non-mentored students to have found employment independently, and demonstrated greater assertiveness in their job search (which, as discussed earlier, is itself an important contributor to employment outcomes). Certainly, access to successful blind individuals as mentors will provide clients seeking employment with positive role models who can share first-hand experiences and practical advice and support.

The development of these skills is best achieved through efficient and effective vocational rehabilitation programming. Kirchner et al. (1997) explored the key facilitators and barriers to the achievement of employment outcomes for clients of the Illinois Bureau of Blind Services, and identified five strategies that could help to improve these outcomes. First, effective communication between the rehabilitation agency and employers, clients and rehabilitation professionals is required. This should include, for example, referring clients to consumer organisations that may be able to provide supplementary resources, and implementing feedback and evaluation-gathering activities to continually monitor programme performance. Second, a greater emphasis on data-derived placements and career orientations (including tie-ins to the state's general employment assistance systems) would better enable clients and their counsellors to explore potential employment opportunities. Third, vocational rehabilitation services must address the full gamut of job readiness skills including literacy (reading and writing using, as appropriate, braille, large type, computers, CCTVs, etc.), orientation and mobility and independent living skills. Fourth, rather than adopting a one-size-fits-all approach, service providers must be prepared and equipped to deliver a variety of specialised vocational rehabilitation services as appropriate: job retention to maintain existing employment, job placement to find new employment, transition assistance for students or those changing careers and career advancement for those seeking upward mobility. Finally, service providers should incorporate the first-hand expertise of successfully employed blind and visually impaired adults in different career domains to inform their service provision strategies.

Conclusion

Notwithstanding all the existing research on employment of the blind and visually impaired, to say nothing of the efforts of governments, advocates, community organisations and vision rehabilitation professionals, employment rates of the blind remain alarmingly low across age groups and across countries. Part of the reason for this may be that much of the existing literature is focused on identifying real or perceived problems, rather than on developing evidence-based solutions to those problems. In devising future research protocols, three recommendations arise from these observations. First, researchers must consider that as the population ages so significantly, there has been and will continue to be a significant rise in the number of people with adventitious vision loss who are seeking re-employment and whose vocational rehabilitation needs are vastly different from those of the congenitally blind. Second, the often-cited employment rates do not adequately account for the significant comorbidities that appear to exist for blind and visually impaired individuals (see Chapter 27 by Wittich and Simcock), and it is not at all clear from the research that blindness *alone* is the determining factor of employment outcomes. Finally, while much research has been done on employment rates, little is reported on the employment readiness or job-searching skills of those individuals. This makes it very difficult to unravel or pinpoint the myriad of internal and external factors that could determine those outcomes. Future research on employment, underemployment and unemployment rates of the blind must do more to consider these conflating concerns. Economic and political instabilities that influence the employment market affect us all but an argument can be made that individuals with disabilities are more vulnerable to these effects. As part of the ongoing efforts to improve the situation of persons with visual impairments, additional efforts will need to be made in order to strengthen their ability to be gainfully employed and to find fulfilment in the work they conduct. Such stability will provide a framework for persons with a visual impairment to self-direct and self-control their lives, thereby improving their ability to participate in society on an equal footing with others.

References

Adam, R. and Pickering, D. 2009. Where are all the clients? Barriers to referral to low vision rehabilitation. *Vision Impairment Research*, 9(2–3), 45–50.

Ajuwon, P. and Oyinlade, O. 2008. Educational placement of children who are blind or have low vision in residential and public schools: A national study of parents' perspectives. *Journal of Visual Impairment and Blindness*, 102(6), 325–339.

American Foundation for the Blind. n.d. *CareerConnect for job seekers who are blind or visually impaired* [e-publication]. Accessed July 2018. www.afb.org/info/living-with-vision-loss/for-job-seekers/12.

Antonelli, K., Steverson, A. and O'Mally, J. 2018. College graduates with visual impairments: A report on seeking and finding employment. *Journal of Visual Impairment and Blindness*, 112(1), 33–45.

Arim, R. 2015. *Canadian survey on disability, 2012: A profile of persons with disabilities among Canadians aged 15 years or older, 2012*. Ottawa, ON: Statistics Canada.

Australian Bureau of Statistics. 2016a. *Average weekly earnings, Australia, Nov. 2016* [e-publication]. Accessed January 2018. www.abs.gov.au/AUSSTATS/abs@.nsf/allprimarymainfeatures/F92AC28F348B112B CA25817E00140618?opendocument.

Australian Bureau of Statistics. 2016b. *Disability, ageing and carers, Australia: Summary of findings, 2015* [e-publication]. Accessed January 2018. www.abs.gov.au/ausstats/abs@.nsf/Latestproducts/4430.0Main %20Features452015?opendocumentandtabname=Summaryandprodno=4430.0andissue=2015andnum= andview=.

Barnes, C., Mercer, G. and Shakespeare, T. 1999. *Exploring disability: A sociological introduction*. Chichester: Wiley.

Bell, E. 2012. Mentoring transition-age youth with blindness. *Journal of Special Education*, 46(3), 170–179.

Bell, E. and Mino, N. 2013. Blind and visually impaired adult rehabilitation employment survey: Final results. *Journal of Blindness Innovation and Research*, 3(1). http://dx.doi.org/10.5241/2F1-35.

Bell, E. and Mino, N. 2015. Employment outcomes for blind and visually impaired adults. *Journal of Blindness Innovation and Research*, 5(2). http://dx.doi.org/10.5241/5-85.

Bjorkmann, A. 2008. Of course I'm going to work! [presentation]. *Proceedings of the 9th International Conference on Low Vision: Vision 2008*. Montréal, Québec.

Brown, D.K. 2001. The social sources of educational credentialism: Status cultures, labor markets, and organizations. *Sociology of Education*, 74, 19–34.

Campbell, N. 1999. *The decline of employment among older people in Britain*. London: Centre for Analysis of Social Exclusion.

Capella-McDonnall, M. 2005. Predictors of competitive employment for blind and visually impaired consumers of vocational rehabilitation services. *Journal of Visual Impairment and Blindness*, 99(5), 303–315.

Capella-McDonnall, M. 2013. Employer attitudes toward blind or visually impaired employees: Initial development of a measurement instrument. *Rehabilitation Counseling Bulletin*, 20(10), 1–18.

Capella-McDonnall, M. and Crudden, A. 2009. Factors affecting the successful employment of transition-age youths with visual impairment. *Journal of Visual Impairment and Blindness*, 103(6), 329–341.

Caprani, N., O'Connor, N.E. and Gurrin, C. 2012. Touch screens for the older user. In F.A. Cheein (ed.), *Assistive technologies* (pp. 95–118). IntechOpen [e-publication]. Accessed February 2018. www. intechopen.com/books/assistive-technologies/touch-screens-for-the-older-user.

Centers for Disease Control and Prevention. 2016. Employment status by disability status and types. *Disability and Health Data System* [e-publication]. Accessed February 2018. https://dhds.cdc.gov.

Chu, R.J.-C. and Tsai, C.-C. 2009. Self-directed learning readiness, Internet self-efficacy and preferences towards constructivist Internet-based learning environments among higher-aged adults. *Journal of Computer Assisted Learning*, 25(5), 489–501.

Clarke, J.H. 1980. Adults in the college setting: Deciding to develop skills. *Adult Education*, 30(2), 2–100.

Clement, D., Silver, W. and Trottier, D. 2012. *The evolution of human rights in Canada*. Ottawa, ON: Canadian Human Rights Commission.

Collin, C. 2008. *Measuring poverty: A challenge for Canada*. Ottawa, ON: Library of Parliament.

Crudden, A. and Fireison, C.K. 1997. *Employment retention after vision loss: intensive case studies*. Starkville, MS: Mississippi State University.

Crudden, A., McBroom, L., Skinner, A.L. and Moore, J.E. 1998. *Comprehensive examination of barriers to employment among persons who are blind or visually impaired*. Starkville, MS: Mississippi State University.

Crudden, A., Sansing, W. and Butler, S. 2005. Overcoming barriers to employment: Strategies of rehabilitation providers. *Journal of Visual Impairment and Blindness*, 99(6), 325–335.

Deloitte Access Economics Pty Ltd. 2016. *Socioeconomic impact of low vision and blindness from paediatric eye disease in Australia.* Sydney, Australia: Save Sight Institute.

Dixon, J. 1983. Attitudinal barriers and strategies for overcoming them. *Journal of Visual Impairment and Blindness*, 77(6), 290–292.

Doering, M., Rhodes, R. and Schuster, M. 1983. *The aging worker: Research and recommendations.* London: Sage.

Donohue, B., Acierno, R., Van Hasselt, V. and Hersen, M. 1995. Social skills training in a depressed, visually impaired older adult. *Journal of Behavior Therapy and Experimental Psychiatry*, 26(1), 65–75.

Duquette, J. and Baril, F. 2013. *Factors influencing work participation for people with a visual impairment.* Longueuil, Quebec: Institut Nazareth and Louis-Braille [e-publication]. Accessed March 2018. www.inlb.qc.ca/wp-content/uploads/2015/01/Factors-influencing-work-participation-in-persons-with-VI.pdf.

Erickson, W., Lee, C. and von Schrader, S. 2017. *Disability statistics from the American community survey (ACS)* [e-publication]. Accessed July 2018 www.disabilitystatistics.org.

Feather, N.T. and O'Brien, G.W. 1987. Looking for employment: An expectancy-valence analysis of job-seeking behavior among school-leavers. *British Journal of Psychology*, 78(2), 251–272.

Fichten, C., Asuncion, J. and Scapin, R. 2014. Digital technology, learning, and postsecondary students with disabilities: Where we've been and where we're going. *Journal of Postsecondary Education and Disability*, 27(4), 369–379.

French, S. 2017. *Visual impairment and work: Experiences of visually impaired people.* Abingdon, UK: Routledge.

Galer, D. 2014. *"Hire the handicapped!" Disability rights, economic integration and working lives in Toronto, Ontario 1962–2005.* Toronto, ON: University of Toronto.

Garvia, R. 1996. The professional blind in Spain. *Work, Employment, and Society*, 10(3), 491–508.

Goetz, Y.H., Lierop, B.A.G.V., Houkes, I. and Nijhuis, F.J.N. 2010. Factors related to the employment of visually impaired persons: A systematic literature review. *Journal of Visual Impairment and Blindness*, 104(7), 404–418.

Golub, D.B. 2006. A model of successful work experience for employees who are visually impaired: The results of a study. *Journal of Visual Impairment and Blindness*, 100(12), 715–725.

Greenland, C. 1976. *Vision Canada: The unmet needs of blind Canadians.* Toronto, ON: Canadian National Institute for the Blind.

Hagenmoser, S.D. 1996. The relationship of personality traits to the employment status of persons who are blind. *Journal of Visual Impairment and Blindness*, 90(2), 134–144.

Hartman, R.O. and Betz, N.E. 2007. The five-factor model and career self-efficacy: General and domain-specific relationships. *Journal of Career Assessment*, 15(2), 145–161.

Herie, E. 2005. *Journey to independence: Blindness – the Canadian story.* Toronto, ON: Dundurn.

Hersen, M., Kabacoff, R.I., Van Hasselt, V.B., Null, J.A., Ryan, C.F., Melton, M.A. and Segal, D.L. 1995. Assertiveness, depression, and social support in older visually impaired adults. *Journal of Visual Impairment and Blindness*, 89(6), 524–530.

Hewett, R. and Keil, S. 2016. *Investigation of data relating to blind and partially sighted people in the quarterly labour force survey: October 2012–September 2015.* London: RNIB.

Hill, K., Davis, A., Hirsch, D., Padley, M. and Smith, N. 2015. *Defining a minimum income standard for people who are sight impaired.* London: Thomas Pocklington Trust.

Historic England, n.d. *The impact of the First World War* [e-publication]. Accessed February 2018. https://historicengland.org.uk/research/inclusive-heritage/disability-history/1914-1945/war.

Jenkins, S.P. and Rigg, J.A. 2003. *Disability and disadvantage: Selection, onset and duration effects.* London: London School of Economics.

Jo, S.-J., Chen, R.K. and Kosciulek, J.F. 2010. Employment outcomes among individuals with visual impairments: The role of client satisfaction and acceptance of vision loss. *Journal of Applied Rehabilitation Counseling*, 41(3), 3–8.

Joseph, M.-A. and Robinson, M. 2012. Vocational experiences of college-educated individuals with visual impairments. *Journal of Applied Rehabilitation Counseling*, 43(4), 21–28.

Keegan, D.L., Ash, D.D.G. and Greenough, T. 1976. Blindness: Some psychological and social implications. *Canadian Psychiatric Association Journal*, 21(5), 333–340.

Kirchner, C., Johnson, G. and Harkins, D. 1997. Research to improve vocational rehabilitation: Employment barriers and strategies for clients who are blind or visually impaired. *Journal of Visual Impairment and Blindness*, 91(4), 377–392.

Kirchner, C., Schmeidler, E. and Todorv, A. 1999. *Looking at employment through a lifespan telescope: Age, health, and employment status of people with serious visual impairment.* New York: American Foundation for the Blind.

Kirchner, C. and Smith, B. 2005. Transition to what? Education and employment outcomes for visually impaired youths after high school. *Journal of Visual Impairment and Blindness*, 99(8), 499–504.

Koestler, F.A. 2004. *The unseen minority: A social history of blindness in the United States* [e-publication]. Accessed March 2018. www.afb.org/unseen/book.asp?ch=Koe-00toc.

La Grow, S. 2004. Factors that affect the employment status of working-age adults with visual impairments in New Zealand. *Journal of Visual Impairment and Blindness*, 98(9), 546–559.

La Grow, S.J. and Daye, P. 2005. Barriers to employment identified by blind and vision-impaired persons in New Zealand. *Social Policy Journal of New Zealand*, 26, 173–185.

Lacey, J.N. amd Crosby, O. 2004. Job outlook for college graduates. *Occupational Outlook Quarterly*, 48(4), 15–27.

Lee, I.S. and Park, S.K. 2008. Employment status and predictors among people with visual impairments in South Korea: Results of a national survey. *Journal of Visual Impairment and Blindness*, 102(3), 147–159.

Lepofsky, D. and Graham, R. 2009. Universal design in legislation: Eliminating barriers for people with disabilities. *Statute Law Review*, 30(2), 97–122.

Loretto, W., Duncan, C. and White, P. 2000. Ageism and employment: controversies, ambiguities, and younger people's perceptions. *Aging and Society*, 20, 279–302.

Lorimer, P. 2000. Origins of braille. In *Braille into the next millennium* (pp. 18–39). Washington, DC: National Library Service for the Blind and Physically Handicapped.

Mochizuki, C. 2013. *Working for equality: Activism and advocacy by blind intellectuals in Japan, 1912–1995*. Kansas, MO: University of Kansas.

Mueller, J. 1999. Assistive technology and universal design in the workplace. *Assistive Technology*, 10, 37–43.

Nijhuis, F.J.N., van Lierop, B. and van de Toren, K. 2008. Surviving in employment: The use of compensation strategies in the working situation [oral presentation]. *Proceedings of the 9th International Conference on Low Vision: Vision 2008*. Montréal, Québec.

O'Day, B. 1999. Employment barriers for people with visual impairments. *Journal of Visual Impairment & Blindness*, 93(10), 627–642.

O'Mally, J. and Antonelli, K. 2016. The effect of career mentoring on employment outcomes for college students who are legally blind. *Journal of Visual Impairment and Blindness*, 110(5), 295–307.

Overbury, O., Wittich, W. and Ferraresi, P. 2008. Barriers to vision rehabilitation: A new starting point. *Proceedings of the 9th International Conference on Low Vision: Vision 2008*. Montréal, Québec [e-publication]. Accessed March 2018. www.mabmackay.ca/librairies/sfv/telecharger.php?fichier=1288&menu=7&sousmenu=66.

Pearce, J.L. 2012. Not for alms but help: Fund-raising and free education for the blind. *Journal of the Canadian Historical Association*, 23(1), 131–155.

Ponchillia, P.E. and Ponchillia, SV. 1996. *Foundations of rehabilitation teaching with persons who are blind or visually impaired*. New York: American Foundation for the Blind.

Presley, I. and D'Andrea, F.M. 2009. *Assistive technology for students who are blind or visually impaired: A guide to assessment*. New York: American Foundation for the Blind.

Reymann, R. 2008. Blind people into work: lessons from an awareness raising campaign [presentation]. *Proceedings of the 9th International Conference on Low Vision: Vision 2008*. Montréal, Québec.

Rodolfo, C. 2009. *The employment of blind and partially-sighted persons in Italy: A challenging issue in a changing economy and society*. Paris, France: European Blind Union Commission on Rehabilitation, Vocational Training and Employment.

Ryles, R. 1996. The impact of braille reading skills on employment, income, education, and reading habits. *Journal of Visual Impairment and Blindness*, 90(3), 219–226.

Santuzzi, A.M., Waltz, P.R, Finkelstein, L.M. and Rupp, D.E. 2014. Invisible disabilities: Unique challenges for employees and organizations. *Industrial and Organizational Psychology*, 7(2), 204–219.

Schmit, M., Amel, E. and Ryan, A.M. 1993. Self-reported assertive job-seeking behaviors of minimally educated job hunters. *Personnel Psychology*, 46(1), 105–124.

Schriner, K. and Roessler, R. 1991. Public policy, work, and disability: Toward an agenda for action. In *The social organization of disability experiences* (pp. 41–46). Salem, OR: Willamette University and the Society for Disability Studies.

Shaw, A. and Gold, D. 2011. Development of a tool for the assessment of employment preparedness specifically for persons who are blind or partially sighted. *Work*, 39(1), 49–62.

Shaw, A., Gold, D. and Wolffe, K. 2007. Employment-related experiences of youths who are visually impaired: How are these youths fairing? *Journal of Visual Impairment and Blindness*, 101(1), 7–21.

Slade, J. and Edwards, R. 2015. *My voice 2015: The views and experiences of blind and partially sighted people in the UK, Version 1.1*. London: RNIB [e-publication]. Accessed March 2018. www.rnib.org.uk/sites/default/files/My%20Voice%202015%20-%20Full%20report%20-%20Accessible%20PDF_0.pdf.

Slade, J., Edwards, E. and White, A. 2017. *Employment status and sight loss*. London: RNIB [e-publication]. Accessed February 2018. www.rnib.org.uk/sites/default/files/Employment%20status%20and%20sight%20loss%202017.pdf.

Slade, J. and Simkiss, P. 2008. Work focus: Creating an employment marketplace for blind and partially sighted people. *Proceedings of the 9th International Conference on Low Vision: Vision 2008*. Montréal, Québec.

Smith, D. 2016. *Disability in the United Kingdom 2016: Facts and figures*. Cambridge: Papworth Trust.

Southall, K. and Wittich, W. 2012. Barriers to low vision rehabilitation: A qualitative approach. *Journal of Visual Impairment and Blindness*, 106(5), 261–274.

Statistics Canada. 2016a. *Canadian survey on disability: Seeing and hearing disabilities*. The Daily, 29 February [e-publication]. Accessed February 2018. www150.statcan.gc.ca/n1/daily-quotidien/160229/dq160229c-eng.htm.

Statistics Canada. 2016b. *Seeing disabilities among Canadians aged 15 years and older, 2012* [e-publication]. Accessed February 2018. www.statcan.gc.ca/pub/89-654-x/89-654-x2016001-eng.htm

Stats NZ. 2016. *NZ social indicators: Employment – Table 2 (annual employment)*, s.l.: Stats NZ [e-publication]. Accessed March 2018. http://archive.stats.govt.nz/browse_for_stats/snapshots-of-nz/nz-social-indicators/Home/Labour%20market/employment.aspx.

Thoms, P., Moore, K.S. and Scott, K.S. 1996. The relationship between self-efficacy for participating in self-managed work groups and the big five personality dimensions. *Journal of Organizational Behaviour*, 17(4), 349–362.

Turcotte, M. 2014. *Insights on Canadian society: Persons with disabilities and employment*. Ottawa, ON: Statistics Canada.

Tuttle, D.W. and Tuttle, N.R. 2004. *Self-esteem and adjusting with blindness: The process of responding to life's demands*. Springfield, IL: Charles C. Thomas.

United Nations. (n.d.). *Convention on the rights of persons with disabilities (CRPD)* [e-publication]. Accessed February 2018. www.un.org/development/desa/disabilities/convention-on-the-rights-of-persons-with-disabilities.html.

UPIAS. 1976 *Fundamental principles of disability*. London: Union of the Physically Impaired Against Segregation.

Varma, R., Vajaranant, T. and Burkemper, B. 2016. Visual impairment and blindness in adults in the United States: Demographic and geographic variations from 2015 to 2050. *Journal of the American Medical Association: Opthalmology*, 134(7), 802–809.

Villaneuva, I. and Di Stefano, M. 2017. Narrative inquiry on the teaching of STEM to blind high school students. *Education Sciences*, 7(89). doi:10.3390/educsci7040089

Visier, L. 1998. Sheltered employment for persons with disabilities. *International Labour Review*, 137(3), 347–365.

Wanberg, C.R., Watt, J.D. and Rumsey, D.J. 1996. Individuals without jobs: An empirical study of job-seeking behaviour and reemployment. *Journal of Applied Psychology*, 81(1), 76–87.

Wittich, W., Watanabe, D., Scully, L. and Bergevin, M. 2013. Development and adaptation of an employment-integration program for people who are visually impaired in Quebec, Canada. *Journal of Visual Impairment and Blindness*, 107(6), 481–495.

Wolffe, K. 1996. Career education for students with visual impairments. *Re: View*, 28(2), 89–93.

Wolffe, K. 2008. Career preparation: Research and practical implications for professionals [presentation]. *Proceedings of the 9th International Conference on Low Vision: Vision 2008*. Montréal, Québec.

Wong, C.-K. and Wong, H. 2004. The case for an expenditure-based poverty line for the newly industrialized East Asian societies. *Issues and Studies*, 40(2), 187–205.

World Health Organization. 2001. *International classification of functioning, disability and health (ICF)*. Geneva: Author.

World Health Organization. 2011. *World report on disability*. Geneva: Author.

Wright, S.E., McCarthy, C.A., Burgess, M. and Keefe, J.E. 1999. Vision impairment and handicap: The RVIB employment survey. *Australian and New Zealand Journal of Ophthalmology*, 27(3–4), 204–207.

27

Aging and combined vision and hearing loss

Walter Wittich and Peter Simcock

The problems of deafness are deeper and more complex, if not more important, than those of blindness. Deafness is a much worse misfortune. For it means the loss of the most vital stimulus – the sound of the voice that brings language, sets thoughts astir and keeps us in the intellectual company of man.

(Keller, 1933, p. 68)

Introduction

Any discussion of aging with a visual impairment would be incomplete without placing it in context of one of its common co-morbidities: hearing loss. This chapter begins with a description of the various current definitions and nomenclature of deafblindness /dual sensory impairment and how these relate to older individuals with combined vision and hearing loss. The next section reviews the literature on prevalence and incidence, with a particular focus on older people, across different geographic locations, as well as different subpopulations. The third section focuses on aetiology, noting both congenital and acquired conditions, and their development throughout the lifespan, followed by a brief overview of the history of deafblindness research. It then reviews the psychosocial impact of deafblindness on older people, and includes the priorities of older adults and how these link to the current development or offer of relevant services. Finally, the chapter concludes with a view of the future of deafblindness rehabilitation for older adults, and important gaps in the literature, outlining priorities for the research, policy and practice communities.

Definitions and nomenclature of deafblindness/dual sensory impairment/combined vision and hearing loss

Terminology in the field of combined vision and hearing loss remains complex and confusing, in part due to several historical, clinical and inter-professional reasons. Historically, the terms *deaf* and *blind* were combined and hyphenated when referring to individuals that had both sensory impairments; however, the non-hyphenated term *deafblind* was then proposed in order to reflect the unique properties of the combined impairment, not just the addition of one and the other (Lagati, 1995). The umbrella use of *deafblindness* in the clinical, service and rehabilitation context implies two interesting restrictions, whereby professionals assume that the sensory impairments are more severe (e.g. total absence of vision and hearing) and that the population described is made up of children or individuals with congenital impairment (Wittich et al., 2013). Meanwhile, non-clinical stakeholders, such as researchers or administrators reported that they lean towards the use of the term dual sensory impairment, which softens the description of this population and is potentially more inclusive, specifically when communicating with and about older adults with acquired sensory loss, who neither identify with nor want to seek services for blind and deaf individuals.

The classification and its terminology have been well described in its complexity by Dammeyer (2014) who breaks down the population categories based on whether each impairment is congenital or acquired and each ranging from mild to total. Ask Larsen and Damen (2014) took this approach further in the context of congenital aetiology, adding the dimensions of diagnostic/medical definitions, whether onset time preceded the development of communication abilities and ability as it relates to mobility and access to information, as well as onset order relative to chronological age. Such work develops the earlier identification of four distinct groups of deafblind people (Deafblind Services Liaison Group, 1988), which also considered the timing and order of onset of each impairment. The UK Department of Health (1997), in their good practice guidelines for health and social care services, added a fifth distinct group and applied the classifications specifically to older deafblind people: (1) those whose deafblindness has been acquired and developed in old age; (2) older people who have lived with sight impairment and subsequently acquire a hearing loss; (3) older deafened or hearing impaired people who have used speech to communicate, who subsequently acquire visual impairment; (4) older culturally Deaf people who use sign language, who subsequently acquire visual impairment; and (5) older people who have been deafblind for all or the majority of their life. The majority of deafblind people fall into the first of these groups.

In the context of the present chapter, this large variety and variability among terms and dimensions provides both a challenge and an opportunity because older adults with combined vision and hearing loss may be part of any and all the groups described above. Therefore, for the sake of continuity and simplicity within this chapter, we largely utilise the term *deafblindness* when referring to this population, independently of when or how the sensory losses occurred or how severe they are. We do, however, want to highlight that the great variability within this population is reflected in the great variability of their unique and specific needs, even though a single label may give the impression that this population is easily summarised within one term (Simcock, 2017b).

Prevalence and incidence

Obtaining accurate estimates of deafblindness prevalence is important in order to plan the allocation of resources, the education and preparation of the next generation of health and social care professionals, as well as the initiation of efforts for prevention, detection, treatment and rehabilitation. However, determining deafblindness prevalence is challenging because of the lack of a consistent definition for the phenomenon, limitations inherent to self-reported assessments of impairment, disability or handicap, in addition to communication difficulties in completing formal assessments and the comparatively small size of the population. Several efforts have been made to estimate the prevalence of age-related or acquired deafblindness, with specific focus on subgroups such as community-dwelling older individuals (Bazargan, Baker and Bazargan, 2001; Chia et al., 2006; Keller et al., 1999), those with intellectual disabilities (Evenhuis et al., 2001), those hospitalised for hip fractures (Grue, Kirkevold and Ranhoff, 2009; Lieberman, Friger and Lieberman, 2004), veterans (Lew et al., 2011; Smith, Bennett and Wilson, 2008), seniors receiving nursing home or long-term care (Guthrie et al., 2018; Guthrie et al., 2016; Yamada et al., 2015), as well as participants in large population-based epidemiological studies (Dawes et al., 2014; Gopinath et al., 2013; Kwon et al., 2015; Parfyonov et al., 2016). The overall consensus is that the prevalence of deafblindness increases with increasing age, and that great variability exists in prevalence among the subgroups. For example, using objective measures of vision and hearing, the proportion of older individuals with deafblindness has been reported as high as 20% in residential care or day centres (Roets-Merken et al., 2014) and up to 30.1% in hip fracture patients (Grue et al., 2009). When using subjective questionnaire measures of sensory loss, estimates have been as high as 26% in nursing home residents (Yamada et al., 2015), 33.9% in long-term care residents (Guthrie et al., 2016), and 37.6% among centenarians (Cimarolli and Jopp, 2014).

Estimates of the number of older people with congenital or early-onset deafblindness are not currently available. The closest approximations come from studies that describe specific deafblind populations, such as a study from Denmark that reported that 9 of their 190 congenitally deafblind participants (4.7%) were over the age of 60 (Dammeyer, 2010). Similarly, the portrait of the deafblindness rehabilitation population in Montreal, Canada (Wittich, Watanabe and Gagne, 2012) described that 69% of individuals receiving rehabilitation services for combined vision and hearing loss were reported to be over the age of 64; at the same time, within that the same population, 49% were categorised as having a diagnosis of any age-related or adult-onset sensory condition. These numbers indicate that 20% of the older adults in this population were receiving services for the rehabilitation of congenital or progressive illnesses, such as Usher syndrome or more rare conditions such as Charcot-Marie-Tooth syndrome (Evers, Barber and Wittich, 2012). One methodological challenge in interpreting these large differences may lie in differences in how congenital deafblindness is defined, reflecting what is perhaps an artificial distinction between congenital and acquired deafblindness (Möller, 2003), and whether individuals with Usher syndrome are included in such groupings or not. Arguably, Usher syndrome is a *congenital* condition resulting in *acquired* deafblindness. In the Montreal sample, this population is likely larger than elsewhere, given a reported Founder effect in the French-Canadian population (Ebermann et al., 2007). Incidence of deafblindness among older adults has only been examined in one population-based study (Schneider et al., 2012), which reported that, over a period of five years, there was a 1.6% incidence among individuals without sensory impairment, and a 11.3% incidence among those already affected with one sensory impairment. However, the authors mention that statistical power was low to identify specific risk factors due to survivor bias and the small sample that progressed to deafblindness within the study period.

Aetiology

This brings us to some of the most prevalent causes of deafblindness, an impairment known to have a "range of aetiologies" (Bodsworth, Clare and Simblett, 2011, p. 7). This range may be best demonstrated in Table 27.1, which provides diagnostic groupings and frequency counts for the data published by Wittich et al. (2012). It does not come as a surprise that one-third of individuals were diagnosed with the two most common age-related sensory impairments, namely age-related macular degeneration and presbycusis, affecting vision and hearing respectively. It becomes apparent that most age-related/acquired causes for vision loss (e.g. glaucoma or diabetic retinopathy) are independent of those causes reported for hearing loss (e.g. noise exposure),

Table 27.1 Diagnostic groupings and frequency counts of deafblindness.

Frequency	Description	Total
1. Hereditary/chromosomal syndromes and disorders		
1	Leber's congenital amaurosis	
1	Ataxia Charlevoix-Saguenay	
1	Leber's hereditary optic neuropathy (LHON) aka Leber's optic atrophy	
2	Retinitis pigmentosa; no hearing diagnosis	
1	Alstrom syndrome	
2	Charcot-Marie-Tooth syndrome	16
1	Cornelia de Lange syndrome	
2	CHARGE syndrome	
1	Jacobson syndrome	
1	Kearns-Sayre syndrome	
2	Norrie syndrome	
1	Refsum syndrome	
84	Usher's syndrome (undifferentiated)	
4	Usher's syndrome (Type 1)	95
5	Usher's syndrome (Type II)	
2	Wolfram syndrome (DIDMOAD)	
2	Mixed diagnosis (1–2)	11
9	Mixed diagnosis (1–3)	
	Total	122
2. Pre-natal/congenital complications		
3	Congenital rubella	
1	Neurometabolic disorder	5
1	Microcephaly (Seckel syndrome)	
1	Mixed diagnosis: congenital cataracts – neuropsychological impairment	
2	Mixed diagnosis: congenital cataracts – unspecified congenital condition	
1	Mixed diagnosis: cortical blindness – cerebral palsy	6
1	Mixed diagnosis: optic nerve coloboma – unspecified congenital condition	
1	Mixed diagnosis: optic nerve hypoplasia cerebral palsy	
3	Mixed diagnosis (2–1)	5
2	Mixed diagnosis (2–3)	
	Total	16
3. Post-natal/non-congenital complications		
1	Stroke	
2	Encephalitis	
2	Meningitis	13
1	Severe accidental head injury	
1	Sjögren's syndrome	
6	Tumor (e.g. craniopharyngioma, meningioma, rhabdomyosarcoma)	

(continued)

Table 27.1 (continued)

Frequency	Description	Total
3	Mixed diagnosis: diabetic retinopathy –adult-onset diabetes	
1	Mixed diagnosis: diabetic retinopathy – juvenile diabetes	
1	Mixed diagnosis: diabetic retinopathy –meningitis	
1	Mixed diagnosis: diabetic retinopathy –Ménière's disease	
1	Mixed diagnosis: direct trauma to eye and/or ear – severe head injury	12
1	Mixed diagnosis: optic atrophy secondary to stroke – severe head injury	
1	Mixed diagnosis: retinal detachment –perforated eardrum	
1	Mixed diagnosis: serpiginous choroiditis – traumatic noise exposure	
1	Mixed diagnosis: tumor – infection	
1	Mixed diagnosis: uveitis – infection(s)	
	Total	25

4. Related to prematurity

2	Complications of prematurity	2
	Total	2

5. Undiagnosed

1	No determination of etiology – age of onset unknown	1
1	Mixed diagnosis (5–1)	
2	Mixed diagnosis (5–2)	
1	Mixed diagnosis (5–3)	
4	Mixed diagnosis (1–5)	30
2	Mixed diagnosis (2–5)	
6	Mixed diagnosis (3–5)	
2	Mixed diagnosis (5–6)	
12	Mixed diagnosis (6–5)	
	Total	31

6. Age-related vision and hearing diagnoses

15	ARMD (atrophic/dry) – presbycusis	
23	ARMD (exudative/wet) – presbycusis	
87	ARMD (undifferentiated) – presbycusis	142
14	Glaucoma – prebycusis	
1	Maculopathy – presbycusis	
2	Retinopathy – presbycusis	
2	Mixed diagnosis (6–2)	
25	Mixed diagnosis (6–3)	
11	Mixed diagnosis (1–6)	60
1	Mixed diagnosis (2–6)	
21	Mixed diagnosis (3–6)	
	Total	202
	Grand total	398

except that each of their prevalence increases with increasing age. Another noteworthy complexity is the variability of combinations whereby one impairment may be acquired, whereas the other may be congenital. What complicates the picture further is that some of the diagnostic categories are associated with limited life span (e.g. Alstrom syndrome, CHARGE syndrome or Kearns-Sayre syndrome) whereas other are not (e.g. Charcot-Marie-Tooth syndrome); therefore, older adults with deafblindness are an extremely heterogeneous population as some of them have simply aged with a congenital condition. Similarly, Dammeyer (2010) provided a detailed description of aetiologies of congenital deafblindness, where the most frequent causes among those that lived into adulthood included Rubella (28.3%), Down's syndrome (7.9%) and complications related to prematurity (7.1%), in addition to 24.4% whose aetiologies were undetermined or unknown. Even though their sample age extended all the way to 80 years, a breakdown of aetiology for older adults was not available.

History of deafblindness research

The origins of deafblindness campaigning organisations are often found in shared concern about the needs of deafblind children. "Deafblind International", an international, not-for-profit membership organisation working to promote awareness of deafblindness and to influence appropriate service development globally, began its life in the 1950s as the *International Association for the Education of Deaf-Blind* (www.deafblindinternational.org/). At this time, its work centred on improving education for deafblind children. The UK charitable organisation *Sense* also began in the 1950s, with the campaigning work of ten families of children with congenital rubella syndrome. Similarly, the research community initially focused on deafblind children and their educational and rehabilitation needs (Wittich, Jarry et al., 2016). It was not until the 1980s that organisations became explicitly concerned with the needs of other groups of deafblind people. In particular, Wittich, Jarry et al. (2016) note emerging consideration of the rehabilitation needs of older people with acquired deafblindness. This decade also saw a broadening of the age range of deafblind persons included in research activity. Much of this work was undertaken in the United States (Rönnberg and Borg, 2001), following amendments to the Rehabilitation Act 1973, which increased the mandate of the newly created National Institute of Handicapped Research (Wittich, Jarry et al., 2016). A 2001 review of the behavioural and communicative research on deafblind individuals during the 1980s and 1990s highlighted increased inclusion of diverse subgroups of deafblind people in research activity (Rönnberg and Borg, 2001). However, the authors noted that "[f]rom an international perspective, the population of deafblind [had] received little research attention" (p. 74). They go on to critique some of the included studies for failing to make explicit the particular subgroup of deafblind people under investigation. As a highly heterogeneous population, such omission has resulted in limited generalisability and difficulties in synthesising research findings; Dammeyer (2015) argues that this is one of the reasons for research in deafblindness remaining in its infancy, and calls on researchers to offer thorough definitions of the study population concerned.

As a result of changes in the demographic profile in developed countries, research into the needs of those with late-life acquired deafblindness has however increased and gained visibility. A systematic review of the literature on comorbidities and outcomes associated with deafblindness in older adults (Heine and Browning 2015) identified 42 papers concerned with this population. The papers report on research adopting a range of methodologies, including cross-sectional design and longitudinal studies, and the reviewers note the use of varying methods of vision and hearing assessment and a variety of terminology for deafblindness in this work. Such variation was also observed in Tiwana, Benbow and Kingston's (2016) systematic review of the impact of acquired deafblindness on everyday competence; the reviewers note how this problematises attempts to draw conclusions from the body of research.

While research on late-life acquired deafblindness has increased, there is a dearth of research on older people who have aged with deafblindness. This reflects the observation of Jeppsson Grassman and colleagues (2012) that little is known about the experiences of people ageing with a range of impairments. Though these are a much smaller subpopulation of older deafblind people than those with late-life acquired deafblindness, the need for further research has been noted (Simcock, 2017a). There have been calls for further study on changing clinical needs (Dalby et al., 2009) and on those of specific groups, for example, individuals born with congenital rubella syndrome during the 1960s rubella pandemic (Armstrong and O'Donnell, 2004) and those with Usher syndrome (Damen et al., 2005; Miner, 1995). Themes identified in a 2016 systematic review of the experiences of those ageing with deafblindness (Simcock, 2017a) were similar to those of adults ageing with other impairments: ongoing change and the resultant need for enduring adaptation; a particular relationship between ageing and impairment, with one exacerbating the other; a sense that while one can learn adaptive strategies having lived with impairment for a long time, it does not necessarily get easier. However, just as Heine and Browning (2015) and Tiwana et al. (2016) observe, Simcock (2017a) notes that both definitional variation and a failure of study authors to offer clarity in reporting on the particular deafblind population concerned, rendered synthesis of the identified material problematic.

The psychosocial impact of deafblindness on older people

Our understanding of the psychosocial impact of deafblindness on older people is adversely affected by the paucity of research on the consequences of the impairment (Brennan and Bally, 2007). Schneider et al. (2011) observe inconclusive findings relating to the presence of and nature of any additional or interactive impact of dual over single sensory impairment, albeit that "intuitively [deafblindness] may be expected to have additional impacts" (p. 1319). This has implications for future research priorities, which are considered later in this chapter. However, studies have identified various psychosocial consequences, which have been described as both serious (Heine and Browning, 2004) and wide-ranging (Brennan and Bally, 2007) and have the potential to impact on individuals' well-being (Dean et al., 2017).

Although they are a highly heterogeneous population, what deafblind people have in common is deprivation in use of the distance senses (sight and sound) (McInnes, 1999), resulting in difficulties with communication, accessing information and mobility (Department of Health, 1997). There is a recognised link between sensory impairment and communication difficulties (Heine and Browning, 2004); Erber and Scherer (1999) highlight that such difficulties can be severe and, for older people, are often complicated by co-morbidities common in later life such as dysarthria, depression and cognitive impairment. Responding to the limited evidence on the experience of communicative challenges associated with dual sensory loss, Heine and Browning (2004) undertook a systematic study involving in-depth qualitative interviews with ten older adults with sensory loss, four of whom had deafblindness. Participants reported frequent episodes of "communication breakdown", particularly in social and other group situations; these breakdowns often resulted in embarrassment, anxiety and fatigue. In their secondary analysis of two large datasets and case studies of 20 older adults with acquired deafblindness, Pavey, Douglas and Hodges (2009), similarly found communication difficulties to be "an extremely strong theme to emerge from the research" (p. 7). Participants reported feeling socially isolated, in part as a result of communication difficulties. The experience of social isolation among older deafblind people is noted elsewhere in the literature (see for example

Bodsworth et al., 2011; Cook, Brown-Wilson and Forte, 2006; Göransson, 2008; LeJeune, Steinman and Mascia, 2003; Schneider et al., 2011) and as such, ongoing human contact has been recommended in order to sustain the psychosocial well-being of this population (Erber and Scherer, 1999). Nonetheless, in their UK based study of the experiences of deafblind people using British Sign Language, Kyle and Barnett (2012) highlight that participants did not describe high levels of social isolation. However, as the authors acknowledge, participants in this study were "more confident", "already in contact with organisations" and "those who have friends who were also Deafblind" (p. 42). Furthermore, no participants over the age of 65 were recruited, and all participants identified as members of the Deaf community. These contrasting findings are illustrative of diverse experiences and differing psychosocial needs among the heterogeneous deafblind population.

While communication difficulties may result in diminished psychosocial well-being for some older deafblind people (Erber and Scherer, 1999), reflecting earlier research, Heine and Browning (2004) observed that their participants developed and adopted their own strategies for managing communication breakdown. Such strategies often involve making adjustments to communication methods and techniques; indeed, some older deafblind people have described how they have needed to learn new methods of communication over their entire life course (Göransson, 2008; Gullacksen et al., 2011; Spring, Adler and Wohlgensinger, 2012). This need may be associated with changes in residual hearing and vision or other age-related physical changes (Damen et al., 2005; Oleson and Jansbøl, 2005; Yoken, 1979). However, while communication training programmes have been recommended for both older deafblind people and their communication partners (Heine et al., 2002), Hersh (2013b) notes that the corresponding need for communication partners to adapt to such changes is not always acknowledged or explored in the literature; this impacts on our understanding of the psychosocial impact of communication difficulties associated with deafblindness.

Although sensory impairments have been described as "stable" conditions (Kelley-Moore, 2010; Shakespeare and Watson, 2001), older deafblind people report experiencing changes in both their hearing and vision in a number of studies (see for example Göransson, 2008; Gullacksen et al., 2011; LeJeune, 2010; Oleson and Jansbøl, 2005) and in personal accounts (see for example Pollington, 2008; Stiefel, 1991; Stoffel, 2012; Yoken, 1979). For those deafblind as a result of Usher syndrome, changes in vision in particular are noted, owing to the nature of retinitis pigmentosa progression (Damen et al., 2005; Miner, 1995, 1997). One reported consequence of such physical change is the need to make adjustments, particularly adjustment to progressive loss (Brennan and Bally, 2007), albeit that these changes are not always deteriorative in nature (Stoffel, 2012). Brennan and Bally (2007) observe that for many older people, loss of vision and hearing occurs alongside other losses or disengagements, such as retirement, widowhood and reduced social networks, impacting on the process of adaptation. Older people experience both physical and environmental change (Göransson 2008; Heine and Browning 2004) and a model of individual adjustment is therefore inadequate as an interpretative model. Göransson (2008) and Gullacksen et al. (2011) adopt a "life adjustment model" to interpret their interview and focus group data. This model acknowledges that adjustment is not just an individual response to impairment, but that people also need the social environment and service providers to adjust as they age.

It is not just those with late-life acquired deafblindness that experience such changes in hearing and vision. A survey collecting information on the ageing process completed by 58 congenitally deafblind adults in Denmark identified that some of these changes resulted from the original aetiology of deafblindness and their potential late manifestations; others were attributed to other disorders, including age-related conditions (Laustrup, 2004). Similarly, older adults who have aged with deafblindness are reported to experience the need to make a range of consequent adjustments (Simcock 2017a). This appears to support the conclusion of Göransson (2008) that "deafblindness can never be regarded as something static" (p. 16), irrespective of the age and timing of onset of the impairment.

Several studies report that single sensory impairment adversely impacts on the everyday competence and independence of older people (Lupsakko et al., 2002; Tiwana et al., 2016). Conversely, much less is known about how late-life acquired deafblindness affects such "everyday competence", defined as the ability to complete both activities of daily living (ADL) and instrumental activities of daily living (IADL) (Brennan, Su and Horowitz, 2006; Lupsakko et al., 2002; Roets-Merken et al., 2018; Tiwana et al., 2016). Even less is known about the impact of deafblindness on the independence of those ageing with the impairment, albeit that some older people report that living with deafblindness over a period of time does not make maintaining independence any easier (Damen et al., 2005; Simcock, 2017a).

A 2002 Finnish study found that older deafblind people had greater difficulty with ADL and IADL compared to those with either no or single sensory impairment (Lupsakko et al., 2002). Analysis of quantitative data in the UK identified that older deafblind people had increased difficulty with independent living skills; feelings of loss of independence were likewise evident in the qualitative data (Pavey et al., 2009). In their systematic review exploring the impact of late life acquired deafblindness on everyday competence, Tiwana et al. (2016) identified studies similarly reporting that the impairment adversely impacted on the ability to maintain independence (see, for example, Brennan, Horowitz and Su, 2005; Grue et al., 2009; Harada et al., 2008). Tiwana et al. (2016) also note that older people with deafblindness appear to have greater difficulty completing both ADL and IADL than those with single sensory loss. However, the authors highlight limitations of the studies included, such as varying definitions of deafblindness, reliance on self-reported sensory impairment, and small samples consisting of older people known to specialist organisations. Furthermore, older deafblind people may have additional age-related impairments and health problems that can impact on the maintenance of independence (Pavey et al., 2009) and Tiwana et al. (2016) acknowledge that "[i]t may be difficult to tease out the role of sensory impairments, physical illnesses and advancing age when people have difficulties with everyday tasks in later life" (p. 204). There have therefore been calls for further research, including recommendations for more qualitative studies, to explore the experiences of older deafblind people in relation to everyday competence (Schneider et al., 2011; Tiwana et al., 2016).

The negative impact of single sensory impairment on older people's quality of life has been observed in various studies (Bodsworth et al., 2011; Tay et al., 2007) and each impairment has been described as having a "unique detrimental effect" (Heine and Browning, 2015, p. 1). Less is known about the effect of deafblindness on quality of life (Bodsworth et al., 2011), though deafblind people have been observed as reporting reduced quality of life (Heine and Browning, 2014; Tseng et al., 2018). Brennan and Su (2003) and Dean et al. (2017) maintain that there is an increasing body of evidence that deafblindness has a negative impact on quality of life. Chia et al. (2006) and Dean et al. (2017) focus specifically on health-related quality of life (HRQOL) in their Australian and UK-based studies with deafblind people. Chia et al. (2006) observed that dual sensory impairment was associated with poorer HRQOL than single sensory loss; this association was evident irrespective of the aetiology of sensory impairment. Dean et al. (2017) undertook a survey-based study with 90 people with Usher syndrome, identifying a link between psychosocial well-being and HRQOL.

In addition to reduced HRQOL, older people with deafblindness have self-reported poorer health (Crews and Campbell, 2004; Tiwana et al., 2016). Congenitally deafblind people are identified as being at risk of further physical health problems in later life, in part owing to late manifestations of the original aetiology (Gullacksen et al., 2011). They have also been identified as being at greater risk than non-deafblind people of various emotional, psychological and mental health difficulties (Simcock, 2017a; Wickham, 2011), with higher risk of acute confusion in long-term residential care (Cacchione et al., 2003) and high levels of psychological distress (Bodsworth et al., 2011; Pavey et al., 2009). In their examination of delirium in older people admitted to a district hospital in the United States, George, Bleasdale and Singleton (1997) observed significantly higher levels of dual sensory impairment in those admitted with the condition. While psychological assessment of deafblind people is complex (Bodsworth et al., 2011), such findings do suggest that those with dual sensory loss are at increased risk of emotional, psychological and mental health problems.

However, whether deafblind people are at greater risk than the general population is difficult to determine. For example, when considering the research relating to depression among deafblind people, both Chou (2008) and Hersh (2013b) highlight mixed findings. Studies adopting both self-reporting and objective measures of impairment and health status have noted greater frequency of depressive symptoms or increased risk of depression among deafblind people than those without the impairment, even after controlling other significant covariates for the condition (Brennan and Bally, 2007; Cosh et al., 2017; Guthrie et al., 2016; Han et al., 2018; Schneider et al., 2011; Tiwana et al., 2016). However, Lupsakko et al. (2002) observed that while depressive symptoms were common in older deafblind people, major depression was not. Analysing data from the English Longitudinal Study of Ageing (ELSA), Chou (2008) observed that, once health indicators were controlled for, the association between deafblindness and depression was not maintained, while sight loss remained a clear predictor of depression. Volden and Saltnes (2010) note that depression among deafblind people may result from a number of complex, inter-related factors. For older deafblind people, the risk factors related to depression in later life, such as a move to residential care and increasing difficulty with ADL/IADL, may also be significant (Lupsakko et al., 2002; McDonnall, 2009).

Mixed findings are also evident in research on sensory loss and cognitive impairment (Tiwana et al., 2016). A Spanish study exploring the impact of deafblindness on cognition of older people found that those with deafblindness had poorer cognition than those single sensory impaired or with no sensory impairment (Vazquez et al., 2012). Similar to the Australian study of Gopinath et al. (2013) and the Icelandic study of Fisher et al. (2014), Guthrie and colleagues (Guthrie et al., 2018; Guthrie et al., 2016) observed higher rates of cognitive impairment among older deafblind people. However, in their US based quantitative study, Lin et al. (2004) found that deafblindness doubled the risk of cognitive decline over a period of four years, when compared to no sensory impairment, but not when compared with vision impairment alone, which posed a comparable level of risk. Led by the University of Manchester, UK, the European Sense Cog Project (www.sense-cog.eu) is seeking to develop our understanding of the relationship between age-related sensory impairment and cognitive and mental health functioning. A team of clinicians and researchers across Canada within Team 17 (Interventions at the Sensory-Cognitive Interface) of the Canadian Consortium on Neurodegeneration and Aging (http://ccna-ccnv.ca/en) are undertaking a range of experimental studies and interventions, qualitative interviews and analyses of large databases such as the Canadian Longitudinal Study on Aging (www.clsa-elcv.ca) to develop our understanding of the relationships between sensory and cognitive loss in older adults, specifically those who are at risk of dementia. Even though the assessment of dementia in the deafblind remains difficult (Bruhn and Dammeyer, 2018), such large-scale research projects will enhance our understanding and have the potential to inform interventions aimed at improving quality of life, care and support for the older deafblind population. Research-informed interventions are of particular importance in this context, as the risk of mental health difficulties among the deafblind population is exacerbated by the paucity of specialist services (Bodsworth et al., 2011; Mar, 1993; Wickham, 2011). The risk of misdiagnosis of mental health conditions, as a result of miscommunication or misinterpretation of the effects of deafblindness, has also been noted (Hersh, 2013a; Miner, 1997; Sauerburger, 1993).

The psychosocial consequences of deafblindness are not limited to the individual with the impairment. Lehane, Wittich and Dammeyer (2016) highlight that "[a]cquired sensory loss of one family member can have a significant impact on the well-being of the entire family, especially the spouse" (p. 34). However, although the impact of an individual's single sensory loss on their family has been extensively researched, Brennan and Bally (2007) maintain that much less is known about the impact of deafblindness on family members. While literature reviews have reported on the adverse impact of single sensory loss on older couples' psychosocial well-being (Lehane, Dammeyer and Elsass, 2016), Westaway, Wittich and Overbury (2011) found no significant differences between spouses of people with deafblindness and those with single sensory impairment, in relation to depression levels or caregiver burden, a conclusion likely limited by their small sample size.

Responding to the dearth of literature on this topic, particularly in relation to sexuality, Lehane et al. (2017) undertook the first known study to examine older couples' sexual activity where one spouse has acquired deafblindness. This survey-based study, adopting a cross-sectional design, involved 45 couples aged 50 years or over. Couples were asked about their sexual desire, sexual activity and satisfaction with their sex lives. Data identified reduced sexual activity among couples living with acquired deafblindness, which was associated with reduced desire and lower levels of sex life satisfaction. The study authors suggest therefore that "the experience of [acquired deafblindness] may have an impact on older couples' sexual relationships" (p. 9), and call on practitioners to pay careful attention to the importance of sexuality in their work with older deafblind people. A recent and, at the time of writing, on-going international online longitudinal study of couples' experiences of sensory loss, named the *International Study of Support and Sensory Loss Project (Project ISSSL)*, seeks to identify the most effective methods of support and coping for couples living with single and dual sensory loss; this study will further contribute to our understanding of the wider psychosocial impact of deafblindness.

The future of deafblindness rehabilitation and research

The current demographic trends are likely a driving force in how the field of deafblindness will develop over the coming decades (Christensen et al., 2009). In the demographic profile of deafblindness rehabilitation clients, Wittich et al. (2012) pointed out that the majority of service users in 2010 were over the age of 65, with over 43% being over 85, thereby representing the parents of the baby boomers. These proportions were similar to those reported in Denmark (Dammeyer, 2013), and their distribution is a good indicator of likely research and service provision priorities. Potential future directions and current gaps have been described from three different perspectives: older adults with deafblindness themselves (LeJeune, 2010), researchers working with this population (Saunders and Echt, 2007, 2011) as well as their clinical service providers (Wittich, Jarry, et al., 2016).

The study by LeJeune (2010) provided particularly rich data because the sample that participated in the nine focus groups consisted of all possible members of the aging deafblind community, including those who grew old with congenital impairments, as well as those with one or both acquired sensory losses, and those that communicated either orally or via sign language (as an aside, the challenges of conducting focus groups with deafblind sign language users have been described elsewhere (Arndt, 2011) and are worth reflection). LeJeune (2010) provided an insightful qualitative description of the client perspective on topics such as feeling abandoned by service delivery programmes, because many professionals traditionally trained and working with one sensory impairment were overwhelmed and unqualified to provide their services when a second sensory loss was present. Clients reported a lack of available information about assistive devices, and saw this lack reflected in the knowledge of their service providers as well. For culturally Deaf individuals, acquired vision loss becomes a communication disorder in addition to the impairments that are traditionally associated with visual impairment, such as mobility constraints. Participants reported that they faced ageist stereotypes and needed to overcome preconceived perceptions about older adults using assistive technologies in the presence of sensory loss (also see Fraser et al., 2016; Hersh, 2013b). Many of these challenges made them concerned about their future, initiating psychosocial and psychological fears of loneliness, depression and isolation (Mick et al., 2018). Finally, finding herself separated from life through her sensory losses, one participant pointedly expressed her lack of cognitive stimulation with the statement: "There is nothing to help my mind think" (LeJeune, 2010, p. 151), highlighting the possible effects of sensory deprivation.

From the perspective of clinical researchers in dual sensory impairment and aging, Saunders and Echt (2007) discussed research priorities. As far as service provision was concerned, they first pointed towards a need for training to detect acquired deafblindness and the development of screening tools that are suitable for older adults, an effort that is currently underway (McGilton et al., 2016; Wittich et al., 2018). Furthermore, they discussed the need for suitable and specific measurement techniques and tools because current evaluation and outcome measures in vision or hearing were designed for only one sensory impairment, not both. Since then, Dalby and colleagues (2009) have reported on the development of the Deafblind Supplement to the interRAI Community Health Assessment as an evaluation tool specifically designed for deafblindness (Hirdes et al., 2007); however, this supplement is linked to the administration of a detailed overall health assessment, and is not intended to be administered separately. Once deafblindness is detected, needs shift towards improved communication abilities between service providers and clients in order to ensure optimal adherence to treatment and intervention protocols. In the context of assistive technologies, the authors discussed three specific aspects of development priorities: improved communication, enhanced environmental awareness, as well as greater device usability. In the context of communication, the authors suggest increasing the combination of visual and auditory cues, in order to provide redundancy to increase signal over noise. Environmental awareness could potentially be improved through the enhancement of localisation cues, and the continued development of devices that are designed specifically for the deafblind (e.g. Vincent et al., 2014). Finally, Saunders and Echt (2007) suggested that interconnectivity of information may increase access to assistive technologies. Further, general accessibility and ergonomics will need to be improved; however, this direction of research has so far only received little attention (Evers et al., 2012; Wittich, Southall et al., 2016).

When pooling opinions from clinical and rehabilitation service providers, Wittich and colleagues (Wittich, Jarry et al., 2016) were able to separate which future directions were specific for rehabilitation versus research in deafblindness, and which overlapped. Common themes that have also been reflected in the previous work by LeJeune (2010) as well as Saunders and Echt (2007) included the need for improved assistive technologies, better communication services and strategies, as well as an overall more integrated interdisciplinary approach to this field. The results highlighted the importance of maximising the use of the remaining sensory abilities, and the need to work collaboratively, in order to avoid isolation of professional expertise. With regard to unique research priorities, participants echoed the need for more specific measurement tools, especially those that could capture the clinical outcomes of rehabilitation interventions, in order to provide better evidence to guide practice. Finally, there was a call for more systematic data tracking (e.g. client registries for accurate incidence and prevalence reports) and cost-analysis evaluation (e.g. for quantification of early intervention outcomes). This shift towards providing data likely reflects a transition of this field towards a domain rooted in a strong evidence base. All parties involved will need to contribute to this goal, including clinicians, health professionals, administrators and all other stakeholders.

Conclusion

Looking into the future of research in aging and deafblindness, one of the central challenges as well as opportunities is the need to consider the complexity and diversity of this population. The present chapter is a first attempt to combine knowledge and perspectives on aging with deafblindness across two main populations: those with congenital and those with acquired impairments. However, even this description is too simplified to do all our clients justice, given their heterogeneity. This diversity has other effects for our work, because the scientific literature is not centralised or easily accessible in one peer-reviewed journal, but widely distributed across many professional domains (Wittich et al., 2013). The *Journal of Deafblind Studies on Communication* (http://jdbsc.rug.nl) has become a focal point for research in this field; however, the central topics focus on communication acquisition and development in congenitally deafblind children. There is currently no comparable journal in aging. Resource access has taken important steps forward through online tools such as the Swedish database containing over 3,500 articles on deafblindness, hosted by the *Nationellt kunskapscenter för dövblindfrågor* (http://nkcdb.se/research-overview, interface available in Swedish and English) as well as an online Community of Practice on Deafblindness, *La communauté de pratique en surdicécité*, in Canada (http://cdpsurdicecite.org, interface available in French, translation into English is ongoing) and resources available through organisations such as the *Hellen Keller National Centre for Deaf-Blind Youths and Adults* (www. helenkeller.org/hknc). Still, challenges remain to elevate much of the available online information to a peer-reviewed level that can withstand the rigour of scientific standards.

One of the more philosophical challenges that remain to be investigated and validated in detail is the concept that deafblindness is a multiplicative impairment that goes beyond the addition of vision loss plus hearing loss, but creates a new and more severe entity because the absence of the second sense impairs the capacity to compensate. Luey (1994) describes how this phenomenon of "the combined loss of both hearing and vision creates a whole new world – muffled, blurred, and disorienting" (p. 213). Other authors such as Hersh (2013b) mention the additive or multiplicative effects of deafblindness in order to justify the complexity and severity of this impairment, but without further explanation or investigation of its multiplicative nature. Saunders and Echt (2012) took an important step when reviewing evidence spanning from the psychosocial effects and the functional limitations all the way to audio-visual integration and the neuroanatomical overlap between the two senses, demonstrating how the combined impairment (often) results in larger functional effects; however, these results are not always consistent and likely depend on the type of task or situation in which the measurements and observations are made. Establishing this "breaking point" where one sense cannot compensate for the other anymore is a challenge that continues to elude researchers.

The preparation of professionals working with the deafblind clientele (aging or otherwise) has been a point of discussion for some time (McInnes, 1999). More recently, other allied health care professions, such as occupational therapists, find themselves in need of training and expertise working with older adults that are affected by sensory impairment, but they find themselves lacking where their training is concerned (Wittich et al., 2015; Wittich et al., 2017).

This interest reflects a general underlying need for more information about deafblindness in the context of aging, which is further reflected in the recent inclusion of a chapter on sensory factors relevant to the design of assistive technologies for older adults in a textbook on gerontechnology (Wittich and Gagné, 2016). There remain numerous opportunities to raise awareness about deafblindness, at the level of front-line health and social care, as well as further up in the hierarchy of health and social care administration and policy. Some researchers may shy away from deafblindness as an area of investigation because of the perception that this type of work may be loaded with methodological challenges, and potential difficulties in obtaining funding and producing high-impact publications; however, in the context of geriatrics and gerontology this could be said about many aspects of the study of aging. As our field moves forward, the need for complexity and a tolerance for uncertainty and variability is essential in order to understand a world layered in the same complexity as its research topics.

References

Armstrong, N. and O'Donnell, N. 2004. Rubella: 40 years after the epidemic. *American Journal for Nurse Practitioners*, 8(4), 51–56.

Arndt, K., 2011. Conducting interviews with people who are deafblind: Issues in recording and transcription. *Field Methods*, 23(2), 204–214. https://doi.org/10.1177%2F1525822X10383395.

Ask Larsen, F. and Damen, S. 2014. Definitions of deafblindness and congenital deafblindness. *Research in Developmental Disabilities*, 35(10), 2568–2576. www.ncbi.nlm.nih.gov/pubmed/25016162.

Bazargan, M., Baker, R.S. and Bazargan, S.H. 2001. Sensory impairments and subjective well-being among aged African American persons. *Journals of Gerontology. Series B, Psychological Sciences and Social Sciences*, 56(5), 268–278.

Bodsworth, S.M., Clare, I.C.H. and Simblett, S.K. 2011. Deafblindness and mental health. *British Journal of Visual Impairment*, 29(1), 6–26. http://journals.sagepub.com/doi/10.1177/0264619610387495.

Brennan, M. and Bally, S.J. 2007. Psychosocial adaptations to dual sensory loss in middle and late adulthood. *Trends in Amplification*, 11(4), 281–300. http://journals.sagepub.com/doi/10.1177/10847138 07308210.

Brennan, M., Horowitz, A. and Su, Y. 2005. Dual sensory loss and its impact on everyday competence. *Gerontologist*, 45(3), 337–346. www.ncbi.nlm.nih.gov/entrez/query.fcgi?cmd=Retrieve&db=PubMed &dopt=Citation&list_uids=15933274.

Brennan, M. and Su, Y. 2003. Incidence and prevalence of dual sensory impairment in adults 70 years and older over 5 years. Poster presented at the *Annual Scientific Meeting of the Gerontological Society of America*. San Diego, CA.

Brennan, M., Su, Y. and Horowitz, A. 2006. Longitudinal associations between dual sensory impairment and everyday competence among older adults. *Journal of Rehabilitation Research and Development*, 43(6), 777–792. http://proquest.umi.com/pdf/aa98e7564dc143294d52930f4c381ba6/1292975847//share3/ pqimage/pqirs101v/201012211827/18091/24631/out.pdf.

Bruhn, P. and Dammeyer, J. 2018. Assessment of dementia in individuals with dual sensory loss: Application of a tactile test battery. *Dementia and Geriatric Cognitive Disorders Extra*, 8(1), 12–22. www.karger.com/ Article/FullText/486092.

Cacchione, P.Z., Culp, K., Dyck, M.J. and Laing, J. 2003. Risk for acute confusion in sensory-impaired, rural, long-term-care elders. *Clinical Nursing Research*, 12(4), 340–355. http://search.ebscohost.com/ login.aspx?direct=true&db=rzh&AN=2004031254&site=ehost-live.

Chia, E.-M., Mitchell, P., Rochtchina, E., Foran, S., Golding, M. and Wang, J.J. 2006. Association between vision and hearing impairments and their combined effects on quality of life. *Archives of Ophthalmology*, 124(10), 1465–1470. http://archopht.ama-assn.org/cgi/reprint/124/10/1465.pdf.

Chou, K.-L. 2008. Combined effect of vision and hearing impairment on depression in older adults: Evidence from the English Longitudinal Study of Ageing. *Journal of Affective Disorders*, 106(1–2), 191–196.

Christensen, K., Doblhammer, G., Rau, R. and Vaupel, J.W. 2009. Ageing populations: the challenges ahead. *Lancet*, 374(9696), 1196–1208. http://dx.doi.org/10.1016/S0140-6736(09)61460-4.

Cimarolli, V.R., Jopp, D.S. 2014. Sensory impairments and their associations with functional disability in a sample of the oldest-old. *Quality of Life Research: An International Journal of Quality of Life Aspects of Treatment, Care and Rehabilitation*, 23(7), 1977–1984.

Cook, G., Brown-Wilson, C. and Forte, D. 2006. The impact of sensory impairment on social interaction between residents in care homes. *International Journal of Older People Nursing*, 1(4), 216–224. http://dx.doi.org/10.1111/j.1748-3743.2006.00034.x

Cosh, S., von Tanno, T., Helmer, C., Bertelsen, G., Delcourt, C., Schirmer, H. and the SENSE-Cog Group. 2017. The association amongst visual, hearing, and dual sensory loss with depression and anxiety over 6 years: The Tromsø Study. *International Journal of Geriatric Psychiatry*, October, 1–8.

Crews, J.E. and Campbell, V.A. 2004. Vision impairment and hearing loss among community-dwelling older Americans: Implications for health and functioning. *American Journal of Public Health*, 94(5), 823–829.

Dalby, D.M., Hirdes, J., Stolee, P., Strong, J.G., Poss, J., Tjam, E.Y., Bowman, L. and Ashworth, M. 2009. Characteristics of individuals with congenital and acquired deaf-blindness. *Journal of Visual Impairment and Blindness*, 103(2), 93–102.

Damen, G.W., Krabbe, P.F., Kilsby, M. and Mylanus, E.A. 2005. The Usher lifestyle survey: Maintaining independence: a multi-centre study. *International Journal of Rehabilitation Research*, 28(4), 309–320. www.ncbi.nlm.nih.gov/entrez/query.fcgi?cmd=Retrieve&db=PubMed&dopt=Citation&list_uids=16319556.

Dammeyer, J. 2010. Prevalence and aetiology of congenitally deafblind people in Denmark. *International Journal of Audiology*, 49(2), 76–82. http://ovidsp.ovid.com/ovidweb.cgi?T=JS&CSC=Y&NEWS=N&PAGE=fulltext&D=emed9&AN=20151880.

Dammeyer, J. 2013. Characteristics of a Danish population of adults with acquired deafblindness receiving rehabilitation services. *British Journal of Visual Impairment*, 31(3), 189–197. http://jvi.sagepub.com/content/31/3/189.abstract.

Dammeyer, J. 2014. Deafblindness: A review of the literature. *Scandinavian Journal of Public Health*, 42(7), 554–562. www.ncbi.nlm.nih.gov/pubmed/25114064.

Dammeyer, J. 2015. Deafblindness and dual sensory loss research: Current status and future directions. *World Journal of Otorhinolaryngology*, 5(2), 37–40. www.wjgnet.com/2218-6247/full/v5/i2/37.htm.

Dawes, P., Dickinson, C., Emsley, R., Bishop, P.N., Cruickshanks, K.J., Edmondson-Jones, M., McCormack, A., Fortnum, H., Moore, D.R., Norman, P. and Munro, K. 2014. Vision impairment and dual sensory problems in middle age. *Ophthalmic & Physiological Optics: The Journal of the British College of Ophthalmic Opticians (Optometrists)*, 34(4), 479–488. www.ncbi.nlm.nih.gov/pubmed/24888710.

Deafblind Services Liaison Group. 1988. *Breaking through: Developing services for deafblind people*. London: Royal National Institute for the Deaf.

Dean, G., Orford, A., Staines, R., McGee, A. and Smith, K.J. 2017. Psychosocial well-being and health-related quality of life in a UK population with Usher syndrome. *BMJ Open*, 7(1), e013261. http://ovidsp.ovid.com/ovidweb.cgi?T=JS&PAGE=reference&D=prem&NEWS=N&AN=28082366.

Department of Health. 1997. *Think dual sensory: Good practice guidelines for older people with dual sensory loss*. London: Author.

Ebermann, I., Lopez, I., Bitner-Glindzicz, M., Brown, C., Koenekoop, R.K. and Bolz, H.J. 2007. Deafblindness in French Canadians from Quebec: A predominant founder mutation in the USH1C gene provides the first genetic link with the Acadian population. *Genome Biology*, 8(4), R47.

Erber, N.P. and Scherer, S.C. 1999. Sensory loss and communication difficulties in the elderly. *Australian Journal of Aging*, 18(1), 4–9.

Evenhuis, H.M., Theunissen, M., Denkers, I., Verschuure, H. and Kemme, H. 2001. Prevalence of visual and hearing impairment in a Dutch institutionalized population with intellectual disability. *Journal of Intellectual Disability Research*, 45(5), 457–464.

Evers, P., Barber, P. and Wittich, W. 2012. Telephone accessibility for dual sensory impairment: A case study. *Journal of Visual Impairment & Blindness*, 106(1), 43–46.

Fisher, D., Li, C.-M., Chiu, M.S., Themann, C.L., Petersen, H., Jonasson, F., Jonsson, P.V., Sverrisdottir, J.E., Garcia, M., Harris, T.B., Launer, L.J., Eiriksdottir, G., Gudnason, V., Hoffman, H.J. and Cotch, M.F. 2014. Impairments in hearing and vision impact on mortality in older people: The AGES-Reykjavik Study. *Age and Ageing*, 43(1), 69–76. http://apps.webofknowledge.com.proxy2.library.mcgill.ca/full_record.do?product=WOS&search_mode=AdvancedSearch&qid=9&SID=3AfCcpA4VdHzWa9gkaT&page=1&doc=4&cacheurlFromRightClick=no.

Fraser, S.A., Kenyon, V., Lagacé, M., Wittich, W. and Southall, K.E. 2016. Stereotypes associated with age-related conditions and assistive device use in Canadian media. *The Gerontologist*, 56(6), 1023–1032. www.ncbi.nlm.nih.gov/pubmed/26220417.

George, J., Bleasdale, S. and Singleton, S.J. 1997. Causes and prognosis of delirium in elderly patients admitted to a district general hospital. *Age and Ageing*, 26(6), 423–427. www.ncbi.nlm.nih.gov/pubmed/9466291.

Gopinath, B., Schneider, J.M., McMahon, C.M., Burlutsky, G., Leeder, S.R. and Mitchell, P. 2013. Dual sensory impairment in older adults increases the risk of mortality: a population-based study. *PloS one*, 8(3), e55054. http://apps.webofknowledge.com.proxy2.library.mcgill.ca/full_record.do?product= WOS&search_mode=AdvancedSearch&qid=9&SID=3AfCcpA4VdHzWa9gkaT&page=6&doc=56&cac heurlFromRightClick=no.

Göransson, L. 2008. *Dövblindhet i ett livsperspektiv. Strategier och metoder för stöd*. Finspång, Sweden: Mo Gårds Förlag.

Grue, E.V., Kirkevold, M. and Ranhoff, A.H. 2009. Prevalence of vision, hearing, and combined vision and hearing impairments in patients with hip fractures. *Journal of Clinical Nursing*, 18(21), 3037–3049. www.ncbi.nlm.nih.gov/entrez/query.fcgi?cmd=Retrieve&db=PubMed&dopt=Citation &list_uids=19732248.

Gullacksen, A.-C., Goransson, L., Henningsen Ronnblom, G., Koppen, A. and Jorgensen, A.R. 2011. *Life adjustments and combined visual and hearing disability/deafblindness: An internal process over time*. Slotsgade, Denmark: Nordic Centre for Welfare and Social Issues.

Guthrie, D.M., Davidson, J.G.S., Williams, N., Campos, J., Hunter, K., Mick, P., Orange, J.B., Pichora-Fuller, M.K., Phillips, N.A., Savundranayagam, M.Y. and Wittich, W. 2018. Combined impairments in vision, hearing and cognition are associated with greater levels of functional and communication difficulties than cognitive impairment alone: Analysis of interRAI data for home care and long-term care recipients in Ontario. *PLOS ONE*, 13(2), e0192971. http://dx.plos.org/10.1371/journal.pone.0192971.

Guthrie, D.M., Declercq, A., Finne-Soveri, H., Fries, B.E. and Hirdes, J. 2016. The health and well-being of older adults with dual sensory impairment (DSI) in four countries. *PLOS ONE*, 11(5), e0155073. http://dx.plos.org/10.1371/journal.pone.0155073.

Han, J.H., Lee, H.J., Jung, J. and Park, E.-C. 2018. Effects of self-reported hearing or vision impairment on depressive symptoms: A population-based longitudinal study. *Epidemiology and Psychiatric Sciences*, 1–13. www.cambridge.org/core/journals/epidemiology-and-psychiatric-sciences/article/effects-of-selfreported-hearing-or-vision-impairment-on-depressive-symptoms-a-populationbased-longitudinal-study/ACB0BAE8170F539C43D93D74AA9A972B.

Harada, S., Nishiwaki, Y., Michikawa, T., Kikuchi, Y., Iwasawa, S., Nakano, M., Ishigami, A., Saito, H. and Takebayashi, T. 2008. Gender difference in the relationships between vision and hearing impairments and negative well-being. *Preventive Medicine*, 47(4), 433–437. www.ncbi.nlm.nih.gov/entrez/query.fcgi?cmd=Retrieve&db=PubMed&dopt=Citation&list_uids=18619483.

Heine, C. and Browning, C. 2004. The communication and psychosocial perceptions of older adults with sensory loss: a qualitative study. *Ageing and Society*, 24(1), 113–130. http://journals.cambridge.org/download. php?file=/ASO/ASO24_01/S0144686X03001491a.pdf&code=14325aac7c2b38f6589a28152cc6112a.

Heine, C. and Browning, C. 2014. Mental health and dual sensory loss in older adults: a systematic review. *Frontiers in Aging Neuroscience*, 6(May), 83. www.pubmedcentral.nih.gov/articlerender.fcgi?artid=40301 76&tool=pmcentrez&rendertype=abstract.

Heine, C. and Browning, C. 2015. Dual sensory loss in older adults: A systematic review. *The Gerontologist*, 55(2006), p.gnv074. www.ncbi.nlm.nih.gov/pubmed/26315316.

Heine, C., Erber, N.P., Osborn, R. and Browning, C.J. 2002. Communication perceptions of older adults with sensory loss and their communication partners: implications for intervention. *Disability and Rehabilitation*, 24(7), 356–363.

Hersh, M.A. 2013a. Deafblind people, communication, independence, and isolation. *Journal of Deaf Studies and Deaf Education*, 18(4), 446–463.

Hersh, M.A. 2013b. Deafblind people, stigma and the use of communication and mobility assistive devices. *Technology & Disability*, 25(4), 245–261.

Hirdes, J., Dalby, D.M., Curtin-Telegdi, N., Poss, J.W., Stolee, P., Strong, G., Tjam, E. and Bowman, L. 2007. *interRAI deafblind supplement to CHA: Guide for use of the interRAI deafblind supplement assessment form (Canadian version 9)*. Washington, DC: interRAI.

Jeppsson Grassman, E., Holme, L., Taghizadeh Larsson, A. and Whitaker, A. 2012. A long life with a particular signature: Life course and aging for people with disabilities. *Journal of Gerontological Social Work*, 55(2), 95–111. www.tandfonline.com/doi/abs/10.1080/01634372.2011.633975.

Keller, B.K., Morton, J.L., Thomas, V.S. and Potter, J.F. 1999. The effect of visual and hearing impairments on functional status. *Journal of the American Geriatric Society*, 47(11), 1319025.

Keller, H. 1933. *Helen Keller in Scotland: A personal record written by herself*. J. Kerr Love (ed.). London: Methuen.

Kelley-Moore, J. 2010. Disability and ageing: The social construction of causality. In D. Dannefer and C. Phillipson (eds), *The SAGE handbook of social gerontology* (pp. 96–110). London: Sage.

Kwon, H., Kim, J., Kim, Y., Kwon, S. and Yu, J. 2015. Sensory impairment and health-related quality of life. *Iranian Journal of Public Health*, 44(6), 772–782.

Kyle, J. and Barnett, S. 2012. *Deafblind worlds*, Bristol: Deaf Studies Trust and Sense.

Lagati, S. (1995). "Deaf-blind" or "Deafblind"? International perspectives on terminology. *Journal of Visual Impairment & Blindness*, 89(3), 306.

Laustrup, B. 2004. The ageing process and the late manifestation of conditions related to the cause of congenitally deafblind adults in Denmark. *DbI Review*, 33(January–June), 4–7.

Lehane, C.M., Dammeyer, J. and Elsass, P. 2016. Sensory loss and its consequences for couples' psychosocial and relational wellbeing: An integrative review. *Aging & Mental Health*, 7863(August), 1–11. http://dx.doi.org/10.1080/13607863.2015.1132675.

Lehane, C.M., Dammeyer, J., Hovaldt, H.B. and Elsass, P. 2017. Sexuality and well-being among couples living with acquired deafblindness. *Sexuality and Disability*, 35(2), 135–146. http://link.springer.com/10.1007/s11195-016-9470-8.

Lehane, C.M., Wittich, W. and Dammeyer, J. 2016. Couples' experience of sensory loss: A research and rehabilitation imperative. *The Hearing Journal*, 69(8), 34–36.

LeJeune, B.J. 2010. Aging with dual sensory loss: Thoughts from consumer focus groups. *AER Journal: Research and Practice in Visual Impairment and Blindness*, 3(4), 146–152.

LeJeune, B.J., Steinman, B. and Mascia, J., 2003. Enhancing socialization of older people experiencing loss of both vision and hearing. *Generations*, 27(1), 95–97.

Lew, H.L., Pogoda, T.K., Baker, E., Stolzmann, K.L., Meterko, M., Cifu, D.X., Amara, J. and Hendricks, A.M. 2011. Prevalence of dual sensory impairment and its association with traumatic brain injury and blast exposure in OEF/OIF veterans. *Journal of Head Trauma Rehabilitation*, 26(6), 489–496. www.ncbi.nlm.nih.gov/pubmed/21386715.

Lieberman, D.D., Friger, M. and Lieberman, D.D. 2004. Visual and hearing impairment in elderly patients hospitalized for rehabilitation following hip fracture. *Journal of Rehabilitation Research & Development*, 41(5), 669–674. www.ncbi.nlm.nih.gov/entrez/query.fcgi?cmd=Retrieve&db=PubMed&dopt=Citation&list_uids=15558396.

Lin, M.Y., Gutierrez, P.R., Stone, K.L., Yaffe, K., Ensrud, K.E., Fink, H.A., Sarkisian, C.A., Coleman, A.L. and Mangione, C.M. 2004. Vision impairment and combined vision and hearing impairment predict cognitive and functional decline in older women. *Journal of the American Geriatrics Society*, 52(12), 1996–2002. www.ncbi.nlm.nih.gov/entrez/query.fcgi?cmd=Retrieve&db=PubMed&dopt=Citation&list_uids=15571533.

Luey, H.S. 1994. Sensory loss: A neglected issue in social work. *Journal of Gerontological Social Work*, 21(4), 213–223.

Lupsakko, T.A., Mantyjarvi, M.I., Sulkava, R.O. and Kautiainen, H.J. 2002. Combined functional visual and hearing impairment in a population aged 75 and older in Finland and its influence on activities of daily living. *Journal of the American Geriatrics Society*, 50(10), 1748–1749. www.ncbi.nlm.nih.gov/entrez/query.fcgi?cmd=Retrieve&db=PubMed&dopt=Citation&list_uids=12366637.

McDonnall, M.C. 2009. Risk factors for depression among older adults with dual sensory loss. *Aging & Mental Health*, 13(4), 569–576. http://pdfserve.informaworld.com/997035_770885140_913256147.pdf.

McGilton, K.S., Höbler, F., Campos, J., Dupuis, K., Labreche, T., Guthrie, D., Jarry, J., Singh, G. and Wittich, W. 2016. Hearing and vision screening tools for long-term care residents with dementia: protocol for a scoping review. *BMJ Open*, 6(7), e011945. http://bmjopen.bmj.com/lookup/doi/10.1136/bmjopen-2016-011945.

McInnes, J. 1999. *A guide to planning and support for individuals who are deafblind*. Toronto, ON: University of Toronto Press.

Mar, H.H. 1993. Psychosocial services. In J.W. Reiman and P.A. Johnson (eds), *National symposium on children and youth who are deaf-blind* (pp. 42–60). London: Teaching Research Publications.

Mick, P., Parfyonov, M., Wittich, W., Phillips, N. and Pichora-Fuller, M. 2018. Associations between sensory loss and social networks, participation, support, and loneliness. *Canadian Family Physician*, 64(1), 33–41.

Miner, I.D. 1995. Psychosocial implications of Usher syndrome, Type 1, throughout the life cycle. *Journal of Visual Impairment & Blindness*, 89(3), 287–296.

Miner, I.D. 1997. People with Usher syndrome, Type 2: Issues and adaptations. *Journal of Visual Impairment & Blindness*, 91(6), 579–589.

Möller, C. 2003. Deafblindness: Living with sensory deprivation. *Lancet*, 362 (Suppl. December), 46–47. www.ncbi.nlm.nih.gov/pubmed/14698128.

Oleson, B. and Jansbøl, K., 2005. *Experiences from people with deafblindness: A Nordic project*. New York: Information Center for Acquired Deafblindness.

Parfyonov, M., Mick, P., Pichora-Fuller, M. and Wittich, W. 2016. Association between sensory loss and social outcomes: A preliminary report. *Canadian Acoustics*, 44(3), 124–125.

Pavey, S., Douglas, G. and Hodges, L. 2009. *The needs of older people with acquired hearing and sight loss*. London: Thomas Pocklington Trust.

Pollington, C. 2008. Always change: The transitions experienced by an older woman with declining sight and hearing. *Talking Sense*, 52(2), 30–33.

Roets-Merken, L.M., Zuidema, S.U., Vernooij-Dassen, M.J.F.J. and Kempen, G.I.J.M. 2014. Screening for hearing, visual and dual sensory impairment in older adults using behavioural cues: A validation study. *International Journal of Nursing Studies*, 51(11), 1434–1440. www.ncbi.nlm.nih.gov/pubmed/24656434.

Roets-Merken, L.M., Zuidema, S.U., Vernooij-Dassen, M.J.F.J., Teerenstra, S., Hermsen, P.G.J.M., Kempen, G.I.J.M. and Graff, M.J.L. 2018. Effectiveness of a nurse-supported self-management programme for dual sensory impaired older adults in long-term care: A cluster randomised controlled trial. *BMJ Open*, 8(1), e016674. http://bmjopen.bmj.com/lookup/doi/10.1136/bmjopen-2017-016674.

Rönnberg, J. and Borg, E. 2001. A review and evaluation of research on the deaf-blind from perceptual, communicative, social and rehabilitative perspectives. *Scandinavian Audiology*, 30(2), 67–77. http://ovidsp. ovid.com/ovidweb.cgi?T=JS&CSC=Y&NEWS=N&PAGE=fulltext&D=med4&AN=11409790.

Sauerburger, D. 1993. *Independence without sight or sound: suggestions for practitioners working with deaf-blind adults*. New York: AFB Press.

Saunders, G. and Echt, K.V. 2007. An overview of dual sensory impairment in older adults: perspectives for rehabilitation. *Trends in Amplification*, 11(4), 243–258. www.ncbi.nlm.nih.gov/entrez/query.fcgi?c md=Retrieve&db=PubMed&dopt=Citation&list_uids=18003868.

Saunders, G. and Echt, K.V. 2011. Dual sensory impairment in an aging population. *ASHA Leader*, 16(3), 5–7. http://search.ebscohost.com/login.aspx?direct=true&db=rzh&AN=2010978320&site=ehost-live.

Saunders, G. and Echt, K.V. 2012. Blast exposure and dual sensory impairment: An evidence review and integrated rehabilitation approach. *Journal of Rehabilitation Research & Development*, 49(7), 1043–1058. www.ncbi.nlm.nih.gov/pubmed/23341278.

Schneider, J.M., Gopinath, B., McMahon, C., Leeder, S., Mitchell, P. and Wang, J.J. 2011. Dual sensory impairment in older age. *Journal of Aging and Health*, 23(8), 1309–1324. www.ncbi.nlm.nih.gov/pubmed/21596997.

Schneider, J.M., Gopinath, B., McMahon, C., Teber, E., Leeder, S.S.R., Wang, J.J. and Mitchell, P. 2012. Prevalence and 5-year incidence of dual sensory impairment in an older Australian population. *Annals of Epidemiology*, 22(4), 295–301. www.ncbi.nlm.nih.gov/pubmed/22382082.

Shakespeare, T. and Watson, N. 2001. The social model of disability: An outdated ideology? In S.N. Barnartt and B.M. Altman (eds), *Exploring theories and expanding methodologies: Where we are and where we need to go* (Research in Social Science and Disability, vol. 2, pp. 9–28). Bingley, UK: Emerald.

Simcock, P. 2017a. Ageing with a unique impairment A systematically conducted review of older deaf-blind people's experiences. *Ageing & Society*, 37(8), 1703–1742.

Simcock, P. 2017b. One of society's most vulnerable groups? A systematically conducted literature review exploring the vulnerability of deafblind people. *Health and Social Care in the Community*, 25(3), 813–839.

Smith, S.L., Bennett, L.W. and Wilson, R.H. 2008. Prevalence and characteristics of dual sensory impairment (hearing and vision) in a Veteran population. *Journal of Rehabilitation Research and Development*, 45(4), 597–610. www.ncbi.nlm.nih.gov/entrez/query.fcgi?cmd=Retrieve&db=PubMed&dopt=Citati on&list_uids=18712645.

Spring, S., Adler, J. and Wohlgensinger, C. 2012. *Deafblindness in Switzerland: Facing up to the facts. A publication on the study "The living circumstances of deafblind people at different stages of their lives in Switzerland."* Zurich, Switzerland: Swiss National Association of and for the Blind (SNAB).

Stiefel, D. 1991. *The madness of Usher's coping with vision and hearing loss (Usher syndrome Type II)*. Corpus Christi, TX: The Business of Living Publications.

Stoffel, S. 2012. *Deaf-blind reality: Living the Life*. Washington, DC: Gallaudet University Press.

Tay, T., Wang, J.J., Lindley, R., Chia, E.-M., Landau, P., Ingham, N., Kifley, A. and Mitchell, P. 2007. Sensory impairment, use of community support services, and quality of life in aged care clients. *Journal of Aging and Health*, 19(2), 229–241.

Tiwana, R., Benbow, S.M. and Kingston, P. 2016. Late life acquired dual-sensory impairment: A systematic review of its impact on everyday competence. *British Journal of Visual Impairment*, 34(3), 203–213. http://jvi.sagepub.com/cgi/doi/10.1177/0264619616648727.

Tseng, Y.-C., Liu, S. H.-Y., Lou, M.-F. and Huang, G.-S. 2018. Quality of life in older adults with sensory impairments: a systematic review. *Quality of Life Research*, 27(8), 1957–1971. http://link.springer.com/10.1007/s11136-018-1799-2.

Vazquez, M.C., Gigirey, L. M., del Oro, C.P. and Seoane, S. 2012. Is dual sensory loss a risk factor of cognitive decline? *Journal of Aging and Physical Activity*, 20(s1), S63.

Vincent, C., Routhier, F., Martel, V., Mottard, M.-È., Dumont, F., Côté, L. and Cloutier, D. 2014. Field testing of two electronic mobility aid devices for persons who are deaf-blind. *Disability and Rehabilitation. Assistive Technology*, 9(5), 414–420. www.ncbi.nlm.nih.gov/pubmed/24266810.

Volden, M. and Saltnes, H. 2010. Norway's new ways with mental health. *Talking Sense*, Summer, 201.

Westaway, L., Wittich, W. and Overbury, O. 2011. Depression and burden in spouses of individuals with sensory impairment. *Insight: Research and Practice in Visual Impairment & Blindness*, 4(1), 29–36.

Wickham, K. 2011. Depression in the deafblind community: Working from a social work perspective. *DbI Review*, 46(January), 56–58.

Wittich, W., Barstow, E. A., Jarry, J. and Thomas, A. 2015. Screening for sensory impairment in older adults: Training and practice of occupational therapists in Quebec. *Canadian Journal of Occupational Therapy*, 82(5), 283–293. http://cjo.sagepub.com/content/early/2015/02/19/0008417415573076.full.

Wittich, W. and Gagné, J. 2016. Perceptual aspects of gerotechnology. In S. Kwon (ed.), *Gerotechnology: Research, practice, and principles in the field of technology and aging* (pp. 13–34). New York: Springer.

Wittich, W., Höbler, F., Jarry, J. and McGilton, K. 2018. Recommendations for successful sensory screening in older adults with dementia in long-term care: A qualitative environmental scan of Canadian specialists. *BMJ Open*, 8(1), e019451. www.hefce.ac.uk/rsrch/oa.

Wittich, W., Jarry, J., Barstow, E. and Thomas, A. 2017. Vision and hearing impairment and occupational therapy education: Needs and current practice. *British Journal of Occupational Therapy*, 80(6), 384–391. http://journals.sagepub.com/doi/10.1177/0308022616684853.

Wittich, W., Jarry, J., Groulx, G., Southall, K. and Gagné, J.-P. 2016. Rehabilitation and research priorities in deafblindness for the next decade. *Journal of Visual Impairment & Blindness*, 110(July–August), 219–231.

Wittich, W., Southall, K. and Johnson, A. 2016. Usability of assistive listening devices by older adults with low vision. *Disability & Rehabilitation: Assistive Technology*, 11(7), 564–571. www.ncbi.nlm.nih.gov/pubmed/25945610.

Wittich, W., Southall, K., Sikora, L., Watanabe, D.H. and Gagne, J.-P. 2013. What's in a name: Dual sensory impairment or deafblindness? *British Journal of Visual Impairment*, 31(3), 198–207. http://jvi.sagepub.com/content/31/3/198.short.

Wittich, W., Watanabe, D.H. and Gagne, J.P. 2012. Sensory and demographic characteristics of deafblindness rehabilitation clients in Montreal, Canada. *Ophthalmic & Physiological Optics: The Journal of the British College of Ophthalmic Opticians (Optometrists)*, 32(3), 242–251. www.ncbi.nlm.nih.gov/pubmed/22348651.

Yamada, Y., Denkinger, M.D., Onder, G., Henrard, J.-C., van der Roest, H.G., Finne-Soveri, H., Richter, T., Vlachova, M., Bernabei, R. and Topinkova, E. 2015. Dual sensory impairment and cognitive decline: The results from the Shelter Study. *Journals of Gerontology Series A: Biological Sciences and Medical Sciences*, 71(1), 1–7. http://biomedgerontology.oxfordjournals.org/cgi/doi/10.1093/gerona/glv036.

Yoken, C. 1979. *Living with deaf-blindness: Nine profiles*. Washington, DC: Gallaudet University Press.

Index